Clinical Electrophysiology

Electrotherapy and Electrophysiologic Testing

Third Edition

EDITION 3

Clinical Electrophysiology

Electrotherapy and Electrophysiologic Testing

ANDREW J. ROBINSON

Professor
Department of Physical Therapy
Ithaca College
Ithaca, New York

LYNN SNYDER-MACKLER

Professor
Department of Physical Therapy
University of Delaware
Newark, DE

Wolters Kluwer | Lippincott Williams & Wilkins
Health

Philadelphia • Baltimore • New York • London
Buenos Aires • Hong Kong • Sydney • Tokyo

Acquisitions Editor: Peter Sabatini
Managing Editor: Andrea M. Klingler
Marketing Manager: Allison M. Noplock
Production Editor: Julie Montalbano
Designer: Doug Smock
Compositor: International Typesetting and Composition

First Edition, 1989
Second Edition, 1995

351 West Camden Street
Baltimore, MD 21201

530 Walnut Street
Philadelphia, PA 19106

9 8 7 6

Printed in the United States of America

Library of Congress Cataloging-in-Publication Data

Robinson, Andrew J., Ph. D.
Clinical electrophysiology : electrotherapy and electrophysiologic testing / Andrew J. Robinson and Lynn Snyder-Mackler. — 3rd ed.
p. ; cm.
Includes bibliographical references and index.
ISBN-13: 978-0-7817-4484-3
ISBN-10: 0-7817-4484-9
1. Electrotherapeutics. 2. Electrodiagnosis. 3. Electrophysiology. I. Snyder-Mackler, Lynn. II. Title.
[DNLM: 1. Electric Stimulation Therapy. 2. Electric Stimulation. 3. Electrodiagnosis. WB 495 R658c 2008]
RM872.S68 2008
615.8'45—dc22

2007022715

DISCLAIMER

Care has been taken to confirm the accuracy of the information present and to describe generally accepted practices. However, the authors, editors, and publisher are not responsible for errors or omissions or for any consequences from application of the information in this book and make no warranty, expressed or implied, with respect to the currency, completeness, or accuracy of the contents of the publication. Application of this information in a particular situation remains the professional responsibility of the practitioner; the clinical treatments described and recommended may not be considered absolute and universal recommendations.

The authors, editors, and publisher have exerted every effort to ensure that drug selection and dosage set forth in this text are in accordance with the current recommendations and practice at the time of publication. However, in view of ongoing research, changes in government regulations, and the constant flow of information relating to drug therapy and drug reactions, the reader is urged to check the package insert for each drug for any change in indications and dosage and for added warnings and precautions. This is particularly important when the recommended agent is a new or infrequently employed drug.

Some drugs and medical devices presented in this publication have Food and Drug Administration (FDA) clearance for limited use in restricted research settings. It is the responsibility of the health care provider to ascertain the FDA status of each drug or device planned for use in their clinical practice.

To purchase additional copies of this book, call our customer service department at **(800) 638-3030** or fax orders to **(301) 223-2320.** International customers should call **(301) 223-2300.**

Visit Lippincott Williams & Wilkins on the Internet: http://www.lww.com. Lippincott Williams & Wilkins customer service representatives are available from 8:30 am to 6:00 pm, EST.

To our parents,

—Arthur W. Robinson, Jr., and Doris E. Robinson

A.J.R.

—Richard and Loraine Snyder

L. S-M.

They were the role models for our lives who showed us how contributions to the greater good require effort, time, and dedication. They were also always there when they were needed.

Foreword

When reviewing the contents of this textbook, it seems to me that everyone—students, academicians, clinicians, and third-party payers—should be excited about the use of electrical stimulation and biofeedback as clinical modalities. There is no question that I am biased in favor of their use; there is evidence to support application for a variety of impairments, the devices often provide some indication of change in function, and they are fun to use. Because of my bias in favor of this equipment and its clinical application, I cannot understand the gap between what the literature suggests is "best" practice, or at least "better" practice, and actual practice in which electrical stimulation is not a routine modality. In my opinion, there is adequate evidence to support claims for reimbursement.

Each of the chapters in this book reviews the relevant literature in a very thoughtful way using the research findings to support or refute claims of effectiveness. The body of literature keeps growing and includes randomized, controlled trials and systematic reviews. For example, comparison between this new edition and the second edition shows that the number of references increased from 48 to 116 in the chapter on electrical stimulation for pain modulation (Chapter 5), and from 67 to 105 citations in the chapter on electrical stimulation for muscle (Chapter 6). It is clear that Andrew Robinson made a decision to narrow the broad category of tissue healing and focus on the use of electrical stimulation for chronic wound healing, where there is evidence to support its effectiveness. I am delighted to see the chapter on the use of electrical stimulation or electromyographic feedback for genitourinary dysfunction. This is an area where additional research is necessary, and I hope that this well-conceived chapter will help establish appropriate protocols for the needed scholarship.

In reading this book after spending time in class teaching the neuroscience content to physical therapist students, I was reminded once again that the use of electrical modalities as described throughout this textbook might actually enhance neural reorganization. It is well accepted that muscle fibers are capable of change in response to decreased or increased activity (i.e., they are mutable). Moreover, there is research that suggests that particular doses of electrical stimulation alter skeletal muscle properties. The evidence for neural plasticity, however, is more recent. Interventions to optimize "good" reorganization have received a lot of attention in the current research literature. The constraint-induced training in people with chronic upper extremity impairments following a stroke, and of locomotor training using body-weight support and a treadmill in people with incomplete spinal cord injury, are examples of attempts to restore function rather than to compensate by adopting new strategies. The assumption underlying this research is that the nervous system is capable of reorganizing in response to training. There is also evidence that the brain reorganizes in accomplished athletes and musicians, as well as in people with chronic pain or in those who have sustained an amputation, traumatic brain injury, or stroke. One principle that is emerging emphasizes the need for an adequate dose of training over a longer period of time. Another principle is specificity of training. Isn't that what this book is all about? I would like to think so.

I thank the authors for their sustained efforts to promote the proper use of electrical stimulation and biofeedback for intervention and diagnosis. They have done an excellent job describing potential mechanisms as well as good-practice principles. The cases and self-study questions clearly test the reader's comprehension of the chapter. I hope that others enjoy reading this book as much as I did.

Rebecca L Craik, PT, PhD, FAPTA
Department of Physical Therapy
Arcadia University (formerly Beaver College)
Glenside, Pennsylvania

Preface

This third edition of *Clinical Electrophysiology* has been written by a combination of recognized, experienced authorities, and a number of other contributors who may well represent the next generation of practitioners and researchers in the field of clinical electrophysiology. Several new contributors to the third edition with established records of accomplishments include Kathleen A. Sluka, PT, PhD; Rebecca Stephenson, PT, DPT; and Beth Shelly, PT, BCIA-PMDB. Dr. Sluka has contributed a completely new chapter on the physiology of pain and pain modulation by electrotherapeutic interventions. She is a well-respected and highly published researcher and educator who has coupled her knowledge of pain mechanisms and pain control interventions with her years of experience in the classroom to create a chapter that clinicians and students alike will find directly applicable to the use of electrical stimulation for pain control in the clinic.

This new edition includes a new chapter addressing electrical stimulation and electromyographic biofeedback for the treatment of urogenital disorders. Written by two seasoned clinicians, Rebecca Stephenson and Beth Shelly, this chapter clearly describes a framework for understanding urogenital impairments and outlines a variety of stimulation and biofeedback techniques designed to manage these impairments. Much of this chapter addresses clinical disorders, including urinary incontinence and pelvic pain.

Several new and younger authors have been recruited to contribute some fresh perspectives to topics in this third edition. Scott Stackhouse, PT, PhD, has written the new chapter on neuromuscular electrical stimulation for the control of posture and movement disorders. This chapter addresses topics ranging from neuromuscular electrical stimulation (NMES) for glenohumeral subluxation, to implanted NMES systems for movement control in central nervous system dysfunction. Tara Jo Manal , PT, OCS, SCS, has co-authored a revised chapter on electrical stimulation for pain control with editor Lynn Snyder-Mackler. The focus of this chapter is on the decision-making process in implementing electrical stimulation for pain control and the evidence from clinical trials regarding treatment efficacy. Sara Farquhar, PT, MPT, has also co-authored the updated chapter on NMES for muscle strengthening with Dr. Snyder-Mackler. Jennifer Bushey, PT, OCS, has rewritten and updated the chapter on electromyographic biofeedback for motor control with the author of this chapter in the second edition, Dr. Stuart Binder-Macleod.

In general, an objective of each of the authors of the clinical application chapters was to include clear and concise discussion of the evidence underlying clinical intervention, especially the results of randomized, controlled trials.

Features of the second edition that were particularly well-received have been retained. Self-study questions appear at the end of each chapter and have been revised and updated from the second edition. Answers to these questions appear in Appendix B. Case studies appear in each intervention chapter and provide examples of how electrotherapeutic interventions may be safely and effectively applied based on the available clinical evidence. Laboratory exercises have been added to this edition in these chapters. Key terms are italicized in each chapter to help students recognize important concepts. Additionally, both the quantity and quality of the figures throughout this new edition of *Clinical Electrophysiology* have been increased.

This book is truly a blend of something old and something new with respect to both the writers and the content. Our highest hope for the book is that it may contribute to the ongoing development of clinical practice, and ultimately allow those who receive the interventions discussed in this new and revised edition of *Clinical Electrophysiology: Electrotherapy and Electrophysiologic Testing* better function and an improved quality of life.

Contributors

Andrew J. Robinson, PT, PhD
Professor
Department of Physical Therapy
School of Health Sciences and Human Performance
Ithaca College
Ithaca, New York

Kathleen A. Sluka, PT, PhD
Associate Professor
Graduate Program in Physical Therapy and Rehabilitation Science
University of Iowa
Iowa City, Iowa

Tara Jo Manal, PT, MPT, OCS, SCS
Clinic Director/Orthopedic Residency Director
Department of Physical Therapy
University of Delaware
Newark, Delaware

Lynn Snyder-Mackler, PT, ScD, SCS, FAPTA
Professor
University of Delaware
Department of Physical Therapy
Newark, Delaware

Sara Farquhar, MPT
Department of Physical Therapy
University of Delaware
Newark, Delaware

Scott Stackhouse, PT, PhD
Assistant Professor
Department of Physical Therapy
Arcadia University
Glenside, Pennsylvania

Rebecca G. Stephenson, PT, DPT, MS
Coordinator of Women's Health Physical Therapy
Brigham and Women's Hospital
Boston, Massachusetts

Elizabeth R. Shelly, PT, BCIA-PMDB
Women's Health Specialist
Quad City Physical Therapy and Spine
Davenport, Iowa

Charles D. Ciccone, PT, PhD
Professor
Department of Physical Therapy
School of Health Sciences and Human Performance
Ithaca College
Ithaca, New York

Stuart A. Binder-Macleod, PT, PhD, FAPTA
Professor
Department of Physical Therapy
University of Delaware
Newark, Delaware

Captain Robert Kellogg, PT, PhD
Commanding Officer
United States Navy Hospital
Guam

Jennifer A. Bushey, PT, OCS
Physical Therapist
Towson Sports Medicine
Towson, Maryland

Contents

CHAPTER 1

Basic Concepts in Electricity and Contemporary Terminology in Electrotherapy

Andrew J. Robinson

Electricity is a form of energy, and it can produce significant effects on biological tissues. This chapter briefly reviews basic concepts of electricity and electromagnetism that form a foundation for understanding therapeutic electrical stimulation. Equations describing electrical phenomena are kept to a minimum, and frequent analogies are used to allow the reader to visualize what may happen in human tissues as electrical stimulation is applied. The focus of the chapter is the conceptualization of relevant electrical phenomena rather than memorization. This chapter also introduces the terminology used to qualitatively and quantitatively describe electrical currents employed in clinical applications. These terms will be used throughout the text to ensure the clear, unambiguous, and consistent communication of the technical details of stimulation procedures. Those readers who have recently completed study in the physics of electricity may want to forgo the first section on fundamental concepts in electricity and begin reading the section "Language of Electrotherapeutic Currents."

FUNDAMENTAL CONCEPTS OF ELECTRICITY

Electric Charge

Electric charge (or simply "charge") is a fundamental physical property in the same way that "mass" and "time" are fundamental physical properties. The problem in attempting to explain charge is that charge is operationally defined. That is, one cannot ever see a charge, but one can see through experimentation how charge is manifest. For example, a physics instructor may demonstrate how rubbing cloth on amber (a yellowish fossil resin) allows the amber to attract lightweight substances such as bits of paper. Early scientists described this property of amber as static electricity, which is nothing more than a manifestation of the electromagnetic force of attraction exerted by the charged particles within the amber. Amber becomes charged by exchanging electrons with those in the atoms of the cloth. As a result, both the cloth and the amber show the ability to attract or repel a variety of other charged objects.

Charge is the property of matter that is the basis of electromagnetic force. Experiments designed to characterize the properties of electric charge have shown that two types of electric charge, positive and negative, exist (1). At the simplest level, charge is carried by the electrons (negative charge) and the protons (positive charge) of atoms. Like charges repel each other, and opposite charges attract each other. Charge can be transferred from one object to another (charges may be separated), but charge can be neither created nor destroyed. The concept of electric charge is not limited to the subatomic level of matter. An electrically neutral atom is one that contains an equal number of protons and electrons. If an atom of an element loses electrons without changing the number of protons in the nucleus, it becomes positively charged. If an atom gains electrons, it becomes negatively charged. Atoms of elements with either an excess or a deficiency of electrons are called *ions*. Atoms that are positively charged are referred to as *cations*, and negatively charged atoms are called *anions*.

Objects or substances may also become electrically charged. Consider the charges on the terminals of a simple dry-cell battery. As a consequence of the chemical reactions taking place within the battery, one metal terminal (the *cathode*) gains electrons and becomes *negatively* charged, while the other metal terminal (the *anode*) loses electrons and becomes *positively* charged. The anode and cathode of a battery are sometimes referred to as the poles of the battery. The term *polarity* is used to indicate the relative charge (positive or negative) of the terminals or two essential leads of an electrical circuit at any one moment in time.

The force exerted between two electrical charges can be determined experimentally and is expressed in coulombs (C). The Coulomb force (F) between two stationary charges, ($q1$) and

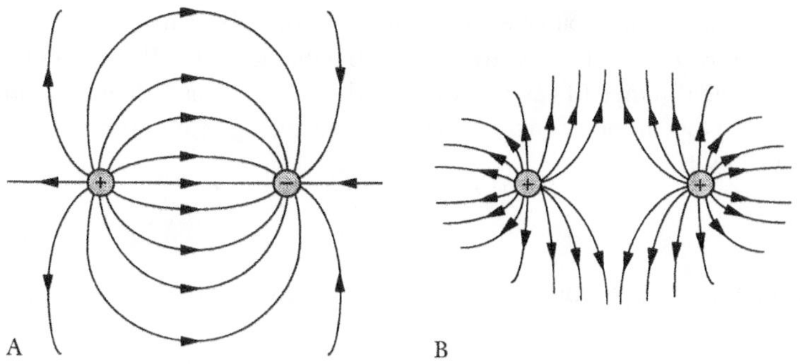

Figure 1.1. Electric field lines around oppositely charged particles **(A),** and two like charges **(B).** Configuration of the field lines reflects the attraction of oppositely charged particles and repulsion between similarly charged particles.

($q2$), is proportional to the magnitude and sign of the charges and is inversely proportional to the square of the distance (r) between them, as expressed by Coulomb's law:

$$F \propto (q1 \times q2)/r^2 \cdot$$

Coulomb's law simply states that the larger the respective charges or the closer the two charges, the larger the attractive (or repulsive) force between them. The coulomb forces of electrons and protons are equal in magnitude but opposite in sign. The Coulomb force for a single electron is 1.6×10^{-19} C. Consequently, to produce a charge of 1 C requires the presence of 6.24×10^{18} electrons.

Electric Field

The electric force of charged particles is carried to other charged particles by the *electric field* (E) that each charge creates. Charges transmit force through an electric field in a manner analogous to the way the earth's force of gravity is transmitted via gravitational fields. The characteristics of electric fields created between two oppositely charged substances and two substances of the same charge are illustrated in Figure 1.1.

Voltage

To understand the concept of voltage, consider the situation diagrammed in Figure 1.2. Large charged substance A is brought close to small similarly charged substance B. As the two charged

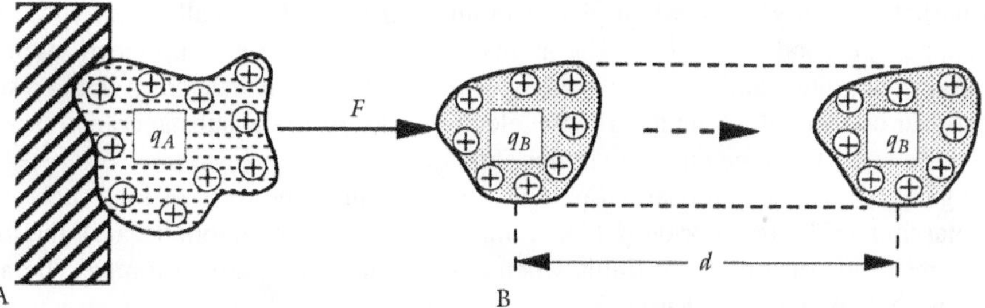

Figure 1.2. The effect of approximating two similarly charged objects (having charges *q*A and *q*B). **A:** Fixed position. **B:** The Coulomb force (*F*) of repulsion between the two objects will tend to separate the objects by some distance (*d*).

masses are approximated, the repulsive Coulomb force of A is transmitted through A's electric field and is "felt" by B, raising B's electrical potential energy (PE). If free to move, B will shift to a new position some distance (d) away from its original position. When B is moved, substance A has done work (W) that amounts to the product of the average Coulomb force applied to B and the distance moved by B; that is,

$$W = F \times d.$$

As substance B moves, the potential energy initially gained by interaction with A is lost in doing the work. Thus,

$$W = \Delta\text{PE}.$$

Because the work done is directly proportional to the charge on B, and because the change in potential energy is also directly proportional to the charge on B (q_B), the voltage (V) is defined as

$$V = \Delta\text{PE}/q_B$$

Voltage is the change in electrical potential energy between two points in an electric field per unit of charge and is synonymous with the term *electrical potential difference*. From a more practical standpoint, voltage represents the driving force that makes charged particles move and is often referred to as *electromotive force* (emf). Voltages are produced when oppositely charged substances are separated, when like-charged substances are approximated, or when charged particles within a system are not evenly distributed. The standard unit for voltage is the volt (V). One volt is equal to a 1 J (joule) change in energy per Coulomb of charge:

$$1\ \text{V} = 1\ \text{J}/1\ \text{C}.$$

The range of voltages used in electrotherapeutic applications may be as small as the millivolt (mV, 10^{-3} V, thousandths of a volt) range or as high as several hundred volts (applied over an extremely short time).

Conductors and Insulators

Charged particles, such as electrons in metals or ions in solution, will tend to move or change position as a result of their interactions with other charged particles. In other words, charged particles will tend to move in matter when electrical potential differences exist. For charged particles to move when subjected to a voltage, they must be free to move. Those substances in which charged particles readily move when placed in an electric field are called *conductors*. Metals such as copper are good conductors. The atoms of metals tend to give up electrons from their outer orbital shell quite readily when placed in an electric field. If a negatively charged substance is brought near one end of a long metal wire, electrons closest to the substance will be displaced along the wire away from the mass of similar charge.

Biological tissues contain charged particles in solution in the form of ions such as sodium (Na^+), potassium (K^+), or chloride (Cl^-). Human tissues are conductors because the ions there are free to move in aqueous body fluids when exposed to electromotive forces. The ability of ions to move in human tissues varies from tissue to tissue. Muscle and nerve are good conductors, whereas skin and fat are poor conductors.

In contrast to substances that allow easy movement of charged particles in an electric field, *insulators* are substances that do not tend to allow free movement of ions or electrons. Rubber and many plastics are good insulators.

Electrical Current

The properties of electric charges in motion are more important to the understanding of therapeutic electrical stimulation than are the properties of charges at rest. The movement of charged particles through a conductor in response to an applied electric field is called *current* (I). The conduction of electrical charge through matter from one point to another is the transfer of energy that brings about physiological changes during the clinical application of electrical stimulation.

Producing electrical current requires (a) the presence of freely movable charged particles in some substance, and (b) the application of a driving force to move the particles. In metal circuits, electrons are the movable charged particles, whereas in biological systems, ions in body fluids (electrolytic solutions) are the charged particles. The forces that induce current in biological fluids are the applied voltages. The magnitude of current induced in a conductive medium is directly proportional to the magnitude of the applied voltage:

$$\text{Current} \propto \text{Voltage} \qquad (I \propto V).$$

Current is defined as the amount of charge (q) moving past a plane in the conductor per unit time (t), or

$$I = \Delta q/\Delta t.$$

The standard unit of measurement for current is the ampere (A). One ampere is equal to the movement of 1 C of charge past a point in 1 second. Currents used in electrotherapeutic applications are very small and are generally measured in milliamperes (mA, 10^{-3} amperes, thousandths of an ampere), or in microamperes (μA, 10^{-6} amperes, millionths of an ampere).

Resistance and Conductance

The magnitude of charge flow is determined not only by the size of the driving force (voltage), but also by the relative ease with which electrons or ions are allowed to move through the conductor. This characteristic of conductors may be described in two ways. The property of conductors called *resistance* (R) describes the relative opposition to movement of charged particles in a conductor. Conversely, the property called *conductance* (G) describes the relative ease with which charged particles move in a medium. For metals, resistance is dependent on the cross-sectional area (A), length (L), and resistivity (ρ) of the conductor by the formula

$$R = \rho\left(\frac{L}{A}\right).$$

The standard unit of resistance is the ohm (Ω). The magnitude of the current induced in a conductor is inversely proportional to the resistance of the conductor:

$$I \propto 1/R.$$

An alternative way to describe the ability of charged particles to move in conductors, conductance, is inversely related to resistance:

$$R = 1/G.$$

The standard unit of conductance is the siemens (S; the mho is no longer used).

The resistance of electrical conductors is analogous to the opposition to fluid movement that occurs in hydraulic systems. Just as the resistance to fluid movement increases as the diameter of pipe decreases (or the length of pipe increases), the resistance to electrical current increases as the diameter of the conductor decreases (or the length of conductor increases).

Ohm's Law

The relationship between voltage and resistance that determines the magnitude of current (I) is expressed in Ohm's law:

$$I = V/R \qquad \text{or} \qquad V = I \times R.$$

Ohm's law simply states that the current induced in a conductor increases as the applied driving force (V) is increased or as the opposition to charge movement (R) is decreased. Alternatively, Ohm's law may be expressed in terms of conductance (G) rather than resistance:

$$I = V \times G \qquad \text{or} \qquad V = I/G.$$

Capacitance and Impedance

In order to understand current in biological tissues, two other electrical concepts must also be introduced. *Capacitance* is the property of a system of conductors and insulators that allows the system to store charge. Currents produced in biological tissues are influenced not only by tissue resistance but also by tissue capacitance.

An electrical circuit device, the capacitor, is made up of two thin metal plates separated by an insulator (or dielectric; Fig. 1.3A). If a fixed voltage is applied across the capacitor, current does not pass through the device because of the presence of the insulating material. However, the potential difference between the two plates of the capacitor exerts a force on the molecules within the insulator, raising the potential energy within these molecules (Fig. 1.3B). If the applied voltage is removed, the stored energy (electrical potential difference across the capacitor) remains until the capacitor is discharged through some conductive pathway.

A capacitor stores electrical energy in a manner similar to that of an elastic impermeable membrane placed in a hydraulic system. Consider the situation illustrated in Figure 1.3C, where a thin rubber membrane is placed in the base of an inelastic tube. A piston is used to produce a driving force on the fluid—no fluid actually passes through the membrane (no current is produced); the driving force causes the membrane to distend (Fig. 1.3D). The membrane stores energy by virtue of its distended shape. If the valve in the tube is closed and then the piston pressure is released, the membrane will remain in the distended, energy-storing position until the valve is reopened (Fig. 1.3E). If the valve is reopened, the recoil of the membrane will produce a movement of the fluid (current) that will continue until the membrane returns to its original, resting position. Thus, the elastic membrane in the hydraulic circuit stores energy that induces a fluid current, just as a capacitor stores electrical energy that induces an electrical current. Notice that the membrane in the tube blocks fluid flow (current) through the tube when a constant, unidirectional piston pressure is applied, just as a capacitor blocks electrical direct current when a constant voltage is applied. Although capacitive systems tend to block direct currents, they tend to allow alternating currents to pass. For a system at a particular capacitance, the higher the frequency of alternating current, the more effectively the current will pass through the system.

The capacitance of a capacitor or any similarly constructed system of conductors and insulators is expressed in farads (F); 1 F is the magnitude of capacitance as 1 C of charge is stored when 1 V of potential difference is applied.

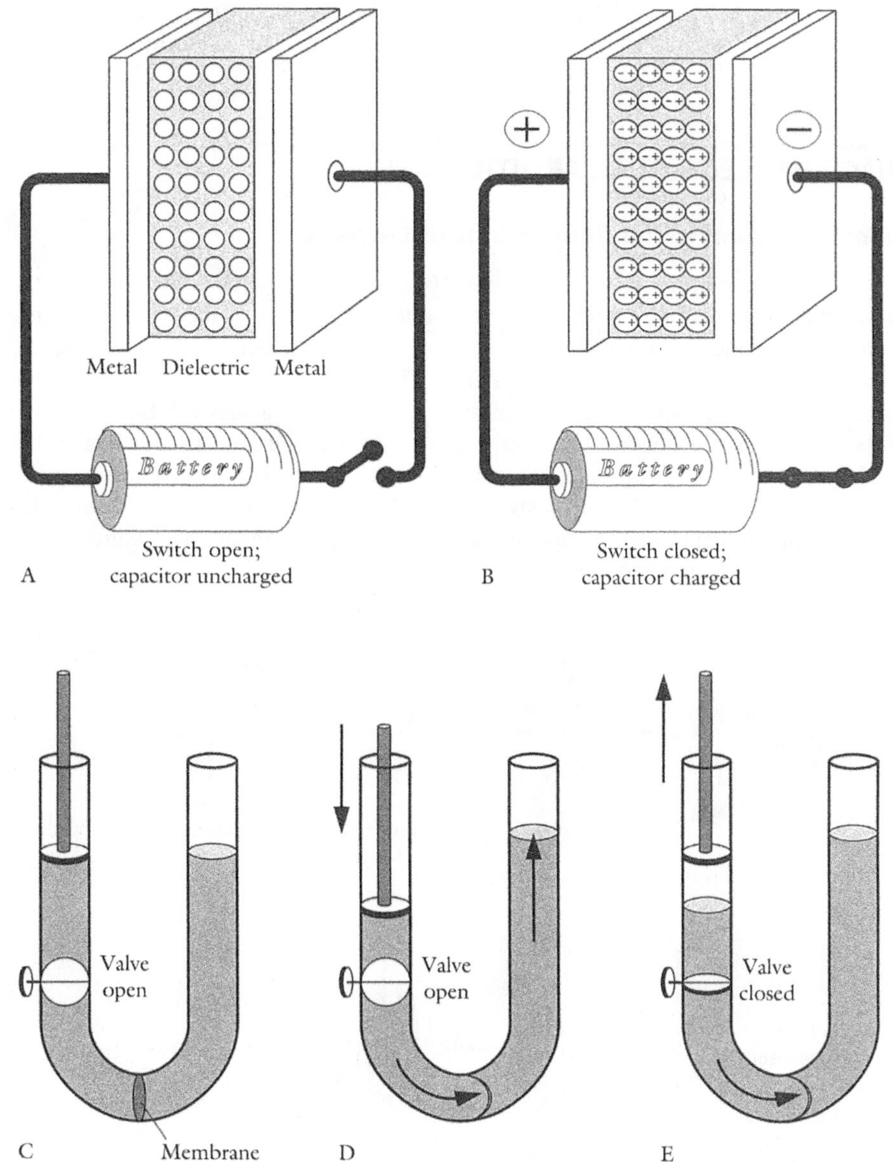

Figure 1.3. Diagrammatic representation of a capacitor in a simple electrical circuit in uncharged **(A)** and charged **(B)** states. A capacitor stores electric energy by the deformation of dielectric molecules. A hydraulic analog of an uncharged capacitor **(C),** charging capacitor **(D),** and charged capacitor with charging force removed **(E).** Energy is stored in the deformation of an impermeable elastic membrane.

The term *impedance (Z)* describes the opposition to alternating currents, analogous to the way resistance describes the opposition to direct currents. Impedance takes into account both the capacitive and resistive opposition to the movement of charged particles. When dealing with clinical electrical stimulation, it is more appropriate to express the opposition to current in terms of impedance, because human tissues are better modeled as complex resistor and capacitor (R-C) networks. Because impedance depends on the capacitive nature of biological tissues, its magnitude depends on the frequency of applied stimulation. In general, the higher the frequency of stimulation, the lower the impedance of tissues. The standard unit of impedance is the ohm.

LANGUAGE OF ELECTROTHERAPEUTIC CURRENTS

Traditional and Commercial Designations of Currents

Electrical currents have been used for therapeutic purposes for hundreds of years. With the development of different forms of electrical generators during this century, the types of electrical currents used in therapeutic applications have proliferated. The introduction to the health-care market of many different types of stimulators producing different forms of electrical currents has led to substantial confusion regarding the characteristics of the currents generated. Before 1990, no system had been developed to standardize descriptions of electrical currents used in electrotherapy.

Characterization of electrotherapeutic currents was often driven by historical developments or by the commercial sector. Figure 1.4 shows a number of the various types of currents used in the early years of clinical electrotherapy and their traditional designations. Figure 1.5 illustrates several commercially designated current (or voltage) waveforms.

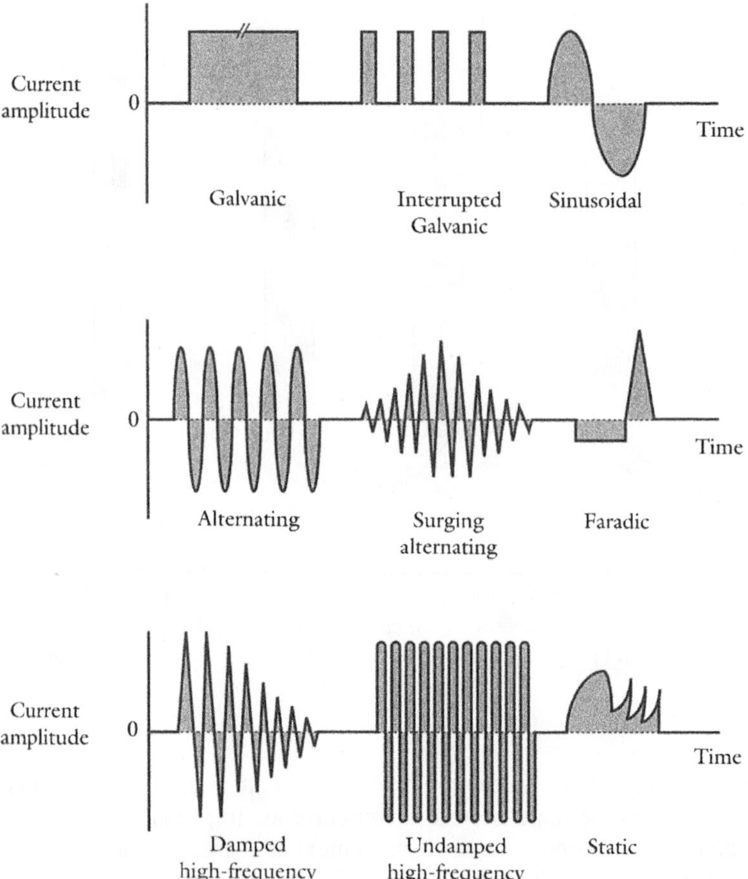

Figure 1.4. Traditional designations of selected electrical currents used historically in clinical practice. Each graph shows changes in current amplitude over time.

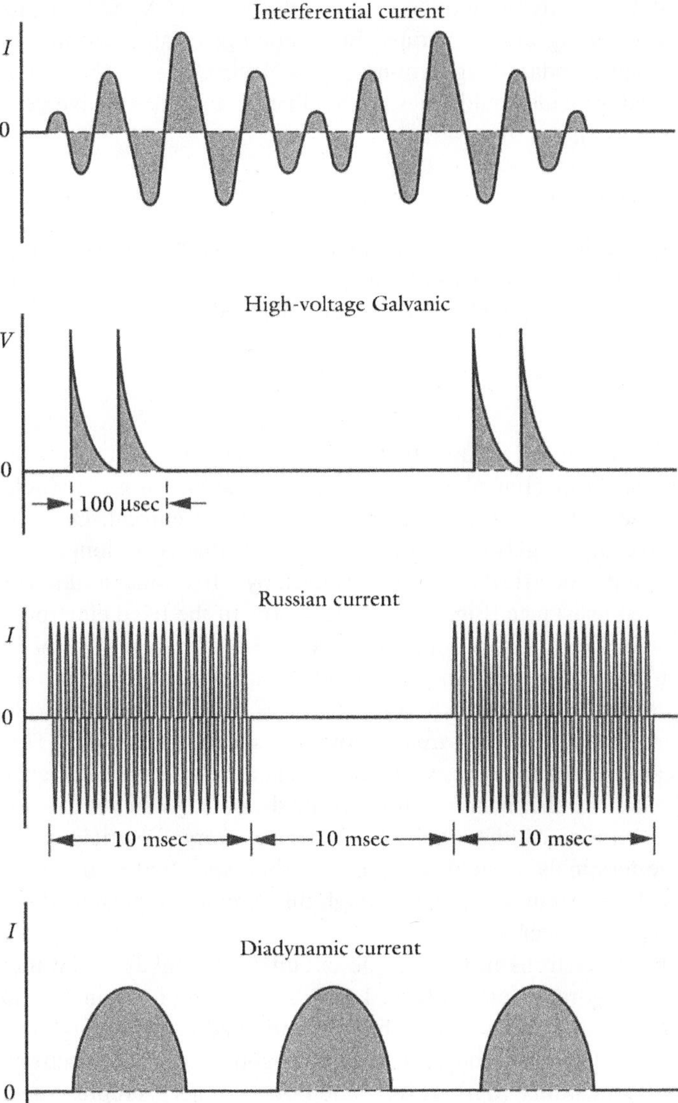

Figure 1.5. Commercial designations of selected electrical currents available from certain contemporary stimulators. Graphs show either changes in current amplitude over time or changes in voltage amplitude over time.

Differentiation among these traditional and commercial types of currents was often based on only a single current characteristic, such as the amplitude of voltage or the frequency of stimulation. Such one-dimensional distinctions led to dichotomous designations, such as "low-volt versus high-volt" or "low-frequency versus medium-frequency" stimulators, that persist even today. An appreciation by practicing clinicians for the traditional and commercial designations of electrotherapeutic currents is important because literature published through the 1980s used traditional or commercial terminology and clinicians educated during this era continue to use this terminology.

In the mid-1980s, the Section on Clinical Electrophysiology (SCE) of the American Physical Therapy Association recognized that such arbitrary descriptions of electrotherapeutic currents, along with the proliferation of commercial designations of currents, fostered confusion in communication regarding electrotherapy. In an attempt to alleviate the problem, the SCE developed a monograph standardizing terminology in electrotherapy. The monograph, which has recently been updated, provides guidelines for qualitative and quantitative descriptions of electrotherapeutic currents (2).

Types of Electrotherapeutic Currents

Electrical currents used in contemporary clinical electrotherapy can generally be divided into three types: direct current, alternating current, and pulsed (or pulsatile) current. This section of the chapter differentiates among these types of current based on their qualitative and quantitative characteristics.

DIRECT CURRENT

The continuous or uninterrupted unidirectional flow of charged particles is defined as *direct current* (DC). In the context of clinical applications, the flow of charged particles must continue uninterrupted for at least 1 second to be considered as direct current. Direct current has traditionally been referred to as "galvanic" current; however, this is no longer the preferred term. Direct current in a simple electrical circuit is produced by a fixed-magnitude voltage applied to a conductor with a fixed resistance (Fig. 1.6A). The source of the fixed electromotive force is the battery, where chemical reactions produce an excess of electrons on one pole (cathode) and a deficiency in electrons on the opposite pole (anode). The opposition to current in the circuit is represented as a resistor. When a switch in the circuit is closed, electrons flow from the area of high concentration (cathode) to the area of low concentration (anode). This flow, which is impeded by the resistance of the wire, will continue until the charge difference between terminals is eliminated when the chemical reactions within the battery can no longer provide free electrons to the negative terminal. Although the movement of charged particles in this circuit is from negative to positive terminals, current is, by convention, specified as moving from positive to negative terminals. The current that flows through this circuit is represented in Figure 1.6C as a graph of current amplitude over time.

The movement of electrons in this simple circuit is analogous to the movement of water molecules in a simple hydraulic circuit (Fig. 1.6B). The driving force in this fluid model is represented as the pressure difference created by the pump and is analogous to the voltage difference across the battery. The water molecules are analogous to the free electrons in the electrical circuit. The *hydraulic resistance* (opposition to the flow of water) is represented primarily by the narrowing of the tubing halfway through the circuit and is analogous to the resistance of the wire in our simple electrical circuit. The fluid will flow in the circuit as long as the pump maintains a pressure difference, just as electron flow will continue as long as the battery maintains an electrical potential difference. The volume of fluid that passes by a point in the fluid circuit per unit of time (current) will remain constant as long as the pressure gradient is kept constant and the geometry of the tubing is maintained. A drop in either the pressure gradient or the diameter of the tube will reduce fluid flow, just as a drop in voltage or an increase in circuit resistance will reduce electron flow.

Direct current induced in an electrolytic aqueous solution containing both positively and negatively charged ions (cations and anions, respectively) is associated with the movement of these two types of ions in opposite directions. Figure 1.7 illustrates the ionic movements in an electrolytic solution when the solution is exposed to a constant-voltage electric field. As shown in the figure, anions move toward the anode, and cations migrate toward the cathode. The movement of each type of ion in the solution occurs at a fixed rate as long as the battery voltage is constant. The migration of ions or electrically charged molecules according to their charge when exposed to a

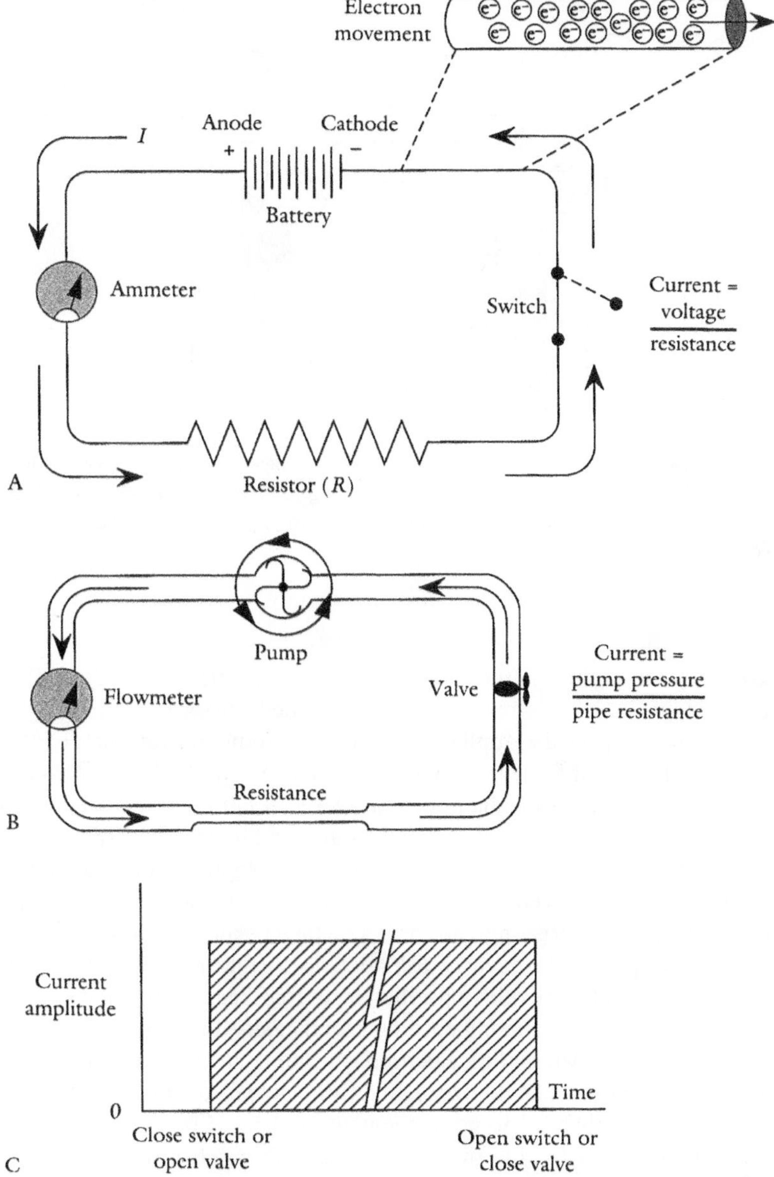

Figure 1.6. Diagram of a simple electrical circuit showing the unidirectional movement of electrons in response to a constant driving force **(A).** Hydraulic analog of a simple electrical circuit showing unidirectional movement of fluid in response to constant pressure produced by a pump **(B).** Graphical representation of direct current on a current amplitude versus time plot **(C).**

fixed emf is called *electrophoresis* and is the basis of *iontophoresis*, a therapeutic technique used to drive electrically charged medications through the skin (see Chapter 10). Figure 1.7 also illustrates the liberation of gases near the electrodes, which often accompanies DC effects on electrolytic solutions. In this case, a reduction reaction occurs at the cathode to produce hydrogen gas (H_2), and an oxidation reaction occurs at the anode to yield oxygen gas (O_2). The use of electric energy to produce such chemical reactions is called *electrolysis*.

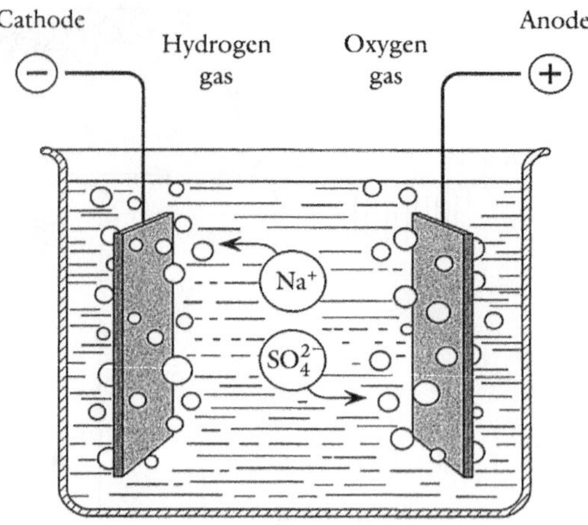

Figure 1.7. An example of ionic movements in a solution with negatively charged ions (anions) moving toward the anode and positively charged ions (cations) moving toward the cathode when exposed to a fixed electromagnetic field. In aqueous solutions (water as solvent), hydrogen gas is liberated from the cathode, and oxygen is released from the anode.

ALTERNATING CURRENT

Alternating current (AC) is defined as the continuous or uninterrupted bidirectional flow of charged particles. To produce this type of current, the voltage applied across a simple circuit oscillates in magnitude, and the polarity of the applied voltage is periodically (at least once per second) reversed. Electrons in the circuit first move in one direction. When the electric field is reversed, the electrons move back toward their original position. An alternating current may be produced by rotating a fixed voltage source in the circuit, as illustrated in Figure 1.8A. The alternating current that flows through this circuit is represented in Figure 1.8C, a graph of current amplitude over time. Alternating currents are characterized by the frequency (f) of oscillations and the amplitude of the electron or ionic movement. Alternating current frequency is expressed in hertz (Hz) or in cycles per second (cps). The reciprocal of frequency ($1/f$) defines a value, known as the *period*, that is the time between the beginning of one cycle of oscillation and the beginning of the next cycle.

A better understanding of alternating currents can be gained if one considers the forces and flows in a fluid-filled system. Alternating electrical current is analogous to fluid in a closed system moving first in one direction and then back in the opposite direction. Consequently, for many types of alternating current, there is no net movement of charged particles when the alternating electric field is withdrawn. For fluid to move back and forth in a hydraulic system, the pressure gradient must first be in one direction, then fall for an instant to zero, and then reverse direction. In the case of the hydraulic pump in Figure 1.8B, the pump rotates back and forth, much like the agitator in a washing machine. The oscillating pressure produced by the pump produces a back-and-forth movement of the fluid.

Alternating voltages applied to electrolytic solutions (as opposed to a metal conductor) produce cyclical movements in anions and cations in the solution. For some period of time, these ions experience an anode and cathode oriented in one fashion, and then the polarity of the electrodes in the solution switches. Consequently, the ions in solution move back and forth in solution, just as electrons move back and forth in metals when exposed to an alternating voltage.

Alternating currents are used in a number of electrotherapeutic applications. The most common contemporary clinical use of AC is in *interferential* electrical stimulation, where two circuits each producing sinusoidal AC are applied simultaneously for the management of problems such as pain.

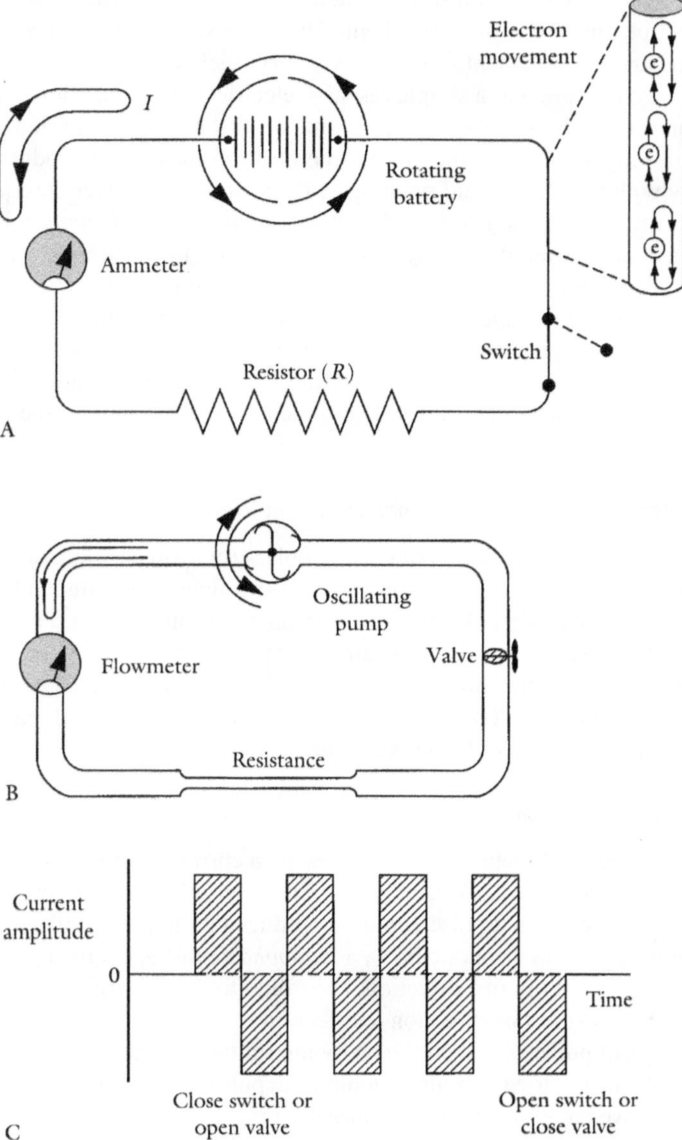

Figure 1.8. Simple electrical circuit in which a battery rotates at constant speed and regularly changes the direction of the driving force (voltage) acting on the electrons in the conductor **(A).** Note the back-and-forth movement of electrons. Hydraulic analog circuit of the electrical circuit in **(A)** illustrating the back-and-forth movement of the pump that produces the alternating movement of fluid within the system **(B).** Graphical representation of the alternating current produced in **(A)** on a current amplitude versus time plot **(C).**

PULSED CURRENT

Pulsed current (pulsatile, or interrupted, current) is defined as the unidirectional or bidirectional flow of charged particles that periodically ceases for a brief, finite period of time. A description of this type of current may not be found in basic physics textbooks, but the term is important because it describes the most commonly used form of current in clinical applications of electrical stimulation. Physicists and engineers might refer to pulsed current as either *interrupted DC* or *interrupted AC.* Pulsed current is characterized by the features of an elemental unit of this type of current, called a *pulse*. A single pulse is defined as an isolated electrical event separated by a brief, finite period of time from the next event. That is, a single pulse represents a very brief period of charged particle movement followed by a very brief cessation of movement.

If a fixed voltage is applied to a simple resistive electrical circuit as shown in Figure 1.6A, a unidirectional current will be induced in the conductor. If the circuit is periodically interrupted by opening and closing a switch in the circuit, the electron movement produced will start and stop in synchrony with the closing and opening of the switch. The current produced is intermittent and in one direction only and is referred to as *monophasic pulsed current.*

In a similar manner, if an alternating voltage is applied to the simple electrical circuit as shown in Figure 1.8, and the circuit is interrupted on completion of each cycle of the alternating voltage, the electrons in the conductors will briefly move back and forth, stop, and then begin to oscillate again. The current produced is intermittent, and the charged particle movement is bidirectional. Such a current is called a *biphasic pulsed current*. The changes in amplitude of the biphasic pulsed current for each pulse are determined by the changes in the amplitude of the applied voltage.

Descriptive Characteristics of Pulsed or Alternating Current Waveforms

The qualitative and quantitative features of current pulses (or a single cycle of AC) are most easily understood by examining a graph of the current (or voltage) amplitude changes that occur over time. The shape of a single pulse or AC cycle on a current versus time (or voltage versus time) plot is called the *waveform*. Some examples of waveforms produced by commercially available clinical electrical stimulators are illustrated in Figures 1.4 and 1.5. A single pulse or cycle of AC may be characterized by its amplitude- and time-dependent characteristics, as well as by a number of other descriptive features (Table 1.1).

NUMBER OF PHASES IN A WAVEFORM

The term *phase* refers to unidirectional current flow on a current/time plot. A pulse that deviates from the zero-current line (baseline) in only one direction, like that shown in Figure 1.9A, is referred to as monophasic. Such a pulse could be produced by intermittently interrupting a constant voltage source applied to a conductor. In a *monophasic pulse*, charged particles in the conductive medium move briefly in one direction, according to their charge, then stop. A pulse that deviates from baseline first in one direction and then in the opposite direction is called *biphasic* (Fig. 1.9A). This type of pulse can be produced by intermittently interrupting an alternating voltage source applied to an electrical circuit. In a biphasic pulse, charged particles move first in one direction and then move back in the opposite direction.

Waveforms with three phases are called *triphasic*, and those with more than three are called *polyphasic*. Some commercially produced waveforms that have been referred to by other authors as polyphasic may in fact be an uninterrupted series of biphasic waveforms when reduced to the simplest common electrical event.

Table 1.1. Descriptive Characteristics of Pulsed and Alternating Current Waveforms

Characteristic	***Common Designations***
Number of phases	Monophasic, biphasic, triphasic, polyphasic
Symmetry of phases	Symmetric, asymmetric
Balance of phase charge	Balanced, unbalanced
Waveform or phase shape	Rectangular, square, triangular, sawtooth, sinusoidal, exponential

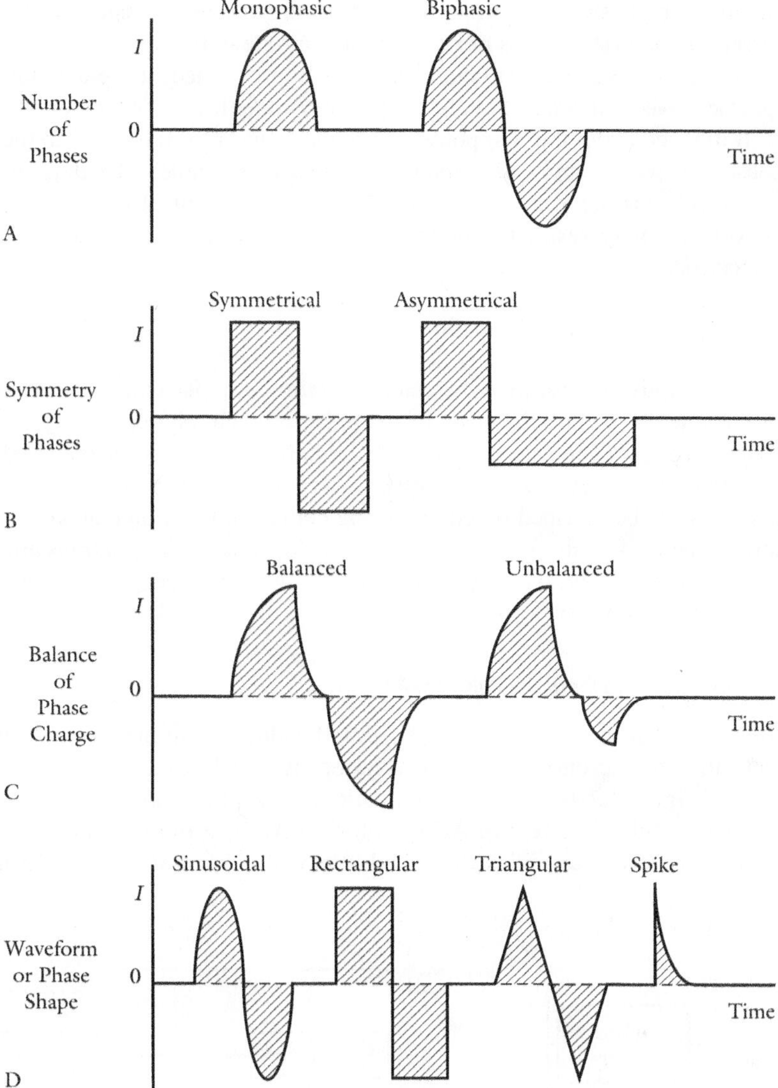

Figure 1.9. Characteristics of pulsed or alternating current waveforms.

SYMMETRY IN BIPHASIC WAVEFORMS

For biphasic pulses or AC cycles, the manner in which charges move back and forth may or may not be the same. If the way in which current amplitude varies over time for the first phase of a biphasic waveform is identical in nature but opposite in direction to that in the second phase, the biphasic waveform is described as *symmetrical* (Fig. 1.9B). That is, a waveform is described as symmetrical if the first phase is the mirror image of the second phase of a biphasic pulse or single cycle of AC. A waveform is referred to as *asymmetrical* if the way in which current amplitude varies in the first phase of a biphasic pulse is not the mirror image of the second phase (Fig. 1.9B).

CHARGE BALANCE IN BIPHASIC WAVEFORMS

For symmetrical biphasic waveforms, the total amount of current for one phase is equal to the absolute value of the total current flowing in the second phase. This condition may or may not be true for asymmetrical biphasic waveforms. If for an asymmetrical biphasic waveform the time integral for current in the first phase is not equal in magnitude to the time integral in the second phase, then the waveform is called *unbalanced*. More simply stated, if the area under the first phase of a biphasic waveform is not the same as the area under the second phase, the waveform is unbalanced. If the area under the first phase of a biphasic waveform is equal to the area under the second phase, the waveform is described as *balanced*. Examples of balanced and unbalanced biphasic waveforms are shown in Figure 1.9C. From a clinical perspective, the use of unbalanced waveforms may result in noticeable differences in the sensation of stimulation under surface electrodes.

WAVEFORMS

A very common descriptive approach to the characterization of pulsed and AC waveforms is the use of terms to denote the geometric shape of the pulse or cycle phases as they appear on the graph of current (or voltage) versus time. Shape designations frequently encountered in the professional and commercial literature include *rectangular*, *square*, *triangular*, *sawtooth*, and *spike*. Alternatively, shapes can be ascribed based on the mathematical function that would give rise to a graph (or portion thereof) of similar shape. Two examples of such designations are waveforms based on *sinusoidal* or *exponential* changes in current (or voltage) over time. Figure 1.9D illustrates several of the common waveforms.

Combining Qualitative Terms to Describe Pulsed or Alternating Currents

The descriptive terms defined above are of limited value for improving communication regarding electrotherapeutic currents unless a system is developed to link these terms in a consistent manner. Figure 1.10 shows an organizational chart that can be used to assign qualitative descriptions to pulsed current or AC waveforms. After examining the waveforms, one first decides which type of current is displayed. Next, the number of waveform phases is

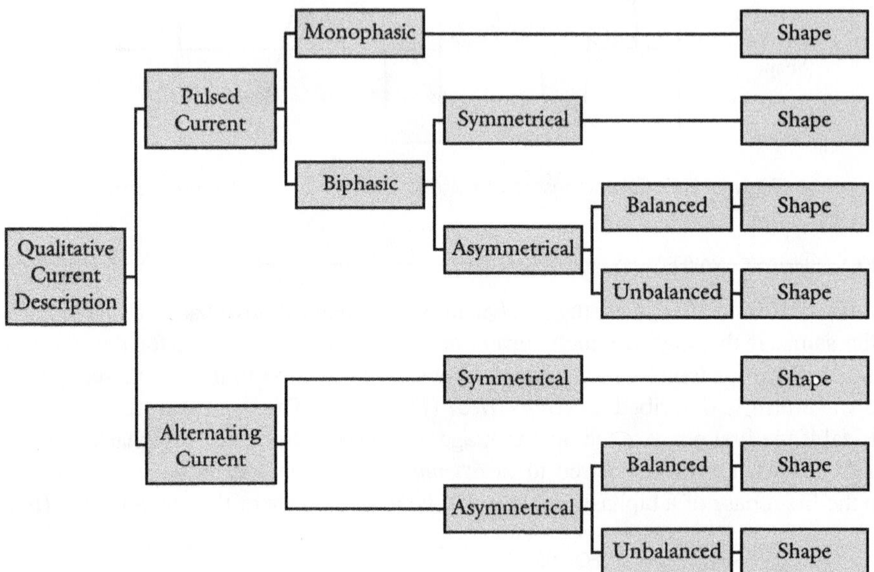

Figure 1.10. Diagram of the system for combining descriptive current designations in naming alternating or pulsed current waveforms.

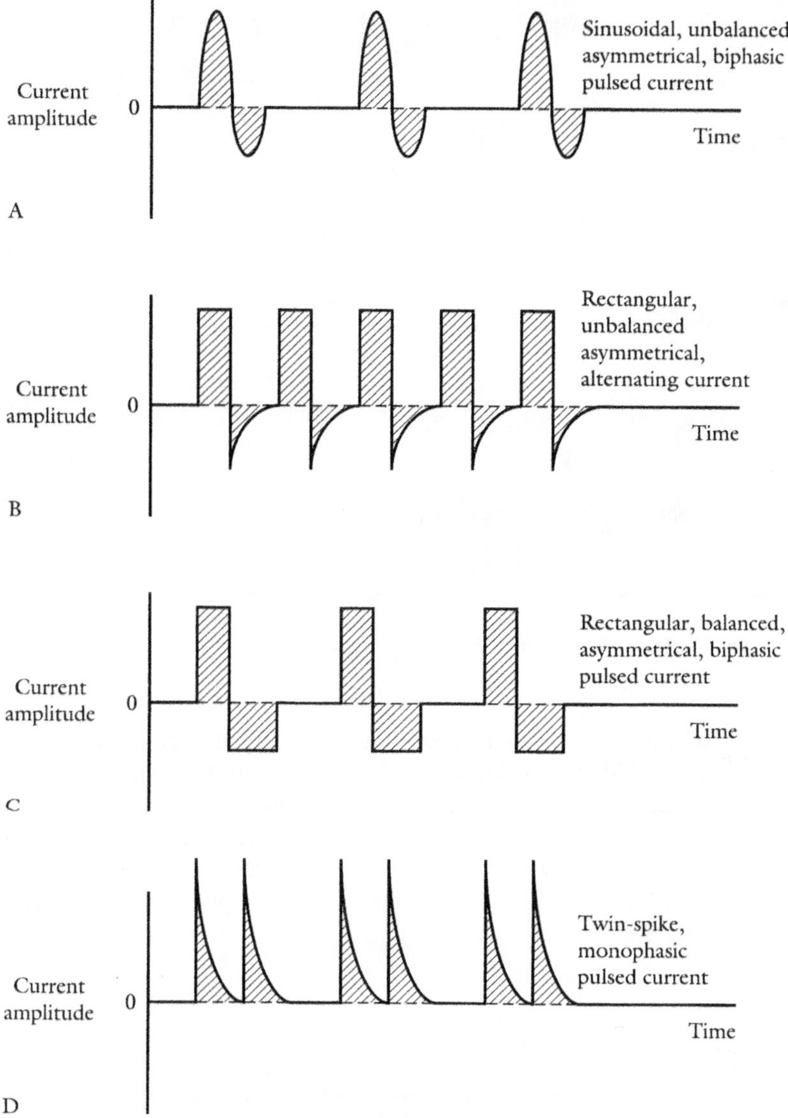

Figure 1.11. Graphical representation of several common forms of pulsed current labeled with appropriate *descriptive* designations. Waveforms represented in **(B)** and **(D)** have previously been called high-voltage pulsed galvanic and faradic, respectively.

determined, followed by the symmetry and balance of charge for biphasic waveforms. Finally, a shape designation may be assigned either to the entire pulse or, often, to the first phase of biphasic pulses.

The naming of the current waveform then proceeds from right to left along the chart. Figure 1.11 shows several current waveforms and indicates the qualitative description of these currents using the system shown in Figure 1.10. Note that this proposed system for naming electrotherapeutic currents may not be sufficient for describing all possible types of currents, but it does allow therapists and other practitioners to consistently describe most of the currents used in contemporary practice.

Table 1.2. Quantitative Characteristics of Pulsed and Alternating Currents

Amplitude-dependent characteristics
Peak amplitude
Peak-to-peak amplitude
Root-mean-square amplitude
Average amplitude
Time-dependent characteristics
Phase duration
Pulse duration
Rise time
Decay time
Interpulse interval
Intrapulse interval
Period
Frequency
Amplitude- and time-dependent characteristics
Phase charge
Pulse charge

Quantitative Characteristics of Pulsed and Alternating Currents

CHARACTERISTICS OF SINGLE PULSES

Pulsed current or AC waveforms may be quantitatively characterized by their amplitude- and time-dependent features (Table 1.2). Amplitude is a measure of the magnitude of current with reference to the zero-current baseline at any one moment in time on a current versus time graph (Fig. 1.12A). Alternatively, the amplitude may be a measure of the driving force (voltage) applied to induce a current when a waveform is plotted as a voltage versus time graph. Amplitude-dependent properties of current pulses (or voltage pulses) can be characterized by the measurement of the following:

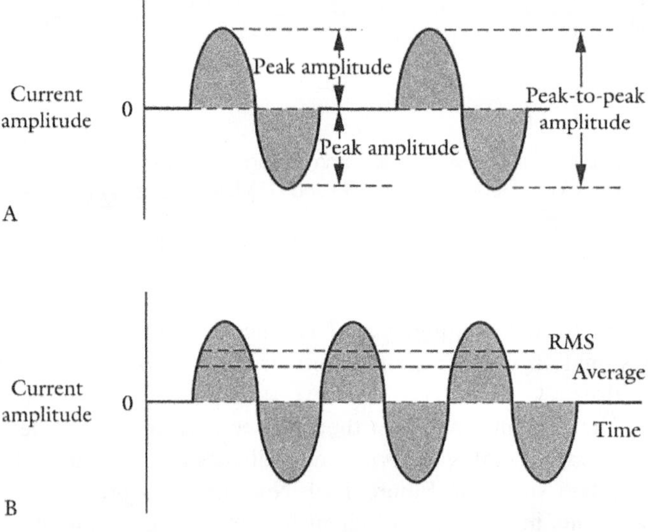

Figure 1.12. Sinusoidal AC waveforms and their amplitude-dependent characteristics. Amplitudes may be expressed as either peak amplitudes for each phase or peak-to-peak pulse amplitude **(A).** Alternatively, root mean square (RMS) or average amplitudes can be used to describe the magnitude of currents or voltages **(B).**

Peak amplitude: the maximum current (or voltage) reached in a monophasic pulse or for each phase of a biphasic pulse.

Peak-to-peak amplitude: the maximum current (or voltage) measured from the peak of the first phase to the peak of the second phase of a biphasic pulse.

Of these two methods of measuring current (or voltage) amplitude, peak amplitude of each phase is recommended. Other ways to describe current amplitude, such as *root mean square* (RMS, or effective) amplitude or *average current* per unit time, depend on the particular waveform examined. For instance, the RMS value for a pure sinusoidal waveform equals about 70% of the peak amplitude value, whereas the average current for the same waveform is about 64% of the peak value. Illustrations of these measures of current amplitude are given in Figure 1.12. Average current and RMS current measures take pulse shape into account and may more accurately reflect the stimulating power of the waveform than do peak amplitude measures.

The amplitude of currents applied using clinical stimulators is sometimes referred to as the *intensity of stimulation*. Therefore, controls on clinical generators that regulate the amplitude of induced current (voltage) are often labeled "intensity." Because the term intensity is also frequently used to describe pulse charge, it is recommended that the term intensity *not be used* to describe amplitude characteristics of pulsed current or AC waveforms.

A variety of time-dependent characteristics are used to quantify current pulses (Fig. 1.13). Time-dependent pulse characteristics of currents include the following:

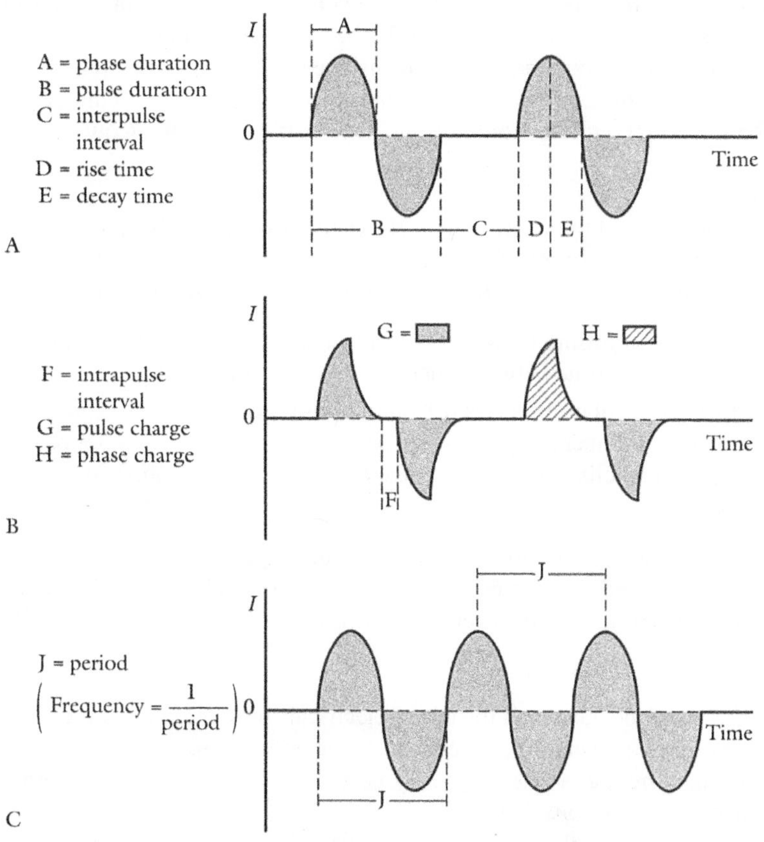

Figure 1.13. Time-dependent characteristics of pulsed or alternating current waveforms.

Phase duration: the elapsed time between the beginning and the end of one phase.

Pulse duration: the elapsed time between the beginning and the end of all phases in a single pulse; on clinical stimulators the pulse duration is often incorrectly labeled "pulse width."

Period: the elapsed time from a reference point on a pulse waveform or cycle of AC to the identical point on the next successive pulse; the reciprocal of frequency (period = $1/f$). For pulsed current, the period is equal to the pulse duration plus the interpulse interval.

Interphase interval: the elapsed time between two successive phases of a pulse; also known as the intrapulse interval.

Rise time: the time for the leading edge of the phase to increase in amplitude from the zero current base line to peak amplitude of one phase.

Decay time: the time for the trailing edge of the phase to return to the zero current base line from the peak or maximum amplitude of the phase.

These time-dependent characteristics of pulses are generally expressed in microseconds (μs, 10^{-6} seconds, millionths of a second) or milliseconds (ms, 10^{-3} seconds, thousandths of a second) when dealing with applications of pulsatile currents in clinical electrotherapy.

One of the most important quantitative characteristics of pulses from a physiologic standpoint is the charge carried by an individual pulse or phase of a pulse. The *phase charge* is defined as the time integral of current for a single phase. That is, the phase charge is represented by the area under a single phase waveform (Fig. 1.13B). As such, the phase charge is determined by both the amplitude of the phase and the duration of the phase. The magnitude of the phase charge will provide an indication of the relative influence a pulse will have in producing changes in biological systems. The *pulse charge* of a single pulse is the time integral for the current waveform over the entire pulse (Fig. 1.13B). For a typical biphasic pulse, the pulse charge is the sum of the area under each phase. For monophasic waveforms, the pulse charge and phase charge are equal. Phase and pulse charges are expressed in Coulombs, and pulse charges commonly found in clinical stimulation fall into the micro-Coulomb (μC, 10^{-6}, millionths of a Coulomb) range.

CHARACTERISTICS OF A SERIES OF PULSES

In addition to the terms used to quantify the features of individual pulses, a number of important terms are used to describe a series of pulses, the usual manner in which electrical currents are induced in biological tissues for their therapeutic effects. Among those terms are the following:

Interpulse interval: the time between the end of one pulse and the beginning of the next pulse in a series; the time between successive pulses (Fig. 1.13A).

Frequency (f): the number of pulses per unit time for pulsed current expressed as pulses per second (pps); the number of cycles of AC per second expressed in cycles per second (cps) or hertz (Hz); often on clinical stimulators the frequency of stimulation control is labeled "rate (Fig. 1.13C)."

Because voltage and current are directly proportional, many of the terms used to describe the amplitude- and time-dependent characteristics of currents may also be used to describe the voltage pulse features that induce these current waveforms.

CURRENT MODULATIONS

Amplitude and Duration Modulations. In the use of electrical stimulation for management of patient problems, current amplitude- and time-related characteristics are often varied in a prescribed fashion. Changes in current characteristics may be sequential, intermittent, or variable in nature and are referred to as *modulations*. Several of the quantitative characteristics of pulsed current and AC are modulated in selected clinical applications. Variations in the peak amplitude of a series of pulses are called *amplitude modulations* (Fig. 1.14A). Regular changes in the time over which

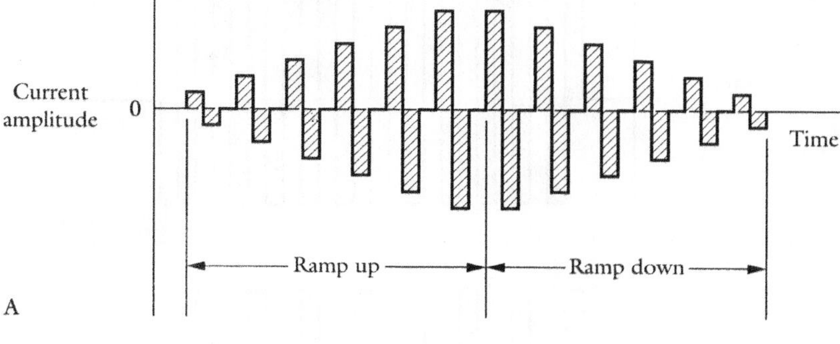

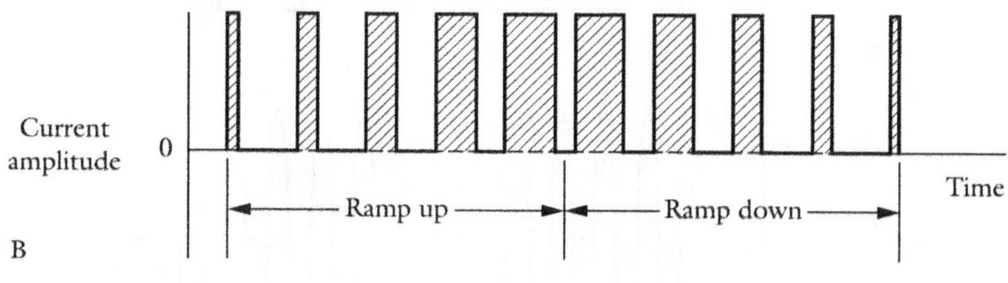

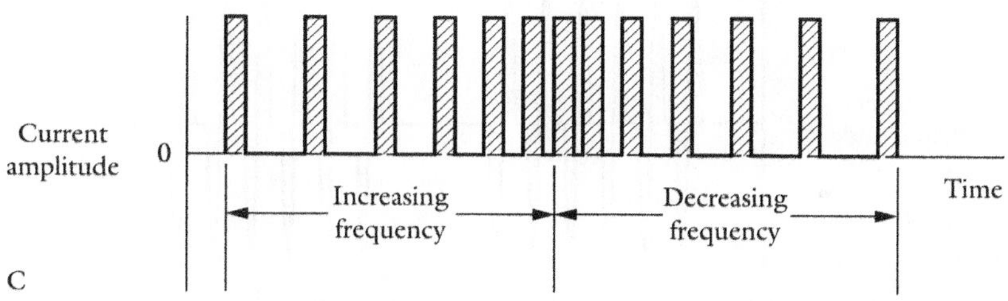

Figure 1.14. Examples of automatic modulations of stimulation characteristics. **A:** Amplitude modulation. **B:** Pulse duration modulation. **C:** Frequency modulation.

each pulse in a series acts are referred to as *pulse* or *phase duration modulations* (Fig. 1.14B). *Frequency modulations* consist of cyclic variations in the number of pulses applied per unit time (Fig. 1.14C). The illustrations of modulations shown in Figure 1.14 occur in a systematic fashion. Modulations in amplitude, pulse duration, or frequency can also be provided randomly.

Another modulation encountered rather frequently in clinical electrical stimulation is *ramp* (*surge*) *modulation*. Ramp modulations are characterized by an increase (ramp up) or decrease (ramp down) of pulse amplitude, pulse duration, or both, over time. In the past, ramp modulations have been referred to as *rise time* and *fall time*. However, these two terms are now used to describe single-pulse characteristics, not the variations in features of a series of pulses.

Timing Modulations. A continuous, repetitive series of pulses (series of pulses at a fixed frequency) or a segment of AC is called a *train* (Fig. 1.15A, B). Systematic variations in the pattern of delivery of a series of current pulses are referred to as *timing modulations*. Several terms are now recognized for describing timing modulations. They include the following:

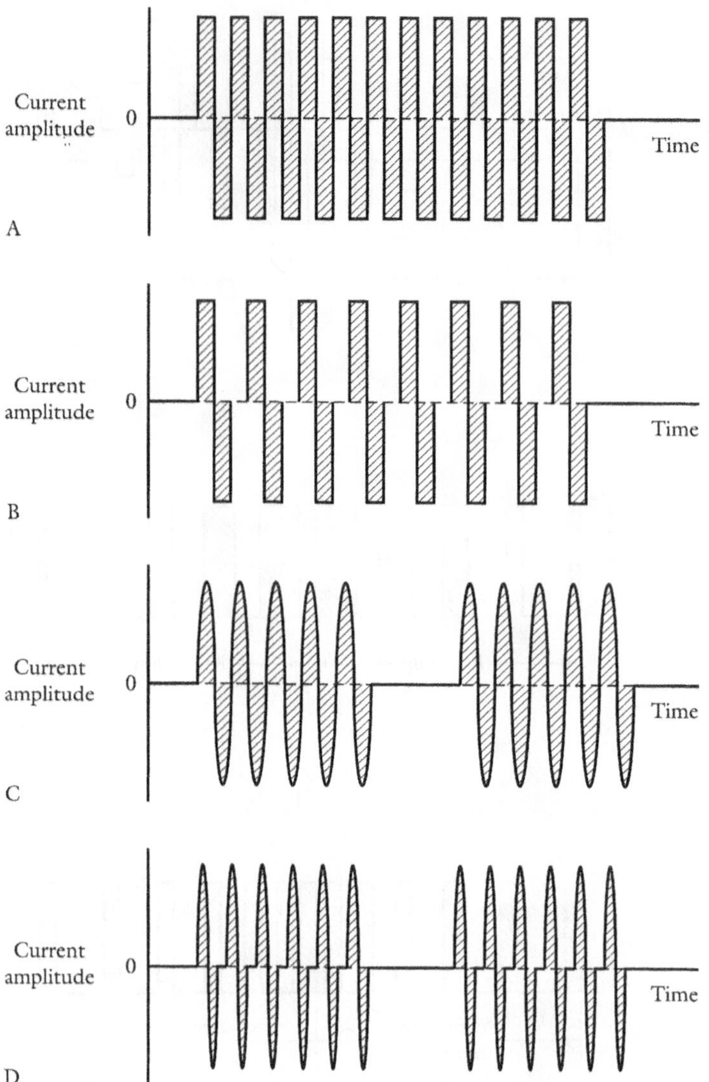

Figure 1.15. Examples of stimulation trains and burst modulations. **A:** Continuous train of rectangular, symmetric, biphasic AC waveforms. **B:** Continuous train of rectangular, symmetric, biphasic pulsed current waveforms. **C:** Burst-modulated, sinusoidal AC waveforms. **D:** Burst-modulated, sinusoidal pulsed current waveforms.

Burst: a series of groups of pulses or groups of alternating current cycles delivered at a specified frequency over a specified time interval (Fig. 1.15C and D) followed by a brief time interval without charged particle movement. The time interval over which the finite series of pulses or AC cycles is delivered is called the *burst duration*. The time period between bursts is called the *interburst interval*. In contemporary clinical applications of such burst modulations, the burst duration and interburst interval are usually on the order of a few milliseconds. The number of bursts delivered per unit of time is called the *burst frequency*.

In some forms of electrotherapy, trains of pulses, trains of AC, or series of bursts are applied to patients without any interruption for the entire treatment period. Such a pattern of stimulation is often described as a *continuous mode* of stimulation. In many other approaches, trains of pulses, trains of AC cycles, or series of bursts are often applied to patients for times ranging from a few seconds to a minute or more, followed by comparable periods of no stimulation before stimulation is resumed. That is, trains or series of bursts are intermittently or regularly interrupted. Such patterns of stimulation are quantitatively characterized by two time intervals, called the *on time* and the *off time*:

On time: the time during which a train of pulses, trains of AC, or a series of bursts is delivered in a therapeutic application.

Off time: the time between trains of pulses, trains of AC, or a series of bursts.

A closely associated characterization of the interrupted patterns of stimulation used in many clinical applications is embodied in the concept of the *duty cycle*. The duty cycle of stimulation is the ratio of on time to the sum of on time plus off time multiplied by 100, expressed as a percentage (Fig. 1.16).

$$\text{Duty Cycle} = \frac{\text{On time}}{(\text{On time} + \text{Off time})} \times 100\%$$

For example, if the on time equals 10 seconds and the off time equals 30 seconds, the duty cycle for such a pattern of stimulation would be 25% (Fig. 1.16A). A very different pattern of stimulation with an on time of 5 seconds and an off time of 15 seconds yields the same 25% duty cycle (Fig. 1.16B). For this reason and because in some cases the duty cycle has erroneously been equated with the simple ratio of on time divided by off time, confusion has arisen from the use of the term duty cycle. For clear documentation of stimulation patterns, specific on times and off times of stimulation should be specified rather than using the duty cycle or on/off ratios.

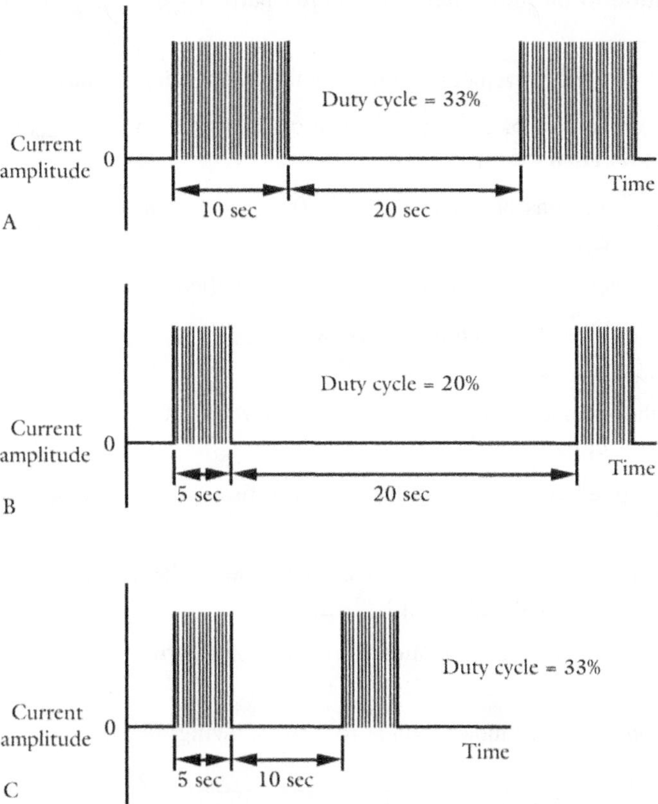

Figure 1.16. Examples of on times and off times of stimulation and the concept of duty cycle, with 2-pulse per second monophasic pulsed currents at fixed amplitude. **A:** 10-second on time and 20-second off time. **B:** 5-second on time and 20-second off time. **C:** 5-second on time and 10-second off time.

SUMMARY

This chapter has presented fundamental concepts in electricity and standardized terminology associated with the application of electrotherapeutic currents. The review of basic electrical concepts was included to refresh the reader's memory of physical entities and principles that form a foundation for understanding the electrical and chemical events associated with clinical applications of electricity. Standardized qualitative and quantitative terminology was presented to facilitate clear communication among researchers, clinicians, students, and manufacturers involved in the use and development of clinical electrotherapy. To this end, the standardized terminology is used throughout the rest of the book. The various quantitative characteristics defined in this chapter represent the features of electrical stimulation that must be either selected or regulated by therapists or other practitioners to safely and effectively use electrotherapy to achieve therapeutic outcomes.

SELF-STUDY QUESTIONS

For answers, see Appendix B.

1. The driving force that makes charged particles move is called ____(a)____, ____(b)____, or ____(c)____.
2. The movement of charged particles in a conductor is called a ________.
3. The opposition to the movement of charged particles in an electrical circuit is called ________.
4. The opposition to the movement of ions in biological systems is called ________.
5. The negative pole of a battery or electrical circuit is called ____(a)____, and the positive pole is called the ____(b)____.
6. Positively charged ions are called ____(a)____, and negatively charged ions are called ____(b)____.
7. Anions are attracted to the [*cathode/anode*] and repelled from the [*cathode/anode*].
8. Ohm's law describes the relationship between ____(a)____, ____(b)____, and ____(c)____.
9. The larger the voltage applied to an electrical circuit, the larger the ________ produced in the circuit.
10. For a fixed applied voltage, if the impedance of tissue is decreased, the magnitude of the current will ________.
11. The three types of current used in contemporary electrotherapy are ____(a)____, ____(b)____, and ____(c)____.
12. The shape of the visual representation of currents on a current amplitude versus time graph is called a ________.
13. Give the standard unit of measurement for the following:

    a. current ________

    b. electromotive force ________

    c. resistance ________

    d. capacitance ________

e. impedance ______________________________

f. conductance ______________________________

g. pulsed current frequency ____________________

h. AC frequency ______________________________

i. peak amplitude (current) ____________________

j. pulse duration ______________________________

k. phase charge ______________________________

l. on time/off time ____________________________

14. Use the flowchart in Figure 1.10 to assign qualitative descriptions to the currents diagramed below.

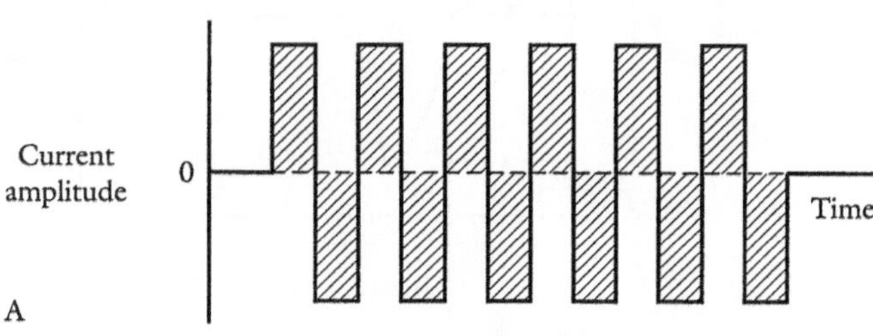

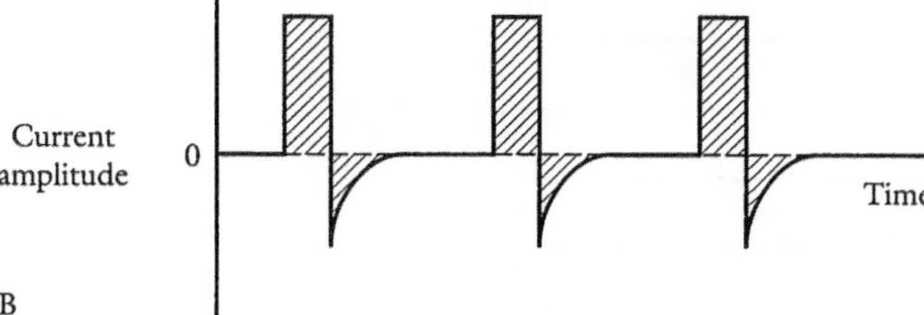

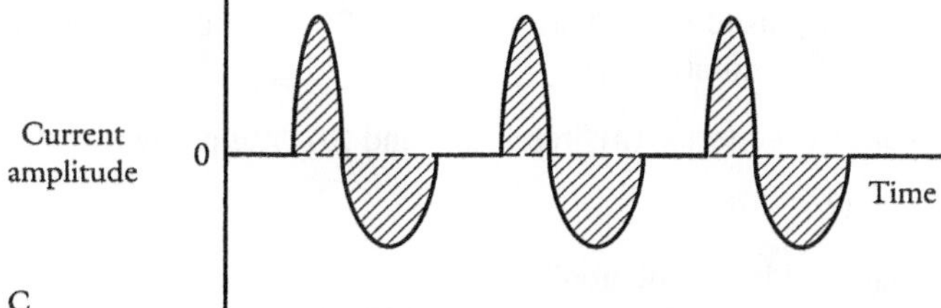

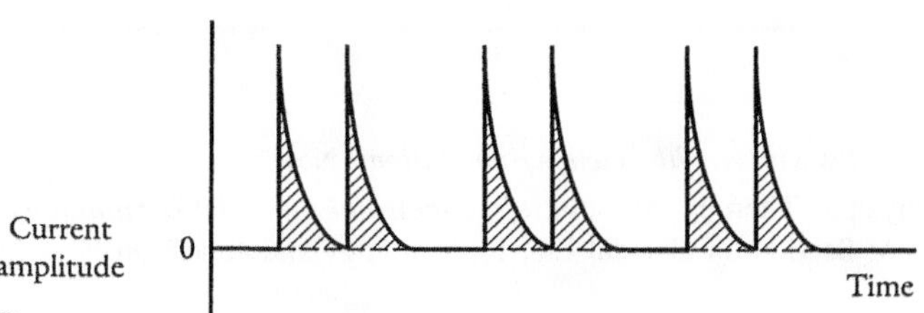

15. Draw examples of the following types of currents on current amplitude versus time graphs.

a. Triangular, symmetrical, biphasic pulsed current

b. Rectangular, balanced, asymmetrical, biphasic pulsed current

c. Sinusoidal, unbalanced, asymmetrical alternating current

d. Square, monophasic pulsed current

16. For the pulsed current waveforms shown, provide labels for the lettered amplitude- and time-dependent characteristics.

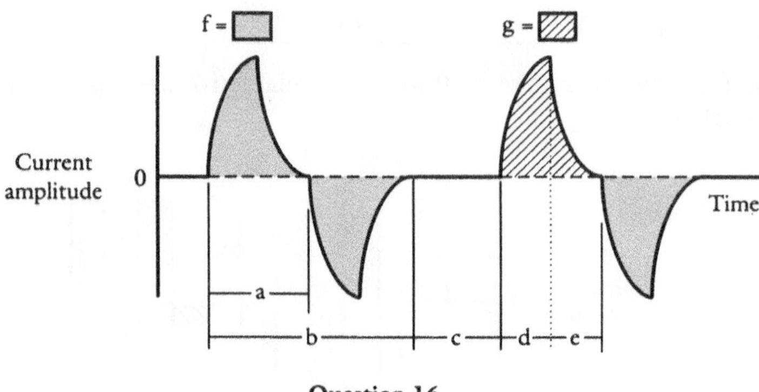

Question 16

a. ______________________________

b. ______________________________

c. ______________________________

d. ______________________________

e. ______________________________

f. ______________________________

g. ______________________________

17. If the on time of pulsed current stimulation is 20 seconds and the off time is 60 seconds, the duty cycle of stimulation is ________________.

18. What is meant by the terms (a) "ramp up" and (b) "ramp down"?

19. What is a burst?

20. What is an amplitude modulation?

REFERENCES

1. Urone, P.P. *Physics with Health Science Applications.* New York: Harper and Row; 1986:264–343.
2. American Physical Therapy Association. *Electrotherapeutic Terminology in Physical Therapy.* Alexandria, VA: Section on Clinical Electrophysiology and American Physical Therapy Association; 2001.

CHAPTER 2

Instrumentation for Electrotherapy

Andrew J. Robinson

A wide variety of devices are commercially available for electrotherapeutic applications. Instrumentation in electrotherapy is evolving because of advances in engineering, developments in electrotherapy research, and a broader range of problems managed by electrotherapy. A clear understanding of the components and operating principles of electrical stimulation devices is essential for safe and effective clinical applications. This chapter describes (a) design features and general principles for operating electrical stimulators; (b) typical controls to regulate parameters of stimulation; (c) common types and features of commercially available stimulators; and (d) types of electrodes and general considerations in the selection and application of electrodes. The objective of this chapter is to provide a description of electrotherapeutic stimulators available to the practitioner, rather than to provide a detailed presentation suitable only to the biomedical engineer. Discussion of commercial classes of stimulators is not intended to include specific descriptions of each manufacturer's stimulator features. Instead, the intention is to present the characteristics and features of devices generally marketed within a particular class. Such information may also be of value to those responsible for the acquisition of electrical stimulators for clinical applications. In the final section of the chapter, issues related to electrical safety in the selection and clinical utilization of stimulators are discussed.

DESIGN FEATURES OF STIMULATORS FOR ELECTROTHERAPEUTIC APPLICATIONS

Electrotherapeutic devices are used to induce electrical currents in body tissues. When electrotherapy has been determined to be an appropriate therapeutic intervention, the first question faced by the clinician is, What stimulator do I use to achieve the desired outcome? The choice of a stimulator for a particular application is determined by a number of design-related factors, including the following:

1. Does the stimulator produce the specific parameters of electrical stimulation required to bring about the desired effect? Are the waveform, output frequency range, output channel timing, and so forth, sufficient for the particular application?
2. Does the stimulator have sufficient maximum output amplitude to achieve the desired effect?
3. Does the stimulator have a sufficient number of output channels for the application?
4. Does the stimulator have appropriate controls to make any necessary adjustments of stimulation parameters during treatment?
5. Can stimulation parameters be adjusted while stimulation is being provided, or does the instrument need to be turned off?

6. Is a battery-operated stimulator appropriate for the application, or should a line-powered stimulator be selected?
7. Is the stimulator preprogrammed, or should the stimulation parameters be adjusted separately for each type of application?
8. Are important safety features included in the stimulator design?

Questions such as these related to stimulator design are important considerations in the planning of an electrotherapy program. Clinicians who use electrotherapy need to be aware of the different design features of stimulators, as well as the potential advantages and disadvantages of each. If the clinician has a clear understanding of the output characteristics and control features of a stimulator, he or she need not understand the operation of internal circuitry or discrete electronic components (e.g., oscillators, transformers, rectifiers) to be able to safely and effectively use the stimulator.

Portable, Battery-Operated versus Line-Powered Stimulator Designs

Depending on the stimulation characteristics applied, that is, the magnitude and duration of the stimulation required, the power requirements of stimulation devices may be small or large. Those therapeutic interventions that require relatively high stimulator output for long periods dictate the use of standard, line-powered (115 V, sinusoidal AC) devices. One advantage of line-powered stimulators is that stimulation parameters should remain at set levels for as long as treatment is provided, given no interruption in the power supply. The main disadvantage of the line-powered devices is that they can only be applied when clients can remain stationary during stimulation.

When an electrotherapeutic intervention does not require relatively high device output and/or prolonged periods of stimulation, battery-powered (1.5 V to 9.0 V) stimulators are often selected. Battery-operated stimulators in general have much lower peak output amplitudes than line-powered units. Portable, battery-driven devices have the advantage of allowing stimulation while a client is moving, as in the stimulation of muscle during ambulation or stimulation for pain control while a patient is on the job. The performance of portable stimulators depends on battery life, which is in turn determined by the particular stimulation procedure used. Suffice it to say that the higher the amplitude requirements or the more frequently the stimulator is used, the greater the power consumption and the shorter the battery life. In most uses of battery-operated therapeutic stimulators, batteries should be either recharged (nickel–cadmium batteries) or replaced (alkaline batteries) frequently because the power drain is substantial even in short-term applications, and an undesirable drop in the output amplitude may result as treatment is continued. Carbon batteries are generally not suitable for use in portable stimulators because of their short operating life and the potential for leakage of corrosive chemicals that may damage the stimulator.

Analog Control versus Digital Control Stimulator Designs

Analog control stimulators allow the adjustment of stimulation parameters primarily through the use of rotary knobs or dials. Because these stimulator controls are mechanical in nature (e.g., potentiometers), analog-controlled stimulators may also be referred to as "hardware controlled." Digital control stimulators, in contrast, allow adjustment through the use of push buttons or pressure-sensitive switches. In general, devices with a digital control design include some form of visual display (e.g., an LCD) that allows one to select from a menu of available stimulation parameters. Today's digital design stimulators are generally microprocessor-based and are also called "software-controlled." Figure 2.1 illustrates two portable neuromuscular stimulators, one with more traditional analog controls and one of a newer design with digital control.

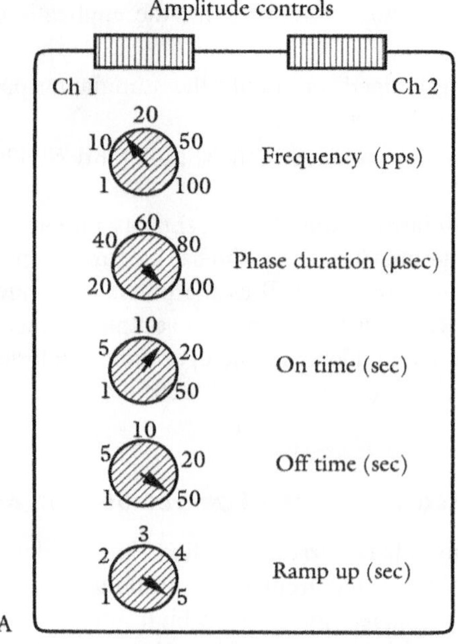

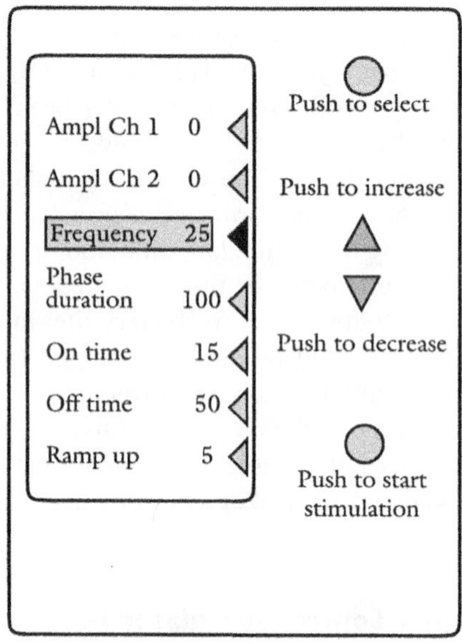

Figure 2.1. Control panel of portable stimulator with analog controls **(A)** and digital controls **(B).**

Both analog and digital instruments have advantages and disadvantages. The primary advantage of analog controls is the ability to continuously adjust many of the stimulation parameters, thus allowing the knowledgeable user to make fine adjustments in stimulation characteristics while the treatment is occurring. In contrast, digital controls often allow only incremental adjustment of parameters. This disadvantage can be minimized if the size of the increments from one setting to the next is made as small as possible. For example, frequency adjustment in increments of 1 pps (pulse per second) as opposed to increments of 10 pps would enhance the user's ability to precisely control the pattern of stimulation for a variety of applications. In addition, modification of stimulation characteristics with digital devices often requires the user to scroll through menu options. This control approach is time-consuming if changes are desired during the course of treatment. Analog controls may be more user friendly in the hands of those who were grew up with analog-controlled radios and televisions; whereas those who have been regularly exposed to digitally controlled electronics (e.g., computer games) may be more comfortable with digital stimulators.

Some digital devices have a memory capability that allows the user to store a set of stimulation parameters for later use. Preprogrammed patterns of stimulation (protocols) may be useful to clinicians who are less familiar with the electrotherapy literature; such preprogrammed patterns make stimulator use easier. The use of preprogrammed protocols assumes that the stimulator manufacturer has selected stimulation characteristics that are effective and safe for a particular application. Note that this may not always be the case. Analog-controlled stimulators usually do not have preprogrammed memory, although some would argue that the positions in which the knobs and switches are left constitutes memory; at least a memory of the last treatment. In general, stimulators with primarily analog controls require the user to be more knowledgeable regarding electrotherapy and to be aware of the expected consequences of stimulation parameter adjustment.

Some contemporary stimulators incorporate both analog control and digital control technology in their design and hence take advantage of the benefits of each approach.

CONTROLS TO REGULATE THE CHARACTERISTICS AND PATTERN OF ELECTRICAL STIMULATION

Although an understanding of the function of the internal components of electrical stimulators may be of interest to the user, this knowledge is not critical for one to use electrical stimulators in the clinic. In contrast, knowledge of the types of current produced, the waveform characteristics, and how the stimulation parameters are regulated is essential for the safe and effective application of electrotherapy. The specific output parameters that can be adjusted, selected, or set by users of electrical stimulators vary from device to device. The parameters are adjusted with analog or digital controls, usually located on one main control panel of the stimulator. In some cases (e.g., portable stimulators) these controls are located in covered or hidden compartments. Such a design reduces the chance that the user will inadvertently or intentionally change the stimulus parameters and cause an unintended pattern of stimulation to be applied. Controls located in hidden compartments are often initially set and/or adjusted only by the health care professional responsible for implementing the stimulation.

No industry standard exists for the types of stimulator controls that every type of stimulator should possess. The stimulator controls common to many units currently used in clinical practice are discussed below. The focus of the following discussion is on analog as opposed to digital controls.

Waveform Selection Controls

The proliferation of commercially available stimulation devices has been accompanied by the development of numerous types of current (or voltage) waveforms that can be used in clinical electrotherapy. Most devices designed before the early 1980s included waveform generators capable of producing only one type of waveform from a single instrument. Today, many commercially available stimulators are capable of producing several distinct waveforms. One of the first steps in applying stimulation clinically is to select a suitable waveform. This is achieved in some stimulators by a

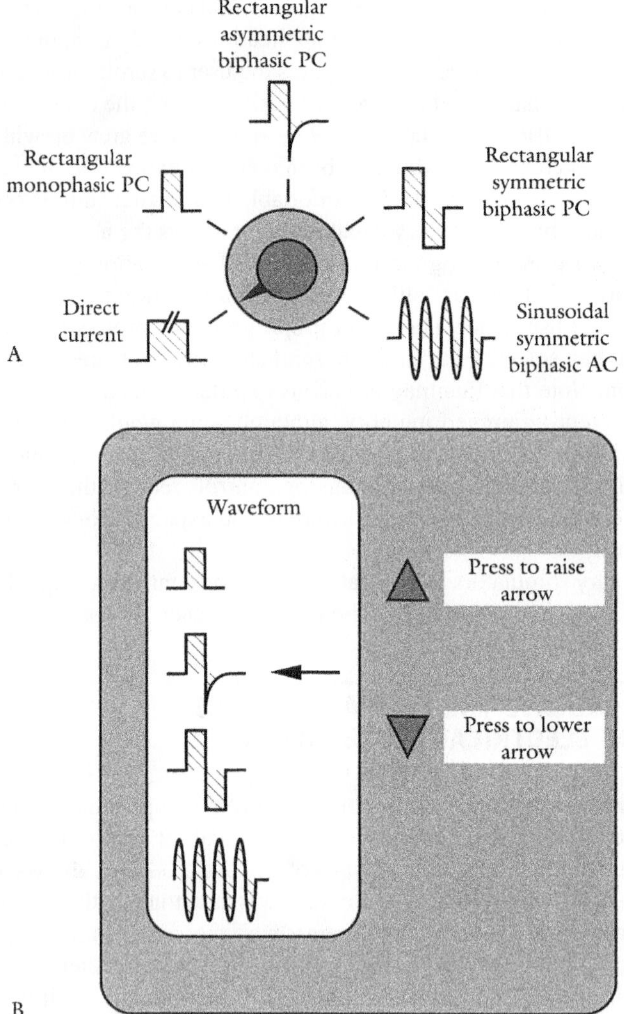

Figure 2.2. Waveform selector control illustrating the options available for treatment applications. **A:** Analog control. **B:** Digital control.

control generically referred to as a *waveform selector*. Waveform selectors may be rotary switches, pressure-sensitive switches, or other types of controls labeled with small diagrams of the available waveforms (Fig. 2.2). In some microprocessor-based stimulators, waveforms can be selected from a menu on the display screen. The choice of the "most appropriate" waveform for a particular outcome should be based on findings or recommendations from the scientific or professional literature. Information on waveform selection for specific applications is given in subsequent chapters that address the types of clinical impairments that may be managed with electrotherapy.

Amplitude Controls

The *amplitude controls* on stimulators allow the user to adjust the magnitude of the output voltage or current from the output amplifier circuit. On direct current generators the amplitude controls regulate the magnitude of current and generally do not allow the current to exceed 5 mA (milliamperes) at maximum settings. On AC or pulsed current generators, amplitude controls allow

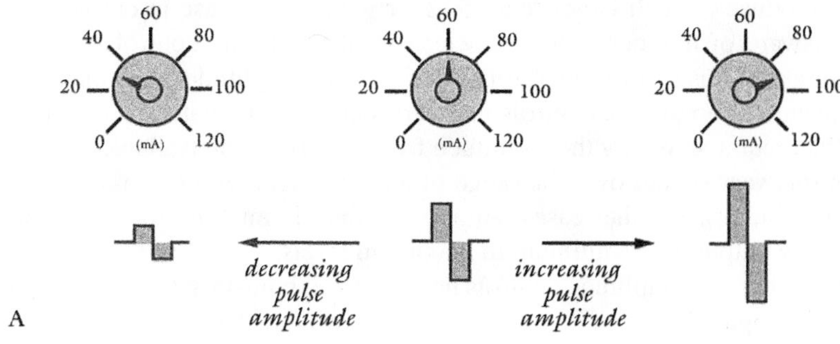

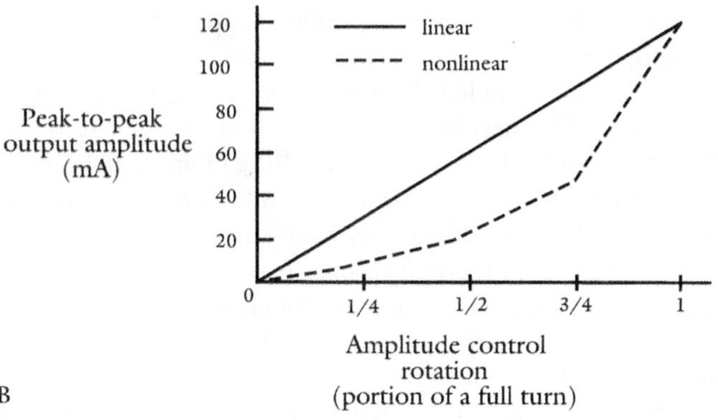

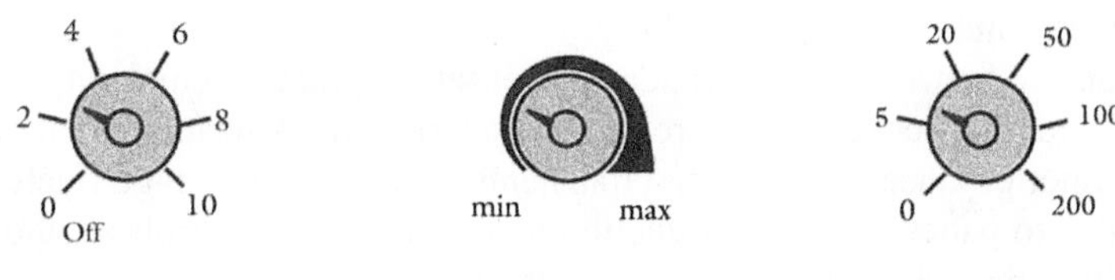

Figure 2.3. Amplitude controls. **A:** The effect of changes in dial setting on pulse amplitude. **B:** The relationship between the amplitude control setting and peak-to-peak pulse amplitude. **C:** Examples of the amplitude control labeling used on commercial stimulators.

the practitioner to adjust the peak amplitude or peak-to-peak amplitude of AC cycles or pulses (Fig. 2.3A). Depending on the specific stimulator, either output current or voltage are regulated, and amplitudes usually do not exceed peak values of 100 to 200 mA or 500 V, respectively.

Analog amplitude controls are variable resistors, or potentiometers. Ideally, these potentiometers should be linear. In a linear potentiometer, every increment of rotation of the potentiometer dial produces an equal change in stimulator output amplitude (Fig. 2.3B). For instance, a one-quarter turn of the dial would change the resistance by 25% and correspondingly would alter the output amplitude by 25%. Commonly, however, the amplitude controls are nonlinear (1,2). In such cases, a one-quarter turn of the dial may produce only a small (e.g., 5%) rise in amplitude in the initial range of rotation, whereas a one-quarter turn at the end of the range of rotation might produce a much larger (e.g., 50% or greater) increase in output amplitude. The user who is unaware of this common characteristic of amplitude controls may inadvertently deliver a startling stimulus to a patient during the course of amplitude adjustment.

Another feature of amplitude controls that varies among stimulators is the number of revolutions of the dial required to vary the amplitude from 0 to 100% of available output. Most often amplitude controls vary output over the range of a single clockwise turn (actually about three-quarters of a revolution). In other cases, amplitude controls must be rotated several complete revolutions to vary output from minimum to maximum levels.

In some instances, the amplitude controls have a switch built-in at the beginning of the range of rotation. Such amplitude dials (Fig. 2.3C) must be switched to the "off" position before the stimulator can be turned on in subsequent sessions. This is a valuable safety feature designed to prevent the output circuits of the stimulator from being "powered up" when the amplitude control is left at a level other than zero output. This design of output controls is intended to prevent unexpected stimulation to the patient.

On digital or microprocessor-based stimulators, output amplitude is usually adjusted in incremental steps by depressing pressure-sensitive switches.

Amplitude controls are frequently labeled "intensity" or "voltage," and numbers ranging from 1 to 10 indicate the lowest to highest level of stimulation output. Users of stimulation devices should be aware that the numerical labels often bear little relation to the actual or relative amplitude of stimulation being applied to an individual. In other cases, controls may have no numerical labeling related to output amplitude, or may have labeling that reflects the nonlinear characteristics of the control (Fig. 2.3C). Precise information on relative output changes in current or voltage as amplitude controls are adjusted may be obtained only by observing the analog or digital meters available on some devices or by monitoring stimulator output using an oscilloscope. No industry standards exist for monitoring or displaying the amplitude of either monophasic or biphasic current waveforms in stimulators. Furthermore, the absolute amplitude of stimulation does not bear a consistent relationship to evoked response (e.g., muscle contraction level) from subject to subject or from session to session in the same subject. In actual clinical stimulation sessions, one of the best indicators of the amplitude is the patient's subjective perception of the stimulation.

The relationship between the amplitude control setting and the actual output of the stimulator should be periodically checked to ensure proper functioning. Adjustments of analog amplitude controls should not produce large voltage transients (unexpected voltage fluctuations) that may be uncomfortable to patients. Any malfunctioning of amplitude controls should be immediately corrected by either replacing or cleaning the controls.

Ideally, independent amplitude controls should be available for each output channel. On some devices, however, only one amplitude control is present for changing amplitude on two output channels simultaneously. In some cases, the single-output amplitude control for two channels is accompanied by a dial called a *balance control*. Adjustment of the balance control shifts the relative amplitude of stimulation from one channel to another (Fig. 2.4). The balance control increases the amplitude on one channel and simultaneously decreases it on the other. Such a design is more difficult to use than one having independent amplitude controls on each channel. When the balance control is initially set to equally divide the stimulator output and the amplitude control is gradually advanced, the amplitude increases by the same amount on each output channel. If amplitude control is set at a particular level and the balance control is adjusted, the amplitude of stimulation increases on one output channel and simultaneously decreases on the other. Such an arrangement can be problematic when, in a two-channel application, the desired amplitude is reached on the first channel but is insufficient on the second. In order to reach desired stimulation levels on each channel, the balance control is adjusted to raise the relative amount of stimulation to the second channel. This change decreases the stimulation of the first channel, which must then

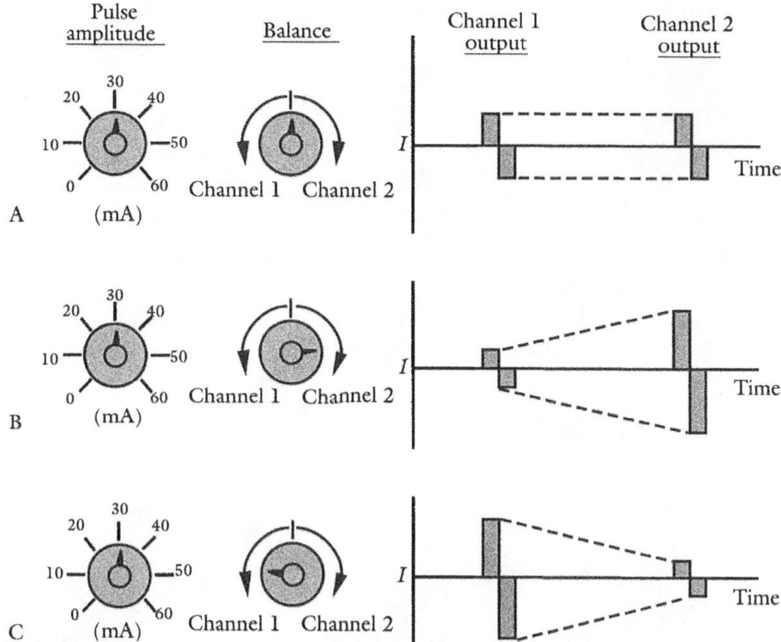

Figure 2.4. Effects of balance control adjustment on pulse amplitude for each of two stimulation channels. **A:** Output amplitude balanced between two channels. **B:** Output amplitude increased on channel 2 while decreased on channel 1. **C:** Output amplitude increased on channel 1 while decreased on channel 2.

be compensated for by another amplitude adjustment. A number of such adjustments may be required before the desired level of stimulation is reached on each channel.

The maximum output amplitude of electrical stimulators has been used as a basis for categorizing these devices. The common differentiation of stimulators based on output amplitudes is "low volt" and "high volt." Low-volt devices are those that produce peak amplitudes of less than 100 to 150 V, whereas high-volt devices produce peak amplitudes of more than 150 V. Differentiation among stimulators based on output amplitudes alone is not recommended, because such a system does not take into account many of the other important characteristics of stimulation, such as the output frequencies or the phase (or pulse) durations. In addition, the high-volt devices are capable of producing low-voltage output when the amplitudes are adjusted within the low range of the device capability.

Phase Duration and Pulse Duration Controls

Phase duration controls adjust the duration of a single phase of biphasic pulses, usually the first phase of the pulse. *Pulse duration controls* regulate the total duration of individual waveforms in pulsed-current stimulators (Fig. 2.5). Such controls are common on portable, battery-operated stimulators designed for pain reduction, and they are becoming more common in recent designs of 60-Hz AC-powered devices for neuromuscular stimulation applications. Phase and pulse duration controls are not found on most AC stimulators because the cycle duration is determined by the frequency of stimulation.

Phase and pulse duration controls are often labeled "pulse width" or "width." Such designations are not recommended because phase and pulse durations are measured in units of time (generally milliseconds or microseconds), not in units of length. A numerical-scale labeling of analog phase (or pulse) duration controls in equal increments from 1 to 10 is common. Like that

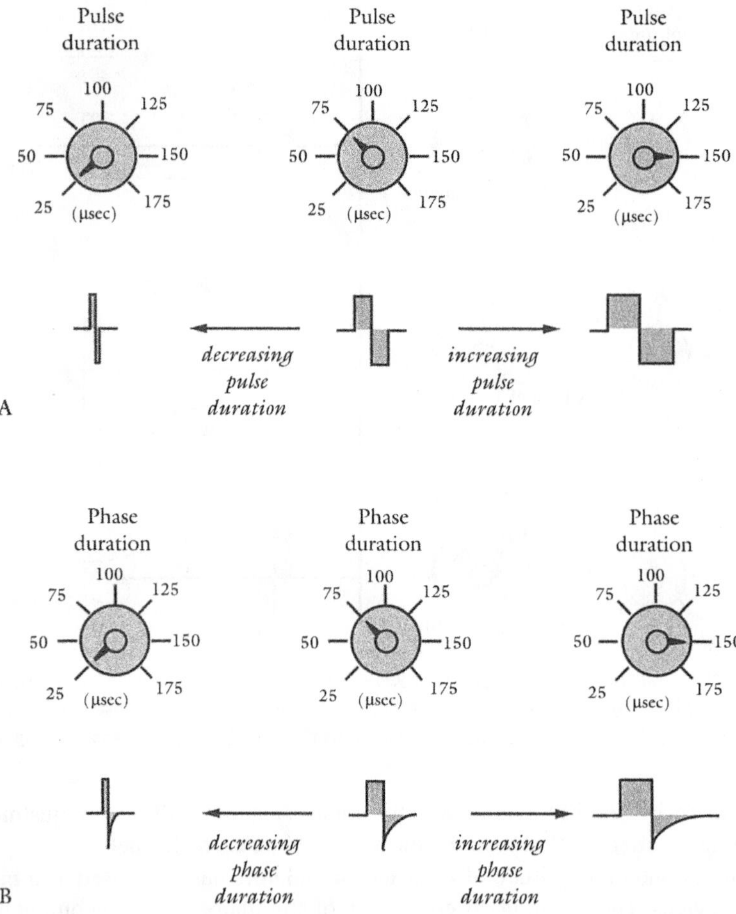

Figure 2.5. A: Pulse duration controls showing the effect of changes in dial setting on the pulse duration. **B:** Phase duration controls showing the effect of changes in dial setting on the duration of the first phase of a rectangular, asymmetric, biphasic pulse.

for analog amplitude controls, such labeling may not reflect relative changes in phase (or pulse) duration as the duration dial is rotated. Similarly, the adjustment of phase duration dials may not produce linear changes in phase duration (1). In some stimulator designs, the phase duration control is a rotary switch rather than a smoothly rotating potentiometer. Often in such cases, the phase duration control will allow the user to select the specific phase or pulse duration shown on the dial label. In digital stimulator designs, phase durations can be selected from screen menu options or can be adjusted in preset increments by using pressure-sensitive switches. On most commercially available pulsed-current stimulators, one phase (or pulse) duration control adjusts this parameter for all output channels. This configuration appears to be adequate for most contemporary electrotherapy protocols.

The adjustment of amplitude and phase or pulse duration controls changes the phase and/or pulse charge of each waveform applied. Increasing the amplitude, the phase (or pulse) duration, or both increases the net charge per stimulus and induces a larger current in biological tissues. That is, the stimulus is "stronger" as either amplitude or phase duration is increased. Because increasing either amplitude or phase duration increases the phase charge, these controls regulate what has been traditionally referred to as the *intensity* or *strength* of stimulation. As discussed in Chapter 3, these two parameters of stimulation determine the number of nerve or muscle fibers activated in response to stimulation.

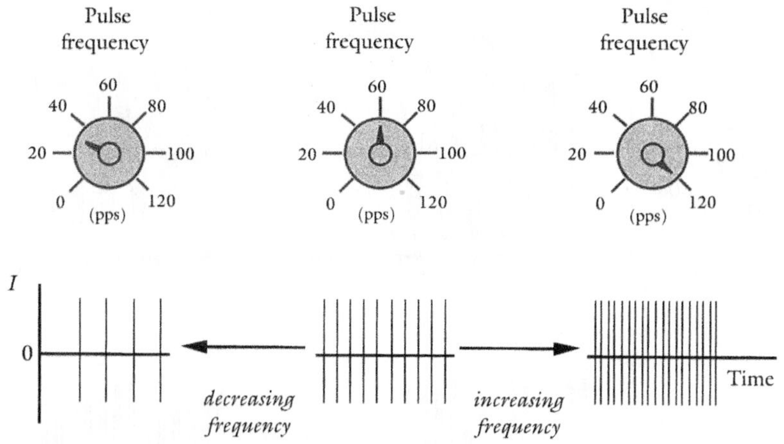

Pulse frequency (pps): 0, 20, 40, 60, 80, 100, 120

I, 0, Time

decreasing frequency

increasing frequency

Figure 2.6. Pulse frequency controls showing the effect of changes in dial setting on the frequency of pulses produced.

Frequency Controls

Frequency controls are provided on electrical stimulators to allow users to set the number of pulses (or AC cycles) delivered through each channel per second (Fig. 2.6), the number of bursts applied per second (Fig. 2.7), or the frequency of pulses within a burst (Fig. 2.8). Frequency

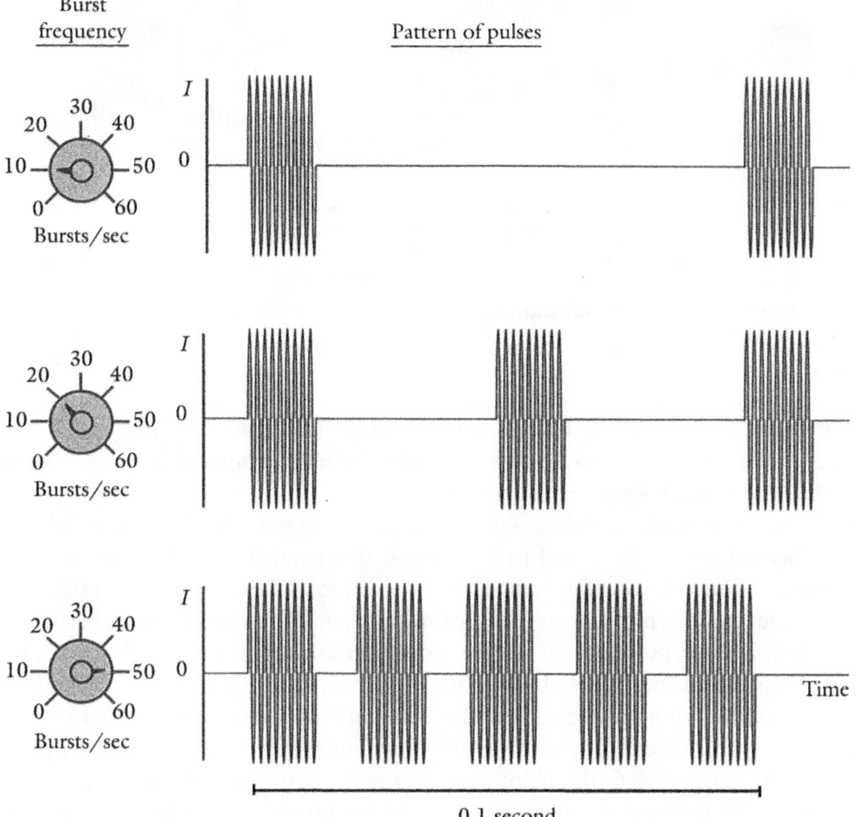

Figure 2.7. Burst frequency controls showing the effect of changes in dial setting on the frequency of bursts produced.

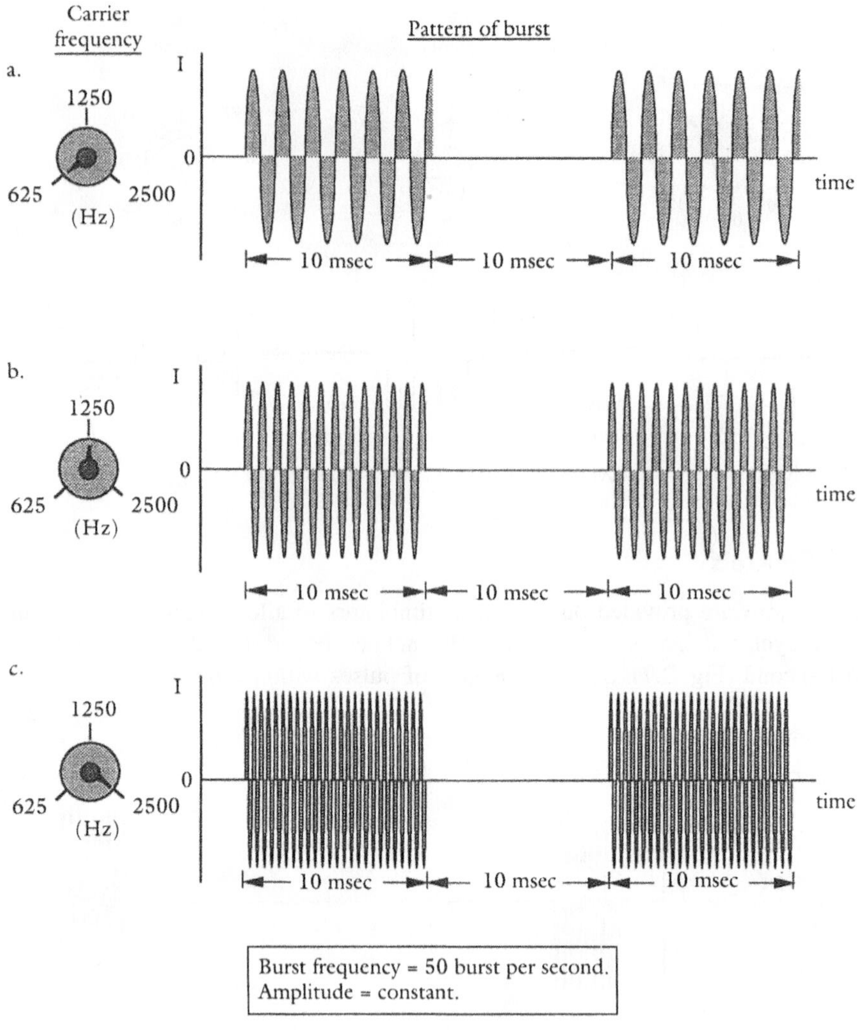

Figure 2.8. Carrier frequency controls showing the effect of changes in dial setting on the frequency of AC within each burst.

controls on stimulators are usually labeled simply "rate," "pulse rate," or "burst rate," depending on which parameter of stimulation is to be regulated. On many commercially available stimulators, more than one type of frequency control is present.

As with pulse amplitude and phase duration controls, rotating the frequency dial to a particular setting may not reflect the actual pulse or burst frequency delivered. Similarly, as the frequency dial is adjusted, incremental changes in the position of the dial may not reflect equivalent changes in frequency. This more imprecise type of frequency control is present on some portable stimulators designed for protocols to reduce pain (transcutaneous electrical nerve stimulation devices), where an exact frequency of activation is not as critical to achieving effective stimulation (1). The portable stimulators designed for the activation of innervated muscles (referred to as functional electrical stimulation devices) usually have more accurately labeled frequency controls. On microprocessor-based stimulator designs, the frequency of stimulation is often selected by controls linked to a digital frequency display, which provides an accurate indication of the frequency selected.

The frequency of pulsed stimulation commonly ranges from 1 to 1,000 pps, and burst frequency generally ranges from 1 to 100 bursts per second. The frequency of pulses within bursts (carrier frequency) or AC frequencies may range from 1 to 10,000 pulses or cycles per second.

The output frequency characteristics of various stimulators have been used as a basis for their classification: stimulators capable of producing 1 to 1,000 pps have been commonly referred to as *low-frequency* stimulators, those producing 1000 to 10,000 pps have been called *medium frequency*, and those producing pulses at frequencies in excess of 10,000 pps have been designated as *high frequency*. Such a classification scheme is commonly used in literature originating in Europe and Canada as well as in commercial circles. For this reason, those interested in electrotherapy should be aware of the meaning of these frequency designations. However, the differentiation among stimulators on the basis of frequency characteristics alone is not recommended. Some stimulators are capable of producing AC or pulsed currents at frequencies that cross the frequency boundaries just described, and hence they cannot be accurately categorized by a single designation.

On-Time and Off-Time Controls

When intermittent stimulation is required for a particular electrotherapeutic intervention, controls are necessary to set the duration of stimulation and the duration of rest between the periods of stimulation. The controls associated with setting these periods of stimulation and rest are called *duty cycle* or *cycle time* controls. In general, duty cycle controls are labeled "on time" and "off time"; they will adjust periods of stimulation and rest from 1 to 60 seconds. Many devices designed for neuromuscular stimulation include on-time and off-time controls, whereas many portable electrical stimulators designed for pain control do not. Figure 2.9 shows how on time and off time control settings regulate the pattern of a pulsed current.

Some stimulators allow the timing of stimulation on a channel to be manually controlled by the use of a remote switch. Some remote switches begin stimulation when the switch is depressed and stop stimulation when the switch is released; others operate in the opposite way. This timing-control approach is often found on devices used in neuromuscular stimulation applications, especially those used to produce contractions of muscle during functional activities.

Ramp-Up and Ramp-Down Controls

In order to automatically increase or decrease the phase or pulse charge in a pattern of stimulation, *ramp modulation controls* are included in several types of commercially available stimulators. These controls allow the therapist to set the number of seconds over which the amplitude (or phase/pulse durations) will gradually increase (or decrease) to (or from) the maximum value set by the amplitude control (Fig. 2.10). Ramp modulations on the leading and trailing ends of a train of pulses provide a more comfortable onset and cessation of stimulation in a variety of applications, especially when very high levels of stimulation are required for a particular therapeutic goal. In neuromuscular stimulation applications, the inclusion of a ramp-up time on the leading edge of a train of pulses or AC allows for the gradual recruitment of motor nerve fibers, and hence the gradual increase in muscle fiber contraction, which results in the smooth increase in muscle force output. The gradual onset of muscle stimulation produces contractions that more closely mimic those produced in functional activities during voluntary muscle activation, and the gradual onset is more comfortable for the individual receiving the stimulation. Ramp controls are usually not available on portable stimulators designed specifically for pain control. Depending on the instrument used, rise time and fall time controls may be labeled "slope time," "surge time," "ramp up," or simply "ramp."

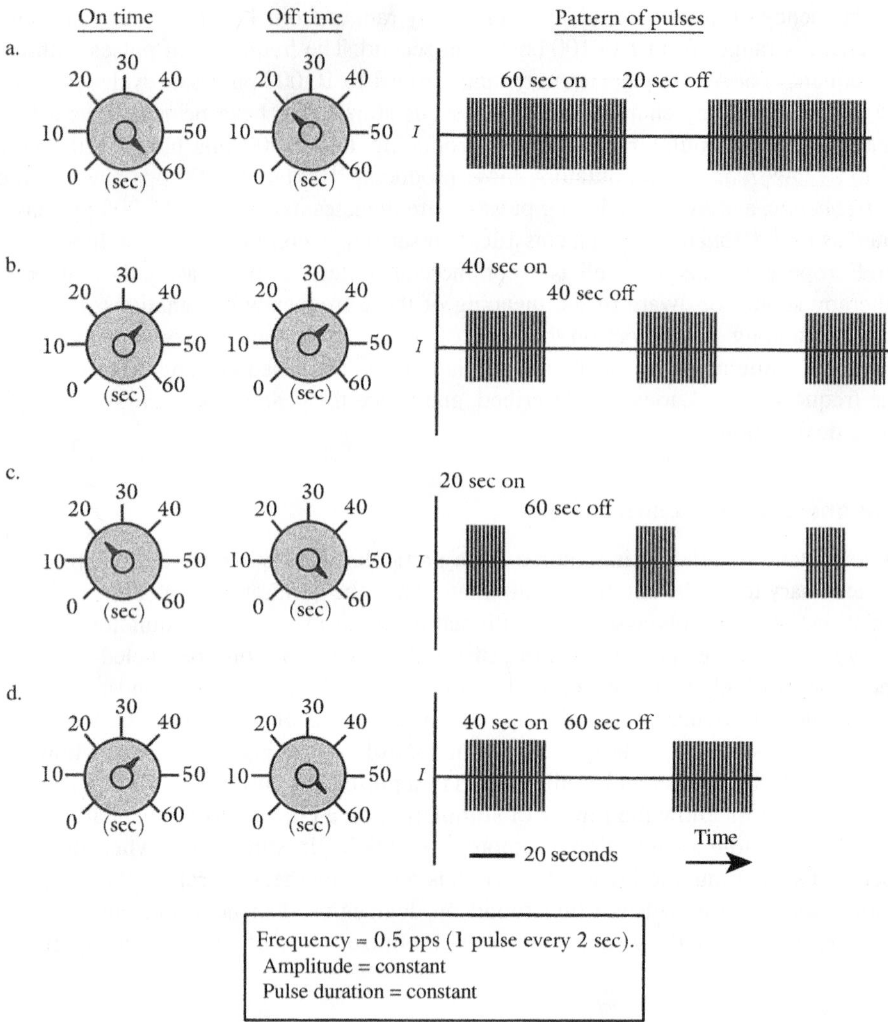

Figure 2.9. On-time and off-time controls showing the effect of changes in dial settings on the pattern of pulses produced.

Although ramp modulations are commonly associated with the automatic regulation of either amplitude or phase duration characteristics, they may also be used to automatically vary the frequency of stimulation.

Programmed Stimulation Pattern Controls

Programmed stimulation controls are available on some stimulation devices. Generally, in analog control devices, these controls are simply slide or rotary switches that allow the health care professional to select from the available stimulation patterns. In digitally controlled stimulators, preprogrammed stimulation can be selected from a menu display. If the option for preprogrammed stimulation is chosen, many of the time-dependent and/or amplitude-dependent characteristics of the stimulation pattern are automatically set or modulated. In some portable stimulators designed for pain control, such preprogrammed patterns of stimulation might be labeled "burst mode," "modulated mode," or even simply "pain." In other devices, designed

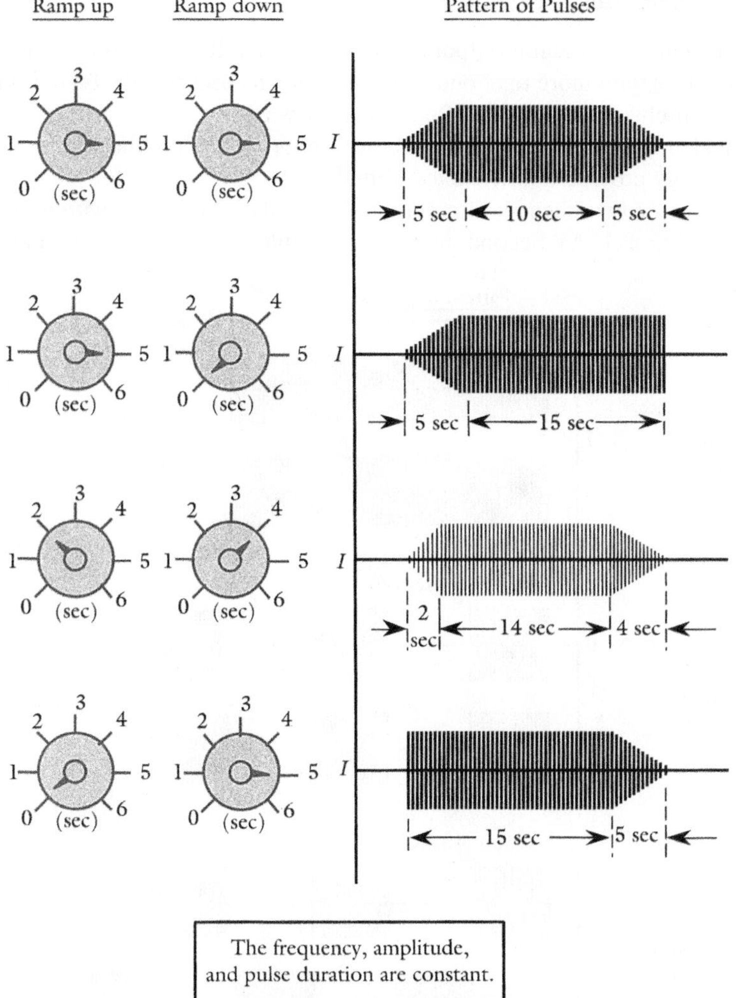

Figure 2.10. Ramp controls showing the effect of changes in dial setting on the time over which the amplitude of pulses is automatically increased (ramp up) or decreased (ramp down) during a 20-second train of pulses.

primarily for the activation of muscle, preprogrammed patterns of stimulation are labeled "muscle stimulation." The option to select a predetermined set of stimulation parameters can be very useful when a patient is taught to use stimulation at home. For example, such preprogrammed parameters are often used in the application of transcutaneous nerve stimulation for pain, for which parameters such as pulse amplitude, pulse duration, or both are automatically modulated. The choices offered by preprogrammed controls, however, may limit the utility of a device for a wide range of applications, especially if the user is unable to program stimulation patterns tailored to a specific application.

Preprogrammed stimulus options should be clearly described in the technical literature of a stimulator so that a user can determine if the pattern of stimulation is appropriate for a particular application. No uniform industry standards exist for the patterns of stimulation produced in the various "modes" of stimulation. The manufacturer's operating manual should be consulted for a description of precisely what stimulation characteristics are automatically modulated in specific predetermined modes of stimulation.

Output Channel Selection Controls

The signal from a single stimulator output amplifier is generally referred to as an *output channel*. Many stimulators with more than one channel allow the user to select the timing of stimulation through each channel. There are four common ways for stimulation to be coordinated when two channels are applied in a single treatment approach. First, the stimulator may be set so that both channels provide uninterrupted stimulation (no off time) for the entire treatment period. This pattern of two-channel stimulation is usually called the *continuous* or *constant stimulation mode* (Fig. 2.11A). Second, many devices may turn stimulation on and off to both

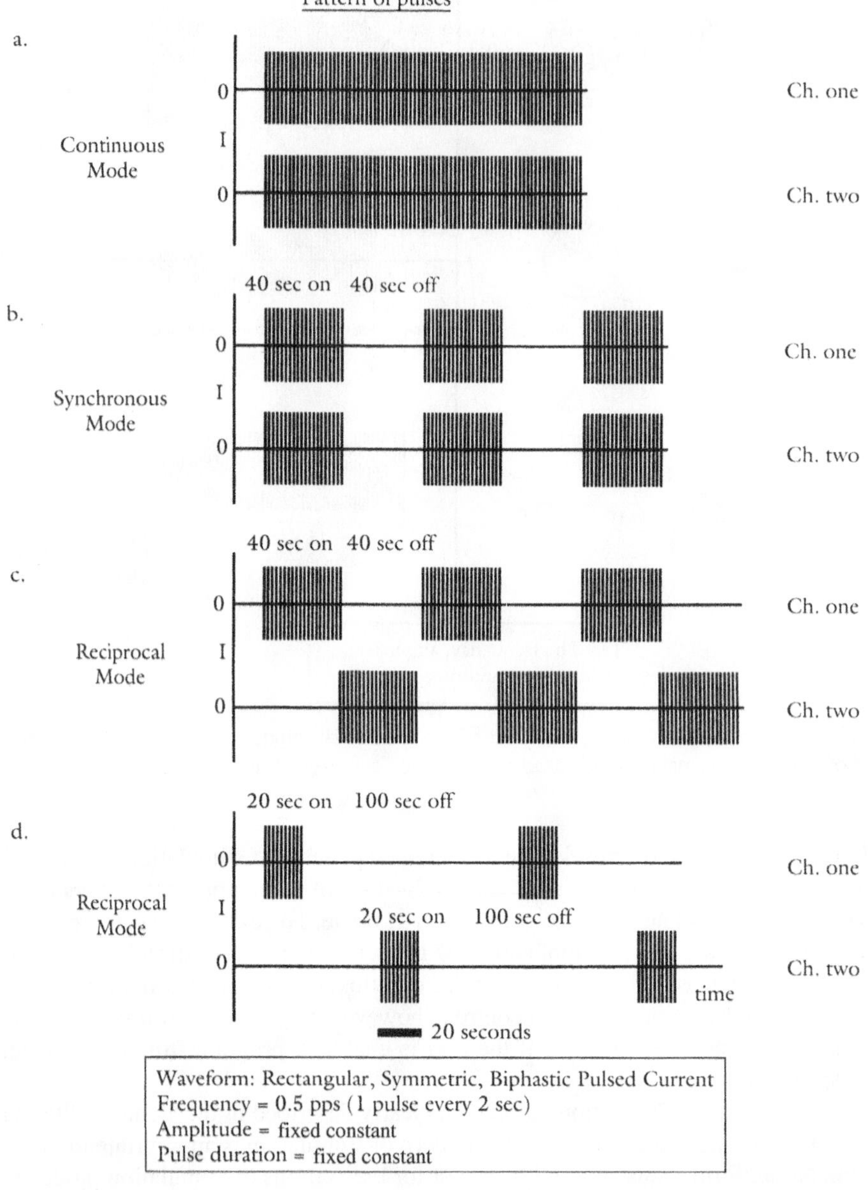

Figure 2.11. Channel-timing output controls showing three of the common patterns of stimulation. **A:** Continuous mode with both channels producing uninterrupted trains of pulses. **B:** Synchronous mode with both channels producing the same pattern of pulses simultaneously. **C** and **D:** Reciprocal mode with each channel producing alternating brief trains of pulses.

channels at the same time (Fig. 2.11B). This mode of stimulation is called *synchronous*, *simultaneous*, or *interrupted mode*. The synchronous and simultaneous designations for this pattern of two-channel stimulation are the less confusing designations. The third way in which the timing of stimulation is regulated in two-channel applications is to alternate stimulation between the two channels. That is, one channel provides stimulation while the second channel is off, and vice versa (Fig. 2.11C, D). This pattern of stimulation on two channels is generally referred to as *alternate* or *reciprocal mode*.

Finally, a few stimulators provide a stimulation pattern on two channels called *delayed mode*. In this mode, stimulation is started on one channel, and the stimulation is delayed on a second channel for periods ranging from one to several seconds. Such control over the timing of stimulation output can be of value in the electrical stimulation of skeletal muscles, when contraction in one muscle group should precede contraction in a second muscle group in order to produce functional limb movement.

When the option to select on times and off times is included in a stimulator, each channel should be linked to a *channel output indicator*. These small lights simply inform the user about when stimulation is being applied through each channel. Channel output indicators allow the user to know at what time during a stimulation program the amplitude of stimulation may be adjusted.

The ability of the health care provider to select the timing of stimulation between two channels is a desirable feature for a stimulator because it allows a broader range of treatment applications than would otherwise be possible. The reader is cautioned that the labeling of controls that regulate the timing of two-channel stimulation has no industry-wide standard. Users should consult the operator's manual for a specific instrument to learn how timing patterns between two channels can be controlled.

Treatment Timer

Many commercially available stimulators include a timing device, called the *treatment timer*, that allows the user to set the time that a pattern of stimulation will be provided for a single treatment session. Timers on many stimulators permit the adjustment of treatment times of up to 60 minutes, and some include timers that extend the treatment time up to 99 minutes. Some timers will trigger an audible signal when the time has expired. Treatment timers automatically turn stimulation off after the selected treatment time has expired. Devices with electromechanical timers as opposed to electronic timers should be periodically checked to ensure that the timer is functioning properly.

Certain types of devices, such as portable stimulators designed for pain control, do not contain treatment timers and will run continuously until turned off or until the batteries powering the unit discharge to the point where they no longer drive the electronics.

ELECTRODE SYSTEMS FOR ELECTROTHERAPY

An electrode is a conductive material that serves as the interface between a stimulator and the body tissues. Electrodes are connected to stimulators by insulated wires called *electrode leads*, *cables*, or *cords*. In most applications, electrodes are attached to the skin (surface electrodes). In other applications, electrodes have been designed to be implanted near tissues such as peripheral nerve or bone (invasive or indwelling electrodes) or in body cavities (internal electrodes). The following discussion is restricted to surface electrodes.

The material from which the electrodes are fabricated, electrode sizes and shapes, the location of the electrodes with respect to relevant tissues, and the orientation of the electrodes with respect to each other, all need to be considered in the development of an electrotherapy plan of care.

Types of Surface Electrodes

Stimulating electrodes used in today's conventional electrotherapy are usually made of a polymer or electrically conductive, carbon-impregnated, silicon rubber. Some electrodes provided with selected stimulators are made of metals such as stainless steel or aluminum foil. Surface-stimulating electrodes require the use of a coupling medium to provide a lower-resistance pathway for the flow of current from stimulator to tissue. For the flexible conductive rubber electrodes, the coupling medium may be an electrolytic paste, gel, cream, or liquid. Some commercially available electrodes are coated with a self-adhesive conductive polymer that serves as the coupling agent. In the case of metal electrodes, sponges soaked with tap water (not distilled water) are most commonly used to provide a pathway for current. The coupling media decrease the impedance at the interface between the electrode and the skin. Skin impedance may be further reduced by properly cleaning the skin with a mild, hypoallergenic soap or by mildly abrading the skin. A number of the commonly available types of surface electrodes are illustrated in Figure 2.12.

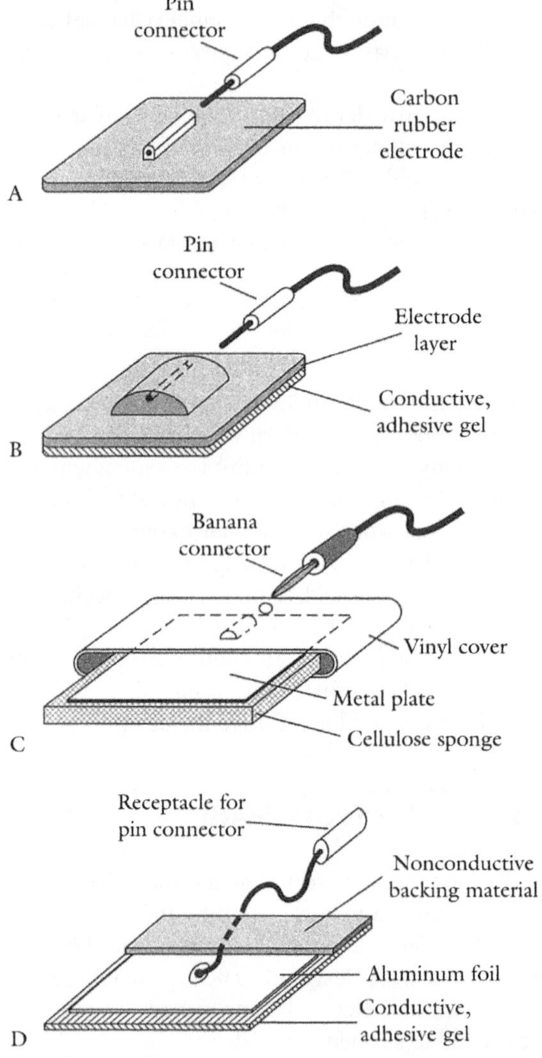

Figure 2.12. Diagrams of common surface electrodes. **A:** Simple conductive rubber electrode. **B:** Conductive rubber electrode bonded to a conductive, adhesive gel. **C:** Metal/sponge electrode. **D:** Foil/conductive adhesive electrode.

Electrodes are available for repeated use, short-term use (2 to 15 days), or for single use. The flexible, conductive rubber electrodes provided by manufacturers with most stimulators are fabricated to provide long-term, repeated use and will generally maintain their conductive properties for many months. After a period of time, however, the conductive rubber electrodes will begin to deteriorate and will not provide uniform current flow over their entire surface. This change in an electrode's ability to uniformly conduct will be accompanied by variations in current density beneath the electrodes and may result in uncomfortably high levels of stimulation in small spots (hot spots), often perceived by patients as a burning sensation. For this reason, flexible, conductive rubber electrodes should be replaced regularly (e.g., every 3 to 6 months). To maintain carbon rubber or similar electrodes, they should be cleaned with a mild soap solution after every use.

Flexible conductive rubber/gel and metal/sponge electrode systems should be securely attached to the skin with elastic straps to ensure uniform contact with the skin. Some manufacturers provide custom-cut adhesive bandages to secure carbon rubber electrodes. For active users of electrotherapy, the adhesive bandages may provide better long-term stabilization of the electrodes.

Disposable electrodes available commercially are designed for short-term use on a single patient. Disposable electrodes are often fabricated with a thin carbon rubber or foil layer and a conductive medium, which acts as the coupling agent. In some cases, the gel also acts as an adhesive, and in other cases, an adhesive bandage surrounds the electrode and secures it to the skin. The foil/adhesive gel electrodes have electrical resistances on the order of 10 to 100 Ω (ohms), whereas carbon rubber/gel systems have resistance values of approximately 1,000 Ω. Some self-adhering electrodes designed for single or short-term use have impedances in excess of several thousand ohms (3).

Different commercially available electrodes made from what appear to be similar materials may not be similar with respect to their ability to conduct (3). The significance of these findings for clinical electrotherapeutic applications remains to be determined.

Significance of Size and Shape of Surface Electrodes

The required contact area of the stimulating electrodes depends in part on the area of excitable tissues to be stimulated. An electrode that is too large or the wrong shape may cause the current to spread to excitable structures other than the nerve or muscle of interest. Electrodes are available in a wide range of sizes and shapes to accommodate the spectrum of electrotherapeutic procedures common to contemporary practice.

With uniform electrode conductivity, the *current density* (amount of current per unit of conduction area) is inversely proportional to the electrode contact area. Therefore, as electrode contact area decreases, current density increases. This means that if the same electrical voltage is applied first across a pair of small electrodes and then across a pair of large electrodes, the amplitude of stimulation will feel greater beneath the smaller pair. If one small and one large electrode are used in a single application, the stimulation will generally be perceived as greater beneath the small electrode.

In documenting electrotherapeutic procedures, it is recommended that the type, size, and shape of electrodes be clearly specified, and that changes made in any of these electrode characteristics be noted in the medical record.

Designation of Electrode Location in Therapeutic Applications

The placement of electrodes in electrotherapy is critical to achieving therapeutic benefits, so the exact location should be clearly recorded. To accurately describe electrode placement, measurements should be made from the center of electrodes to known anatomical landmarks or structures (e.g., 5 cm proximal to the superior edge of the patella over the rectus femoris, or 10 cm distal to

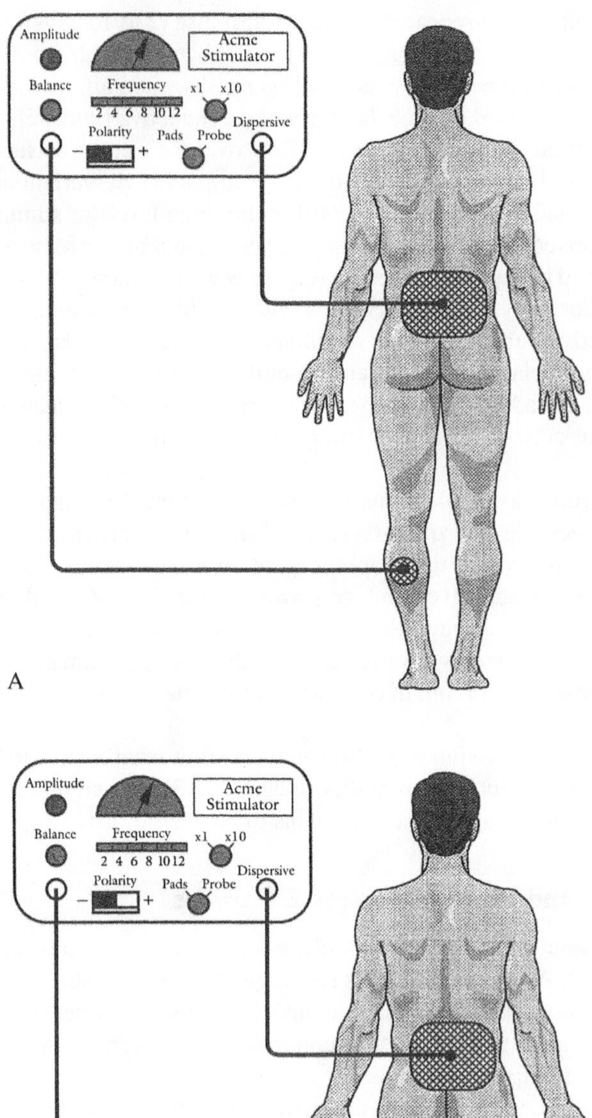

Figure 2.13. Monopolar electrode configurations. **A:** One electrode (the "active" electrode) in the target region (calf) and a second electrode away from target region. **B:** Two electrodes bifurcated from one channel lead (pole) in the target region (posterior calf) and second electrode away from the target region.

the axillary fold in the midaxillary line). These measurements should be recorded after initial treatments, and changes in electrode position should be documented in a similar fashion in the medical record. This quantitative approach is the clearest method to describe electrode location.

Historically, electrode placements have been described in relation to the relative position of the electrodes employed. Three terms, *monopolar*, *bipolar*, and *quadripolar*, have been regularly used to describe electrode orientations (4).

In the simplest *monopolar electrode orientation*, a single electrode is placed over the target area or over the tissue where the greatest effect is desired (Fig. 2.13A). The second electrode of the stimulating circuit is placed at a distance well away from the target area in order to complete the electrical circuit. The electrode placed in the target area is sometimes called the *stimulating*, or *active*, electrode, whereas the electrode placed distant from the target area is often referred to as the *dispersive*, *indifferent*, or *reference* electrode. Referring to the second electrode, away from the target area, as the "ground electrode" is inappropriate because this electrode is not actually connected to earth ground. In the monopolar orientation, the electrode in the target region is generally smaller than the electrode away from the target area. As a result, the smaller "stimulating" electrode commonly elicits activity in excitable tissue before the larger "dispersive" electrode does because the current density beneath the smaller electrode is greater at any particular amplitude of stimulation. The use of the term *active* to describe the smaller electrode is not recommended because it implies to some that the larger electrode is "inactive" and will not elicit any type of physiologic response. Those who have regularly used electrical stimulation in the clinic will attest that this implication is not always true. The large contact area of the larger electrode minimizes the underlying current density, and hence excitation of nerve and muscle by this electrode is less likely to occur. Referring to the large electrode as either "indifferent" or "reference" is also misleading and has no particular value.

In some situations, the single electrode placed in the target region is replaced by two electrodes connected to the same single lead (Figure 2.13B). Even though this electrode placement configuration uses two electrodes in the target area, both are connected to a single output lead (or pole) of the stimulation channel, and hence this pattern of placement is also referred to as *monopolar*.

In the simplest *bipolar electrode orientation*, both surface electrodes from a stimulator channel are placed over the target area (Fig. 2.14A). This pattern of electrode placement provides current that is more limited to the excitable tissue of interest. The electrodes used in the bipolar technique are usually equal in size. In such cases, the relative ability of each electrode to activate nerve or muscle will be equal when symmetric biphasic waveforms are applied. In some instances, the bipolar technique may require that one of the two electrodes be smaller in order to obtain the desired response; in such a case, the smaller of the two electrodes will be relatively more effective in the activation of excitable tissue. Another bipolar configuration of electrode placement that uses more than two electrodes originating from a single channel is shown in Figure 2.14B.

In the *quadripolar electrode configuration*, two electrodes from two separate stimulating circuits are positioned in the primary target area. Two general quadripolar configurations of electrode placement are shown in Figure 2.15. In Figure 2.15A, the four electrodes are positioned such that currents induced by the respective circuits intersect, interact, or interfere with each other. This type of electrode placement has been used in conjunction with the interferential stimulation technique described later in this chapter. In Figure 2.15B, two electrodes from each of two stimulation channels are placed in the target region (low back) in a manner that would not result in an intersection of the currents induced by each channel. This electrode orientation from two channels, shown in Figure 2.15B, might be described as bipolar for channel 1 in the right low back and bipolar for channel 2 in the left low back. In describing electrode locations, the term *quadripolar* simply refers to the placement of four electrodes from two stimulation channels in the target area, whereas the term *interferential* refers to a particular relative orientation of the two sets of electrodes that employs the quadripolar electrode configuration.

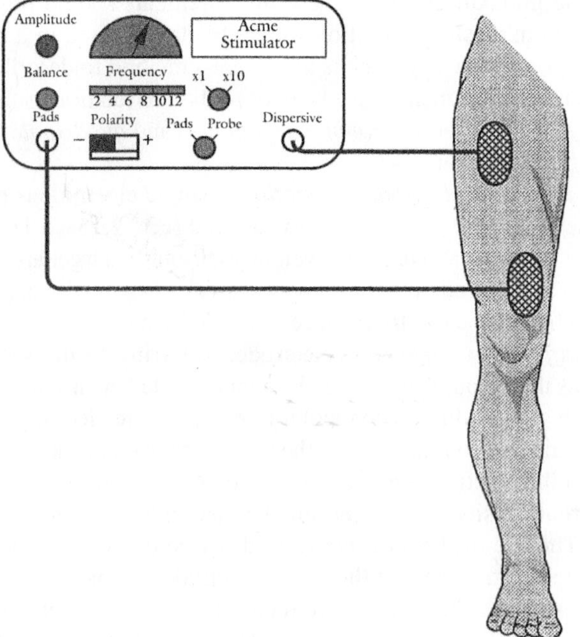

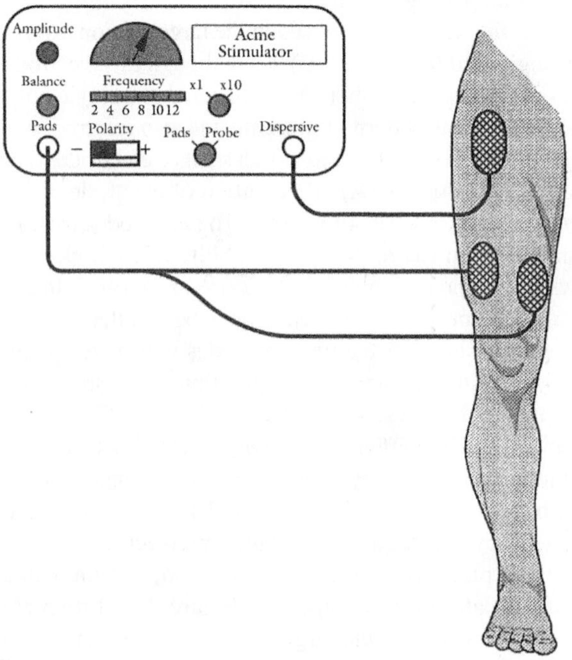

Figure 2.14. Bipolar electrode configurations. **A:** Simple bipolar arrangement with both electrodes from a single stimulator channel in the target region (anterior thigh). **B:** One channel lead bifurcated with two electrodes over lower target region and second lead of the channel with single electrode in target region.

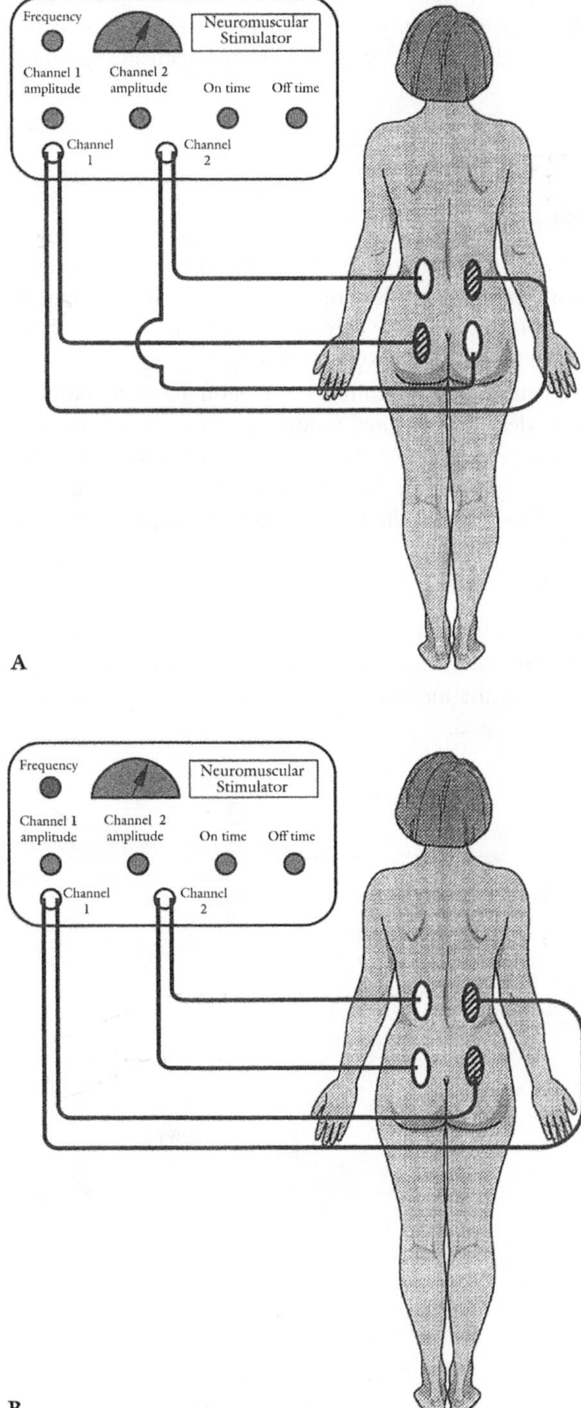

Figure 2.15. Quadripolar electrode configurations in low back target region. **A:** four electrodes from two stimulation channels arranged such that currents produced by channel 1 (shaded electrodes) intersect with currents produced by electrodes of channel 2. **B:** Four electrodes from two channels arranged such that currents produced by the channel 1 electrode (shaded) do not intersect with currents produced by channel two electrodes.

Since the terms *monopolar*, *bipolar*, and *quadripolar* can each be used to represent various combinations of electrode placement, these descriptive terms should be accompanied by an explicit description of each electrode's location, and the electrode types and dimensions should be clearly specified.

Special-Purpose Electrodes

Handheld Probe Electrode

Although simple surface electrodes are the most commonly used electrodes in clinical electrotherapy, a variety of special-purpose electrodes are available. One of the more frequently used special electrodes is the *handheld probe electrode* (Fig. 2.16). Modern versions of these electrodes generally have two controls included in their design: an amplitude control and a switch to control the timing of stimulation. Other parameters of treatment are set on the stimulator to which the electrode is attached. Handheld electrodes were originally developed for use in classical electrophysiological tests such as reaction of degeneration (RD) or strength-duration (S-D) testing. Handheld probe electrodes are now commonly used for locating motor points, for the stimulation of very small muscles, or for the stimulation of very small points such as in electroacupuncture.

Electrodes for Iontophoresis

In traditional iontophoresis (the electrophoresis of charged medications), the treatment electrodes used were either aluminum foil or tin foil placed over an absorbent pad. The pad contained either an aqueous solution of the medication or a simple electrolytic coupling agent. When the

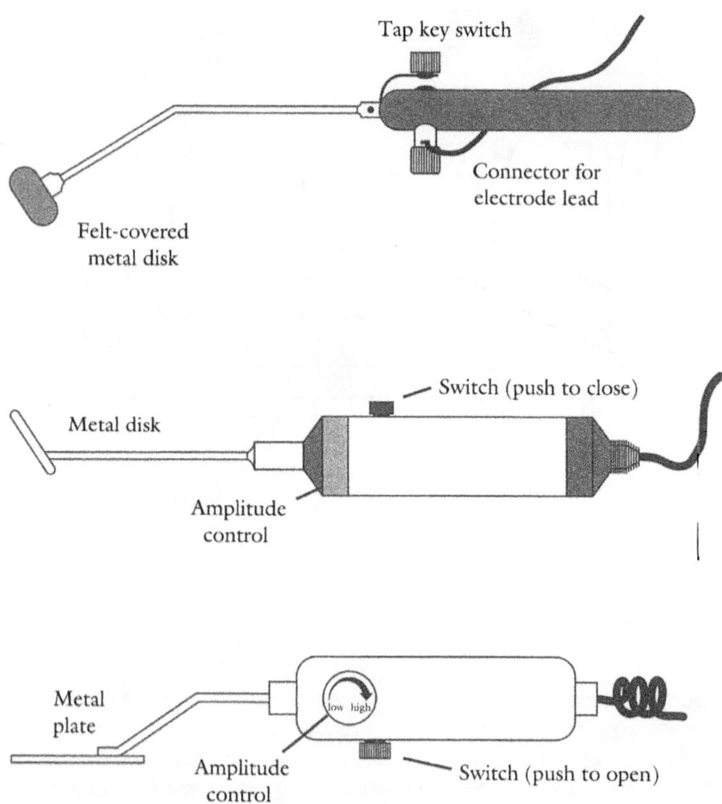

Figure 2.16. Handheld electrodes with different switch configurations.

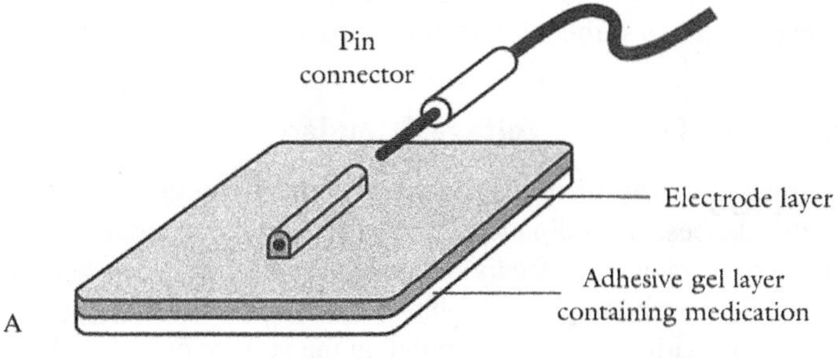

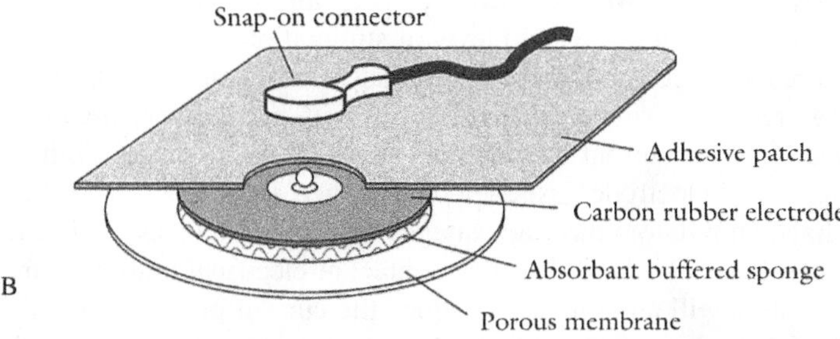

Figure 2.17. Iontophoresis electrodes. **A:** Conductive rubber electrode with medication contained in adhesive gel. **B:** Buffered sponge electrode with medication contained within sponge.

pad contained only the coupling agent, the medication was placed on the skin surface beneath the pad and metal electrode. This traditional iontophoresis electrode system was often difficult to use, and uniform contact of the electrode with the skin surface was hard to achieve. In recent years, manufacturers of stimulators designed for iontophoresis have developed special electrodes that hold or store the medication to be used. The two basic designs provide either (a) the incorporation of the medication into the conductive gel adhesive (Fig. 2.17A) or (b) an absorbent reservoir pad (Fig. 2.17B).

Commercially available iontophoresis electrodes come in a number of sizes and shapes. Iontophoresis electrodes may be designed for single- or multiple-session use. Medication-containing iontophoresis electrodes should not be used on multiple patients.

Electrodes for Internal Applications

A number of unique electrodes have been designed for electrotherapy requiring stimulation within body cavities. Rectal and vaginal electrodes have been developed for the electrical activation of musculature associated with the control of urination, defecation, and ejaculation. Other electrodes have been designed for intraoral stimulation programs for the management of disorders such as temporomandibular joint syndrome. Principles and procedures related to the application of these special electrodes for incontinence are addressed in Chapter 9.

TYPES OF STIMULATORS

Electrical stimulators for therapeutic and diagnostic applications can be generically described by their external power source (battery versus line power) and by the nature of electrical stimulus that is applied to the patient (constant current versus constant voltage). In contrast, commercially available stimulators are usually categorized based on the characteristics of the stimulus waveform or some characteristic related to a stimulation technique associated with the particular stimulator.

Constant Current versus Constant Voltage Stimulators

Constant (or regulated) current instruments provide current that flows at a constant amplitude within a specified range of impedances. According to Ohm's law, the voltage output of the device varies to maintain the current at a constant level as the tissue impedance changes. Constant (or regulated) voltage instruments provide a constant amplitude voltage within a specified range of impedances. The current flow varies inversely with impedance to maintain the voltage output of the device.

Each type of stimulator has potential advantages and disadvantages in clinical applications. During treatment at a particular amplitude setting, constant current stimulators will automatically reduce the driving voltage when electrode contact improves or when electrical transmission increases, thereby maintaining the desired level of stimulation. In cases where electrode contact or transmission is reduced, constant current stimulators will automatically increase the driving voltage, which may result in skin burns as current density rises to very high levels. For this reason, well-designed constant current stimulators often feature a voltage limit, which cannot be exceeded regardless of an electrode/tissue impedance increase.

Constant voltage stimulators have advantages and disadvantages similar to those for constant current devices. In cases where electrode contact or electrical transmission is reduced, constant voltage stimulators will automatically reduce the current produced and thereby lessen the chance of skin burns resulting from increased current density. Conversely, if electrode/tissue contact improves and transmission is better with a constant voltage device, induced currents could significantly increase, resulting in an undesirably high level of stimulation.

Commercial Classes of Stimulators

Transcutaneous Electrical Nerve Stimulation Devices

The resurgence of interest in electrotherapy occurred in the early 1970s with the widespread development and marketing of small (about 2.5 × 4 × 1 inches), lightweight (<200 g), portable stimulators called *transcutaneous electrical nerve stimulation (TENS) units*. The development of these compact stimulators was made possible by two developments: the postulation of the gate-control theory of pain control and the miniaturization of electronic components. Also contributing to TENS development was the ever-increasing incidence of pain related to cumulative trauma disorders (e.g., carpal tunnel syndrome) and the search by health professionals for pain control solutions.

Most devices marketed specifically for pain control applications have common features related to output currents and controls. In general, TENS devices produce a rectangular, asymmetric, biphasic pulsed current. In some early models, the output waveforms were unbalanced in phase charge, but today most stimulation waveforms are balanced.

Today's TENS devices are typically two-channel stimulators with independent amplitude controls for each channel. Pulse duration (also labeled *pulse width*) controls are routinely present and allow the user to vary the pulse duration from low values (20 to 50 μs) to high values (250 to 600 μs). A pulse frequency (also labeled *rate*) control is standard for TENS units and allows adjustment from a low frequency of 2 pps to maximum frequencies ranging from 125 to 200 pps. The pulse duration and pulse frequency are usually the same value on each output channel. Recommendations regarding the stimulation characteristics of TENS devices can be found in the American National Standard for Transcutaneous Electrical Nerve Stimulators, published by the Association for the Advancement of Medical Instrumentation (AAMI) (5).

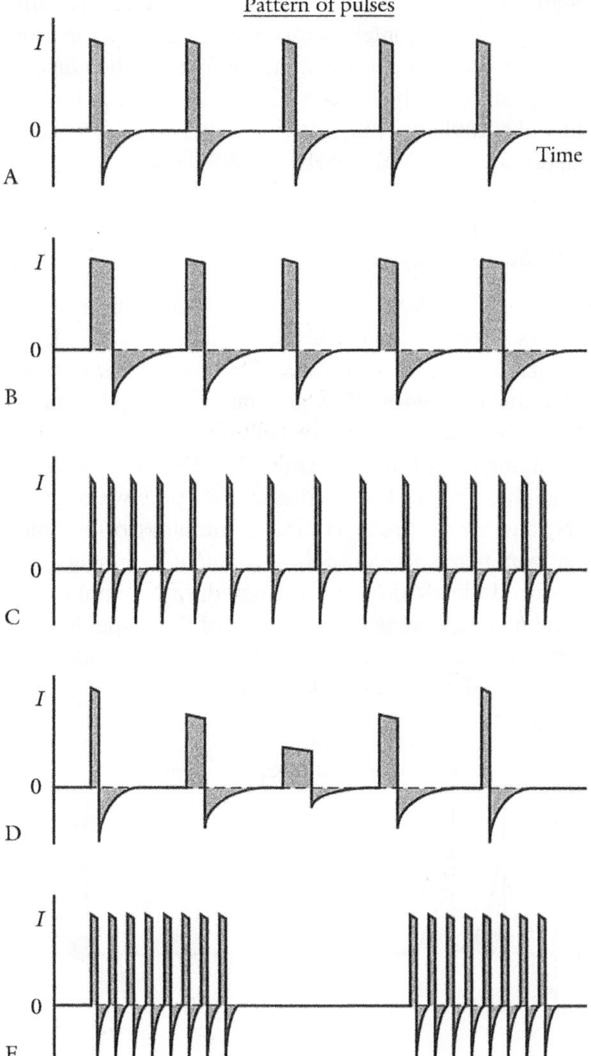

Figure 2.18. Patterns of stimulation commonly produced by transcutaneous electrical stimulation devices. **A:** Normal mode of continuous train of pulses. **B:** Pulse duration mode with automatic modulation of pulse duration to preset level. **C:** Frequency modulation with automatic increase and decrease in frequency to preset level. **D:** Strength duration modulation with automatic reductions of pulse amplitude and increases in pulse duration, followed by increases in pulse amplitude accompanied by decreases in pulse duration. **E:** Burst modulation with regular bursts of pulses.

The feature that distinguishes TENS devices from many other types is the presence of several predetermined stimulation modulation options (Fig. 2.18). These may include systematic modulations to the pulse frequency, pulse duration, both pulse frequency and pulse duration, burst modulation, and amplitude modulation. In each of these modulation modes, the stimulus parameters modulated are systematically lowered from and raised to the maximum setting. Modulation modes were included in the design of TENS devices when clinicians recognized that for certain patterns of stimulation (low amplitude, continuous pulse trains), patients quickly lost the ability to perceive the stimulation. By providing modulation to one or more parameters of stimulation, this reduction in the perception of stimulation is often avoided.

Although the acronym TENS is currently associated with electrical stimulation for pain control, you should be aware that most contemporary electrotherapy for problems other than pain involves transcutaneous stimulation of peripheral nerve fibers. When faced with the management of pain, many clinicians preferentially choose TENS devices for their patients, even though many other types of clinical stimulators may provide a pattern of stimulation analogous to those generated by the commercially available, portable TENS devices.

High-Voltage Pulsed-Current Stimulators

Following the rapid introduction of TENS devices, in the mid-1970s a second commercial class of constant voltage stimulators began to appear in clinics across the United States. This class, the high-voltage pulsed galvanic stimulators {also called *high-volt pulsed-current (HVPC) stimulators*} were actually developed in the mid-1940s. They generate a twin-spike, monophasic pulsed-current waveform (Fig. 2.19A) with peak spike amplitudes of up to 500 V, and pulse durations of about 50 to 200 μs at frequencies ranging from 1 to approximately 120 twin-spike pulses per second. In early models, the ranges of available settings for on time and off time were limited. Designs have been changed over the years, and today many HVPC stimulators offer much more flexibility in the selection of treatment parameters. Because these stimulators produce monophasic waveforms, the output polarity of electrode leads does not change during stimulation. Most HVPC devices allow the user to select and manually switch the polarity of the output leads.

Some twin-spike, monophasic pulsed-current stimulators include a control that adjusts the time between the beginning of the first spike waveform and the beginning of the second

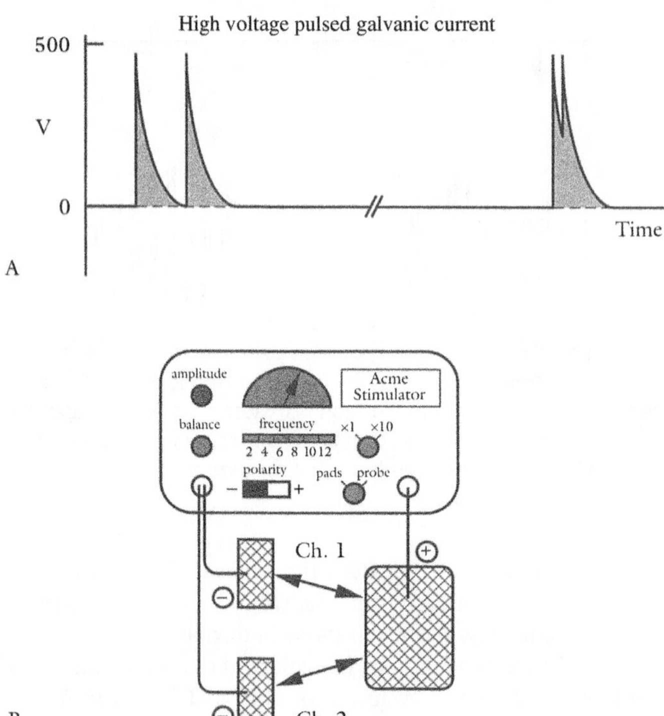

Figure 2.19. High-voltage, pulsed, galvanic current. **A:** Characteristic twin-spike, monophasic waveform with longer and shorter interval between spikes respectively. **B:** Schematic diagram of a typical configuration of output channels and electrodes associated with some commercially available stimulators.

waveform. This time between the two spikes may be reduced such that the two waveforms overlap. During stimulation, as the twin spikes progressively overlap, the stimulation is perceived as being stronger.

One characteristic of high-volt stimulators is the design of the output channel leads. On many of the stimulators in this class, two output leads at one polarity are each used in conjunction with a single lead of opposite polarity (Fig. 2.19B). Such an arrangement of output leads actually reflects the presence of a single channel of stimulation. However, some HVPC devices that use this lead arrangement are labeled as having two channels.

High-voltage pulsed stimulators are now available in both line-operated and battery-operated models, with the major difference being that the peak output voltages are about 100 to 200 V lower in the battery-operated designs.

Neuromuscular Electrical Stimulators

In the latter 1970s after the rapid proliferation of TENS units for pain control, interest in electrotherapy was boosted by research from the Soviet Union suggesting that regular electrical activation of muscle was more effective than exercise in strengthening skeletal muscle in elite athletes. This research resulted in improvements in the development and design of a class of electrical stimulators for *neuromuscular electrical stimulation* (NMES).

Both pulsed and alternating currents are used in NMES devices. The current originally used by the Soviet researchers was a 2500-Hz, sinusoidal, symmetric alternating current that was burst-modulated every 10 ms to provide 50 bursts per second. This form of stimulation has been promoted commercially as "Russian stimulation" (Fig. 2.20A). Today's NMES devices use a variety of waveforms. Most stimulators marketed for NMES produce either (a) the burst-modulated, 2500-Hz AC just described, (b) a rectangular, balanced, symmetric, biphasic pulsed current (Fig. 2.20B), or (c) a rectangular, balanced, asymmetric biphasic pulsed current (Fig. 2.20C). To date, no single waveform has been found to be superior for all NMES applications in all patient populations. Research has demonstrated that individuals may have a preference for particular waveforms used in NMES devices. Selection of the waveform should be based on the ability to evoke the desired level of contraction as well as patient tolerance of the procedure.

Both portable, battery-operated units and line-powered stimulators are available for NMES applications. In general, portable NMES units have lower maximum power output than line-powered ones. For this reason, some portable stimulators may not have enough capacity to maximally activate large muscle groups such as the quadriceps. In addition, portable NMES stimulators, like portable TENS devices, have performance characteristics that are limited by battery life; therefore, batteries should be replaced or recharged frequently. Portable stimulators have a distinct advantage over line-powered models in applications where stimulation evokes functional muscle contraction, such as stimulation of the tibialis anterior and peroneal muscles during the swing phase of gait.

NMES devices usually have two output channels, but some models are available with four channels. Stimulators designed for activation of normally innervated muscle usually have independent amplitude controls for each output channel. Controls are commonly available to provide stimulation on all channels simultaneously (synchronous mode), alternately (reciprocal mode), or such that one or two channels are providing stimulation while the other output channels are off and vice versa. Some NMES units have a "delayed mode," which initiates stimulation on one channel and then begins stimulation on a second channel after a brief delay of from one to several seconds. Usually the output frequency and phase (or pulse) duration controls are common to each channel. Frequency modulation and phase (or pulse) duration modulation are generally not included in NMES stimulators.

The three other features that distinguish stimulators designed for NMES are on-time/off-time controls, ramp controls, and "set output" controls. On-time/off-time controls allow the

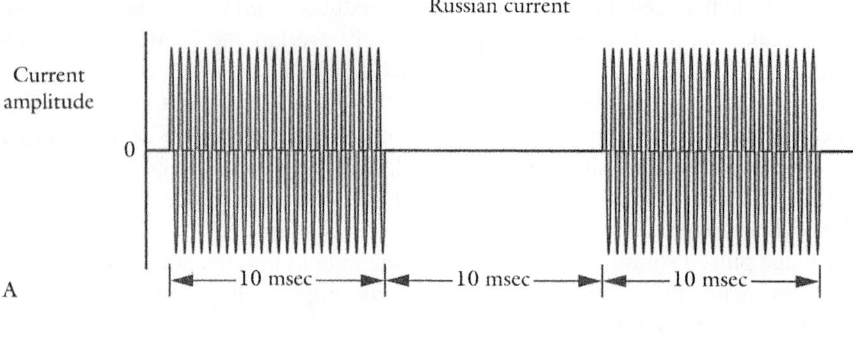

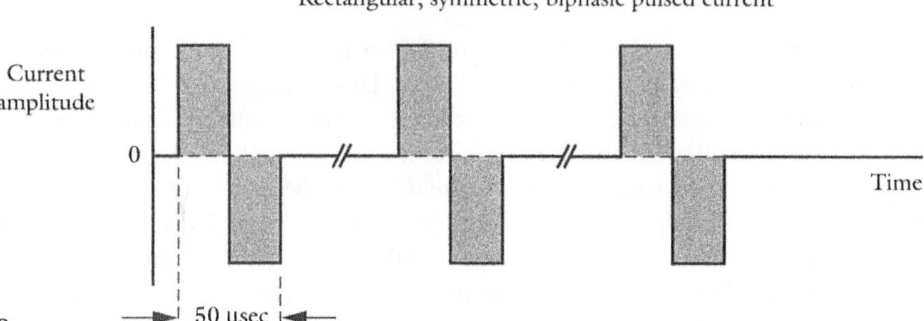

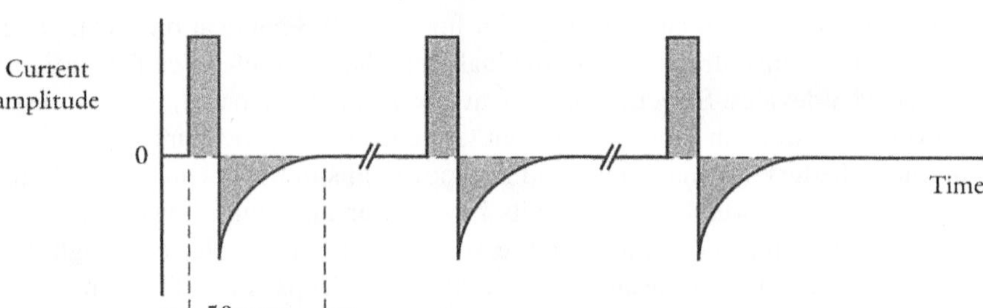

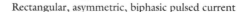

Figure 2.20. Examples of currents used with commercially available stimulators designed for neuromuscular electrical stimulation applications.

user to control the number of seconds of muscle contraction (on time) and the number of seconds of rest (off time). The ramp control adjusts the number of seconds of the on time over which the amplitude gradually reaches the maximum setting (ramp up), or decreases from the maximum setting (ramp down) to zero output. Alternatively, the timing of stimulation can be controlled on many NMES units by a manually operated remote switch (trigger). Such switches are particularly useful in cases where a functional muscle contraction is desired. *Set output* controls allow the user to adjust the amplitude of stimulation to the desired level before switching the device into an on time/off time sequence.

Most line-powered NMES units contain analog or digital meters that reflect some aspect of the amplitude of stimulation. Metering should be available for each output channel and should reflect the actual current applied during stimulation (delivered current). Observation of the meters during the application of stimulation allows the user to know when stimulation begins on an output channel and when stimulation has reached the maximum set value. This information is valuable because the output amplitude should not be adjusted during the ramp up or during the off time, especially when the maximum tolerated levels of stimulation are being reached. On portable NMES units, no output amplitude meter is present. Instead, small lights are used to indicate when stimulation begins and ends. When using such portable NMES instruments, the user must estimate when peak amplitudes of stimulation have been reached before further amplitude adjustment is made. Some NMES units include "channel on" lights as well as output metering.

A final feature common to well-designed NMES devices is the safety switch, which allows the stimulator to be shut off in the event of an unexpected response to stimulation. Often such switches are available to patients during treatment because they are likely to become aware of an unwanted response well before the clinician is.

Recommendations on performance standards and safety requirements for neuromuscular electrical stimulators are being developed by the AAMI (Association of the Advancement of Medical Instrumentation).

Interferential Stimulators

In the early to mid-1980s, another class of stimulators was introduced to the American market, the *interferential stimulators.* These stimulators are generally characterized as two-channel stimulators producing sinusoidal, symmetrical, alternating currents at frequencies of several thousand cycles per second (e.g., 2,000 to 5,000 Hz) on each channel. In clinical applications of the original versions of these devices, both channels are used simultaneously with AC frequencies set at slightly different values, and electrodes are oriented in a quadripolar orientation, as shown in Figure 2.15A. In this or similar electrode placements, the ionic movement in the tissues results from the electromotive forces produced by both channels. In other words, the current that would be produced by one channel interacts with ("interferes with") the current produced by the second channel and produces a net ionic movement different from that produced by either channel alone. Proponents of this form of electrotherapy propose that the resultant current (called *interference current*) is similar to an amplitude-modulated, sinusoidal alternating current with a *beat* frequency that is equal to the difference in AC frequency on the two channels (Fig. 2.21)(6). Such summation of effects to produce an interference current assumes a perfectly homogeneous conductor. Human tissues are not homogeneous in conduction of electrical currents, and the proposed summation of effects across two channels is unlikely to occur precisely as described. Since the frequencies of stimulation using the interferential technique are an order of magnitude higher than those used with pulsed current procedures, proponents claim that tissue impedance is reduced and that currents are induced in deeper tissue levels than those induced by devices generating much lower frequencies. Such claims have been challenged in the literature (7), and the relative effectiveness of interferential stimulation remains to be demonstrated. Nonetheless, interferential therapy has gained a solid foothold in clinics for the management of a wide range of disorders.

An alternative approach to the design of interferential stimulators is to use two channels of stimulation and to have the AC carrier frequency on each channel be the same (e.g., 5,000 Hz) and in phase. This carrier frequency is then burst modulated (1 to 250 bps). In addition, the output of each channel may then be amplitude modulated. This approach is referred to as the *full-field technique* and is purported to increase the volume of tissue exposed to the induced currents.

The types of controls on interferential stimulators vary. Amplitude controls range from a single dial for controlling both channels to independent controls on each channel. In general, controls are available to select the difference in frequency between the two channels (the beat, or interference, frequency). On many units, options are available to continuously modulate the beat frequency. Most instruments contain a metering system for output amplitude. Early interferential stimulator designs often did not incorporate on-time and off-time controls, which meant that

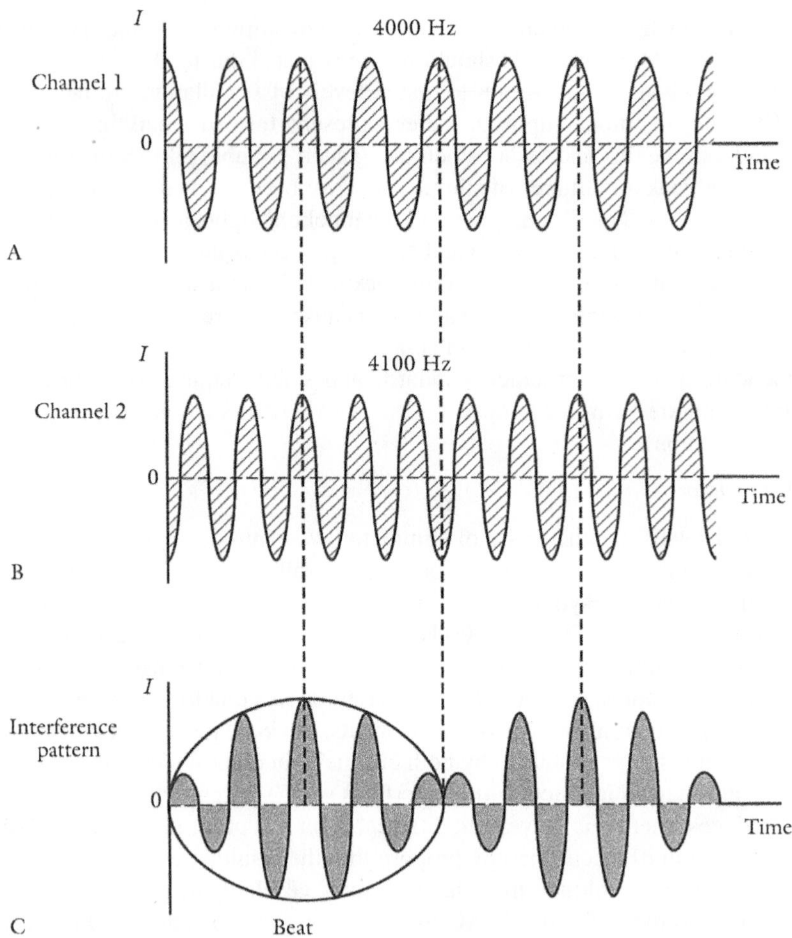

Figure 2.21. Interferential current. **A:** 4000-Hz, sinusoidal AC produced by one channel of the stimulator. **B:** 4100-Hz sinusoidal AC produced by second channel of stimulator. **C:** Amplitude-modulated, sinusoidal AC produced by the "summation" of currents from channels 1 and 2 at point of intersection given a homogeneous medium.

such devices were not ideal for NMES applications. Recent interferential stimulator models include on-time and off-time controls and ramp modulation controls to make them more suitable for NMES applications, although the efficacy of use of interferential current stimulators in NMES applications remains to be demonstrated.

Diadynamic Stimulators

Stimulators classified as *diadynamic devices* are characterized by the production of waveforms derived from the electronic processing of sinusoidal, symmetric, alternating current. The two main types of processing of the AC currents are half-wave rectification and full-wave rectification. Figure 2.22 illustrates the source AC and the alterations produced by half- and full-wave rectification. Briefly, half-wave rectification simply eliminates the second half of each AC cycle and produces a monophasic pulsed current with a pulse duration equal to the interpulse interval and a frequency equal to that of the original AC. This form of diadynamic current (Fig. 2.22B) has been traditionally referred to as *single phase* or *monophasé fixe* (MF).

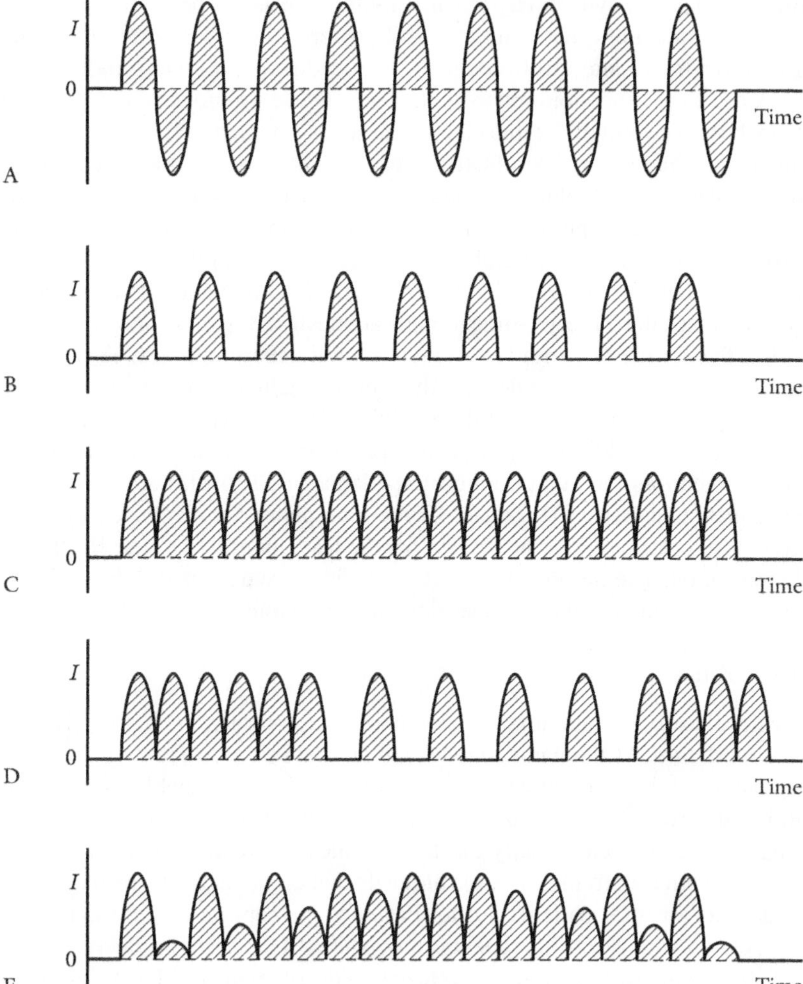

Figure 2.22. Diadynamic current. **A:** Sinusoidal AC, which serves as precursor current. **B:** monophasé fixe, from half-wave rectification of source current. **C:** Diphasé fixe, from full-wave rectification of source current. **D:** Courtes periodes, from alternating periods of full-wave rectification followed by half-wave rectification. **E:** Longues periodes, amplitude modulation of full-wave rectified source current.

Full-wave rectification of sinusoidal AC produces a monophasic pulsed current with no interpulse interval and at twice the original AC frequency. This form of current (Fig. 2.22C) has been called *double-phase* or *diphasé fixe* (DF). Devices that produce these two basic forms of monophasic pulsed currents also modulate the basic waveforms by amplitude and/or time to produce the two other types of diadynamic currents (Fig. 2.22D,E). Diadynamic stimulators may be unfamiliar to many readers in the United States, but these stimulators have been in use in Canada and in Europe for quite some time.

Iontophoresis Stimulators

Iontophoresis, the delivery of medication to subcutaneous tissue by electrical currents, has been used clinically for decades. The devices used for this procedure produce direct current (DC). The fundamental stimulator features required to use this technique are an amplitude control, output current ammeter, and power switch. Historically, iontophoresis has been administered using line-powered electrical stimulators that converted AC power to DC. Very often these devices were designed to perform traditional electrodiagnostic procedures and could produce peak DC currents of 30 mA or more. Since iontophoresis treatments use no more than 5 mA, these devices were not particularly well suited for this electrotherapeutic application.

In recent years, a number of manufacturers have developed portable, battery-operated stimulators designed solely for iontophoresis treatments. These devices are usually powered by a 9-V battery and have maximum output settings of 5 mA. Most are equipped with an accurate ammeter, which provides the user with a reliable indication of the amplitude of the current used on each output channel. Other features include a treatment timer and a low-battery indicator, which alerts the user to replace the battery. Some models are designed with a control system that allows the user to select the dosage of current expressed in milliampere-minutes. This feature may represent an improvement over previous designs that simply included an ammeter to detect the magnitude of current, since the expression of dosage in milliampere-minutes reflects the total charge transfer during treatment. Additionally, new iontophoresis devices also include a sensing circuit that continuously monitors the output circuit impedance and activates an alarm when electrode contact is inadequate to achieve ion transfer. Some iontophoresis units have a switch that allows the polarity (positive or negative) to be chosen for the lead connected to the electrode containing the charged medication. The newer iontophoresis devices are designed to be used with the specially designed drug containment electrodes described previously.

Microcurrent Stimulators

The most recent class of stimulators to appear on the commercial market is referred to as *microcurrent stimulators*. As the name indicates, these devices produce very low amplitude currents (8). The output of these instruments is so small that few are capable of producing 1 mA of total current. For this reason, the electrical output of such constant-current devices is not generally great enough to activate electrically excitable tissues (nerve and muscle). The normal mode of application of the microcurrent devices is at levels that do not activate even cutaneous sensory nerve fibers, and, as a result, patients do not have any perception of the tingling sensation so commonly associated with electrotherapeutic procedures. This form of electrotherapy has been referred to as *subliminal stimulation*. No industry-wide standard has been developed for what types of currents are produced by devices marketed in this class. Figure 2.23 shows an example of the output waveform produced by some microcurrent devices. The individual waveforms are characteristically rectangular, monophasic pulses that periodically reverse polarity. A number of parameter controls related to the delivery of these pulse patterns are typically included.

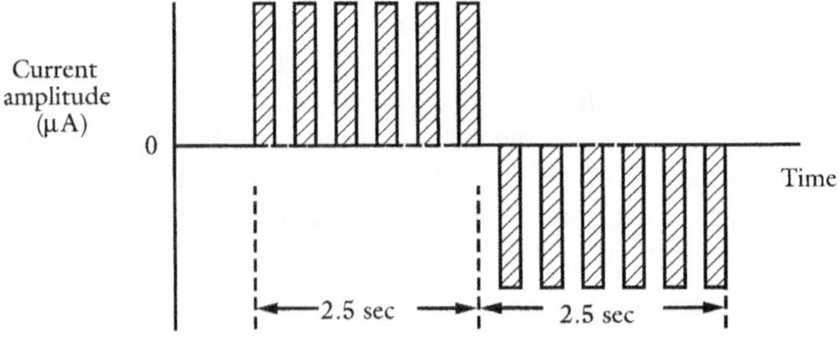

Figure 2.23. Example of one type of current produced by some microcurrent stimulators: rectangular, monophasic pulsed current with regular reversal of electrode polarity.

Amplitude controls allow the adjustment of peak amplitude from 0 to 600 μA. Some microcurrent units provide for an automatic amplitude ramp for the series of pulses delivered. Frequency controls generally allow one to set the frequency of monophasic pulses from 0.1 pps to approximately 1,000 pps. One or two channels of stimulation are commonly available on either line-powered or battery-operated units.

Point Stimulators

Point stimulators are designed to provide noxious-level stimulation to trigger points or acupuncture points. These stimulators typically have one output channel with one lead connected to a conventional surface electrode and the second lead connected to a handheld electrode with a small (1 mm^2) metal tip. Devices in this class consist of two primary components, a stimulator and a point locator. These may produce either rectangular, monophasic pulsed current, or rectangular, symmetrical, biphasic pulsed current. Controls are usually available for the adjustment of pulse amplitude, phase duration, and frequency of pulses. The upper range of phase duration is in excess of 100 ms, a range that is much greater than that of most other classes of stimulators; the range enhances the ability to produce noxious stimulation through the point electrode. Treatment timers on some models have limited ranges (≤1 minute) because treatment times associated with the stimulation of individual trigger or acupuncture points are short.

The point locator associated with point stimulators is a metering system that is used to identify points on the skin with either high conductance or low resistance, a putative characteristic of trigger points and acupuncture points.

SAFETY CONSIDERATIONS FOR ELECTROTHERAPY

Electrical hazards may develop with electrotherapeutic stimulators or may occur when these devices are not used in a safe manner; stimulators can be hazardous to both patients and providers (9–11). This section of the chapter describes common types of electrical hazards that may be associated with the application of electrotherapeutic devices, and it outlines some steps to minimize these hazards.

Sources of Electrical Hazards

Electrical hazards occur when a person comes into contact with a current-carrying conductor. A current-carrying conductor is usually thought of as metal wire that supply electrical power to receptacles, or as the wire within the power-supply cords to electrical devices. Breaks in the insulation on such cables or wires through misuse, normal wear and tear, or deterioration with age expose the conductor. The contact of body tissues with such bare wires may result in shocks with potentially serious consequences.

Less obvious types of potential current-carrying conductors include the metal cases, or other external conductive components on line-powered instruments, that can carry current as a result of contact (electrical short) with internal conductors, inappropriate electrical connections within the device, or other factors. Such currents are commonly referred to as leakage currents. Low levels of leakage current (<1 mA) are routinely found on most line-powered instruments. Normally this current does not present a problem because instrument cases are connected to a wire (safety ground) that provides a low-resistance pathway to ground (Fig. 2.24A). If this pathway does not exist, as when using a line-powered device with a two-prong plug (or "cheater" adapter), or if the wire to the safety ground is broken for any reason, leakage currents can flow to ground through an individual who is touching the device, resulting in electrical shock (Fig. 2.24B).

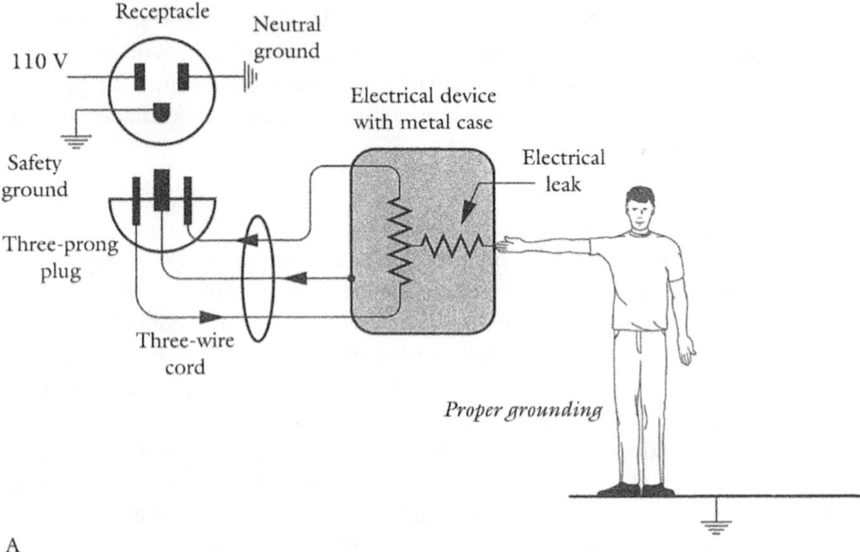

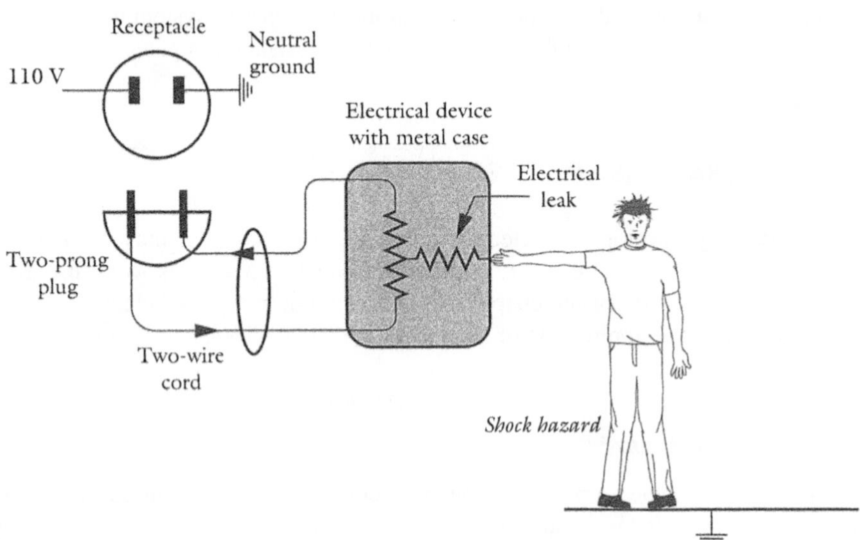

Figure 2.24. A: Pathway to ground of a leakage current in a device with a three-prong plug. **B:** Pathway to ground of a leakage current in a device with a two-prong plug.

Further, care should be taken when an individual is connected to two pieces of equipment simultaneously. If the ground connections in the two devices are separate, current may flow from the higher voltage to the lower voltage machine through the patient, also producing a potentially harmful shock.

The passage of current to ground through pathways other than the power-supply circuit is also called a *ground fault*. An additional approach used to protect against the development of significant ground faults or leakage currents is the use of electrical device called a *ground fault interrupter* (GFI; or sometimes ground fault circuit interrupter). A GFI monitors the amount of current going to and returning from a line-powered device. When the amounts of outgoing and returning currents differ by more than 3 to 5 mA, the GFI opens a switch and instantly cuts the current to the

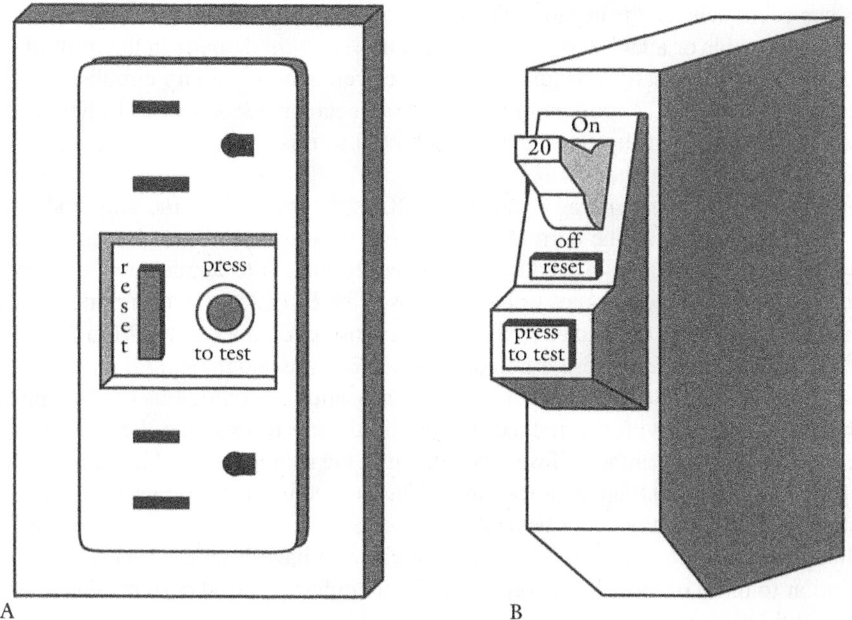

Figure 2.25. Ground fault-interrupt devices. **A:** GFI outlet. **B:** GFI circuit breaker.

device. GFIs are designed to trip in 1/40th of a second. There are two types of GFIs in power-supply circuits (Fig. 2.25): a receptacle GFI, located within a wall outlet and a circuit breaker GFI, located in a circuit breaker box. It is important to note that ordinary circuit breakers are not suitable substitutes for GFI devices on power-supply circuits to areas where line-powered stimulators are used. This has particular significance in those situations where line-powered devices are used for in-home health care. Battery-operated stimulators may be an appropriate alternative for many home treatment programs unless a receptacle GFI is properly installed.

Electrical hazards may also be the result of a misapplication of therapeutic currents. Whether an electrical hazard exists depends on the magnitude of the available current. In physiological systems, high current levels cause damage regardless of the particular type of current.

Potential Adverse Effects of 60-Hz Alternating Current

Currents as low as 1 mA root mean square (RMS; 60 Hz AC applied for 1 second) are perceived as a tingling sensation. The same current applied for 1 second at 16 mA RMS causes muscles to contract so strongly that an individual cannot overcome electrically induced contraction through the volitional contraction of antagonistic muscle groups. Higher levels of electricity can cause tissue damage, respiratory arrest, and cardiac arrest. More than 80 mA RMS of current can cause ventricular fibrillation as well as skeletal muscle contractions that are so rapid and forceful that involuntary jerking can pull the person away from the electrical contact. A startling reaction caused by higher level currents can result in secondary accidents (e.g., falling).

Potential Adverse Effects of Direct Current at Electrotherapeutic Levels

Tissue damage, especially to the skin, can be caused by clinical uses of direct current even at low amplitudes. Skin damage may result from electrolytic reactions that occur when DC passes through the skin. Acidic reactions can occur beneath the positive electrode (anode), and alkaline reactions can occur beneath the negative electrode (cathode) used in DC treatment procedures (12). If the buildup of acids or alkaline by-products is sufficient, skin damage in the form of blistering burns may result. Additionally, coagulation of microcirculation (capillary circulation) may occur beneath the anode of a DC circuit and result in tissue necrosis secondary to ischemia. Although DC clinical applications to the skin have the potential to raise tissue temperature, adverse skin responses are not thought to be thermal burns.

The extent of damage that can result from DC is determined by the amplitude of current applied, the time over which the current is allowed to flow, and the tissue impedance. For these reasons, DC electrotherapeutic procedures are generally limited to applications of current at 5.0 mA or less for periods of 15 minutes or less, and steps are taken to reduce skin impedance before treatment. Electrode sizes are selected so that current densities do not exceed 0.1 to 0.5 mA per cm^2 of electrode surface area. For these treatment parameters, the patient should not report any sensation beneath the electrodes. A report of a tingling sensation as continuous DC is applied should signal the health care provider to reduce the amplitude and re-examine the treatment setup to ensure uniform electrode contact. Close observation of the skin is required in each patient receiving DC stimulation to avoid adverse reactions. This inspection is particularly important due to the anesthetic effect that may occur beneath the electrodes.

Although some forms of pulsed monophasic currents have been reported to have chemical effects similar to those of DC, very short duration monophasic pulsed currents do not apparently produce harmful electrochemical effects on the skin (12).

Steps to Minimize Electrical Shock Hazards

Health care providers using electrical stimulators are responsible for ensuring that such devices do not harm their patients. This section addresses safety considerations relating to three fundamental questions: What are the safety considerations related to the equipment chosen for a clinical procedure? What are the safety considerations with respect to the environment in which electrotherapy is applied? What are the safety considerations related to the actual use of electrical stimulators? The lists of recommendations do not represent all possible steps that can be taken to reduce the shock hazards in clinical electrotherapy.

Suggestions for Equipment Selection

One of the dilemmas facing the health care provider is how to decide which devices to choose for electrotherapeutic applications. In North America, one feature to look for is the approval by a nationally recognized testing laboratory such as Underwriters Laboratories (UL), Canadian Standards Association (CSA), or Electronic Testing Laboratories (ETL). In general, these organizations apply a standard set of tests to electronic equipment when examining the performance of a device. For instance, depending on the type of equipment, leakage currents must be less than 50 to 100 μA to receive approval. The approval assigned by these organizations is for the design of the instrument, not for each stimulator manufactured, and therefore approval does not guarantee performance as instruments age or as they are subjected to heavy use. Safety certification for portable battery-operated devices is currently not required.

NMES devices should meet the AAMI performance standards. Such standards have been developed for TENS devices and are being developed for NMES devices. The standards include the presence of a safety interlock that prevents voltage transients in the patient circuit when a device is powered up or down, and an output interlock that does not allow the device to be powered on unless the amplitude control is first returned to the minimum setting. Instruments for electrotherapy should also be designed such that supply voltage fluctuations do not result in marked increases in stimulator output while in use. In addition, new stimulators should be shielded in such a manner as to protect them from interference from diathermies and other forms of electromagnetic interference.

Forms have been developed to assist in the decision-making process for selection of electrotherapeutic devices (13).

Suggestions for Equipment Inspection and Maintenance

All types of electrical stimulators should be periodically inspected and maintained by a qualified biomedical engineer. There are no standards for how often different types of electrical stimulators should be inspected. Frequency of inspection is generally dictated by frequency of use. Minimally, electrical stimulators should receive an annual inspection. For devices used heavily, inspection should be performed every other month. Any incident such as dropping a stimulator, liquid spills on or near a stimulator, or unexpected electrical shocks to a patient or health care provider should trigger an inspection of the device before use is resumed. New equipment should be inspected before use.

Routine equipment inspections include verification that the output characteristics are consistent with standards provided by the manufacturer, as well as consistent with existing performance standards for particular classes of stimulators.

Preventive maintenance is essential. Any component (switch, dial, meter, lights, connector, lead, electrode, etc.) not in original working order should be replaced or repaired immediately by qualified personnel. Some manufacturers supply service contracts for such equipment maintenance. Records of the results of all safety inspections and routine maintenance should be stored and made available during subsequent inspections.

Although safety inspections are normally performed by qualified biomedical personnel, knowledgeable users of electrical stimulators should be aware of the elements of the inspection because they are in the best position to recognize potential problems with the structure or operation of these instruments. One of the first signs of a developing problem is the intermittent failure of a component during clinical use but that may not occur at the time of inspection. Components that should be checked by the user or qualified personnel include the following:

1. Proper operation of all switches, dials, push buttons, pressure-sensitive switches, or other types of stimulator controls. Dirt in controls or broken controls interfere with stimulator output. Adjustment of malfunctioning controls during a treatment may result in an abrupt change in a stimulation parameter and possibly an uncomfortable stimulus to a patient.
2. Proper function of meters and auditory and visual signals.
3. Loose connections at stimulator or electrode interface.
4. Frayed or broken wires, broken lead insulation, broken power plugs.
5. Worn, old, or otherwise malfunctioning electrodes.

Environmental Factors and Safety in Electrotherapy

Users of electrical stimulators must also be aware of a variety of factors related to the environment in which theses devices are to be used. These environmental factors include the following:

1. Line-powered stimulators should be connected to a power-supply circuit protected by a ground fault-interrupt (GFI) outlet or GFI circuit breaker. As discussed previously, GFIs are designed to shut off the supply circuit if the current provided to the stimulator differs from the current returning from the device by 3 to 5 mA. GFI outlets or GFI circuit breakers should be tested monthly to ensure proper operation. A line-powered stimulator need not be

connected to a GFI-protected power circuit if the stimulator is double-isolated and meets the design standards of Underwriters Laboratories Standard 544. This feature is particularly important for line-powered stimulators used in home settings because many circuits will not be protected by GFI devices.

2. All stimulators should be isolated from the voltage transients (surges) that may occur during power outages or during shifts to emergency power. In hospitals, isolation transformers or other types of surge protection devices are generally included in power supply lines. Such devices may not be available in private homes or in private practice settings. In these cases, a biomedical engineer should be consulted to determine the method of surge protection.
3. Three-prong wall outlets should be tested annually to ensure a secure fit with plugs (pull tension: minimum 4 ounces) and proper grounding. Before initial use of any new supply circuit, the polarity of the circuit should be tested.
4. Use of line-powered electrical stimulators should be avoided in areas where water may accumulate on floors or where individuals can come into contact with grounded conductors such as water pipes, radiators, or cases of other grounded instruments.

Suggestions for Safe Clinical Use of Electrical Stimulators

Once a stimulator has been shown to function according to specification and the power-supply system is safe, the third set of safety considerations relates to the operators' appropriate use of the devices in patient treatment. The following procedures are suggested to minimize risks and undesired responses to patient and clinician.

1. Be sure that the prospective patient does not have any contraindications to the specific electrotherapeutic application considered. Refer to the specific listings of contraindications in subsequent chapters of this book, in professional literature, and manufacturers' operating instructions.
2. Never place line-powered stimulators next to radiator pipes, water pipes, or any other ground pathway within reach of the patient or clinician.
3. To prevent interference or the production of transients in the patient circuit, do not use stimulators within 3 m of short-wave diathermy and microwave devices. Some stimulators may be properly shielded to prevent such interactions.
4. Read and understand the operating manual for the stimulator. If the manual is missing, request a replacement copy. If the precise function of the various components and controls is not clearly specified in the operating manual, the device should not be used until a clear understanding of its operation is obtained from the manufacturer.
5. Apply power to the stimulator before connecting the electrodes to the patient. Never use "cheater" plugs, frayed plugs or cords, or extension cords. Do not remove the ground prong of the power plug to accommodate a two-prong outlet receptacle.
6. Use only the power switch to turn the power on and off.
7. Never disconnect a machine from the wall power outlet with the power turned on.
8. Always turn the output amplitude controls to zero before applying electrodes to the patient.
9. Do not apply or remove surface electrodes while currents are applied to the patient circuit. Use electrodes designed for use with the particular stimulator.
10. Gradually increase stimulation amplitude after all other parameters of stimulation have been set.
11. Do not make major incremental adjustments to stimulation parameters while applying maximally tolerable stimulation.

12. Do not adjust the amplitude of stimulation during the off time.
13. Adjust only one parameter of stimulation at a time.
14. Reduce the output amplitude of stimulation before turning the power off.
15. Only one individual should make changes in stimulation parameters during an electrotherapeutic procedure.
16. Never pull the plug from the socket by pulling on the power cord.
17. Always explain the treatment procedure to the patient; describe what sensations they should expect during stimulation as well as those sensations that are not desired or anticipated.
18. Do not use electrotherapeutic approaches on individuals who are unable or unwilling to clearly communicate.
19. Do not use battery-operated stimulators with a recharger plugged in unless line leakage current is less than 10 μA.

Adverse reactions to the use of electrical stimulation devices should be reported to MedWatch (www.fda.gov/medwatch/), the U.S. Food and Drug Administration's (FDA's) Safety Information and Adverse Event Reporting Program. Reporting of adverse reactions to stimulation treatments may also be made by calling 1-800-FDA-1088. Federal medical device reporting regulations require that health care providers and other users of medical devices report (a) device-related deaths to the FDA and the device manufacturer and (b) device-related serious injuries to the manufacturer, or to the FDA if the manufacturer is not known, within 10 working days of an incident.

SUMMARY

This chapter has described the design features of electrotherapeutic devices, generic stimulator controls, the classes of electrotherapeutic stimulators, and issues related to their safe use. The chapter was intended to provide an introduction to the common features of stimulators to enable the reader to better understand how to operate these machines safely and effectively. This information should enable individuals to make informed decisions regarding instrument selection. Safety considerations were outlined to emphasize that contemporary clinical electrotherapy is not without potential harmful effects. With the information provided here and in subsequent chapters, the informed practitioner should be able to provide clients with electrotherapeutic treatments that can be both safe and of lasting benefit.

SELF-STUDY QUESTIONS

For answers, see Appendix B.

1. Describe the two types of power supplies used in electrotherapeutic stimulators.
2. The component of an electrical stimulator that allows adjustment of the magnitude of the current (or voltage) produced is called the ________________.
3. The two types of electrotherapeutic stimulators based upon the design of the controls to set or adjust stimulation parameters are called ____(a)____ and ____(b)____.
4. Define the function of the following generic stimulator controls:

a. Waveform selector

b. Ramp-up and ramp-down controls

c. On-time and off-time controls

d. Pulse duration control

e. Pulse frequency control

f. Burst frequency control

g. Amplitude control

h. Output channel controls

5. The figure for question 5 shows the controls on a commercially available neuromuscular stimulator. Describe the function of each labeled control.

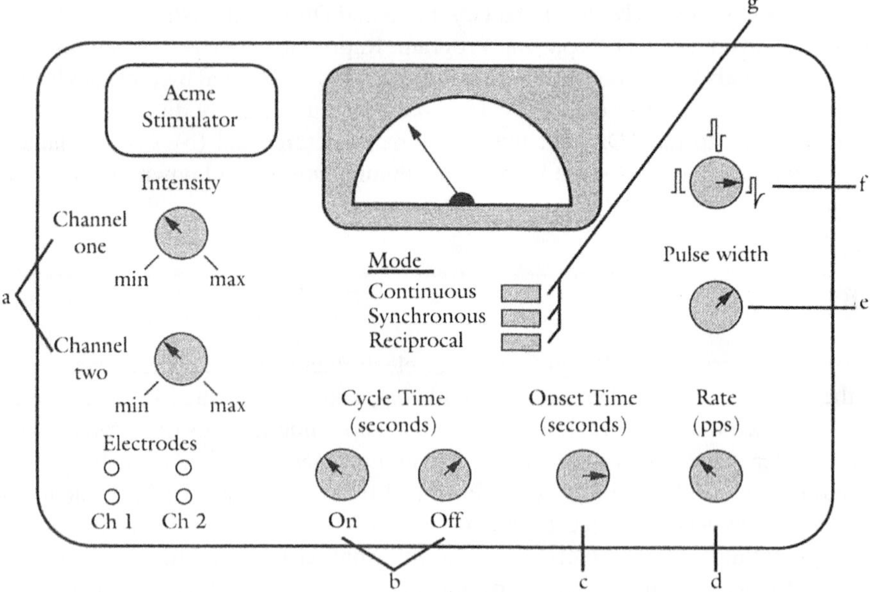

6. What is a surface electrode for electrotherapy? How do the various types of surface electrodes differ?

7. What is the minimum number of electrodes associated with a single output channel of a stimulator?

8. What is meant by monopolar electrode orientation? bipolar electrode orientation? quadripolar electrode orientation? Draw a diagram illustrating examples of these types of electrode placements.

9. Using a tabular format, compare and contrast the common characteristics of a typical TENS device with a typical portable NMES unit.

10. What type of electrical current is produced by common interferential stimulators?

11. What is the waveform produced by a "high volt" stimulator?

12. How does a point stimulator differ from a TENS unit or a portable NMES device?

13. How many channels of stimulation are usually used with an interferential stimulator, and how are the electrodes oriented in the interferential technique?

14. How are iontophoresis devices unique in comparison to other commercial classes of stimulators?

15. What is the difference between a two-prong and a three-prong power-supply plug? Which should be used on medical devices and why?

16. What is a ground fault? Describe the function of a ground fault-interrupt device.

17. What components of electrical stimulators should be routinely inspected by the user to screen the device for electrical safety?

18. How can DC produce skin damage during an electrotherapeutic intervention?

19. Why are electrodes never removed from a patient until after the stimulator has been turned off?

20. Why are electrical stimulators never used in close proximity to short-wave diathermy?

REFERENCES

1. Witters DM, Lapp AK, Hinckley, SM. A descriptive study of transcutaneous electrical nerve stimulation devices and their electrical output characteristics. *J Clin Electrophysiol.* 1991;3:9–16.
2. Campbell JA. A critical appraisal of the electrical output characteristics of ten transcutaneous electrical nerve stimulators. *Clin Phys Physiol Meas.* 1982;1:141–144.
3. Nolan MF. Conductive differences in electrodes used with transcutaneous electrical nerve stimulation devices. *Phys Ther* 1991;71:746–751.
4. American Physical Therapy Association. *Electrotherapeutic Terminology in Physical Therapy.* Alexandria, VA: Section on Clinical Electrophysiology, American Physical Therapy Association; 1990.
5. Association for the Advancement of Medical Instrumentation. American national standard for transcutaneous electrical nerve stimulators. ANSI/AAMI NS4-1985. Arlington, VA: Association for the Advancement of Medical Instrumentation, 1985.
6. Hansjuergens A, May H-U. *Traditional and Modern Aspects of Electrotherapy.* 2nd ed. Monograph Deutsche-Nemectron GMBH, Karlsrule, 1981.
7. Alon G. Principles of electrical stimulation. In: Clinical Electrotherapy, Nelson RM, Currier DP, eds. Norwalk, CT: Appleton and Lange; 1991:48, 58–61.
8. Picker RI. Current-low-volt pulsed microamp stimulation Part 1. *Clin Manage Phys Ther.* 1989;9:10–14.
9. Arledge RL. Prevention of electrical shock hazards in physical therapy. *Phys Ther.* 1978; 58:1215–1217.
10. Berger WH. Electrical shock hazards in the physical therapy department. *Clin Manage Phys Ther* 1985;5:26–31.
11. Roth HH, Teltscher ES, Kane IM. *Electrical Safety in Health Care Facilities.* New York: Academic Press, 1975.
12. Newton RA, Karselis TC. Skin pH following high voltage pulsed galvanic stimulation. *Phys Ther* 1983;63:1593–1596.
13. Nolan TP. Choosing electrotherapeutic devices. *PT Magazine* 1993;July:43–49, 92.

CHAPTER 3

Physiology of Muscle and Nerve

Andrew J. Robinson

Electrical stimulation (ES) has many therapeutic applications. Currently and historically, clinical electrical stimulation has been used primarily to activate electrically excitable tissues—nerve and skeletal muscle. The appropriate use of ES in therapeutic applications requires that clinicians have a clear understanding of the basic structure and function of these tissues, including the mechanisms of their activation by the central nervous system (CNS) and by electrical currents. The primary objective of this chapter is to review the physiology of skeletal muscle and peripheral nerve as it applies to clinical applications of electrical stimulation. The effects of electrical stimulation on other tissues (such as skin) are addressed in Chapter 8.

ELECTRICAL EXCITABILITY OF MUSCLE AND NERVE

Membrane Structure and the Resting Membrane Potential

Structurally, the cell membranes of muscle and nerve cells are similar to those of other cells, consisting of a phospholipid bilayer containing a variety of protein molecules. The proteins in nerve and muscle cell membranes, however, serve several special functions that set these tissues apart from other body tissues. Membrane proteins may serve as (a) *receptor proteins*, which act as binding sites for neurotransmitters or neuromodulators; (b) *channel proteins*, which under certain conditions form a pore through the membrane for the movement of ions such as sodium, potassium, chloride, or calcium; and (c) *transport proteins*, which bind and transfer substances such as sodium and potassium through the membrane, often against concentration gradients (Fig. 3.1). Each of these types of proteins is thought to undergo a change in shape (conformational change) as they perform their respective functions.

By virtue of its structure, the excitable cell membrane functions as a barrier to the movement of substances between the intracellular and extracellular spaces. Substances such as oxygen, carbon dioxide, and water move readily through the phospholipid bilayer. In contrast, ions and

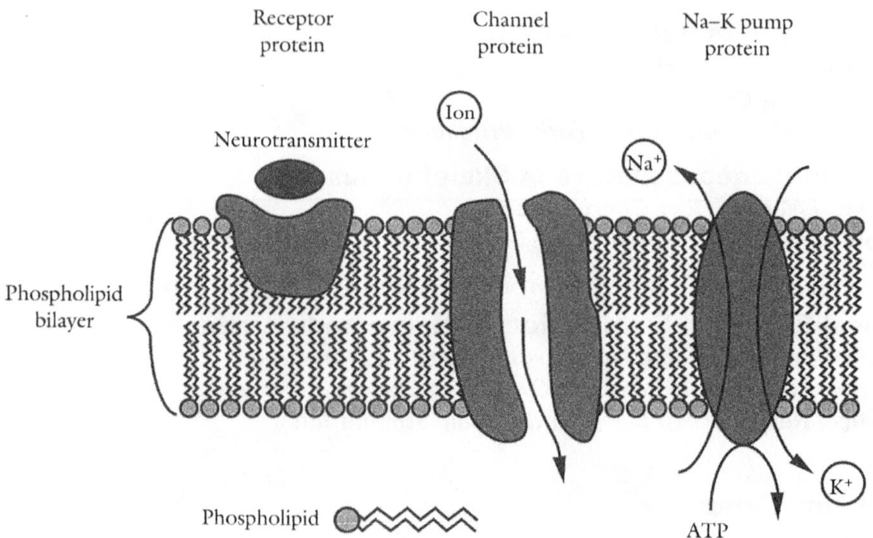

Figure 3.1. Composition of excitable cell membrane, showing phospholipid bilayer and three general types of membrane-bound proteins.

macromolecules such as proteins do not move readily through the membrane. The excitable cell membrane has a differential permeability to different electrically charged particles. In the resting state, when the nervous system is not activating excitable tissues, excitable membranes are readily permeable to potassium ions, slightly permeable to sodium ions, and impermeable to a number of large, negatively charged proteins and phosphates (anions). Because a large number of anions are trapped within the cell and the membrane is readily permeable to potassium, the positively charged potassium ions are drawn into the cell by electromotive forces as the resting state is being established.

Another important property of excitable membranes in the resting state is that they use cellular energy in the form of adenosine triphosphate (ATP) to actively transport sodium and potassium across the membrane. This active *sodium–potassium pump* moves sodium ions out of the cell while moving potassium ions in. An important feature of the sodium–potassium pump is that it is capable of moving the ions against the electrochemical forces tending to oppose their movement in the resting state.

As a consequence of both the selective permeability of the membrane and the membrane pumping mechanisms, the distribution of charged particles across the membrane of electrically excitable cells is not uniform (Fig. 3.2). The concentration of sodium (Na^+) is higher in the fluid surrounding the cells, and the concentration of anions and potassium (K^+) is higher inside. The resulting separation of electrically charged particles gives rise to an electrical potential difference across the membrane. This transmembrane potential difference or voltage is referred to as the *resting membrane potential* (RMP), and hence the excitable cell is described as *polarized.* The RMP exists all along the length of the nerve or muscle cell. For nerve cells, the RMP exists across the membrane cell body, dendrites, and the entire length of the nerve cell axon. The magnitude of the resting membrane potential is approximately –90 mV for muscle and is slightly less, about –70 mV, for peripheral nerve fibers. The absolute RMP values for muscle and nerve of different species vary. Under normal conditions, as long as the membranes of these cells remain intact and ATP can be supplied to the Na^+-K^+ pump, the resting membrane potential of

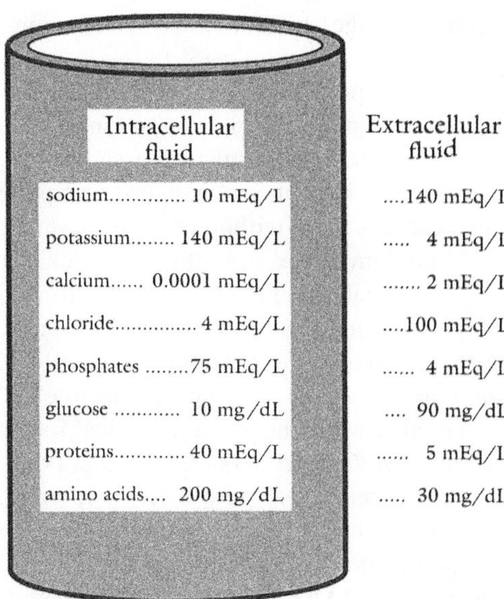

Intracellular fluid
Extracellular fluid
sodium.............. 10 mEq/L
....140 mEq/L
potassium........ 140 mEq/L
..... 4 mEq/L
calcium...... 0.0001 mEq/L
.... 2 mEq/L
chloride.............. 4 mEq/L
....100 mEq/L
phosphates ....75 mEq/L
...... 4 mEq/L
glucose .... 10 mg/dL
.... 90 mg/dL
proteins............. 40 mEq/L
...... 5 mEq/L
amino acids.... 200 mg/dL
..... 30 mg/dL

Figure 3.2. Intracellular and extracellular concentration differences for selected ions and molecules across the membrane of excitable cells.

these cells remains stable. By virtue of the concentration differences of sodium and potassium ions across the membrane and the relative negative charge within the resting membrane, both the chemical and electrical forces acting on sodium are directed into the cell, while the net electrochemical forces acting on potassium are directed out of the cell.

Action Potentials

Muscle or nerve cells are different from other types of body cells because of specialized cell membrane properties that enable them to initiate and propagate action potentials. What are action potentials and why do they occur?

In contrast to the membranes of nonexcitable cells, muscle and nerve cell membranes may quickly and dramatically alter their permeability to ions in response to chemical, electrical, thermal, or mechanical stimuli. When an appropriate stimulus is applied to a small region of the excitable cell (e.g., peripheral nerve fiber), the membrane permeability to sodium and potassium ions transiently increases. Because both the concentration and electrical forces for sodium are directed inward, sodium ions move into the cell, and the transmembrane potential is reduced (approaches zero). This reduction in transmembrane potential, referred to as *depolarization* (Fig. 3.3A), is gradual at first as a small amount of sodium leaks into the cell. When the transmembrane potential reaches a critical voltage level called the *threshold*, voltage-sensitive sodium and potassium channel proteins in the membrane undergo a conformational change and open (Fig. 3.3B). Permeability to sodium abruptly increases as sodium gates open, whereas permeability to potassium increases more slowly because the electrochemical forces acting on potassium ions are initially much lower than those acting on sodium ions. Because both the electrical and chemical forces acting on sodium are initially directed strongly into the cell, sodium rushes in when sodium channels open. As a result, the transmembrane potential rapidly depolarizes as positively charged sodium ions are added to the negatively charged cell interior. If sodium channels remained open for very long, sodium ions would continue to enter the cell until the electrical and chemical forces acting on sodium ions were balanced—(the *sodium equilibrium potential*) which would occur at approximately +60 mV. In fact, sodium influx stops at a point when the transmembrane potential reaches about +35 mV, because at this level the sodium channels close (Fig. 3.3B). At this voltage, the membrane again becomes relatively impermeable to sodium.

When the sodium gates close, the potassium gates remain fully open. Because the inside of the cell is now positively charged and only a few potassium ions have left the cell, both the electrical and chemical forces acting on the intracellular potassium ions strongly force potassium ions out of the cell's interior. The potassium gates remain open, so potassium ions rush out of the cell, thereby removing positive charges from within, and the transmembrane potential becomes progressively more negative. Potassium efflux from the cell quickly makes the transmembrane potential negative again, in a process called *repolarization*. The forces moving potassium out of the cell are so great, and the potassium gates remain open long enough, that the membrane is repolarized slightly past the resting membrane potential, about 10 to 20 mV below RMP. This hyperpolarization of the membrane proceeds until no net electrochemical forces act on potassium. The transmembrane potential at which no electrochemical forces exist to cause potassium ion efflux is called the *potassium equilibrium potential.* At that point in time, potassium gates continue to close, and passive diffusion of ions across the membrane then quickly restores the membrane potential to its original resting level.

The transmembrane voltage changes that occur in response to excitable cell stimulation are collectively called an *action potential* (AP) and are generally completed within 1 ms. These voltage changes occur in response to each stimulus sufficient to raise the transmembrane potential to threshold level. The voltage changes of the AP are simply a reflection of the sodium and

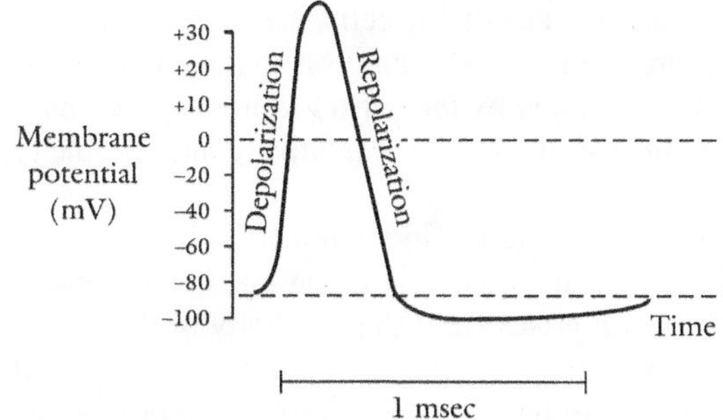

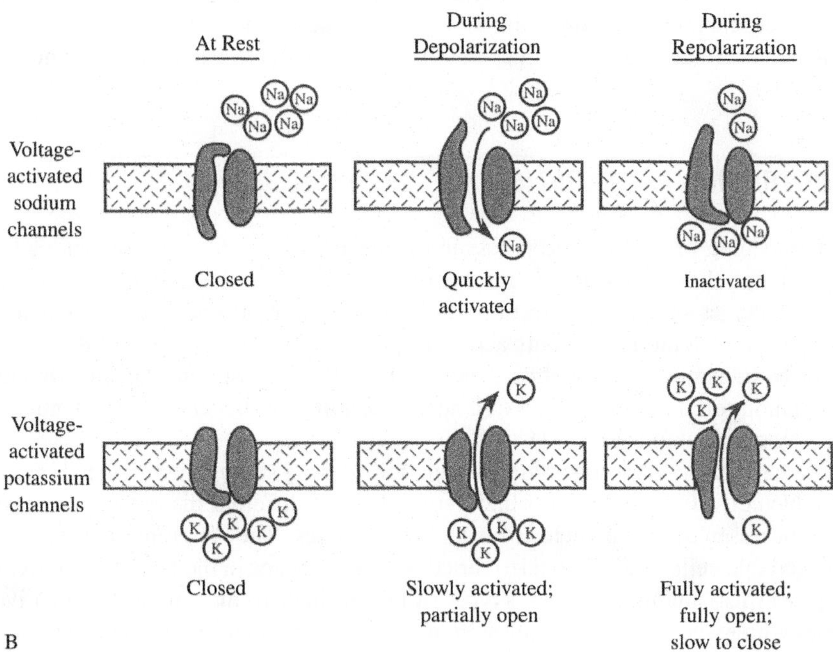

Figure 3.3. A: Intracellular action potential: the transmembrane voltage changes that occur in excitable cells during excitation. **B:** Diagrammatic representation of changes in the voltage-gate sodium and potassium channels during the action potential.

potassium currents that occur over time across the membrane in response to the opening of the sodium and potassium gates. If an excitatory stimulus is large enough to depolarize the membrane to its threshold level, the transmembrane voltage changes that occur by virtue of ion movement happen in precisely the same manner for each stimulus applied. Because the amplitude of voltage changes in response to stimulation is constant from stimulus to stimulus, the AP is described as "all or none." The APs that occur in nerve and muscle cells in response to either normal nervous system activation, the application of sensory stimuli, or electrical stimulation are basically similar.

In monitoring the normal function of peripheral nerve and muscle, single, isolated APs are rarely produced. Usually, volitional activation of nerve and muscle produces series of APs in these cells. The frequency of APs produced in nerve and muscle during normal activities rarely exceeds 60 per second, and ordinary discharge ranges from 5 to 15 impulses per second. In contrast, during electrical stimulation of excitable cells, the AP frequency mirrors the stimulation frequency up to a maximum rate of near 1,000 impulses per second in nerve fibers. This maximum rate of AP generation is determined by the period following the onset of the potential during which the nerve or muscle fiber is absolutely or relatively unexcitable (called the *absolute* or *relative refractory period*).

Where are action potentials initiated? Under normal physiological conditions, action potentials in multipolar neurons, such as those innervating skeletal muscle, begin at the axon hillock, the point at which the axon arises from the cell body of the neuron. In peripheral sensory neurons, APs are normally initiated at the peripheral (distal) end of the sensory axons, often at the point where the axon terminates in a specialized receptor ending. In skeletal muscle fibers, APs are initiated in the region of the neuromuscular junction between the alpha motoneuron and the muscle fiber. Of importance in clinical electrophysiology, APs may be initiated using electrical stimuli at any point along the course of peripheral nerve axons where the electrical stimulus is sufficient to trigger the opening of voltage-gated sodium and potassium channel proteins.

ACTION POTENTIAL PROPAGATION

Although the opening of sodium and potassium gates and resultant action potentials have been discussed as though they occur at one segment of the membrane, the channel opening and associated voltage changes spread to adjacent portions of the nerve or muscle membrane and trigger the same sequence of ionic movements across the membrane. In this manner, the AP is said to propagate, or be transmitted, along the surface of the cell. The resultant transmembrane voltage changes (AP) monitored in one portion of a nerve axon or muscle cell will be identical to those recorded in any other region (Fig. 3.4).

The rate or speed of AP propagation (conduction velocity) along membranes is not the same for all excitable cells. In muscle fibers and nerve fibers of different diameters, the speed of AP propagation increases as the diameter of the fiber increases. The differences in AP conduction velocity in excitable cells of different sizes are due to differences in the passive electrical properties (cable properties) among the various types of fibers. The two most important passive electrical properties with respect to the transmission of ionic currents in nerve and muscle fibers are the *membrane resistance* (r_m) and the *internal (intracellular) resistance* (r_i).

In response to electrical or chemical activation, current spreads within the fiber and becomes attenuated (reduced) with distance. This attenuation occurs because ionic movement longitudinally along an axon is opposed by r_i and because some ions leak out of the fiber through its membrane. The higher the r_i or the lower the r_m, the less the spread of longitudinal currents along the fiber, and hence the lower the propagation speed of AP currents. Small-diameter fibers have relatively high internal resistance compared to large-diameter fibers and consequently have lower conduction velocities than large fibers. In addition, larger diameter peripheral axons have a higher r_m because they are covered along most of their length with an insulating layer of myelin. The transmission of APs along the membrane of both muscle or unmyelinated peripheral nerve fibers occurs in a continuous manner involving every segment of the membrane.

Many types of peripheral nerve fibers, however, are surrounded by *myelin*, an insulating (nonconductive) material. This myelin layer is interrupted at intervals (*nodes of Ranvier*) of about 1 mm, exposing small segments of the axon membrane to the extracellular fluids. In myelinated axons, only those portions of the axon membrane in contact with the extracellular fluid at the nodes of Ranvier undergo the permeability changes and ionic currents associated with the AP. Ionic currents do not occur in those segments of the membrane covered by myelin because the membrane resistance in those regions is extremely high, and areas of membrane beneath the

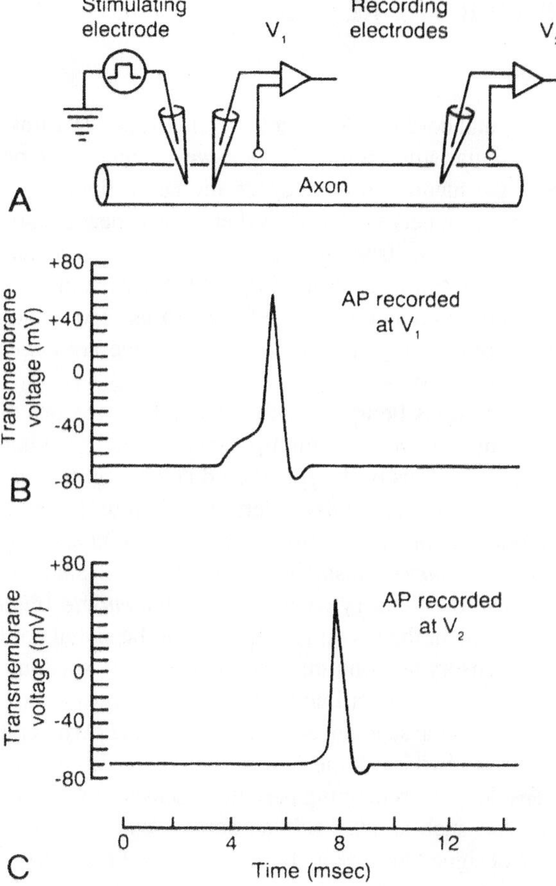

Figure 3.4. A: Experimental setup for examining action potential propagation. **B:** Action potential recorded at V_1. **C:** Action potential recorded at V_2. (Redrawn with permission from Kuffler SW, Nicholls JG. *From neuron to brain: A cellular approach to the function of the nervous system.* Sunderland, MA: Sinauer Associates, Inc.; 1976.)

myelin have relatively few voltage-gated channel proteins. When an AP is initiated by electrical stimulation at one node, ionic currents spread longitudinally until they reach the adjacent node. As a result, current attenuation is less and impulse propagation is more rapid in myelinated axons than in unmyelinated axons.

The AP currents moving along the axon membrane in myelinated axons can be viewed as moving in a stepwise manner from one node to the next. This form of AP propagation in myelinated axons is called *saltatory conduction,* a term derived from the Latin verb *saltare,* which means "to leap." The conduction velocity of myelinated nerve fibers is much higher than that of either unmyelinated axons or muscle fibers because myelinization reduces the amount of membrane involved in the ionic movements of the action potential. Hence, myelinization effectively reduces the amount of axon membrane through which ionic currents must flow.

Action potential propagation occurs in neurons at locations where voltage-gated sodium and potassium ion channel proteins are located. In multipolar neurons these voltage-gated channel proteins are found on the single axon projecting from the cell body. Voltage-gated sodium and potassium channels associated with AP generation are not found on the cell body or the dendrites of multipolar neurons. On unipolar or bipolar neurons, voltage-gated sodium and potassium channel proteins are located on both the peripheral and central processes.

COMPOSITION OF PERIPHERAL NERVES

Peripheral Nerve Fibers

Peripheral nerves link the spinal cord to tissues in the extremities and trunk such as skeletal muscle, skin, joint capsules, vascular smooth muscle and sweat glands. The primary components of peripheral nerves, such as the median or sciatic, are the nerve fibers (axons). Nerve fibers are merely long, thin projections from nerve cell bodies that lie in or near the spinal cord or brainstem. Most peripheral nerves contain axons from three general types of nerve cells: motoneurons, first-order sensory neurons, and autonomic neurons (Fig. 3.5). Because most nerves contain each of these components, most peripheral nerves are referred to as *mixed*. Some peripheral nerves contain axons originating from mainly sensory cells and hence are called *sensory* nerves. No peripheral nerves contain only motor or autonomic fibers.

The cell bodies of motoneurons lie in either the ventral horn regions of the spinal cord or in brainstem motor nuclei of cranial nerves. The multipolar cell bodies of spinal motoneurons project a single axon through the ventral roots of the spinal cord and along the normally well established routes of peripheral nerves. All motoneuron axons terminate in muscle. Functionally, motoneurons can be divided into two groups: *alpha motoneurons*, the cells that innervate ordinary striated skeletal muscle fibers and *gamma motoneurons*, smaller multipolar cells that innervate the special types of muscle fibers contained within a sensory receptor called the *muscle spindle*. The cell bodies of first-order sensory nerve cells lie in the dorsal root ganglia of the spinal cord or in selected cranial nerve sensory nuclei. These sensory neurons are either unipolar (or psuedounipolar) or bipolar cells that project one axon toward the spinal cord and a second axon toward the periphery. The peripheral process of sensory neurons is the segment contained within the peripheral nerve. The peripheral axons of about half of the dorsal root cells terminate as free nerve endings in structures such as skin, muscle, and joint capsules. The remaining peripheral sensory axons end within some specialized type of sensory receptor, such as the Pacinian corpuscles, the Golgi tendon organs, or the muscle spindles, which are designed to respond best to one type of sensory stimulus such as touch, muscle contraction force, or changes in muscle length, respectively.

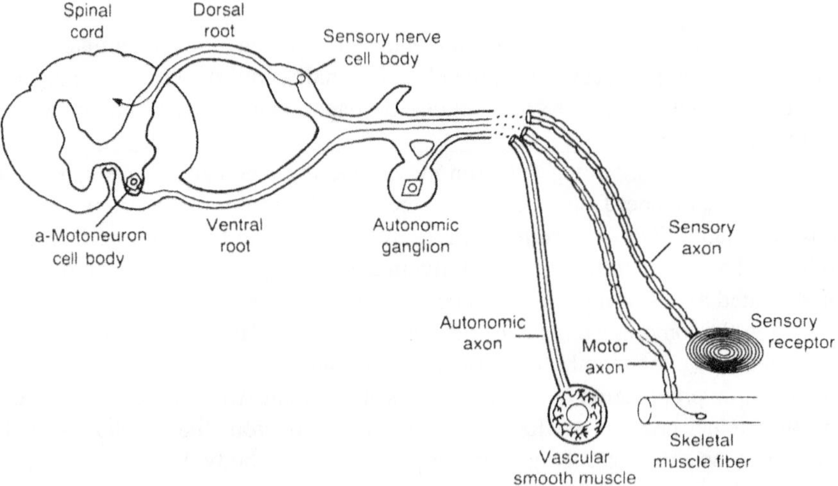

Figure 3.5. Spinal cord cross-section, showing the dorsal and ventral roots and types of axons (sensory, motor, and autonomic) that contribute to the formation of peripheral nerve.

The cell bodies of the autonomic nerve fibers in peripheral nerves are found in the chain ganglia that lie parallel to the spinal cord or in ganglia of the cranial nerves. The axons of autonomic neurons in peripheral nerves terminate in such places as the sweat glands and the smooth muscle in the walls of blood vessels.

Under normal conditions of CNS activation, the motoneurons and autonomic neurons send APs away from the spinal cord and toward the periphery. Conversely, sensory cells of all types normally initiate APs in the periphery in response to stimuli and transmit the information to the spinal cord, whence it can be relayed to higher brain centers. With these primary functions noted, peripheral nerves can be viewed as simply AP transmission pathways. Action potentials are carried along these "two-way streets," and the transmission of signals in one direction along sensory fibers is not impeded by AP transmission in the opposite direction along motor or autonomic fibers. The propagation of APs along axons in the "normal" or "physiologic" direction in a particular type of nerve fiber is referred to as *orthodromic propagation.* Orthodromic transmission for motor and autonomic fibers is away from the spinal cord, whereas orthodromic transmission of sensory fibers is toward the spinal cord. Although peripheral axons normally transmit APs either away from or toward the CNS, all types of peripheral nerve fibers are capable of transmitting APs in both directions from the point of initiation. This can occur, for instance, when electrical stimulation is applied at some point along the course of peripheral fibers. The transmission of APs in the direction opposite the physiological direction is called *antidromic propagation.* Antidromic AP transmission in sensory cells, for example, is directed away from the CNS, whereas antidromic propagation in motoneurons is toward the CNS.

The types of fibers in a peripheral nerve differ in size and structure. In general, the larger the cell body of origin, the larger the diameter of its projecting axon and the higher the AP conduction velocity. The differences in conduction velocity among the various types of fibers in a peripheral nerve have formed the basis for the development of two commonly used nerve fiber classification schemes (Table 3.1). The scheme developed by Gasser and colleagues (1,2) is used to describe all types of axons (motor, sensory, and autonomic) in peripheral nerves, and the Lloyd scheme (3) is restricted to the description of only sensory peripheral nerve fibers. Table 3.1 indicates the distributions of fiber diameters and conduction velocities for axons of specified type. The fiber diameters and conduction velocities were determined in animal nerves and generally exceed those of human peripheral nerve fibers. In spite of this, the relative differences in

Table 3.1. Peripheral Nerve Axon Classification Schemes

Scheme 1[a]	*Scheme 2*[b]	*Diameter (μm)*	*CV (m/sec)*	*Type of Nerve Fiber*
A_α	Ia	12–20	72–120	Muscle spindle primary afferent
	Ib	12–20	72–120	Golgi tendon organ afferent
		12–20	72–120	Skeletal muscle efferent
A_β	II	6–12	36–72	Touch-pressure receptor afferent
		5–12	20–72	Muscle spindle secondary afferent
A_γ		2–8	12–48	Muscle spindle efferent
A_δ	III	1–5	6–30	Pain-temperature afferent
B		<3	2–18	Preganglionic autonomic efferent
C	IV	<1	<2	Pain-temperature afferent
		<1	<2	Postganglionic autonomic efferent

[a]Gasser scheme: all peripheral nerve fibers
[b]Lloyd scheme: sensory fibers only

conduction speed of axons are believed to be similar in human nerves. Large-diameter fibers innervating muscle spindle, Golgi tendon organ, and skeletal muscle conduct much more rapidly than the small-diameter myelinated and unmyelinated pain afferents.

Peripheral Nerve as a Composite of Many Tissues

Although the axons of sensory, motor, and autonomic fibers constitute the primary component of peripheral nerves, many other important types of tissue are contained within nerves. Structures that support peripheral nerve fiber function include Schwann cells, connective tissues, and blood vessels.

All peripheral nerve fibers are surrounded by Schwann cells; they provide several important functions in peripheral nerve, including the formation of myelin. As indicated in the discussion of AP propagation, approximately one-half of the peripheral axons in the average nerve are myelinated. Myelination, the segmented covering of many peripheral axons, increases the velocity of AP conduction. In addition, Schwann cells insulate fibers from each other, which may explain why APs that are propagating distally in motor and autonomic fibers do not interfere with sensory APs traveling centrally.

Peripheral nerve axons are also surrounded by three layers of connective tissue that serve several important roles in relation to nerve transmission (Fig. 3.6).The *epineurium* is a dense sheath of connective tissue that surrounds the entire peripheral nerve and projects inward to enclose and separate bundles of nerve fibers. One role of the epineurium is to protect peripheral axons from compressive forces applied to the nerve. The *perineurium* is a thin sheath of flattened cells layered concentrically around bundles of nerve fiber (fascicles). These perineurial sheaths maintain intrafascicular pressure, act as a bidirectional diffusion barrier, and supply much of the elasticity and tensile strength (passive resistance to stretch) of peripheral nerves. The innermost layer of connective tissue is the *endoneurium*, which is a fine connective tissue matrix surrounding every nerve fiber. The endoneurial layer contains Schwann cells and endoneurial fluid which forms the extracellular environment of each nerve fiber.

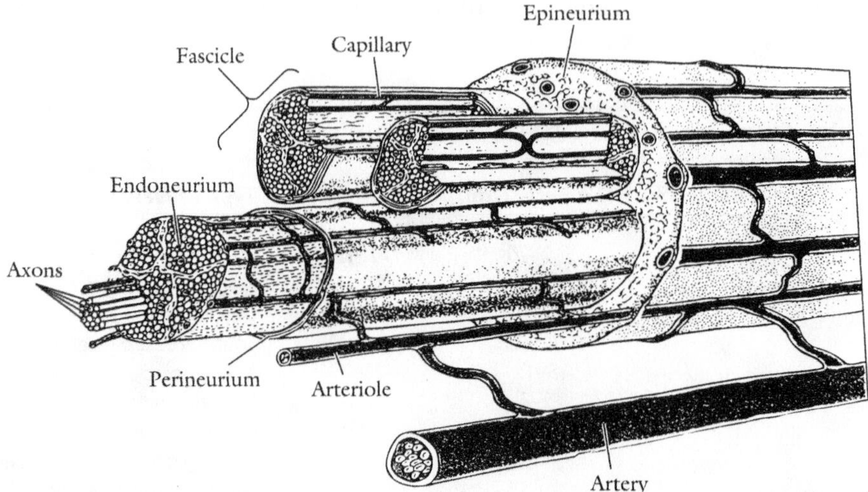

Figure 3.6. Diagram of the components of peripheral nerve: connective tissue layers (epineurium, perineurium, and endoneurium), neural elements (axons contained within nerve fascicles), and vascular (arteries, arterioles, and capillaries). (Reprinted with permission from Lundburg G, Dahlin L.The pathophysiology of nerve compressions. *Hand Clin.* 1992; 8(2):219.)

Peripheral nerves have a well-developed vascular supply (Fig. 3.6). Longitudinally-oriented arterioles and venules are present in the epineurium. These vessels regulate the blood flow to and from the peripheral nerve via sympathetic innervation of the smooth muscle contained within their walls. At regular intervals, epineurial arterioles branch toward the center of the nerve to supply blood flow to one or more nerve fascicles. Smaller diameter, longitudinally-oriented arterioles and venules are also found lying between cells of the perineurium. Branches arise and pass obliquely to form capillary beds within the fascicles. The capillaries of peripheral nerves are relatively large in diameter (approximately twice the size of muscle capillaries), and are contained mostly in the endoneurium within fascicles. The intrafascicular capillary beds are characterized by extensive U-loop anastomoses between capillaries that provide several alternative pathways for blood flow to capillaries that supply the individual nerve fibers.

SKELETAL MUSCLE STRUCTURE

Muscle Cell Structure

The primary component of striated skeletal muscle is the *muscle fiber*. Muscle fibers are cylindrical, elongated cells that have diameters commonly ranging from 50 to 200 μm and lengths that may reach many centimeters. These threadlike cells provide muscle with the electrical and contractile properties that are of special interest to those who study electrotherapy and electrophysiological evaluation. Occupying most of the interior of the muscle cell are bundles of specialized proteins called *myofibrils* (Fig. 3.7). These cylindrical elements are about 1 to 2 μm in diameter and are found throughout the entire length of the muscle fiber. A single large muscle fiber may contain as many as several thousand myofibrils. When a longitudinal section of muscle is viewed with a light microscope, a myofibril has a banded appearance, with alternating light and dark areas. This striated appearance extends along the entire length of the myofibril. On closer inspection, with an electron microscope, the structure of the myofibril becomes clearer (Fig. 3.7D). The repeating pattern of the myofibril is due to the arrangement of a system of contractile proteins, the thick and thin *myofilaments*, contained within the myofibril.

The repeating unit of the myofibril containing light and dark areas is called the *sarcomere* (Fig. 3.7E). A single sarcomere extends between structures known as Z lines. Thick myofilaments are located in the center of each sarcomere, and thin myofilaments extend from each Z line toward the center of the sarcomere and overlap the ends of the thick filaments. The dark bands (A bands) of muscle are made up of thick filaments and overlapping thin filaments. The light bands (I bands) contain only thin myofilaments extending from the centrally located Z line.

Biochemical analysis has revealed that the thick filaments are composed of the contractile protein *myosin*. This protein has a globular head connected to a long, thin tail. Approximately 200 myosin molecules are arranged to make up a single thick filament (Fig. 3.7F). Thin filaments are primarily composed of the contractile protein *actin*. Actin molecules are spherical, and the thin filament is made up of two long chains of actin molecules twisted together, much like a twisted strand of pearls. Included on the thin filament are two other proteins, *troponin* and *tropomyosin*. These regulatory proteins control the interaction between the contractile proteins actin and myosin. Troponin binds free calcium ions and controls the position of tropomyosin. Tropomyosin is a long, thin protein that, by virtue of its position on the thin filaments, interferes with actin–myosin coupling in muscle at rest.

Surrounding each myofibril in a sleevelike fashion is a tubular network called the *sarcoplasmic reticulum* (SR) (Fig. 3.8). The SR is a modified endoplasmic reticulum containing a high concentration of free calcium ions. The SR is divided into units along the length of the muscle fiber, and each unit is made up of three components. The central portion of each SR segment is called the *fenestrated SR*. The tubular network extending from the central region is called the

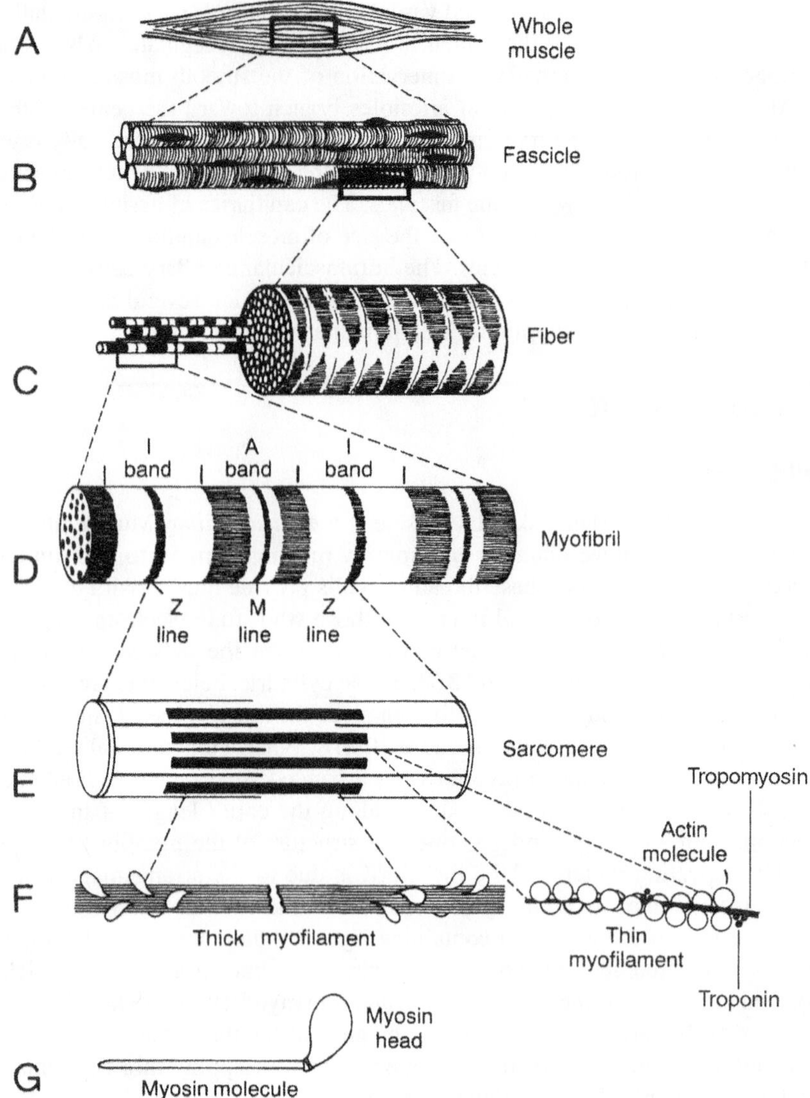

Figure 3.7. Structure organization of skeletal muscle from whole muscle to the molecular level. (Redrawn with permission from Bloom W, Fawcett DW. *A Textbook of Histology*. Philadelphia: W.B. Saunders, 1975.)

longitudinal SR. The longitudinal SR connects to larger cavities called the *lateral* or *terminal cisternae*. The lateral cisternae from adjacent segments of the SR wrap around the *t-tubules*, which are invaginations (central projections) of the surface of the cell membrane.

Just beneath the surface of the cell membrane of each muscle fiber lie the elongated or ovoid *nuclei* of the cell. The nuclei lie along the length of the muscle fiber and are the storage sites for the genetic instructions for cellular activities, such as the production of muscle protein. Since the muscle fibers are so long, it may be that many nuclei are required along their length to efficiently regulate protein synthesis and degradation within the cell.

Another set of internal structures located along the entire length of the muscle fiber are the *mitochondria*. Muscle fiber mitochondria, also known as *sarcosomes*, are rather evenly

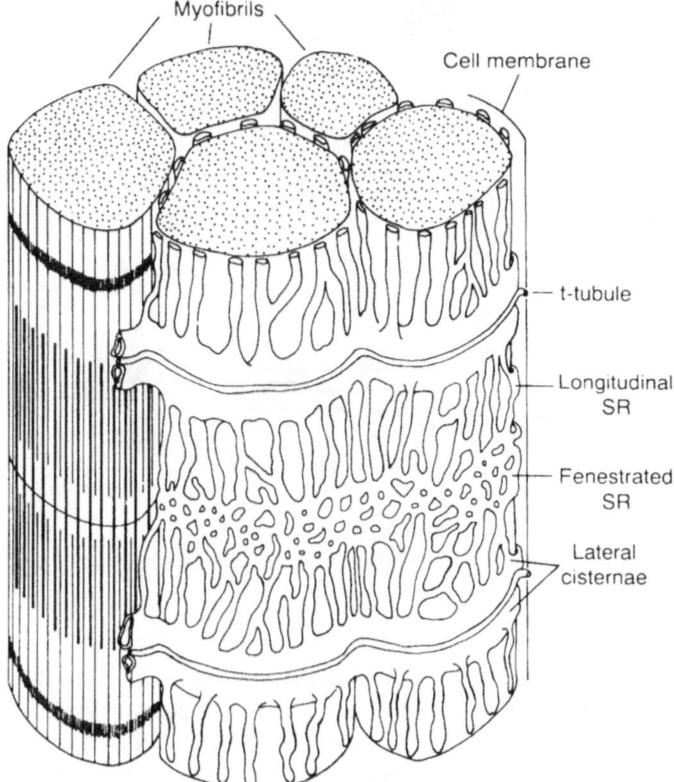

Figure 3.8. Membrane systems of skeletal muscle fiber: sarcoplasmic reticulum surrounding myofibrils and t-tubules extending centrally from the surface. (Redrawn with permission from Ham AW, Cormack DH. *Histology*. Philadelphia: J.B. Lippincott; 1987.)

distributed throughout the volume of the muscle fiber and are commonly found lying between myofibrils. They contain enzymes associated with controlling the oxidative metabolism of muscle fuels such as free fatty acids and glucose. Consequently, sarcosomes are the primary site of ATP production. ATP is required to supply energy for numerous intracellular processes, including protein synthesis, membrane pumps, and muscle contraction.

The last major internal component of muscle cells, which surrounds all of the intracellular structures, is the *cytoplasm*. This intracellular fluid (also called the *sarcoplasm*) is mostly water but contains a variety of other substances critical to the normal function of the muscle cell. The sarcoplasm is the storage site for muscle fuels including free fatty acids, glucose, and a number of nucleotides like ATP. All of the enzymes of glycolysis are located in the cytoplasm, and hence the cytoplasm is the site where glycogen and glucose are anaerobically metabolized to produce ATP. The sarcoplasm is also rich in amino acids, which are the basic building blocks of proteins. Lysosomes are suspended in the cytoplasm for handling of damaged intracellular components. Finally, the cytoplasm contains myoglobin, an oxygen-binding and transport protein, which is essential for the maintenance of oxidative metabolic processes.

The cell membrane of the muscle fiber is called the *sarcolemma*. The membrane regulates those substances that are allowed to enter and leave the cell, maintains the muscle fiber's resting membrane potential, and propagates muscle APs as described previously. The specialized region of the muscle fiber membrane where APs are normally initiated is called the *motor endplate*

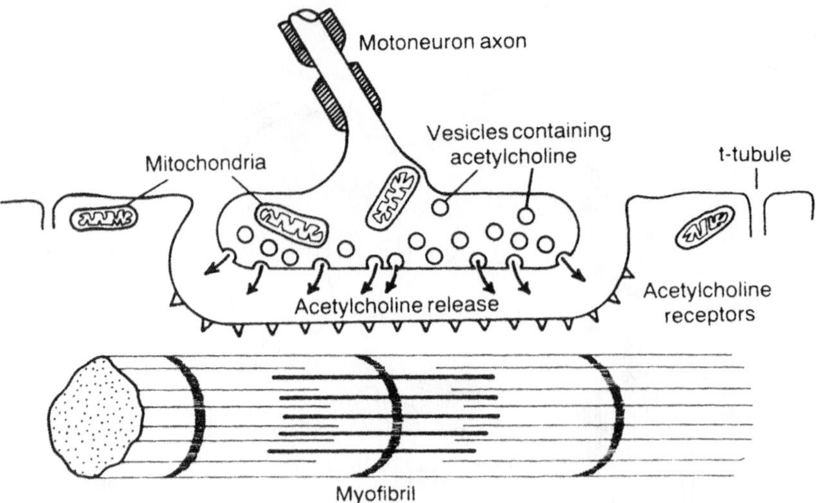

Figure 3.9. Diagrammatic representation of the neuromuscular junction. (Redrawn with permission from Vander AJ, Sherman JH, Luciano DS. *Human Physiology: The Mechanisms of Body Function.* New York: McGraw-Hill; 1990.)

(Fig. 3.9). At the motor endplate, the axon of the nerve cell innervating the muscle fiber, the alpha motoneuron, terminates. This region of the muscle cell contains specialized receptor proteins for the neuromuscular junction transmitter acetylcholine. When acetylcholine is released from the motoneuron terminal and binds to the receptors at the motor endplate, the cell membrane in the region becomes more permeable to sodium ions. So many sodium ions leak into the cell that a muscle AP is initiated each time the motoneuron to the muscle is activated. The normal neuromuscular junction is therefore often described as an *effective synapse.*

Another special feature of the sarcolemma is that at regular intervals the cell membrane is invaginated to form channel-like structures called *t-tubules*, which dive toward the center of the cell (Fig. 3.8). The lumen of each t-tubule is continuous with the extracellular fluid, and the t-tubules provide a pathway for AP propagation to the center of the muscle fiber.

Muscle as a Composite of Many Tissues

In a discussion of the structural features of muscle, it is common to focus primarily on the organization of muscle fiber groups and on the morphological features of individual muscle fibers. Although this is certainly valuable as a basis for understanding, another often overlooked perspective is that of the whole skeletal muscle as a composite of many different types of tissue. Certainly, the primary component of muscle is the muscle fiber or muscle cell. Fiber contraction gives whole muscle the ability to generate and sustain force used to either move or stabilize the skeleton. Several other types of tissue, however, are present within whole skeletal muscle that may significantly influence the muscle's ability to generate or transmit force.

One important component of whole muscle is connective tissue. The connective tissue within whole muscle is subdivided into three main segments. First, the *epimysium* is the dense layer of connective tissue that surrounds the entire muscle. Second, the *perimysium* is the layer of connective tissue that extends from the epimysium and surrounds groups of muscle fibers, called *fascicles*. Finally, the *endomysium* is the fine, lacy, delicate layer of connective tissue extending from the perimysium and composed of collagen fibers and fibroblasts that closely invest each muscle fiber. These three layers of connective tissue account for much of a muscle's resistance to passive stretch. Changes in either the character or amount of connective tissue in muscle can dramatically alter the way in which the contraction force is transferred to the skeletal system.

Another important secondary component is the vasculature of skeletal muscle. As they penetrate the epimysial connective tissue layer, large arteries rapidly branch into complex arteriolar networks in the perimysial layer. The arterioles in muscle are the main blood vessels regulating muscle circulation, and they branch to form elaborate capillary beds. In skeletal muscle, each fiber is served by at least one and usually several capillaries that lie next to the cell membrane in the endomysial layer. At the capillary–muscle cell interface, exchange of fuels and metabolic substrates and by-products occurs. The capillary networks condense to form venules, which drain into larger veins, which in turn exit muscle at the point where the arterial supply entered. The circulatory network of muscle is vital to the normal function of this tissue because muscle is one of the body's largest consumers of oxygen and energy. Without an efficiently operating vascular supply, muscle rapidly loses its ability to sustain contraction, as reflected in the weakness and low fatigue resistance often seen in individuals with circulatory disorders of muscle.

A third component of whole muscles consists of nervous tissue. Skeletal muscles contain both myelinated and unmyelinated nerve fibers. Myelinated nerve fibers innervate not only skeletal muscle fibers, but also numerous types of sensory receptors that monitor muscle activity. Sensory receptors include spindles that monitor muscle length, rate of the change of muscle length, and, under certain conditions, muscle force. Golgi tendon organs are receptors at the musculotendinous junction that monitor the active tension generated by muscle during contraction. In addition, muscle contains numerous free nerve endings that are the terminations of either myelinated or unmyelinated nerve fibers associated with the detection of muscle pain. Other nerve fibers contained within muscle include the larger myelinated axons of alpha motoneurons, which when activated cause the skeletal muscle fibers to contract, and the smaller size axons of the gamma motoneuron system, which regulate the sensitivity of muscle spindles. The remaining nervous system structures in muscle are the fibers of the autonomic nervous system that are primarily involved in the control of muscle circulation by the regulation of the vascular smooth muscle in the walls of arterioles and venules.

All the neural elements within whole muscle play important roles. The alpha motoneuron axon endings in muscle are essential to initiate muscle contraction, as detailed in the following section of this chapter. The sensory receptors in muscle and the sensory afferent fibers that transmit their information to the brain and spinal cord provide valuable information to the central nervous system regarding muscle position and the state of contraction. Such sensory feedback is essential to the regulation of muscle contraction, and hence to the control of posture and movement. Dysfunction of neural components of whole muscle may lead to a reduction in the muscle's ability to produce levels of contraction appropriate to the demands of routine activities.

PHYSIOLOGY OF MUSCLE CONTRACTION

Initiation of Contraction

The series of electrical and chemical events that describes how skeletal muscle is brought to contraction is referred to as *excitation–contraction coupling*. To activate muscle, the central nervous system first initiates action potentials in the axons of alpha motoneurons (Fig. 3.10). Once initiated, the nerve AP passes rapidly along the peripheral axons and finally sweeps over the membrane of the motor nerve terminals. As the nerve APs invade the terminals, acetylcholine, the transmitter substance at the neuromuscular junction (NMJ), is released into the fluid in the region of the motor endplates through a process called *exocytosis*. The acetylcholine moves by diffusion across the gap between the nerve and muscle membranes. When the transmitter reaches the muscle cell membrane, it is rapidly bound to specialized receptor proteins in the endplate region of the

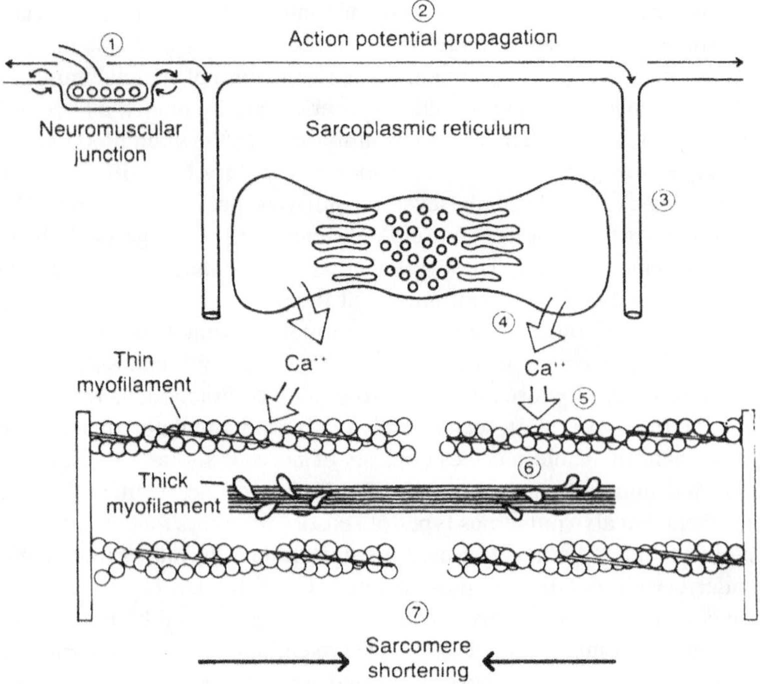

Figure 3.10. Diagrammatic representation of the sequence of events leading to muscular contraction: *1*, Neuromuscular junction activation and initiation of muscle action potential. *2*, Action potential propagation along the muscle membrane. *3*, Action potential conducting along t-tubules. *4*, Calcium release from the sarcoplasmic reticulum. *5*, Calcium binding to troponin and subsequent movement of tropomyosin. *6*, Cross-bridge formation between actin and myosin. *7*, Sarcomere shortening. (Redrawn with permission from Vander AJ, Sherman JH, Luciano DS. *Human Physiology: The Mechanisms of Body Function*. New York: McGraw-Hill; 1990.)

membrane. Immediately on the binding of acetylcholine, the membrane in the region of the receptors increases its permeability to sodium ions by opening sodium channel proteins. Because both electrical and chemical gradients for sodium ions are directed inward, sodium ions move into the muscle cell, and the transmembrane muscle potential is reduced (becomes less negative) as positive charges enter the muscle cells. This reduction in the transmembrane muscle potential can be recorded as an *endplate potential.* In normal muscle, the endplate potential produced in response to the transmitter released from the motor nerve terminal is always great enough to increase the sodium permeability of the muscle fiber membrane just outside the NMJ, thus triggering a *muscle action potential.* Sodium ions rush into the muscle, followed by potassium ions flowing out of the cell in a regenerative process that quickly sweeps over the surface of the entire muscle fiber (see previous discussion on resting membrane potential and AP for further details).

As the processes of the muscle AP pass over the membrane, they encounter the invaginations of the surface membranes called t-tubules. The AP currents invade the t-tubules and are carried along the membrane toward the interior of the cell. As the depolarization is carried along the t-tubule, it triggers the opening of voltage-sensitive calcium channels, and hence an increase in the permeability of the lateral cisternae of sarcoplasmic reticulum to calcium ions. Because the sarcoplasmic reticulum contains a high concentration of calcium ions in comparison to the muscle cell cytoplasm, calcium rapidly diffuses into the cytoplasm. Once released into the sarcoplasm, calcium diffuses away from the sarcoplasmic reticulum into the region of the thick and thin filaments.

On the surface of the thin filaments lies the regulatory protein troponin, which has a very high affinity for calcium ions. Any free calcium in the cytoplasm rapidly binds to any open

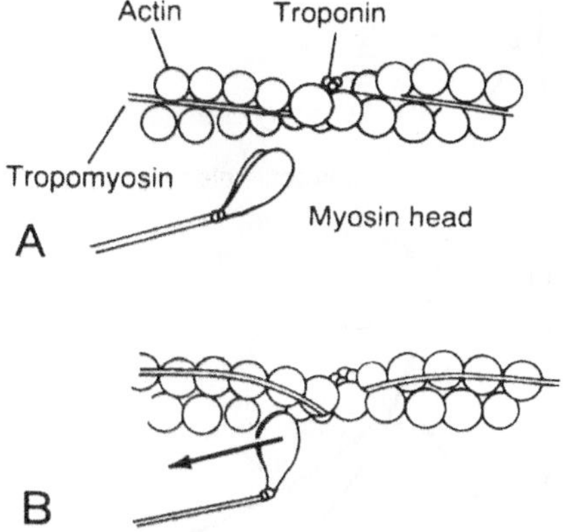

Figure 3.11. Diagrammatic representation of a segment of a thin filament and a myosin head of a thick filament when muscle is at rest **(A)** and contracting **(B).** (Redrawn with permission from Cormack DH. *Ham's Histology*. Philadelphia: J.B. Lippincott; 1987.)

calcium-binding site on the troponin molecule. When calcium binds to the troponin molecules on the thin filaments, a conformational (structural or shape) change of troponin is produced. Troponin is attached to another protein, tropomyosin, as the troponin changes shape, and so it pulls on the tropomyosin and causes an alteration in the position of tropomyosin on the thin filament (Fig. 3.11). Normally, tropomyosin is located in a position on the thin filament covering the site on each actin molecule that has a high affinity or attraction for the heads of the myosin molecules extending from the thick filaments. As troponin draws the tropomyosin away from these binding sites, actin molecules and myosin heads quickly attach. This attachment of myosin heads to the binding sites on actin (cross-bridge formation) immediately triggers a change in shape of the myosin molecules. In effect, the myosin heads swivel and, in so doing, draw the thin filaments toward the center of the sarcomeres. This interaction between actin and myosin, which occurs at literally thousands of sites, is the process that produces the force of muscle contraction.

Cessation of Contraction

The interaction of actin and myosin at any available site will continue as long as sufficient amounts of ATP are available to fuel the swiveling of myosin, and as long as the binding sites on the actin molecules remain unblocked. In response to a single surface muscle AP, a pulse of calcium is released. Some of the calcium binds to troponin, cross-bridges between actin and myosin are rapidly formed, and muscle force generation begins. Almost as soon as it is released from the lateral cisternae, calcium is actively transported back into the SR by ATP-dependent pumps that lie in the wall of the longitudinal cisternae. As the concentration of free calcium falls in the cytoplasm, other bound calcium ions dissociate from the troponin. The troponin thus returns to its original shape and the tropomyosin falls back into its rest position, where it blocks actin-binding sites for myosin. Very rapidly, the number of cross-bridges that can form is reduced, and the force of contraction falls. When all actin-binding sites are blocked by tropomyosin, no thick and thin interaction is possible, and contraction ceases.

Factors Influencing Muscle Force Production

Frequency of Activation

Figure 3.12 shows the force produced within a segment of muscle in response to activation by a single AP when the fibers are held at a constant length. The force produced reaches its maximum value

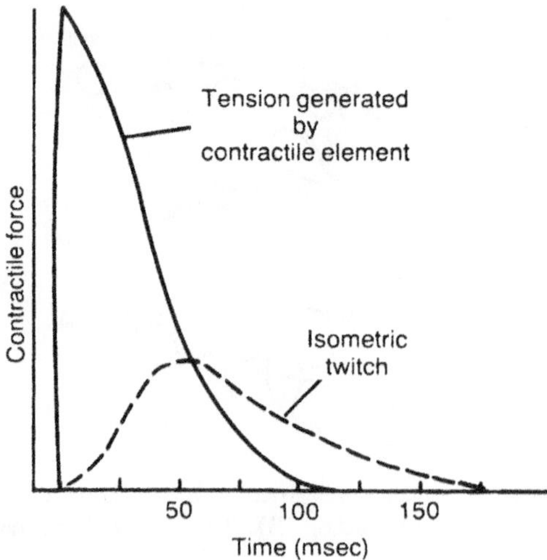

Figure 3.12. Contractile force over time in response to a single action potential. Tension generated by thick and thin filament interaction with the muscle (calculated) is transformed into the isometric twitch response (measured) by a muscle's series elastic elements. (Redrawn with permission from Vander AJ, Sherman JH, Luciano DS. *Human Physiology: The Mechanisms of Body Function.* New York: McGraw-Hill; 1990.)

almost instantaneously, and then gradually falls back to zero. The force pattern generated is a reflection of the rapid formation of many actin and myosin cross-bridges within the muscle, followed by the gradual reduction in the number of cross-bridges as calcium is gradually resequestered into the SR, and myosin-binding sites on actin are covered by the tropomyosin regulatory proteins.

Although in theory this force profile is produced within the muscle segment, the force that can be measured experimentally in response to a single activation is very different in character. Figure 3.12 also shows the isometric force measured from a segment of muscle in response to a single stimulus. In contrast to the force produced within the muscle segment, the force actually measured from the segment rises gradually to an amplitude that is less than that produced by the internal contractile apparatus. This force, measured over time in response to a single activation, is called the *isometric twitch*. For mammalian skeletal muscles, the peak in twitch tension is reached about 20 to 100 msec after the force begins to rise.

Why is the form of the isometric twitch different from that predicted for the internal contractile apparatus of muscle? The answer lies in the way in which the contractile machinery is harnessed to the skeletal system. As discussed previously, the contractile proteins of muscle that produce its force are encircled by elements such as the SR, the muscle cell membrane, and the layers of connective tissue throughout the muscle. The layers of connective tissue within the muscle segment in turn merge at each end of the muscle to form the tendons of muscle. Each of these structures (and possibly others) are elastic in nature. That is, they possess a springlike quality such that applied forces stretch them, but when the force ends, they return to their original size and shape. The force produced within a muscle segment is modified (reduced in amplitude and delayed in time) by the presence of these muscle components, which may account for the form of the measured isometric twitch.

The contractile and elastic elements of muscle can be modeled as shown in Figure 3.13. The force produced by the contractile elements (CE) (i.e., the system of thick and thin filaments) of muscle must be transmitted through the springlike tissue elements, called the *series elastic components* (SEC) of muscle, before it can be measured. When the contractile elements of muscle are activated, some of the force produced is used to stretch out the SEC, while the remainder is transferred through the skeletal system. The amount of force used to stretch out the SEC is equal

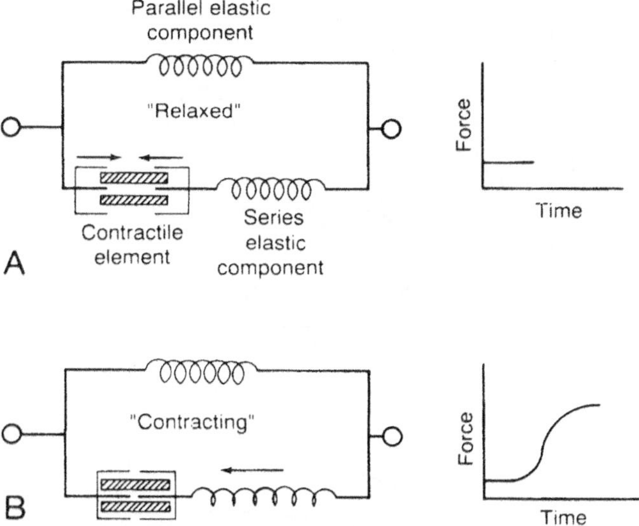

Figure 3.13. Diagrammatic single representation of a muscle's contractile and elastic elements at rest **(A)** and in response to a single action potential under isometric conditions **(B).** Note how contractile activity stretches the series elastic components but does not influence the parallel elastic component length.

to the difference in the peak of the internal force produced and the peak in the isometric twitch tension. The time difference between the contractile element peak force and the peak in measured isometric twitch is due to the fact that some time is required to stretch the SEC. A comparison of the contractile element and twitch forces reveals that twitch tension is a poor indicator of the muscle segment's true ability to generate force.

Thus far, the consequences of muscle activation by only a single, isolated stimulus have been described. During the natural activation of muscle, however, a series of muscle APs is usually produced on the muscle cell membranes. How does such a train of action potentials influence the force produced by the muscle?

In response to the first muscle AP of a train, the contractile element of muscle is activated and the force of a twitch-like contraction is produced. If a second AP is delivered before all of the calcium released by the first AP is resequestered, more calcium from the SR is released, and actin–myosin cross-bridge cycling is allowed to continue. As a result, the force measured from the activated muscle segment rises again. Since the SEC stretched in response to the first AP and it does not have time to fully relax before the second AP, less of the tension generated in response to the second activation is required to stretch out the SEC. Consequently, more tension is transmitted through the springlike harness and can be measured. Subsequent APs in the train produce even further increases in the measured force output of the activated tissue. The profile of force output that appears as oscillations in the tension record is called *unfused tetanus* (Fig. 3.14A). Unfused tetanic contractions are generally elicited in response to activation of the muscle at frequencies from approximately 3 to 20 stimuli per second depending on the particular type of muscle activated.

As the frequency of skeletal muscle activation is increased, the isometric force that can be measured from muscle also increases. In addition, the oscillations in force gradually disappear, and the contraction becomes progressively smoother. Smooth, strong contractions produced in response to the very rapid delivery (>20 to 30 per second) of APs to muscle is a state called *fused tetanus*. Maximum fused tetanic contractions are better indicators of a muscle's contractile capabilities than are twitch contractions.

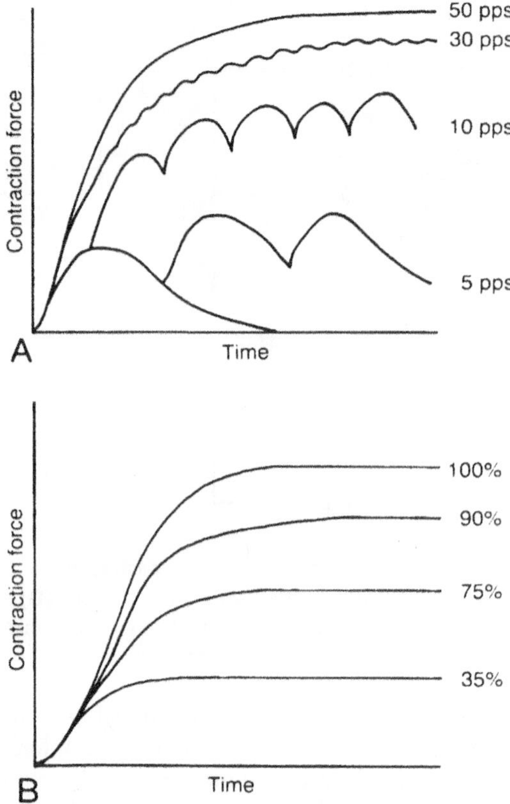

Figure 3.14. Contraction forces recorded from muscle in response to changes in the frequency of activation (rate coding) of a fixed portion of the muscle **(A)** and to changes in the percentage of muscle fibers activated (recruitment) at a tetanic frequency of activation **(B).**

Number of Fibers Activated

A second important factor associated with the regulation of muscle force is the number of muscle fibers activated in a contraction. As the percentage of total muscle fibers activated by motor nerve fibers is increased, the amount of force produced by the muscle at a fixed frequency of activation is increased (Fig. 3.14B). The increase in force as greater numbers of muscle fibers are recruited into contraction simply results from increasing the total number of actin–myosin cross-bridges formed.

Length of Skeletal Muscle

A third factor that determines the active tension that a muscle can produce is the muscle length. The length of muscle at which the maximum number of cross-bridges between thick and thin filaments can be formed is called *rest length.* For many human limb muscles in situ, muscle length can be altered by 20% of rest length (Fig. 3.15A). For example, when the elbow is fully extended, the biceps will be stretched to a length 20% greater than that in midrange. Conversely, if the elbow is fully flexed, the biceps length will be about 20% less than rest length. Muscle generates the maximum amount of tension in the ±10% range of rest length. In biceps for example, the maximum tension is generated by the muscle in the middle 50% of the elbow's range of motion. If the biceps is either lengthened or shortened such that the elbow position is in the middle 50% of its range of motion, biceps tension-generating capacity is reduced.

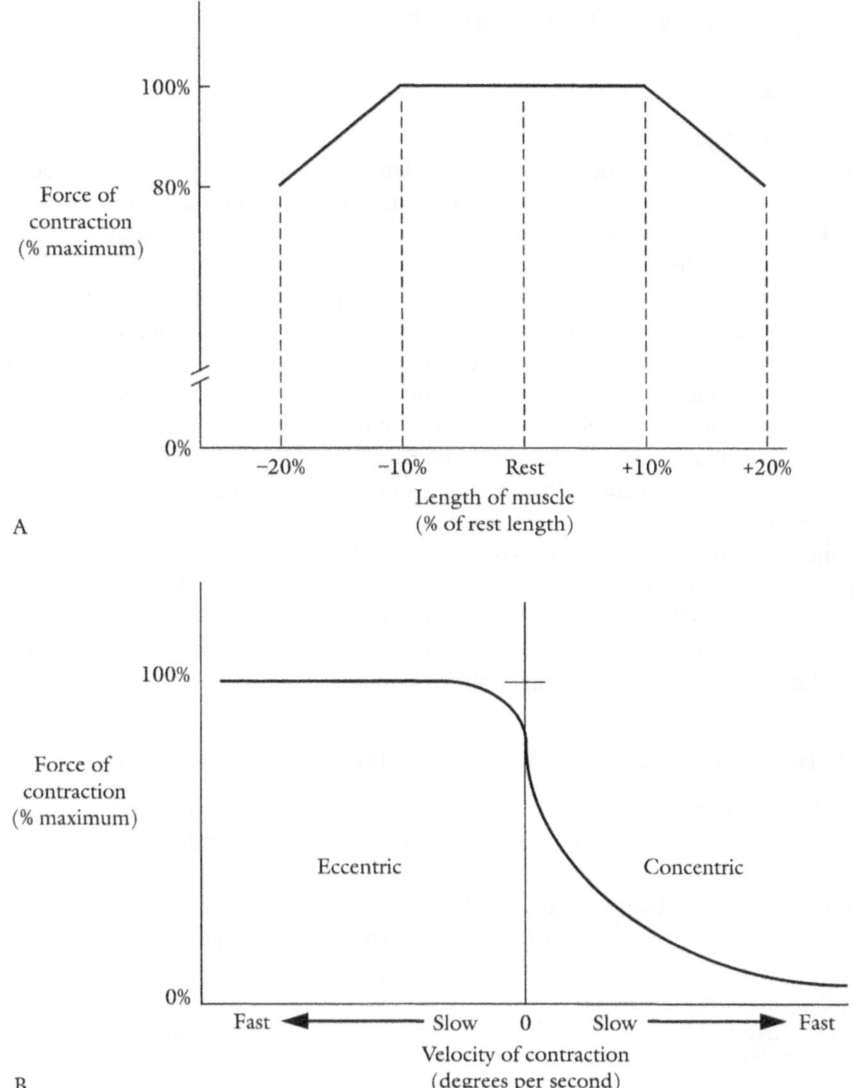

Figure 3.15. Contraction forces produced by muscle as a function of muscle length **(A)** and velocity of concentric isotonic contraction **(B).**

Velocity and Direction of Contraction

Up to this point, muscle contraction has been discussed only under isometric conditions, when the muscle is held at a constant length. If during activation the muscle is allowed to change length, the velocity of shortening becomes a determinant of the amount of force that the muscle can generate. Figure 3.15B shows the force–velocity relationship for concentric (shortening, isometric) and eccentric (lengthening) contractions for skeletal muscle. The graph reveals that the higher forces are produced by muscle under isometric conditions when the velocity of shortening is zero, and progressively declines as the speed of shortening is increased. The graph also illustrates that the highest force levels that a muscle can produce occur in eccentric contractions.

NONHOMOGENEOUS NATURE OF SKELETAL MUSCLE

Skeletal Muscle Fiber Characteristics

In the previous description of the structural and contractile characteristics, skeletal muscle was treated as if all muscles where identical. In fact, it has been known for several hundred years that several different types of skeletal muscle exist and that the differentiation of skeletal muscle appears to be related to how the muscles are used in normal activity. A classical comparison is made between the muscles of the birds of flight and those of domestic fowl.

The breast musculature of chickens is pale in comparison to the dark leg muscles. These barnyard animals rarely use the breast muscles, which move their wings, but use the leg muscles the majority of their waking hours while foraging. In contrast, the breast musculature of migratory birds is dark, while leg muscles are paler in appearance. Such observational findings led early scientists to suspect that there were two types of muscle fibers, light and dark, that made up skeletal muscles. With the advent of microscopic and histochemical techniques in the early and middle part of the twentieth century, we learned that most mammalian skeletal muscles are composed of not two but of three types of muscle fibers.

Over the years, two major classification schemes have been developed to describe the different types of fibers within mammalian striated muscles (Table 3.2). The percentages of these fibers that make up muscle varies from muscle to muscle and from species to species for analogous muscles. In humans, the muscles of the extremities are frequently composed of approximately half fast-twitch muscle fibers and half slow-twitch fibers.

Basic Functional Element of the Neuromuscular System: The Motor Unit

From a structural perspective, skeletal muscle is composed of single muscle fibers of three different types. From a functional perspective, however, muscle contraction does not occur by the isolated activation of single muscle fibers. During normal activities, the force of muscle contraction is produced by the activation of muscle fiber groups acting in concert in response to a stimulus provided by the single nerve cell innervating each fiber in the group. A motoneuron, along

Table 3.2. Classification Schemes and Characteristics of Skeletal Muscle Fibers

	Muscle Fiber Type		
Characteristic	*IIB* *FG*[a]	*IIA* *FOG*[b]	*I* *SO*[c]
Contraction speed	Fast	Fast	Slow
Myofibrillar ATPase	High	High	Low
Fiber diameter	Large	Medium	Small
Capillary supply	Sparse	Rich	Rich
Oxidative enzyme activity	Low	Med-High	High
Mitochondrial content	Low	High	High
Glycolytic enzyme activity	High	High	Low
Glycogen content	High	High	Low
Myoglobin content	Low	High	High

[a]FG = fast twitch, glycolytic
[b]FOG = fast twitch, oxidative, glycolytic
[c]SO = slow twitch, oxidative

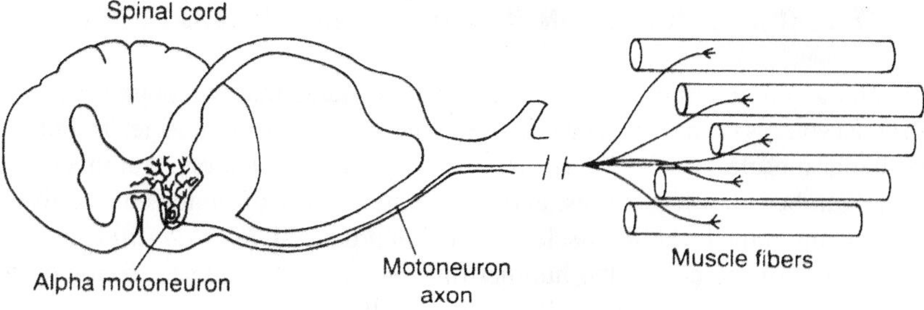

Figure 3.16. Basic functional element of the neuromuscular system, the motor unit.

with the group of muscle fibers it innervates, is called a *motor unit* (Fig. 3.16). The cell body of the multipolar neuron of the motor unit is located in the ventral horn of the spinal cord or in cranial nerve motor nuclei. For motoneurons arising from the spinal cord, large-diameter, myelinated axons project from the cell body, pass through the ventral root of the spinal cord, and subsequently run along peripheral nerves until they reach the target muscle fibers. As motor axons enter muscle, they divide many times into fine branches, which in turn innervate single muscle fibers. The muscle fibers of a single motor unit are usually distributed over a rather large portion of the cross-sectional area of the muscle, and all the fibers of a motor unit are of the same histochemical type. The number of muscle fibers in motor units ranges from about 200 to 300 in hand muscles to more than 1,000 fibers per motor unit in the large muscles of the lower extremities.

Over the past several decades, the properties of single motor units in skeletal muscle have been extensively examined. Nearly all motor units in the muscles studied thus far can be classified into one of three major types. Table 3.3 shows some of the common characteristics of the three major classes of motor units. The presence of varying proportions of motor units of different type provides muscle with the ability to respond appropriately to postural and locomotive demands. Muscles that are required to produce moderate to low levels of tension over long periods of time contain a higher percentage of fatigue-resistant muscle fibers. Muscles required to produce quick, high force levels for brief intervals contain a higher percentage of strong, fast-twitch fatigable units.

Table 3.3. Classification and Characteristics of Motor Units in Skeletal Muscles

Motor Unit Type	FF[a]	FR[b]	S[c]
Muscle Fiber Type	IIb	IIA	I
	FG	FOG	SO
Characteristic			
Contraction speed	Fast	Fast	Slow
Twitch contraction time	Short	Short	Long
Resistance to fatigue	Low	High	V High
Tetanic tension	High	Intermed	Low
Number fibers/unit	Large	Intermed	Small
Frequency of use	Low	Intermed	High
Recruitment order	Last	Intermed	First
Size of unit cell body	Large	Intermed	Small

[a]FF = fast twitch, fatigable
[b]FR = fast twitch, fatigue-resistant
[c]S = slow twitch, very fatigue-resistant

CONTROL OF FORCE GENERATION IN VOLITIONAL CONTRACTION

Studies of voluntary contraction in humans have demonstrated that two main processes are used by the central nervous system to regulate the force output of skeletal muscle. To initiate contraction in a particular muscle, the CNS must first excite alpha motoneurons that innervate the muscle fibers. The number of motoneurons, and hence the number of motor units activated, is one primary determinant of the level of muscle contraction produced. *Recruitment* is the term used to describe the process of increasing the number of motor units brought to excitation to produce increasing levels of muscle contraction. Precisely which motor units are recruited is determined by both descending CNS and peripheral reflex inputs to the alpha motoneurons. If excitatory inputs to the motoneurons sufficiently overwhelm inhibitory inputs to these cells, APs will be produced in the neuron's axon that will evoke contraction.

One question that faced neuroscientists for years was, How does the CNS know which motoneurons to activate in order to produce a particular level of contraction? Available evidence now indicates that motoneurons are recruited in most contractions in an orderly sequence. The CNS command to begin muscle contraction first activates the smallest (highest internal resistance) alpha motoneurons. If more force is required to properly perform an activity, the command signals from the CNS are increased, and progressively larger (lower internal resistance) motoneurons are activated. The recruitment order of motor units into both reflex and voluntary contractions depends on the size of the motoneuron cell body. The small motoneurons require less synaptic current to excite them sufficiently to produce APs. As the size of motoneurons increases, greater amounts of synaptic current are required to excite these cells. The size-dependent recruitment of motor units into contractions is now commonly referred to as the *size principle*. Because the size of the alpha motoneuron is related to the type of muscle fibers innervated by the neuron (Table 3.3), recruitment of motor units in voluntary contractions will generally follow from type S (slow-twitch, fatigue-resistant) motor units to type FR (fast-twitch, fatigue-resistant) units, and finally to type FF (fast-twitch, fatigable) units as the level of contraction increases. Those motor units designed to generate tension for relatively long periods without substantial fatigue (types S and FR) are therefore used most in volitional contractions. Type FF units, which are capable of producing high tension levels for very short periods, are used only occasionally, in high-force-level contractions.

The second way in which the nervous system regulates muscle tension generation is by controlling the rate of motor unit discharge during recruitment. This control process is commonly referred to as *rate coding*. If higher levels of tension are required as a contraction is proceeding, the CNS may simply increase the discharge rate of the motor units already active in the contraction.

As described previously, increasing the firing rate of motor units increases their force output by summation of contraction. Discharge rates of motor units in human voluntary contractions begin at about 8 to 10 per second, and rarely exceed 30 per second. During voluntary muscle contraction, motor units are recruited in an asynchronous manner (Fig. 3.17). That is, motor units are not all activated at the same time. This asynchronous activation has the effect of smoothing the tension output of the whole muscle, even when the individual firing frequencies of motor units may be well below the level at which fused tetanus would occur for the individual units. Discharge frequencies of motor units recruited in voluntary contraction are also not all the same. Some units may be discharging at low steady frequencies, while others may discharge irregularly at higher or lower frequencies.

The relative importance of recruitment and rate coding in the regulation of muscle tension has not been clearly established. Some evidence suggests that in the muscles of the hand, which often produce delicate, controlled movements, rate coding may be the predominant mechanism by which force is regulated. In contrast, in the large muscles of the lower extremity, recruitment may be the dominant mechanism regulating the level of contraction.

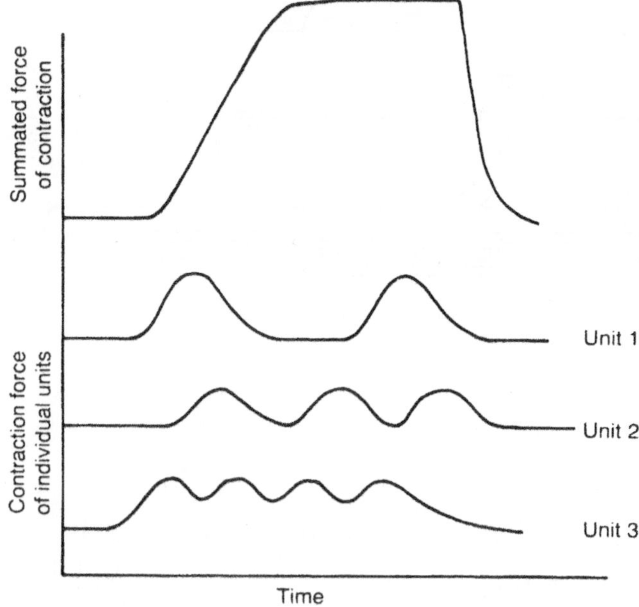

Figure 3.17. Asynchronous activation of motor units results in smooth, summated contraction of whole muscle.

CLINICAL ELECTRICAL STIMULATION OF NERVE AND MUSCLE

In the intact peripheral neuromuscular system, the application of electrical stimulation can induce APs in nerve and muscle that are indistinguishable from those evoked by the normal action of the nervous system. Furthermore, APs evoked by electrical stimulation in peripheral alpha motoneuron axons elicit contraction of skeletal muscle that appears to the uninformed person to be identical to voluntary contraction. In fact, muscle contraction in response to electrical stimulation is very different from that produced by normal physiological mechanisms. One of the objectives of the remaining sections of this chapter is to identify the similarities and differences between the nature of contraction in response to electrical stimulation and normal physiologic activation.

Electrical stimulation may also activate peripheral sensory nerve fibers and the nerve fibers of the autonomic nervous system. The electrical stimulation of sensory fibers gives rise to the characteristic tingling sensation associated with such stimulation and has been found useful in the management of a variety of pain syndromes, but it does not produce patterns of sensory APs like those generated under physiological activation.

Activation of Excitable Tissues with Electrical Stimulation

How does the induction of current in biological tissues bring about the activation of nerve or muscle? Figure 3.18 shows two electrodes of a stimulator circuit applied to the skin directly over a small branch of a peripheral nerve. As stimulation is initiated, one electrode briefly contains an excess of negative charge, and the other electrode is deficient in negative charge. Ions in the region will migrate toward or away from these electrodes according to their charge. The pattern of current induced by the movement of these ions is represented by the lines connecting the electrodes. Some of the ionic movement occurs in the extracellular fluid, and some of the current

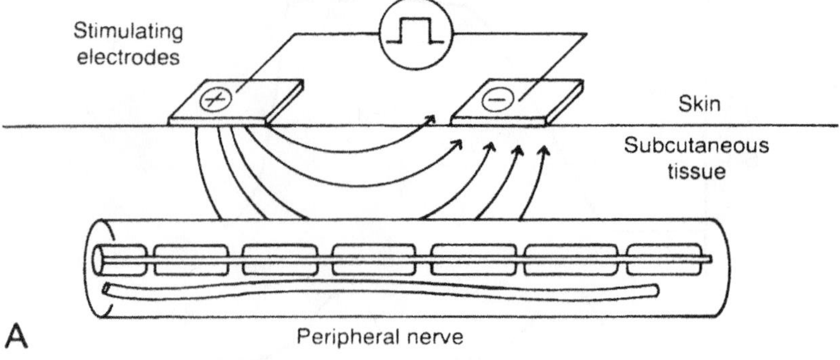

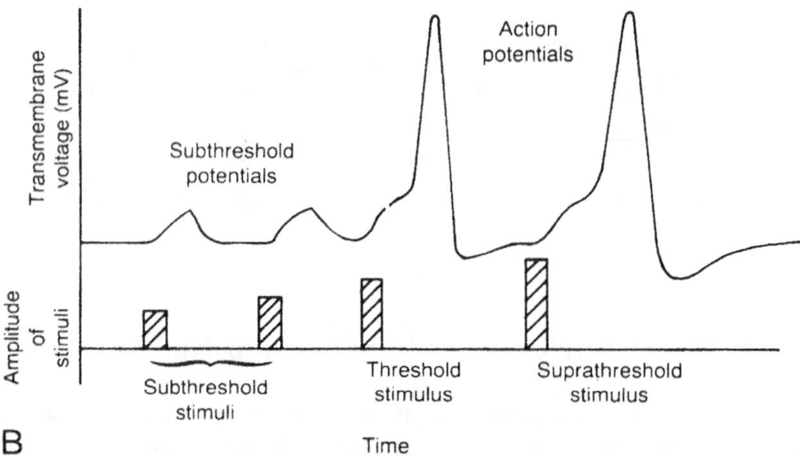

Figure 3.18. A: Surface electrodes placed near a peripheral nerve. **B:** Transmembrane voltage changes in response to stimuli of gradually increasing amplitude.

passes through the nerve membrane. The net effect of this current is a slight depolarization of the nerve membrane. If the brief current induced across the membrane is very small, the change in transmembrane potential will rapidly return to resting membrane potential. If the current induced across the membrane is large enough, voltage-gated sodium and potassium channels will open, and an AP will be evoked and propagated along the membrane. This evoked AP is identical to that produced along the fiber membrane in response to physiological activation.

Action potentials evoked in peripheral nerve are transmitted along the nerve fiber in both directions from the point of initiation. There is conduction in the direction of "normal" propagation (orthodromic) as well as AP propagation in the opposite direction (antidromic). Antidromic conduction is toward the periphery in sensory nerve fibers and toward the CNS in motor nerve and autonomic fibers.

Stimulus Characteristics for Activation of Excitable Tissues

The current induced in biologic tissues must be of sufficient amplitude (strength) and duration to bring excitable cells to a critical transmembrane voltage above the resting membrane potential, called the *threshold*, in order to evoke an AP. For a particular single excitable cell, there is a family of stimulus strength–duration (S-D) combinations that can bring the cell to the level of

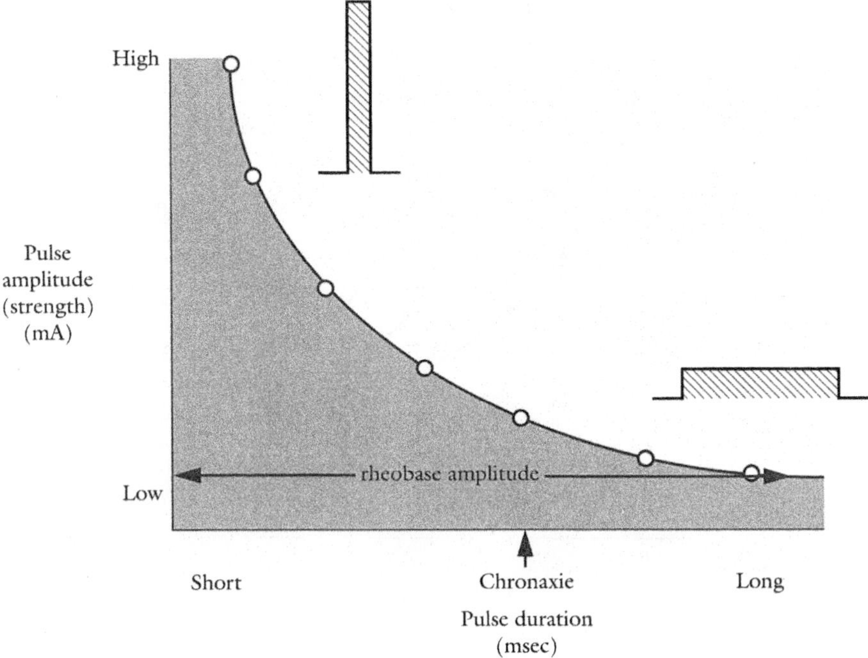

Figure 3.19. Strength–duration curve for a particular excitable tissue showing that an infinite number of amplitude and duration combinations are sufficient to the excite.

depolarization required to trigger the opening of voltage-gated sodium and potassium channel proteins. Plotting the S-D combinations that are sufficient to activate an excitable cell and connecting the points yields a *strength–duration curve* for the threshold of that type of cell (Fig. 3.19). Any stimulus S-D combination that falls below or to the left of this line will not initiate an AP and is described as *subthreshold.* Those stimuli with S-D characteristics above or to the right of the curve are called *suprathreshold* and are always adequate to activate the fiber.

For a particular type of excitable tissue, the minimum amplitude of a stimulus that will activate the tissue at very long stimulus durations is called the *rheobase.* The minimum *duration* of a stimulus at twice the rheobase that is just sufficient to activate the excitable tissue is called the *chronaxie.* In the past, electrical stimulators were used clinically to determine the rheobase and chronaxie values for the peripheral neuromuscular system. The reliability of such techniques is poor. Today, sophisticated electrophysiological evaluation procedures such as nerve conduction velocity studies and electromyography are commonly used to assess peripheral nerve and muscle integrity.

Peripheral nerve fibers are inherently more excitable to electrical stimulation than muscle fibers. Consequently, stimuli with S-D characteristics sufficient to activate peripheral nerve fibers will not be strong enough to activate isolated muscle fibers. Stimuli must have much larger amplitudes and longer durations to initiate APs in denervated muscle fibers. Figure 3.20 shows the S-D curves for three type-A peripheral nerve fibers and isolated (denervated) muscle fibers.

Because nerve fibers contained within a peripheral nerve are not identical in diameter or internal resistance, the relative excitability of these fibers to electrical stimulation varies. When a mixed peripheral nerve is directly stimulated, those fibers with the largest diameter and lowest internal resistance are the most easily excited. When electrical currents are produced in peripheral nerve, the A_α group of nerve fibers are those most likely to be activated based upon their inherent excitability alone. To activate group $A\beta$, $A\delta$, or group C fibers requires stimuli of

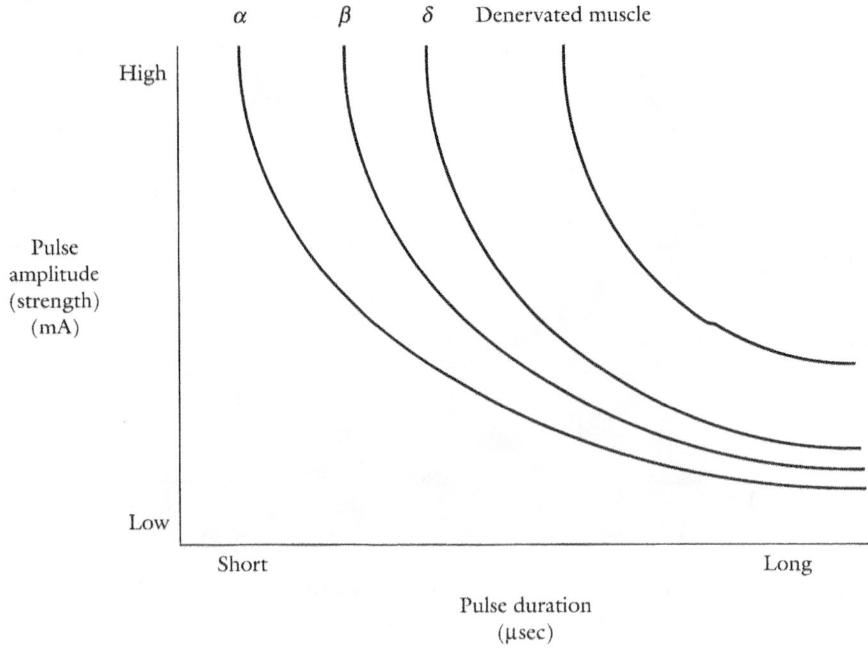

Figure 3.20. Strength–duration curves for three size classes of peripheral nerve fibers (α, β, and δ) and denervated muscle fibers.

progressively larger amplitude and/or duration. The process by which increasing numbers of nerve fibers are activated by progressively increasing the amplitude and/or duration of the stimulus is called *fiber recruitment.* For isolated motor nerve stimulation, the pattern of recruitment tends to be in an order from largest diameter (lowest internal resistance) fiber to smallest diameter fiber (highest internal resistance) in peripheral nerves, which is a pattern opposite to that occurring during volitional activation. In most clinical applications of electrical stimulation to evoke muscle contraction, surface electrodes are used. In such cases, the tendency to recruit larger diameter axons before smaller diameter axons is weak. In fact, a compelling argument has been made that in clinical neuromuscular stimulation, the recruitment pattern of peripheral axons, and hence motor units, is nonselective (4). That is, clinical neuromuscular electrical stimulation recruits both smaller and larger diameter alpha motoneuron axons, and hence recruits both the smaller, slower contracting and larger, faster contracting motor units simultaneously, regardless of the relative magnitude of stimulation.

The effects of inducing currents on nerve and muscle fibers depend not only on the inherent excitability of these tissues, but also on their location with respect to the electrodes used to transfer the current. In general, the closer the excitable tissue is to the electrodes, the more likely it is to be activated by the current. At a fixed intensity of stimulation, small-diameter axons very close to the stimulating electrodes may be activated before large-diameter fibers located farther away (Fig. 3.21). As a result, A_β touch-pressure sensory nerve fibers near the skin are commonly recruited before the more inherently excitable A_α motor and sensory fibers. Because the distance between the electrode(s) and target tissue influences the precise nature of the activation, it is important to position the electrodes as close as possible to the target tissue to achieve optimal activation.

Because both the inherent excitability of nerve fibers and the location influence the order of nerve activation, when ES is applied over a mixed peripheral nerve containing motor, touch-pressure sensory, and pain sensory fibers, ES will normally evoke a pins-and-needles sensory

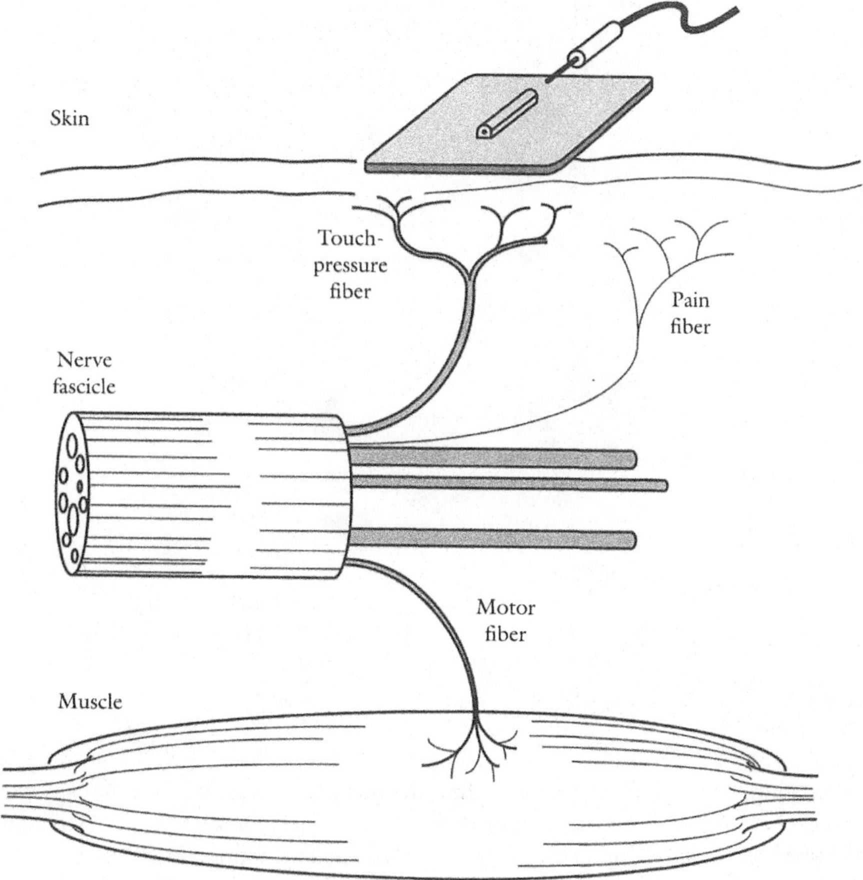

Figure 3.21. Diagrammatic representation of the location of excitable tissue with respect to surface electrodes. Note that sensory fibers are closer than motor fibers.

response before either motor or painful responses (Fig. 3.22). If the amplitude or duration of stimuli is increased sufficiently, motor responses (muscle contractions) will be produced and superimposed on the sensory stimulation. If stimuli amplitudes or durations are increased even more, ES may evoke a painful response, which occurs simultaneously with the sensory and motor responses. In most clinical electrotherapy applications, the pins-and-needles sensation produced by the stimulation of cutaneous touch-pressure afferents will precede motor or painful responses. If stimulation is applied in a region where no alpha motoneuron axons or skeletal muscle fibers exist (e.g., over bony prominences), an increase in stimulation amplitude will likely produce a painful response in the absence of muscle contraction.

Another important consideration in applying ES to activate muscle and nerve is the polarity of the electrodes. This is especially important in the use of monophasic pulsatile currents or asymmetrical biphasic currents. With monophasic waveforms of fixed amplitude and duration, for example, the negatively charged electrode (cathode) is usually slightly more effective in activating excitable tissue than the positively charged electrode (anode).

In the past, when the initiation and cessation of a single pulse were not electronically controlled, pulse durations were relatively long. The application of fixed-amplitude current to motor nerves in this fashion revealed that contractions could occur in response to both closing the stimulating circuit and opening it. In addition, contractions could be elicited by either cathodal or

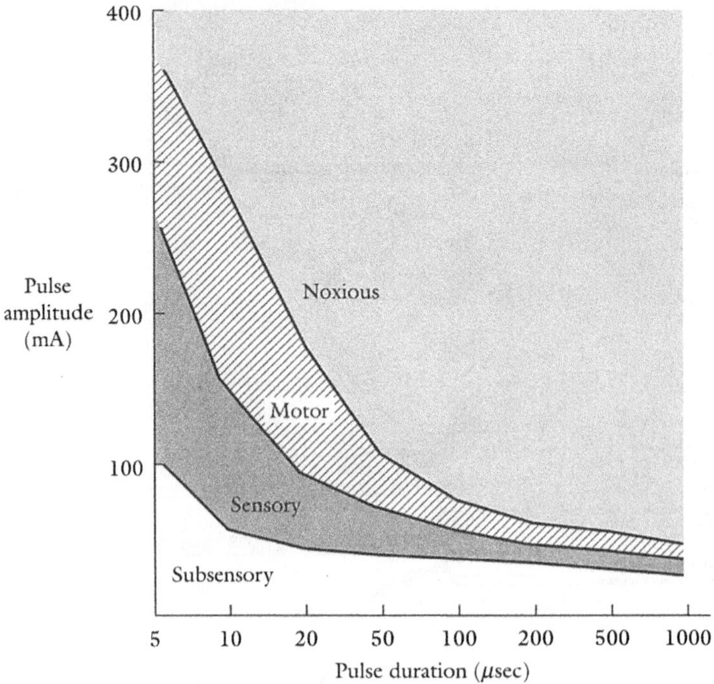

Figure 3.22. Stimulus S-D relationships for the three common clinical levels of electrical stimulation.

anodal stimulation. Overall, the response to the cathode upon closing the circuit (cathode-closing current, CCC) was the most effective approach to neuromuscular stimulation. The contraction response evoked by the anode upon closing the circuit (anode-closing current, ACC) was the next strongest, followed by the contraction beneath the anode upon opening the circuit (anode-opening current, AOC) and the cathode upon opening the circuit (cathode-opening current, COC), respectively. The relationship between anodal and cathodal opening and closing currents has been called *Erb's polar formula*. With the very short-duration pulses used today in electronically controlled stimulation; contractions are not elicited by opening currents during neuromuscular stimulation.

Clinical Responses to Nerve and Muscle Stimulation

Sensory-level Stimulation

When electrodes are placed on the surface of the skin and the amplitude of electrical stimulation is gradually increased, three general forms of response are consistently noted in normal individuals. At relatively low amplitudes, the first response reported by patients is sensory. Commonly, patients identify a pins-and-needles (tingling) sensation if the frequency is greater than a few pulses per second, or a "tapping" sensation if the frequency is set at 1 to 5 pps. This *sensory-level stimulation* is not uncomfortable to most patients and results from the excitation of those sensory nerve fibers that lie in or near the skin in the vicinity of the electrodes where the current density is greatest. As the stimulation amplitude is gradually increased, the sensation becomes stronger and often spreads to the region between the electrodes and deeper into tissues. As can be observed from Figure 3.22, sensory-level stimulation can be achieved by the use of many different amplitude and duration combinations. Whether sensory fibers are activated is independent of the stimulation frequency selected.

If sensory-level stimulation at frequencies greater than about 15 pps is maintained for prolonged periods of time, the subject will generally note a gradual diminution in the ability to sense the stimulation, a phenomenon called *adaptation*. Adaptation may be reduced by intermittently interrupting the stimulation or by varying either its amplitude or frequency.

Motor-level Stimulation

As the intensity of stimulation is gradually increased, the tingling sensation felt by patients increases as progressively greater numbers of sensory nerve fibers are recruited. In addition, the activation threshold of alpha motoneuron axons lying in peripheral nerves innervating skeletal muscle is soon reached. The excitation of alpha motoneuron axons in the intact nervous system that produces muscular contraction is called *motor-level stimulation*. At low levels of motor level stimulation, contraction may only be detected by palpation of innervated muscles. As the amplitude (or pulse duration) is increased, the contraction soon becomes strong enough to produce visible joint movement.

The form and strength of muscular contraction produced by ES are determined by the same two processes, recruitment and rate coding, involved in voluntary contraction. There is progressive activation of greater numbers of alpha motoneuron axons as the amplitude of stimulation is increased (i.e., recruitment). Motoneuron recruitment increases the number of muscle fibers activated (Fig. 3.23), and hence increases the force output of the stimulated muscle.

In voluntary contraction, motor units are recruited from smallest to largest as the requirements for force are increased. In stimulated contraction, recruitment was thought to occur from largest to smallest as the stimulation strength is gradually increased (5). Stimulated contractions were thought to occur by an activation of type FF motor units first, followed by type FR units, and ending with type S units. As indicated previously, this reversed order of motor unit recruitment in electrically induced contractions does not appear to be supported by recent research (4). Rather, it appears as though surface electrical stimulation recruits a combination of FF, FR, and S motor units simultaneously.

Recruitment in stimulated contractions is controlled by varying either the magnitude or the duration of each stimulus or some combination of the two stimulation parameters. Increasing either amplitude or pulse duration increases the phase or pulse charge of each stimulus, increasing the activation "punch" in each waveform.

Figure 3.23C shows the relationship between the amplitude of fixed-duration stimuli delivered at a tetanic frequency and the resultant contraction force of activated muscle. The graph shows that after the motor threshold is exceeded, very small increases in stimulation amplitude produce relatively large increases in the force of muscular contraction, and recruitment increases rapidly. During the use of ES to activate muscle, clinicians must exercise caution in the adjustment of stimulation amplitude to avoid undesirable marked increases in the level of muscle contraction.

On initial exposure to ES for muscle activation, clients frequently exhibit a low tolerance to the stimulation. As a consequence, evoked muscle contraction may not be sufficient to produce either physiologic changes or appropriate joint movements. Repeated exposure to ES is generally accompanied by an increase in client tolerance and associated increases in the force of evoked contraction. Increases in stimulation amplitude may be possible not only from session to session, but also between individual contractions within the same treatment session.

The second primary mechanism regulating the force of contraction in voluntary contraction, rate coding, is also a primary mechanism in regulating stimulated contractions. If the stimulation frequency is low, in a range of 1 to 5 pps, elicited contractions will be twitch-like in character. If the frequency of stimulation is gradually increased, partially fused contractions are formed, followed by fused tetanic contractions as the stimulation frequency rises above a range of 25 to

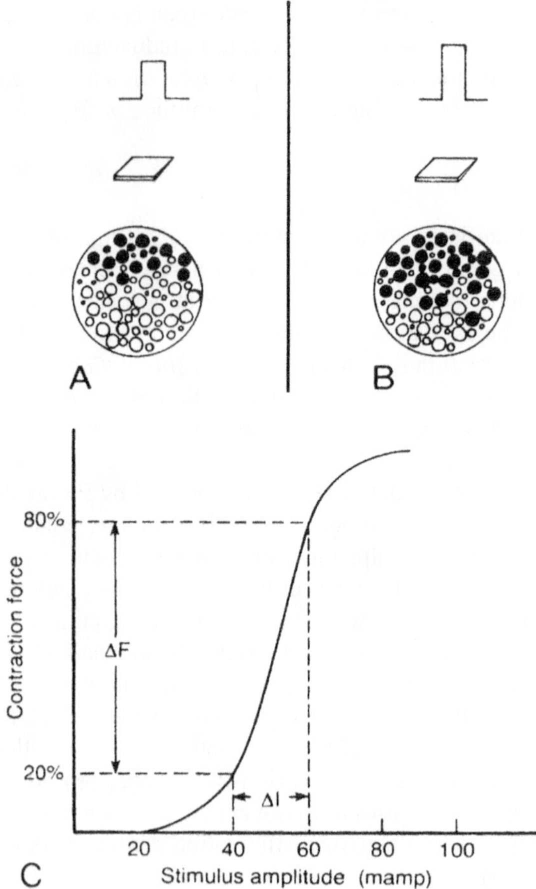

Figure 3.23. A and **B:** Pattern of peripheral axon recruitment in response to stimuli of increasing amplitude. **C:** Relationship between amplitude of stimulation and force of muscular contraction. (Redrawn with permission from Benton LA, et al. *Functional electric stimulation: a practical clinical guide*. Downey, CA: The Professional Staff Association of the Rancho Los Amigos Hospital; 1981.)

30 pps. As in voluntary contraction, as the frequency of motor unit activation rises, the force output of muscle rises.

Another key difference between voluntary and electrically-induced contractions is the synchronous activation of all motor units in stimulated contractions. The initiation of thick and thin filament interaction occurs in all recruited fibers at about the same time.

The previous discussion reveals that electrically elicited contractions are not truly physiological contractions. In spite of this fact, electrical stimulation can be used clinically to produce physiological changes within muscle for strengthening and functional movement, which may allow individuals to function better in their daily activities. Both isometric and isotonic contractions can be produced by the electrical stimulation of muscle. Isometric contractions can be produced by physically blocking the movement about a joint, or by simultaneously stimulating both the agonists and antagonists acting on a joint. Isotonic movements can be evoked by ES when the joint on which the stimulated muscle acts is not stabilized. A common application of an isotonic movement produced by stimulation is ankle dorsiflexion during ambulation to assist in the swing phase of gait. Such stimulation is frequently triggered by a special switching device placed beneath the sole of the foot. In eliciting isotonic contractions, the user must realize that very strong isotonic contractions to the fully shortened position of a muscle may produce severe cramping in the core of the stimulated muscle, and hence such contractions should be avoided in most therapeutic applications.

The application of an uninterrupted train of pulses at an amplitude high enough to elicit muscle contraction will very rapidly induce muscle fatigue. To combat this potential problem in clinical applications, stimulator trains are commonly interrupted at prescribed intervals. When the stimulation is adjusted to a 1:1 on-time to off-time ratio (e.g., 10 seconds on, 10 seconds off), muscle tends to fatigue rapidly. In contrast, 1:5 ratios (e.g., 10 seconds on, 50 seconds off) tend to significantly reduce the onset of muscle fatigue.

Noxious-level Stimulation

The final level of clinical ES is that which is painful to the patient and is referred to as *noxious-level stimulation.* In this situation, the intensity of stimulation is so high that many A_{δ} and C nerve fibers, which normally carry signals associated with painful stimuli, are activated. Action potentials produced in first-order nociceptive afferents in turn activate the spinothalamic pathways leading to the somatosensory cortex and result in the perception of pain. Because the level of stimulation required to activate the small-diameter pain afferents is generally very high, strong muscular contractions often accompany this form of stimulation if motor axons are located close enough to the stimulation electrodes. If noxious stimulation is carried out in a region where no motor axons or muscle fibers are present (e.g., over a bony prominence), a painful response may be elicited without the production of any muscular contraction.

The precise stimulation parameters that evoke a painful response will vary from individual to individual. Other factors such as electrode placement, stimulation waveform, and type or location of sensory fibers in the region of stimulation will also influence the level of stimulation that evokes a noxious response.

SUMMARY

This chapter has reviewed the essential features of nerve and muscle morphology and physiology to provide a foundation for understanding the clinical application of therapeutic electrical stimulation. In addition, volitional and stimulation-induced muscle contraction properties have been compared and contrasted.

Specific techniques commonly used in clinical settings for the management of selected disorders are presented in subsequent chapters. More detailed information on the structure and function of nerve and muscle can be found in comprehensive references and reviews. Astute users of electrotherapy must remain sensitive to the fact that results of ongoing research and clinical studies must be integrated into their knowledge. Such new information may prompt significant changes in the application of electrical stimulation to obtain optimal therapeutic benefit.

SELF-STUDY QUESTIONS

For answers, see Appendix B.

1. (a) What are the two main ions associated with the establishment of the resting membrane potential? (b) What is their relative distribution across the membrane of excitable cells?
2. What is the sodium-potassium pump? What is the function of this pump?

3. The two factors that determine how ions move across the membrane of electrically excitable cell are ________(a)________ and ________(b)________.

4. What components of excitable cell membranes are responsible for the change in membrane permeability when nervous tissue is excited to produce an action potential?

5. Draw a graph of the voltage changes occurring at one point in an excitable membrane when an action potential is produced. Be sure to accurately label axes.

6. What are the three functional types of axons in a mixed peripheral nerve? What functions do these three types of axons control?

7. What is the difference between orthodromic and antidromic action potential propagation in peripheral nerve axons?

8. The speed of propagation of action potentials in peripheral axons is determined by ________(a)________ and ________(b)________.

9. Cell bodies of the motoneurons to limb muscles lie in the ________(a)________, whereas cell bodies of peripheral sensory neurons to the limbs lie in the ________(b)________.

10. What are the connective tissue layers in peripheral nerve? Name one major function of each layer.

11. The primary component of striated skeletal muscle is the ________(a)________. Bundles of contractile proteins are called ________(b)________. The myofilaments are composed of the contractile proteins, ________(c)________ and ________(d)________, along with the two regulatory proteins, ________(e)________ and ________(f)________.

12. What is the function of the mitochondria in nerve and muscle fibers?

13. What is the function of the sarcoplasmic reticulum?

14. What is the purpose of the t-tubule system in skeletal muscle?

15. Define the motor unit. Describe the differences between the three different types of motor units.

16. What is the importance of the strength-duration curve?

17. Describe the excitation-contraction coupling process in a stepwise manner.

18. The two primary factors regulating the force of skeletal muscle contraction in either voluntary or stimulated contractions are ________(a)________ and ________(b)________.

19. The two parameters of electrical stimulation that control recruitment of peripheral axons during therapeutic electrical stimulation are the ________(a)________ and the ________(b)________.

20. The parameter of electrical stimulation that controls "rate coding" is the ________________.

21. Define:

    a. Sensory-level stimulation

    b. Motor-level stimulation

    c. Noxious-level stimulation

22. The class of peripheral axons activated during sensory-level stimulation is called ________________.

23. The sensation produced using sensory level stimulation at very low frequencies (1 to 5 pps) is ________(a)________. The sensation produced during sensory level stimulation at high frequencies (20 to 50 pps) is ________(b)________.

24. The type of muscle contraction produced using motor-level stimulation at low frequencies (1 to 5 pps) is called ________(a)________. The type of contraction produced using motor-level stimulation at high frequencies (20 to 50 pps) is called ________(b)________.

25. Two anatomical factors that determine the order of activation of peripheral nerve fibers in response to electrical stimulation are ________(a)________and ________(b)________.

REFERENCES

1. Erlanger J, Gasser HS. *Electrical Signs of Nervous Activity.* Philadelphia: University of Pennsylvania Press, 1938.
2. Gasser HS, Grundfest H. Average diameters in relation to spike dimensions and conduction velocity in mammalian fibers. *Am J Physiol.* 1939;127:393.
3. Lloyd DPC, Chang HT. Afferent fibers in muscle nerves. *J Neurophysiol.* 1948;11:199–207.
4. Gregory CM, Bickel CS. Recruitment patterns in human skeletal muscle during electrical stimulation. *Phys Ther.* 2005;85(4):358–364.
5. Trimble MH, Enoka RM. Mechanisms underlying the training effects associated with neuromuscular electrical stimulation. *Phys Ther.* 1991;71(4):273–282.

SUGGESTED READING

Cormack DH. *Ham's Histology.* 9th ed. Philadelphia: J.B. Lippincott, 1987.

Nicholls JG, Martin AR, Wallace BG. *From Neuron to Brain.* Sunderland, MA: Sinauer Associates, Inc.; 1992.

Mountcastle VB, ed. *Medical Physiology.* Vol. 1. 14th ed. St. Louis, MO: CV Mosby; 1980.

Vander AJ, Sherman JH, Luciano DS. *Human Physiology: The Mechanisms of Body Function.* 6th ed. New York: McGraw-Hill; 1994.

CHAPTER 4

The Neurobiology of Pain and Foundations for Electrical Stimulation for Pain Control

Kathleen A. Sluka

This chapter reviews the neurobiology of pain and the anatomical and physiological evidence that provides a theoretical foundation for understanding electrical stimulation for pain control. Included is a description of the multidimensional nature of pain and a summary of terminology used to describe pain in the clinical setting. An overview of the fundamental neuroanatomical pain pathway is provided, with a discussion of both the utility and limitations of such simplified concepts in pain transmission. The chapter then provides a more in-depth perspective on the anatomical components and physiological functions of pain pathways that serves as the foundation for understanding the multidimensional nature of pain, the array of responses to pain, and many common clinical pain phenomena. Evidence is presented regarding the existence of endogenous pain-inhibition mechanisms. Finally, common electrical stimulation for pain control interventions are examined in the context of their ability to activate endogenous pain-inhibition mechanisms. An important objective is to present evidence that pain transmission and hence pain perception are modulated by selected electrotherapeutic interventions. For more in-depth information on the neurobiology of pain and pain management, the reader is referred to the following texts: *Sensory Mechanisms of the Spinal Cord*, 3rd edition (1), *The Textbook of Pain*, 5th edition (2), and *Bonica's Management of Pain*, 3rd edition (3). Further, where appropriate, reviews and textbooks are cited to give the reader sources for additional information.

WHAT IS PAIN?

Pain is one of the most common reasons a person seeks medical attention. The management of pain conditions is difficult and challenging, particularly when pain becomes chronic. Pain is defined by the International Association for the Study of Pain as an unpleasant sensory and emotional experience associated with actual or potential tissue damage, or described in terms as such (4). Inherent in this definition is both the subjective nature of pain and the multidimensional nature of pain. Melzack and Casey (5) proposed three dimensions of pain: *sensory–discriminative*, *motivational–affective*, and *cognitive–evaluative*. The sensory–discriminative component of pain is concerned with the quality (e.g., burning, sharp, dull,), location, duration, and intensity (or magnitude). The motivational–affective component of pain is concerned with the unpleasantness of pain (e.g., nauseating, sickening), and motivational tendency toward escape or attack. The cognitive–evaluative dimension is based on past experience and on outcome of different response strategies (annoying, miserable, unbearable). All three dimensions are linked and interact to affect the motor and behavioral consequences responsible for the complex pattern of responses to pain [for review, see *Textbook of Pain* (2). In addition, all three dimensions of pain should be examined during initial evaluations and when the efficacy of clinical interventions is being assessed.

DESCRIPTORS OF CLINICAL PAIN SYNDROMES

Acute versus Chronic Pain

Pain can be acute or chronic. *Acute pain* is protective and serves as a warning sign that the body is experiencing actual or potential tissue damage. Clinically, acute pain is usually the result of an injury that can be pinpointed to time and place, such as being burned, spraining an ankle, or breaking a bone. Acute pain occurs immediately at the time of injury and usually goes away once healing is completed. In contrast, chronic pain is nonprotective and serves no biological purpose. Pain can be considered chronic if (i) pain outlasts normal tissue healing time, (ii) the pain is greater than would be expected from the extent of the injury, and (iii) pain occurs in the absence of identifiable tissue damage (4). Thus, the concept of pain as a symptom, as occurs with acute pain, changes to the concept of pain as a disease, as occurs with *chronic pain.*

Hyperalgesia, Allodynia, and Referred Pain

The terms *hyperalgesia* and *allodynia* are commonly used by clinicians to describe pain behaviors. Hyperalgesia is an increased pain response to a normally noxious (painful) stimulus (6) (Fig. 4.1). When this increased pain response occurs at the site of injury, it is called primary hyperalgesia. Hyperalgesia occurring outside the site of injury is called secondary hyperalgesia. One common example of primary hyperalgesia is the increased pain felt in people with osteoarthritis to external pressure applied to the joint. Secondary hyperalgesia occurs, for example, in people with kidney pain who have tenderness over the lower back. Primary hyperalgesia is thought to reflect changes in the peripheral nervous system, and secondary hyperalgesia is thought to be mediated by changes in the central nervous system (see below). Deep tissues such as muscle, joint, and viscera are commonly associated with secondary hyperalgesia, particularly at sites distant to the injury and in the skin.

Allodynia is defined as pain in response to normally innocuous (nonpainful) stimuli or activities (Fig. 4.1). Allodynia is thought to be mediated by changes in the central nervous system, where activation of a peripherally located non-nociceptor is perceived as painful. Examples

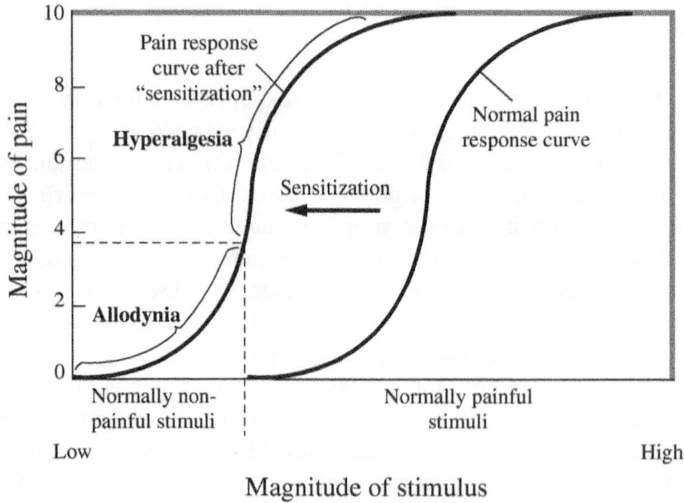

Figure 4.1. Graph of the relationship between the magnitude of applied stimuli and the magnitude of the perceived pain response. The curve to the right illustrates the normal pain response curve. Sensitization of pain pathways shifts the normal curve to the left. This shift produces painful responses to ordinarily nonpainful stimuli (allodynia) and increased pain responses to usually painful stimuli (hyperalgesia). (Cervero F, Laird JMA. Mechanisms of touch-evoked pain (allodynia): a new model. *Pain.* 1996;68:13–23.)

of allodynia include a painful response to gentle touching of the skin after sunburn or pain in patients with nerve injury. In addition, weight bearing on an arthritic joint, muscle contraction in myositis or tendonitis, and joint movement in bursitis may also be examples of allodynia.

Referred pain is pain felt outside the area of injury, but it is not associated with a response to the applied stimuli. Referred pain often arises with diseases or conditions that compromise the function of internal organs. The most common example of referred pain is that of pain in the left shoulder and down the left arm during a heart attack (4). Several common referred pain patterns are illustrated in Figure 4.2 (7). Table 4.1 (8) lists and defines a number of other terms that may be used to describe pain in the clinical setting.

BASIC NEUROANATOMICAL CONCEPTS OF PAIN TRANSMISSION PATHWAYS

A simplified view of pain pathways (Fig. 4.3) is often presented when beginning discussions of pain (8,9). In such a view, the pathway is described as consisting of first-order, second-order, and third-order neurons. The first-order neurons are *nociceptors* that are activated in the peripheral tissue by damaging or potentially damaging (i.e., noxious) stimuli or events. The peripheral terminals of the nociceptors are unencapsulated *free nerve endings* that convert (transduce) noxious stimuli into action potentials that are carried toward the cell body in dorsal root ganglia. The central terminals of this unipolar neuron terminate in the spinal cord dorsal horn, synapsing with a second-order neuron. The second-order neuron is typically referred to as the spinothalamic tract neuron, and it sends projections supraspinally to the ventroposterior lateral nucleus of the thalamus. In the thalamus, the second-order neuron then synapses with a third-order neuron that in turn projects to the somatosensory cortex. Perception of the location and nature of pain occurs when the nociceptive signals reach the cortex.

This simplified three-neuron pain pathway is a valuable concept in clinical neurological examination to assess the ability of individuals to perceive and localize painful stimuli applied to the skin in various areas. The ability to recognize painful stimuli applied to the skin suggests that

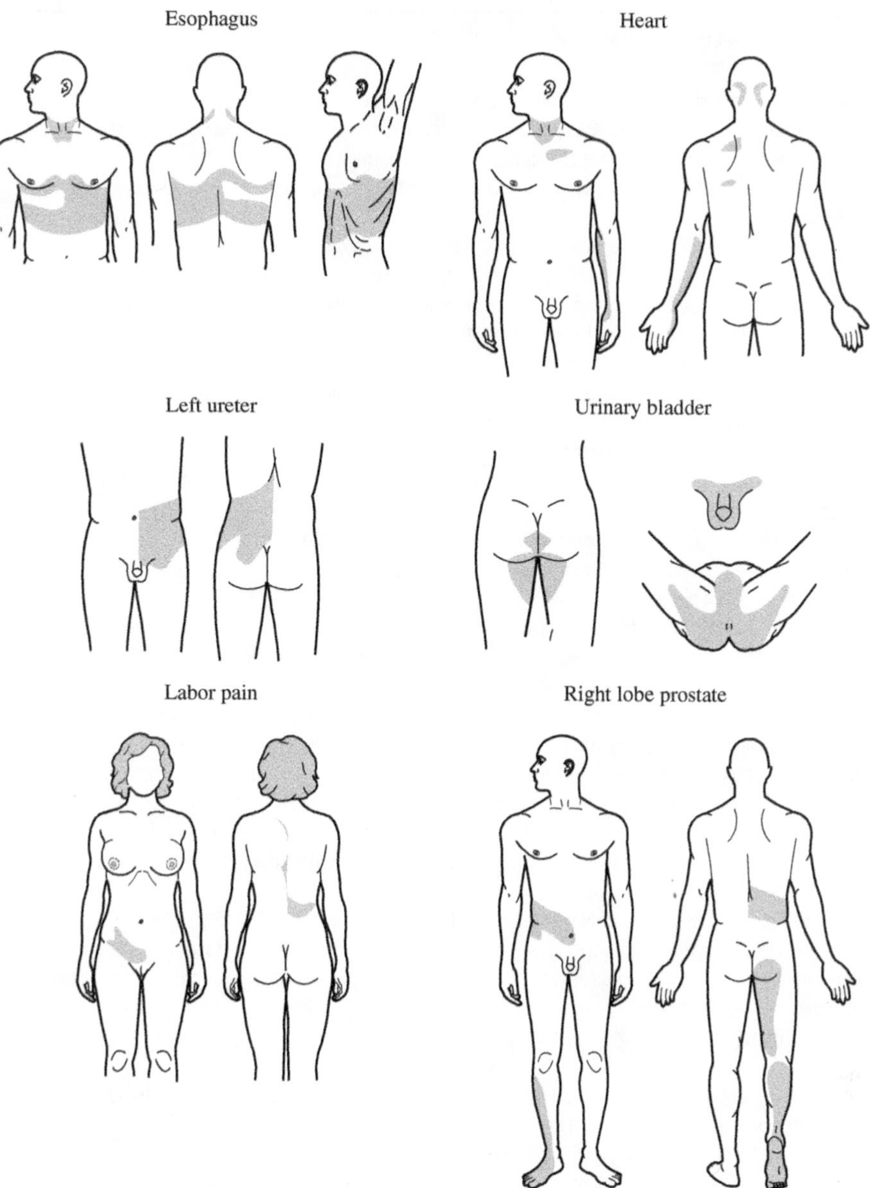

Figure 4.2. Illustrations of referred pain patterns associated with disorders of the esophagus, heart, urinary bladder, left ureter, and the right lobe of the prostate. Note that the referred pain pattern from right lobe prostate disorders is similar to the pain pattern that might arise with lumbosacral nerve root compression or sciatica.

the pain pathway between the site of stimulation and the brain cortex is intact. The inability to perceive skin pinches or pinpricks may be associated with disruption somewhere along the pain pathway. The cutaneous distribution (e.g., peripheral nerve dermatome vs. spinal nerve root dermatome vs. entire limb) of pain perception deficit may assist in identifying the site of a localized lesion in the pathway. Integration of the findings from pain testing with findings from other somatosensory tests (e.g., touch-pressure testing) may further help establish the location and the extent of either peripheral or central nervous system lesions.

Table 4.1. Terms Used to Describe Pain in the Clinical Setting

Allodynia: pain due to a stimulus which does not normally provoke pain (Allodynia is taken to apply to conditions that may give rise to sensitization of the skin, such as sunburn, inflammation, and trauma.)
Analgesia: absence of pain in response to normally painful stimulation
Anesthesia: absence of all cutaneous sensory modalities including pain, touch, joint position, and joint movement
Arthralgia: pain in a joint often due to arthritis or arthropathy
Causalgia: a syndrome of sustained burning pain, allodynia, and hyperpathia after a traumatic nerve lesion, often combined with vasomotor and sudomotor dysfunction and later trophic changes
Central pain: pain initiated or caused by a primary lesion or dysfunction in the central nervous system.
Dysethesia: an unpleasant abnormal sensation, whether spontaneous or evoked
Hyperalgesia: an increased response to a stimulus which is normally painful
Hyperesthesia: increased sensitivity to stimulation, excluding the special senses
Hyperpathia: a painful syndrome characterized by an abnormally painful reaction to a stimulus, especially a repetitive stimulus, as well as an increased threshold (Hyperpathia may occur with allodynia, hyperesthesia, hyperalgesia, or dysesthesia.)
Hypoalgesia: diminished pain in response to a normally painful stimulus
Neuralgia: pain in the distribution of nerves
Neuritis: inflammation of nerves
Neuropathic pain: pain initiated or caused by a primary lesion or dysfunction in the nervous system
Neurogenic pain: pain initiated or caused by a primary lesion, dysfunction, or transitory perturbation in the peripheral or central nervous system
Neuropathy: a disturbance of function or pathological change in a nerve: in one nerve, mononeuropathy; in several nerves, mononeuropathy multiplex; if diffuse and bilateral, polyneuropathy
Nociceptor: a receptor preferentially sensitive to a noxious stimulus or to a stimulus that would become noxious if prolonged (Avoid use of terms such as "pain receptor," "pain pathway," and "pain neuron.")
Noxious stimulus: a stimulus that is damaging or potentially damaging to normal tissues
Pain: an unpleasant sensory and emotional experience associated with actual or potential tissue damage or described in terms of such damage
Pain threshold: the least experience of pain that a subject can recognize
Pain tolerance level: the greatest level of pain that a subject is prepared to tolerate
Peripheral neurogenic pain: pain initiated or caused by a primary lesion or dysfunction or transitory perturbation in the peripheral nervous system
Peripheral neuropathic pain: pain initiated or caused by a primary lesion or dysfunction in the peripheral nervous system
Primary afferent neuron: peripheral sensory neuron that conveys information from its specialized receptor located in peripheral tissue to the central nervous system
Radiculopathy: dysfunction or pathologic change in one or more spinal nerve roots
Radiculitis: inflammation of one or more spinal nerve roots

Adapted from *Pocket Dictionary of Pain.* International Association for the Study of Pain.

To any clinician who has had experience with individuals in pain, it becomes readily evident that the three-neuron pain pathway is inadequate to explain pain experienced by many people and that it does not provide either the structural or functional foundation for noninvasive and pharmacological interventions to manage pain. Table 4.2 lists several of the shortcomings of the simple three-neuron pain transmission concept (9). In response to these shortcomings, the gate-control theory of pain was proposed by Melzack and Wall (10) in 1965. Since then, there has been a wealth of investigation aimed at elucidating the neurobiology of pain and pain control. Subsequent sections of this chapter review anatomical and physiological discoveries to allow the reader to more clearly comprehend clinical pain syndromes and how electrical stimulation can be used to control pain.

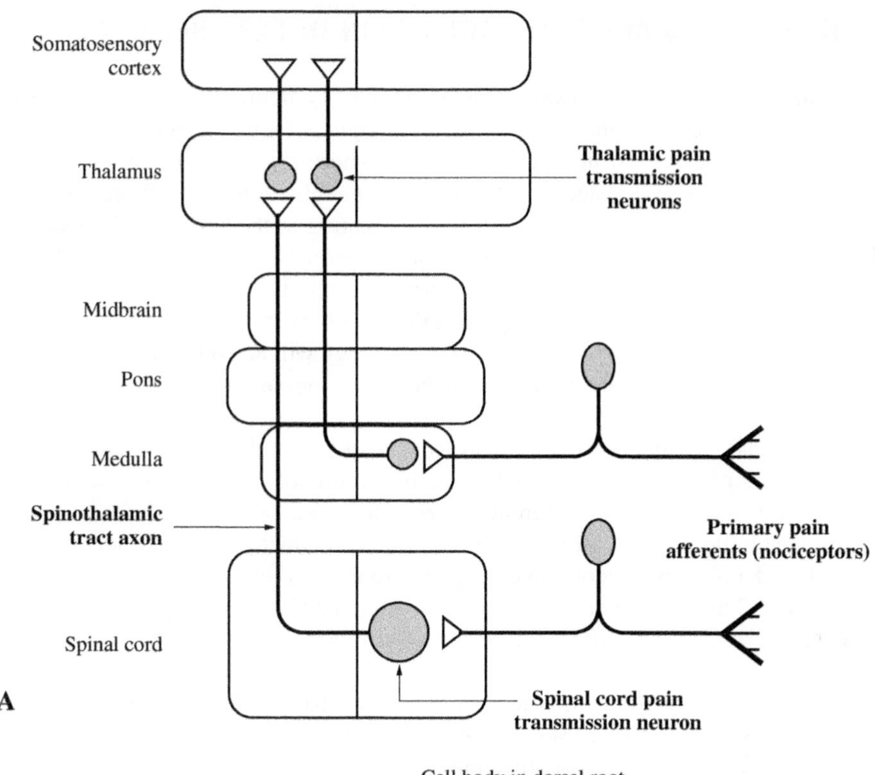

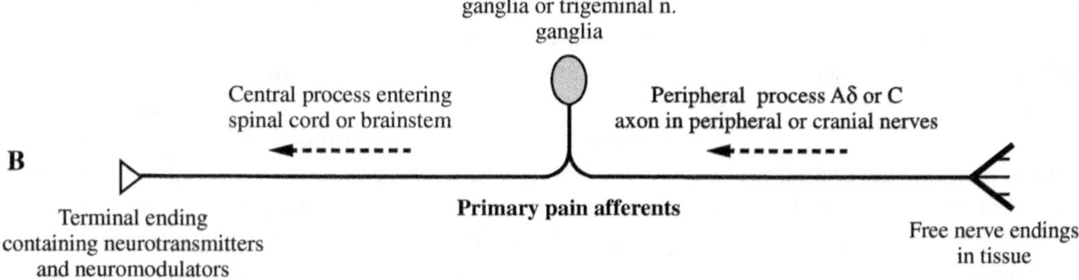

Figure 4.3. Diagrammatic representation of **(A)** basic three-neuron pain pathway and **(B)** components of primary pain afferents (nociceptors).

Table 4.2. Shortcomings of the Simple Three-Neuron Concept of Pain Transmission

The simplified three neuron pathway concept for pain transmission suggests that

1. All first-, second-, and third-order pain transmission neurons are identical in terms of location, inputs, and responses to painful events or conditions.
2. Pain initiation occurs only at the free nerve endings of first-order pain afferents.

The simplified three-neuron pathway concept for pain transmission does not account for

1. Variations in pain perception between individuals in response to painful stimuli
2. Pain in response to lesions within the central nervous system
3. Referred pain syndromes
4. Pain control in response to physical therapeutic interventions

Adapted from Robinson, AJ. Central nervous system pathways for pain transmission and pain control. *J. Hand Ther.* 1997;10:64–77.

PRIMARY PAIN AFFERENTS AND THEIR ACTIVATION IN PERIPHERAL TISSUES

The *first-order neurons* of sensory pathways consist of sensory neurons designed to convert mechanical, thermal, and chemical energy into electrical signals (action potentials) and carry these action potentials to the central nervous system (1). These primary afferent neurons are unipolar neurons with a cell body located in the dorsal root ganglia, a peripheral process innervating the peripheral structures, and a central process terminating in the spinal cord dorsal horn or medulla. For the limbs and trunk, the cell bodies of the sensory neurons are located in the dorsal root ganglia. For the head and face, the sensory neuron cells bodies are located in the trigeminal ganglia. Peripheral terminals of primary afferent fibers terminate peripherally with specialized receptor endings that determine what types of energy will activate the sensory axons. Primary afferent nociceptors terminate in unencapsulated free nerve endings in skin, muscle, joint, and viscera.

The peripheral axons of primary afferent neurons vary in size and are either myelinated or unmyelinated. The speed of conduction is determined by differences in the axon diameter and myelination. Different types of primary afferent neurons therefore conduct at different speeds. For example, muscle spindle primary afferents are the fastest conducting sensory neurons, conducting between 70 and 120 m per second. Nociceptors are either thinly myelinated Aδ or type III, conducting between 2 and 25 m per second, or unmyelinated C-fiber or type IV, conducting <2 m per second. Table 4.3 outlines different types of primary afferent sensory neurons and lists their respective sensory functions.

For primary afferent neurons, two classification schemes exist, one that uses Roman numerals (I, II, III, and IV) (11) and one that uses letters from the English and Greek alphabets (12). Note that, as mentioned above, there are two different types of primary afferent neurons that transmit nociceptive information: thinly myelinated Aδ or type III, and unmyelinated C or type IV. The peripheral terminals of type III and IV nociceptors do not have specialized, encapsulated receptor endings like those primary afferent neurons transmitting nonpainful stimuli such as touch. Rather, nociceptors terminate in tissues as unencapsulated receptors called free nerve endings.

All free nerve endings of primary afferent nociceptors do not respond to all types of painful stimuli. The free nerve endings of cutaneous Aδ and C nociceptors respond to noxious mechanical and/or thermal stimuli. Many cutaneous nociceptors are polymodal, responding to multiple noxious stimuli, including mechanical, thermal, and chemical, and hence are called polymodal nociceptors. A third group of nociceptors has been identified as silent or mechanically insensitive, and are likely activated by inflammatory mediators such as prostaglandins.

The free nerve endings of primary pain afferents (nociceptors) are found in or around most tissues, including skin, muscle, tendons, joint structures, periosteum, intervertebral discs, and even within peripheral nerves (nervi nervorum). Free nerve endings may be activated (produce action potentials) during the activities of everyday living by the application of mechanical, thermal, and chemical stimuli at levels that may produce tissue damage. In addition, tissue inflammation, a normal response to injury, is a condition that commonly produces pain. Many of the substances released from non-neuronal cells at the site of inflammation are capable of activating free nerve endings, ultimately resulting in the perception of pain. Table 4.4 lists a number of chemicals present in and around inflamed tissues that activate free nerve endings.

Sensitization of Primary Afferent Nociceptors

The sensitivity of nociceptors to painful stimuli is modifiable, increasing or decreasing in response to peripherally applied mechanical, thermal, or chemical stimuli. Following tissue injury, particularly joint or muscle inflammation, *sensitization* of primary afferent fibers can

Table 4.3. Classification of Types of Sensory Afferents Located in the Skin, Muscle, or Connective Tissues

Axon Class	Myelinated?	Conduction Velocity	Specialized Ending	Receptor Location(s)	Sensory Function
Ia (Aα)	Yes	70–120 m/s	Muscle spindle	Skeletal muscle	Joint position/movement
Ib (Aα)	Yes	70–120 m/s	Golgi tendon organ	Musculotendinous junction	Muscle contraction force
II (Aβ)	Yes	25–70 m/s	Touch receptors	Skin	Touch/pressure
			Joint receptors	Joint capsule	Joint position/movement
			Muscle spindle secondary	Skeletal muscle	Joint position
III (Aδ)	Yes	2–25 m/s	Free nerve ending	Skin, muscle, connective tissue, tendon, nerve	Fast pain, pricking pain, sharp pain
IV (C)	No	<2 m/s	Free nerve ending	Skin, muscle connective tissue, tendon, nerve	Slow pain, burning pain, dull, achy pain

Table 4.4. Substances Released in Inflamed Tissue That Activate and/or Sensitize Free Nerve Endings

Substance	Source	Activates Nociceptors	Sensitizes Nociceptors
Serotonin	Platelets	+	
Bradykinin	Blood plasma	+	
Substance P	Type IV (C)	+	+
Cytokines	Inflammatory cells	+	+
Prostaglandins	Inflammatory cells		+
Leukotrienes	Inflammatory cells		+
Hydrogen ions	Interstitial fluid	+	+
Potassium ions	Interstitial fluid	+	

occur (13–15). Sensitization of a neuron is characterized by increased spontaneous activity, a decrease in threshold of response to noxious stimuli, an increase in responsiveness to the same noxious stimuli, and/or an increase in receptive field size. By recording the activity of the peripheral nerves before and after induction of acute inflammation, Schaible and Schmidt (13,14) showed increase spontaneous activity and responsiveness to noxious and innocuous joint movement in primary afferent fibers of groups II, III, and IV. Similar changes occur following inflammation of the muscle with carrageenan (15,16) or after ischemia of the muscle (17). In inflammation of a muscle or a joint, there is also an increase in the response of the primary afferents to weak mechanical stimuli, such as innocuous local pressure. Following peripheral inflammation, silent nociceptors begin to respond to both innocuous and noxious stimuli, such as pressure and joint movement. Taken together, there is a general increase in activity of nociceptors. This would increase the number of afferents firing after a peripheral insult and increase input to the central nervous system. This sensitization increases the responsiveness of primary pain afferent nociceptors to noxious stimuli and hence constitutes an explanation for hyperalgesia at the site of injury (i.e., primary hyperalgesia).

For cutaneous pain responses in humans, activation of nociceptors can be described as two distinctly different types of responses called *fast pain* (also known as first pain) and *slow pain* (also knows as second pain). Fast pain arising from free nerve endings in the skin arises at the time of application of a tissue-damaging or potentially damaging stimulus. For example, fast pain is felt at the time the skin is pinched or pricked with a pin. Slow pain of cutaneous origin, in contrast, is lower in magnitude and persists after the painful stimulus is removed. For example, if one touches a hot stove with a finger, a fast pain is experienced at the moment that the finger contacts the stove. Once the finger is withdrawn from the hot surface, a "burning" pain persists. This is slow or second pain. Fast skin pain appears to originate in the Aδ nociceptive afferents, whereas slow pain is thought to originate in type C nociceptive afferents. The ability to detect skin pain is important for protective responses in everyday living and may, in certain diseases or disorders, be the main reason for seeking treatment from a health care provider. More often, however, individuals who seek medical attention have pain that arises from nociceptors in tissues beneath the skin including muscle, tendon, joint structures, and peripheral nerves.

Pain from deep somatic tissues is uniquely different from cutaneous pain. Muscle pain can arise from a variety of disorders, including muscle inflammation (myositis) or tearing of muscle tissue (strain) (18,19). Joint pain occurs acutely after injury to ligaments or the joint capsule, or chronically in conditions such as osteoarthritis or rheumatoid arthritis (20). The quality of pain associated with injury to a muscle or joint differs from that associated with injury to the skin. Injury to deep structures results in diffuse, difficult to localize, aching pain (21,22). Using microneurography, intraneuronal stimulation of muscle nerve fascicles produces only the

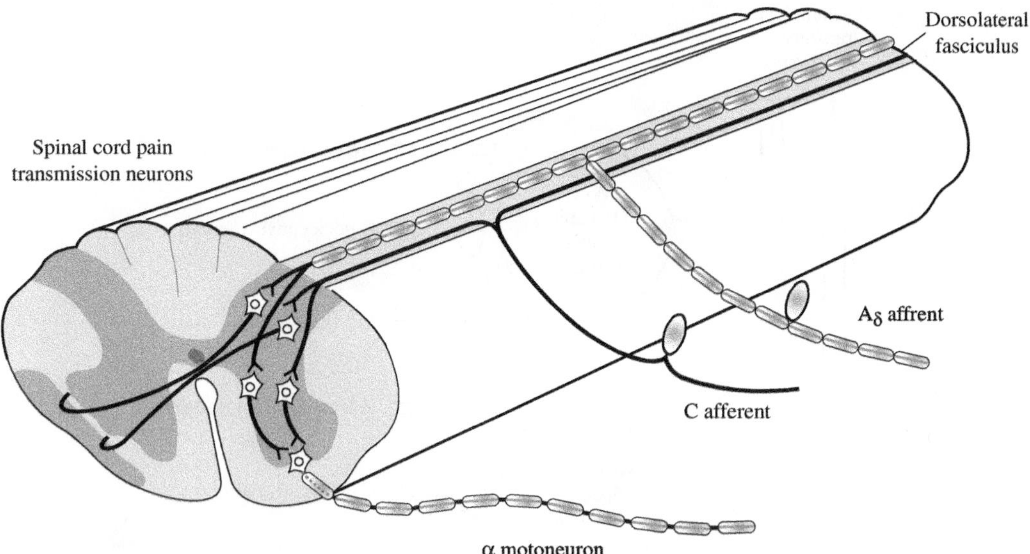

Figure 4.4. Diagram illustrating the location of cell bodies of spinal cord pain transmission neurons, inputs from peripheral nociceptors, and axons that contribute to ascending pain pathways.

sensation of deep, cramplike pain. Stimulation of muscle nociceptors at a low intensity to activate a few primary afferent fibers produces pain that is well localized (22). However, if the stimulus intensity is increased, activating more primary afferent fibers, then the pain is less well localized and spreads to regions outside the area of innervation (23). The spread of muscle pain to areas innervated by different nerves is one type of referred pain. For muscle pain, the size of the area of referred pain correlates with the intensity and duration of the primary muscle pain. In human subjects, painful intramuscular stimulation is rated as more unpleasant than painful cutaneous stimulation, the pain is longer lasting, and referred pain is more frequent (24,25).

Connections of Central Processes of Primary Pain Afferents

The central processes of primary afferent nociceptors enter the central nervous system and synapse on the *pain transmission neurons* (PTNs) in the spinal cord dorsal horn, or trigeminal dorsal horn (Fig. 4.4). The terminals of the central processes contain chemical neurotransmitters that, when released, excite the second-order neurons. Excitatory neurotransmitters released from primary afferent nociceptors are numerous and include glutamate, substance P, and calcitonin gene-related peptide (CGRP). The central terminals of primary afferent nociceptors also contain numerous other substances that are released at the same time as the excitatory neurotransmitters. These substances include adenosine triphosphate (ATP), acetylcholine, nitric oxide, galanin, neuropeptide Y, somatostatin, and vasoactive intestinal peptide (1). These and other chemicals modify nociceptive transmission.

SPINAL CORD PAIN TRANSMISSION NEURONS

The cell bodies of second-order neurons that respond to noxious stimuli are located throughout the dorsal horn of spinal cord at all levels and in the trigeminal nuclei. Two types of neurons that respond to noxious stimuli have been identified (1) (Fig. 4.5). One type of second-order neuron

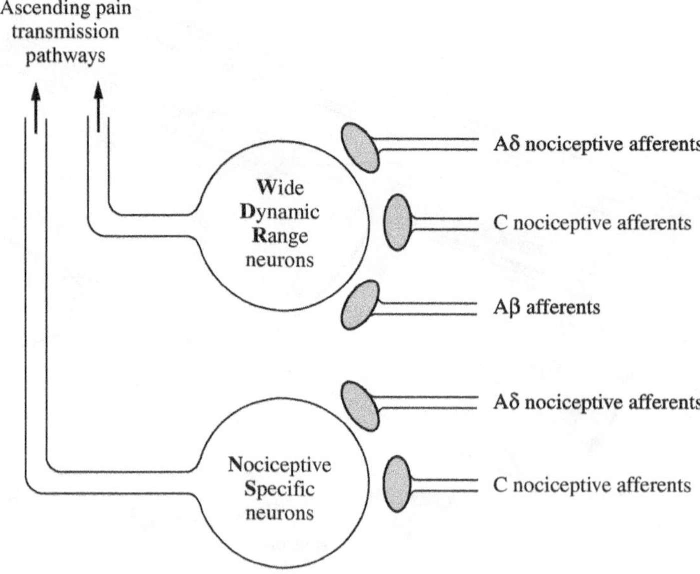

Figure 4.5. Illustration of the two types of spinal cord pain-transmission neurons. Wide dynamic range neurons receive inputs from both nociceptors and sensory afferents associated with nonpainful sensory stimuli (e.g, touch and proprioception). In contrast, nociceptive specific neurons receive sensory input from only nociceptors.

receives input from peripheral nociceptors, but not from any other type of somatosensory afferent, and thus responds only to peripherally applied noxious stimuli. These neurons are called *nociceptive specific* or *high threshold neurons*. In contrast, the second type of second-order neuron receives input from both nociceptive and non-nociceptive primary afferent fibers and thus responds to noxious and non-noxious peripherally applied stimuli. Because activation of these neurons is controlled by many different types of peripheral sensory inputs, these neurons are called *wide dynamic range neurons*. Table 4.5 compares and contrasts nociceptive-specific (NS) and wide-dynamic-range (WDR) pain-transmission neurons.

Individual spinal cord pain-transmission neurons receive convergent input from primary afferent nociceptors arising from both skin and deeper tissues such as muscles, joints, and viscera (Fig. 4.6). This convergence of pain pathways may provide an anatomical basis for referred pain

Table 4.5. Characteristics of the Two Types of Spinal Cord Pain-Transmission Neurons

	Wide Dynamic Range	***Nociceptive Specific***
Highest concentration	In deep dorsal horn	In superficial dorsal horn
Activated by	Aδ and C nociceptors and Aβ primary afferents	Only Aδ and C pain afferents
Output axons contribution to spinothalamic pathways	2/3 of fibers in STT*	1/4 of fibers in STT
Somatotopically organized in dorsal horn?	Yes	Yes
Receptive field size	Large	Small
Pain inputs from	Skin, muscle, joint, and viscera	Skin, muscle, joint, and viscera

*STT, spinothalamic tract.

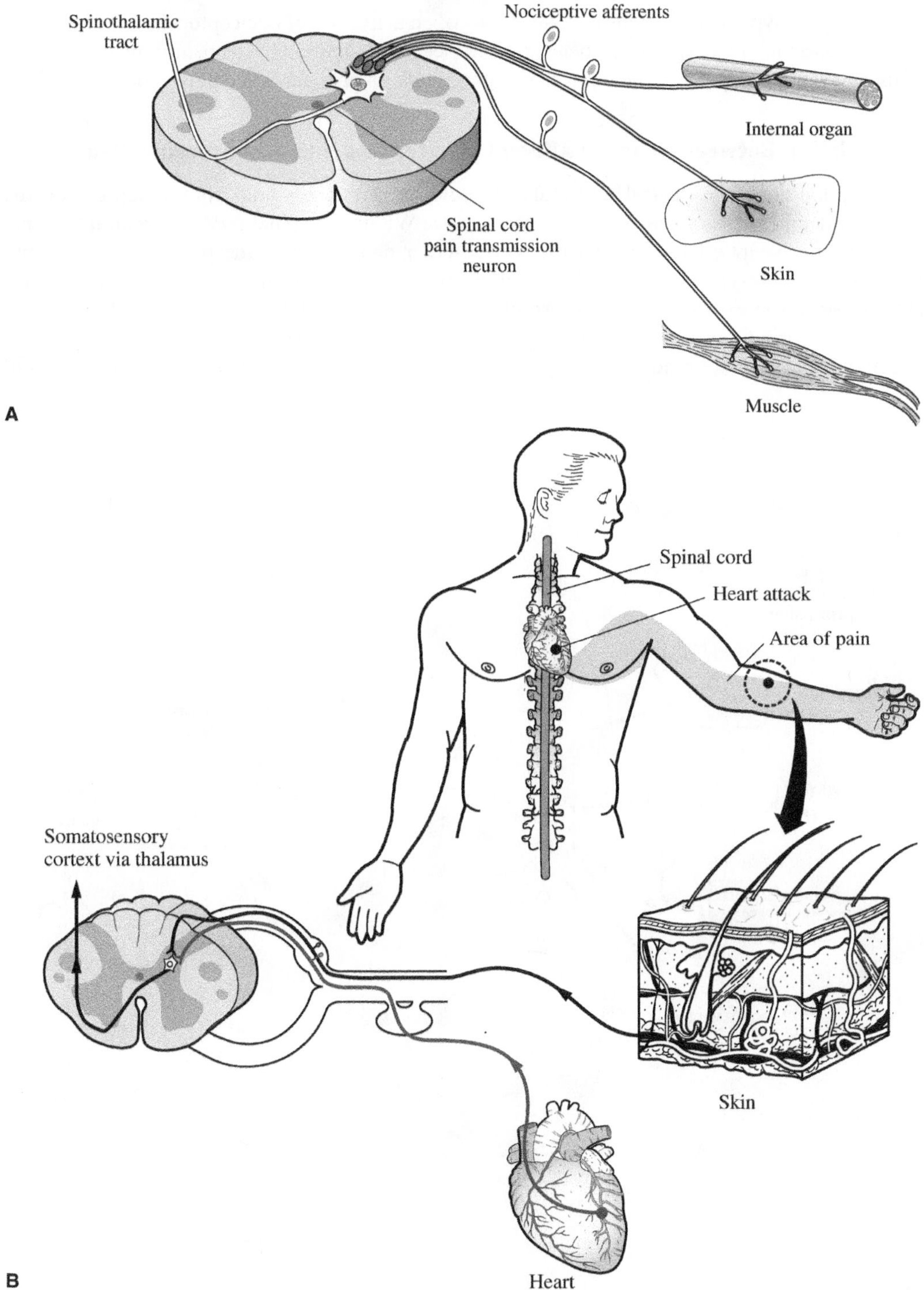

Figure 4.6. A: Illustration of the convergent inputs to spinal pain-transmission neurons from cutaneous (skin), muscle, and internal organ nociceptors. This pattern of convergent input to nociceptors provides one explanation for referred pain to cutaneous and/or muscle with disorders of internal organs. **B:** Illustration of the convergent pain afferents from the heart and the left arm through a nerve root that explains the referred pain pattern to the left arm that may arise at the onset of a heart attack.

and secondary hyperalgesia. Referred pain arises when activation of nociceptors in one type of tissue, such as an internal organ (e.g., heart, gallbladder), is misinterpreted as painful in another type of tissue, such as skin. Thus, the input sent supraspinally is misinterpreted at the cortical level.

Transmission Between Primary Afferent Nociceptors and Second-order Neurons

In the spinal cord, the central terminals of nociceptors in the spinal cord synapse with the second-order dorsal horn neurons in the dorsal horn. Within the spinal cord, the central terminal forms the presynaptic element, and the second-order neuron forms the postsynaptic element. Invasion of the presynaptic element by action potentials depolarizes the central terminal, triggering release of the excitatory neurotransmitters (i.e., glutamate and substance P). These neurotransmitters bind to specific receptors postsynaptically on the second-order neuron (Fig. 4.7). Specifically, glutamate binds to the α-amino-3-hydroxy-5-methyl-4-isoxazole propionic acid

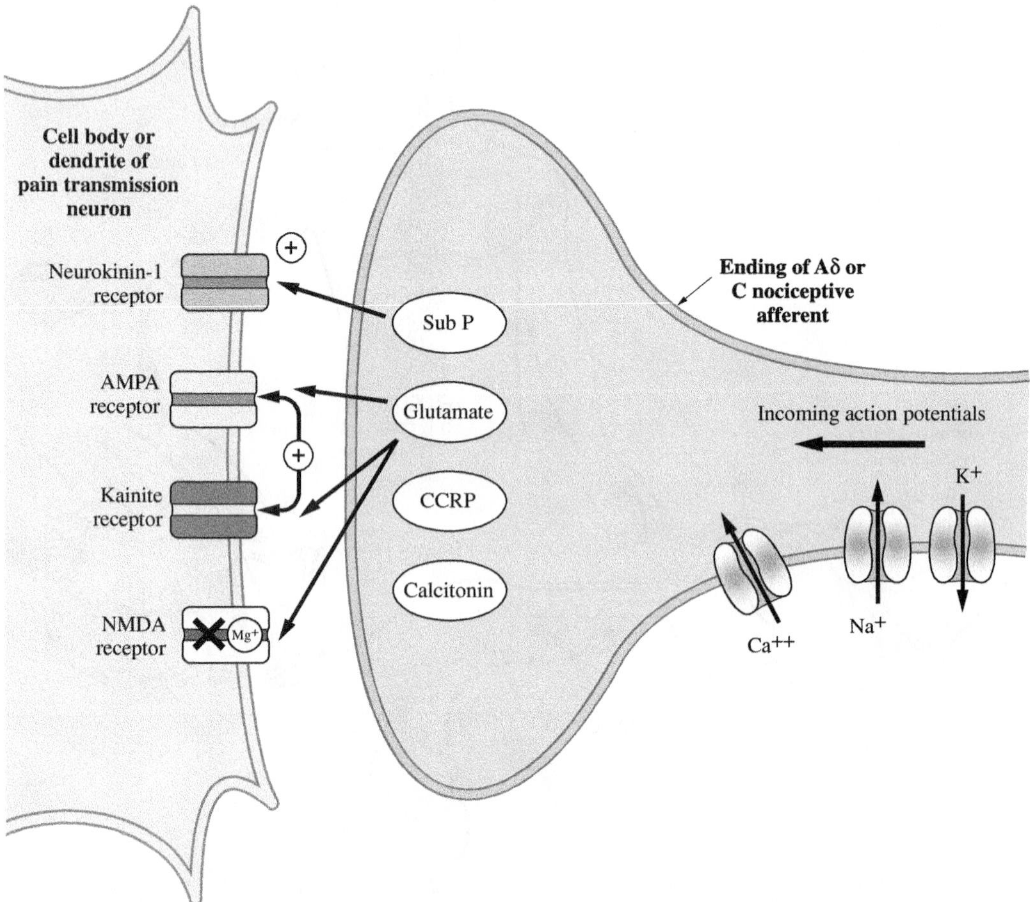

Figure 4.7. Diagram illustrating several of the substances contained within the terminal bouton of nociceptors that are released in response to incoming pain signals. Also illustrated are several of the receptors in the membrane of spinal pain transmission neurons that bind either substance P (neurokinin-1 receptor) or glutamate [α-amino-3-hydroxy-5-methyl-4-isoxazole propionic acid (AMPA), kainite, and/or N-methyl D-aspartate (NMDA) receptors CGRP-calcitonin gene-related peptide]. These neurotransmitters control in part the excitability and subsequent discharge of pain-transmission neurons in the pain pathway.

(AMPA), kainite, *N*-methyl D-aspartate (NMDA), or metabotropic glutamate receptors, and substance P binds to neurokinin 1 (NK1) () receptors. AMPA, kainite, and NMDA receptors are ion channels that open upon binding of glutamate to allow positively charged ions (sodium and/or calcium) to enter the neuron, producing a transient depolarization of the neuron. The NK1 receptor is a G-protein–linked receptor that activates signal transduction pathways when activated by substance P. When painful stimuli are encountered in everyday activities, the transmitter release and the subsequent depolarization of second-order neurons is sufficient to reach the activation threshold and generate action potentials in axons projecting supraspinally. These signals are subsequently conducted through thalamus/cortical and brainstem sites to produce the sensation of pain, along with the associated emotional and autonomic responses to noxious stimuli.

There is substantial evidence that glutamate and substance P play a key role in the spinal cord, transmitting noxious stimuli from nociceptors through dorsal horn neurons to projection neurons. Glutamate mediates excitatory synaptic transmission between primary afferent nociceptors and dorsal horn projection neurons (26,27). The glutamate receptors AMPA and kainite (AMPA/KA) form cation channels that allow passage of sodium ions, but some are also permeable to calcium depending on subunit composition (28). These AMPA/KA receptors are thought to mediate fast excitatory synaptic transmission between primary afferent nociceptors and dorsal horn second-order neurons in response to noxious stimulation. AMPA/KA receptor antagonists inhibit pain associated with peripheral neuropathy, burn injury, inflammation, and incision (29–32).

Substance P and CGRP are located in the central terminals of primary afferent nociceptors with terminals primarily located in laminae I and II [for review, see Millan (33)]. Substance P exerts its effects through activation of the NK1 receptor, located in the superficial dorsal horn, and it may be the neurotransmitter associated with slow pain transmission (34). Activation of the substance P receptor produces pain behaviors and increases activity and responsiveness of dorsal horn pain-transmission neurons (36). In contrast, blockade of NK1 receptors reduces pain associated with tissue injury and reduces sensitization of dorsal horn neurons (37–41). Further loss of NK1-containing neurons in the spinal cord similarly reduces hyperalgesia and sensitization of dorsal horn neurons after tissue injury (42,43). Similarly, administration of CGRP to the spinal cord produces hyperalgesia and sensitizes neurons (44). In contrast, CGRP antagonists reduce hyperalgesia and sensitization of dorsal horn neurons induced by inflammatory tissue injury (45,46). CGRP activates metabotropic receptors that use protein kinases to produce long-lasting excitatory changes (44). CGRP is also released with substance P and slows the degradation of substance P in the spinal cord (47), resulting in a potentiation of the effects of substance P (48). For an extensive review of the neurotransmitters and receptors involved in nociceptive transmission in the spinal cord, see Millan (33).

Sensitization of Spinal Cord Pain Transmission Neurons

After tissue injury, sensitization of both high-threshold NS and WDR neurons may occur. This is manifested as an increase in receptive field size, increased responsiveness to innocuous or noxious stimuli, and/or a decreased threshold to innocuous or noxious stimuli (49–55).

Sensitization of second-order dorsal horn neurons can arise from any or all of three different processes: (i) prolonged synaptic transmission between primary afferent nociceptors and second-order dorsal horn neurons, (ii) a reduction in inhibitory neurotransmitter activity in the dorsal horn, or (iii) the activation of glial cells within the spinal cord dorsal horn (Fig. 4.8).

Sensitization of dorsal horn neurons after increased nociceptor input results in increased release of excitatory neurotransmitters such as substance P and glutamate (56–58). Upon release from primary nociceptor terminals and other dorsal horn neurons, glutamate binds to AMPA/KA receptors to depolarize dorsal horn neurons as well as to NMDA receptors. The NMDA receptor is an ion channel that primarily transmits calcium ions and is normally blocked ("plugged") by

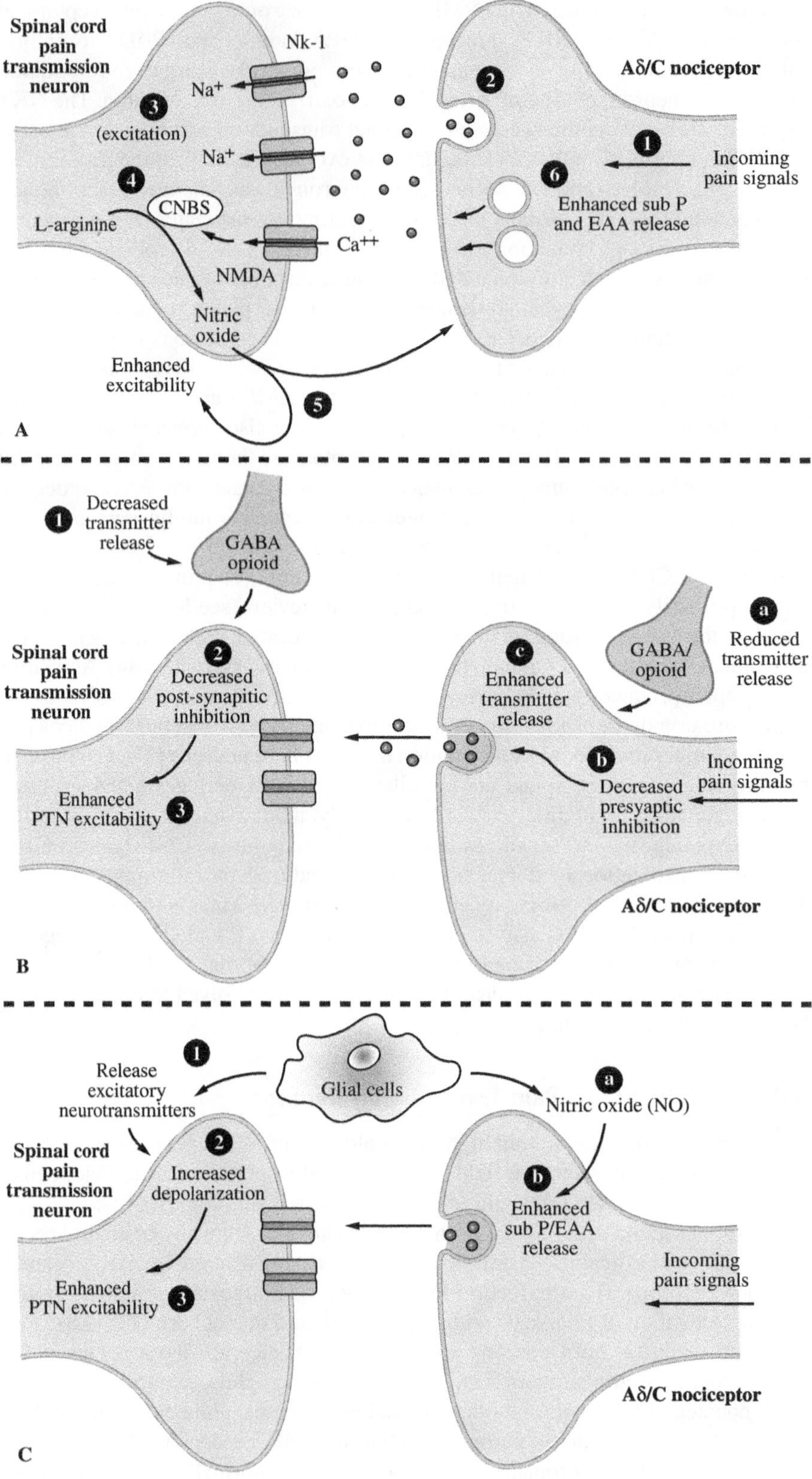
Spinal cord pain transmission neuron
Nk-1
Aδ/C nociceptor
2
Na+
3
(excitation)
1
Incoming pain signals
Na+
6
4
CNBS
Enhanced sub P and EAA release
L-arginine
Ca++
NMDA
Nitric oxide
Enhanced excitability
5
A
1
Decreased transmitter release
GABA opioid
a
Reduced transmitter release
Spinal cord pain transmission neuron
2
Decreased post-synapitic inhibition
c
Enhanced transmitter release
GABA/ opioid
b
Incoming pain signals
Enhanced PTN excitability
3
Decreased presyaptic inhibition
Aδ/C nociceptor
B
1
Release excitatory neurotransmitters
Glial cells
a
Nitric oxide (NO)
Spinal cord pain transmission neuron
2
Increased depolarization
b
Enhanced sub P/EAA release
Incoming pain signals
Enhanced PTN excitability
3
Aδ/C nociceptor
C

magnesium. The magnesium block is removed by depolarization of the neuron, allowing calcium to enter from the extracellular space, further depolarizing the neuron. Calcium also serves as a second messenger and further increases activation of a number of second-messenger pathways, including adenylate cyclase-cyclic adenosine monophosphate, cyclic guanosine monophosphate-nitric oxide, and calcium calmodulin. Activation of these second-messenger cascades, either in the second-order dorsal horn neurons or in the central terminal of primary afferent nociceptors, can have multiple effects, including increased release of neurotransmitters, potentiation of ion channels, and increased transcription of "pain genes." Nitric oxide, a gas, diffuses from the dorsal horn neurons to the terminals of the primary afferent nociceptor, where it enhances the release of excitatory neurotransmitters. This would have the ultimate consequence of increasing excitability of second-order dorsal horn neurons, increasing input to higher brain centers, and ultimately resulting in the perception of pain.

The NMDA receptors are clearly involved in hyperalgesia and the sensitization of dorsal horn neurons that develops after tissue injury. Sensitization of second-order dorsal horn neurons that occurs after joint inflammation or after exposure to formalin, capsaicin, or ultraviolet irradiation is prevented by blocking NMDA receptors (59–61). Spinal application of NMDA glutamate receptor antagonists decreases pain associated with hindpaw inflammation in animal models (62), joint inflammation (63), acid-induced muscle pain (64), formalin injection (65,66), and neuropathic pain models (66,67).

Another possible mechanism for sensitization of PTNs in peripheral neuropathy or inflammation is the reduction of the inhibitory transmitters γ-aminobutyric acid (GABA) or glycine in the dorsal horn of the spinal cord (68). In models of peripheral neuropathy, several studies demonstrate decreases in the number of GABA neurons in the dorsal horn (69–71). In parallel, inhibition of dorsal horn neurons by GABA is significantly reduced in an animal model of neuropathic pain (68). However, several studies show no changes or even increases in GABA content and release in models of peripheral neuropathy (72–74). These discrepancies may depend on the model used (sciatic nerve ligation, spinal nerve ligation), the time after injury (early vs. late), or sampling methodology. After induction of inflammation, GABA and glycine lose their ability to inhibit spinothalamic tract cells (75). The reduction in the inhibitory (hyperpolarizing) influence of GABA and glycine results in increased excitatory responses to noxious stimuli, thus increasing spinothalamic output to supraspinal centers for the perception of pain.

A third component that may contribute to sensitization of second-order dorsal horn neurons is activation of glial cells, astrocytes, and microglia. Structurally, glial cells surround or encapsulate central nervous system synapses, including the synapses between primary pain afferents and spinal cord pain-transmission neurons. Activation of astrocytes and microglia occurs in a number of pain models, including neuropathic and inflammatory models (76–78). Glial cells are activated in response to the release of the excitatory neurotransmitters from the central terminals of primary pain afferents and dorsal horn neurons. This glial cell activation results in the release of

Figure 4.8. Explanation for the sensitization of pain transmission neurons. **A:** Production and release of nitric oxide from pain transmission neurons in response to recurrent pain input from nociceptors. Release of nitric oxide enhances the release or excitatory neurotransmitters from nociceptors that results in increased activity of pain transmission neurons (PTNs). **B:** Reduction in inhibitory neurotransmitter release from spinal interneurons. Reduced release of inhibitory transmitters at axoaxonic synapses between interneurons and nociceptor terminals results in increased substance P and glutamate release to PTNs. Reduced release of inhibitory neurotransmitters from interneurons connecting to PTNs decreases the direct inhibition of these neurons and results in an increased level of responsiveness to excitatory neurotransmitters. **C:** Glial cells release nitric oxide that enhances excitatory neurotransmitter release from nociceptors, and glial cells also release excitatory neurotransmitters that directly activate PTNs. NMDA, *N*-methyl D-aspartate; EAA, excitatory amino acids; GABA, γ-aminobutyric acid; sub P, substance P.

a variety of substances that can then excite pain-transmission neurons (e.g., glutamate, cytokines), enhance pain neurotransmitter release (e.g., second messengers), or sensitize pain-transmission neurons (e.g., cytokines). When administered spinally, proinflammatory cytokines such as those released by glial cells produce nomifensine behaviors and sensitize dorsal horn neurons (79,80), and spinal blockade of proinflammatory cytokines reverses the hyperalgesia in several animal models of pain (81).

Sensitization of second-order dorsal horn neurons may account in part for chronic pain in the absence of any apparent tissue injury, as well as the hyperalgesia and allodynia commonly associated with many chronic pain conditions. This sensitization of dorsal horn neurons may also help explain why clinical interventions aimed at modifying the peripheral terminals of nociceptors often fail to provide pain relief.

ASCENDING PAIN PATHWAYS: TRANSMISSION OF PAIN SIGNALS TO SUPRASPINAL CENTERS

From the spinal cord, pain signals are conveyed to the brain and brainstem via projection neurons that receive inputs from primary afferent nociceptors directly or indirectly through interneurons. There are several ascending pathways that transmit nociceptive information from somatic and visceral tissue (Fig. 4.9) [for review, see Willis and Westlund (82)]. The spinothalamic tract is the main pathway for transmission of nociceptive information to higher centers (relayed through the thalamus) involved in cortical processing and ultimately the perception of pain. The postsynaptic dorsal column pathway transmits nociceptive visceral stimuli to higher centers. The spinomesencephalic and spinoreticular pathways integrate nociceptive information with areas involved in descending inhibition and autonomic responses associated with pain.

Spinothalamic Tract

The pathway considered by many to be most important for the transmission of nociceptive information is the spinothalamic tract [for review. see Willis and Coggeshall (1)]. The spinothalamic tract transmits information to neurons in the ventroposterior lateral (VPL) nucleus and medial thalamic nuclei, which include the central lateral, central medial, parafascicular, medial dorsal, and posterior complex of the thalamus. From here the VPL projects to the somatosensory cortex (SI and SII), and this pathway is thought to be involved in the sensory-discriminative component of pain. Neurons in the VPL receive convergent input from the dorsal column pathway that transmits information regarding touch sensation, and from the spinothalamic tract that conveys information regarding pain and temperature sensation (83,84). Like dorsal horn neurons, there is also convergent input from cutaneous, joint, muscle, and visceral inputs, thus providing another anatomical basis to explain referred pain. Similarly, somatosensory cortex neurons have convergent input from touch and pain sensations, as well as a variety of peripheral structures (85). The ascending projections from the medial thalamic nuclei and the posterior complex are more diffuse and include areas such as the anterior cingulate and insular cortices. Thus, this pathway is thought to be the basis for the motivational–affective component of pain. Because spinothalamic tract cells were considered to signal pain, it was thought that lesioning this pathway could relieve pain by preventing the signal from reaching the brain. In fact, anterolateral cordotomy, which lesions the spinothalamic tract, does cause analgesia. However, in some patients the pain returns after a few months, limiting the usefulness of this procedure. In most cases this procedure is used as a last resort for clients with cancer pain (86).

The spinothalamic tract cells from laminae I project via the lateral and dorsolateral funiculi to the medial thalamic nuclei. These cells respond almost exclusively to noxious thermal and

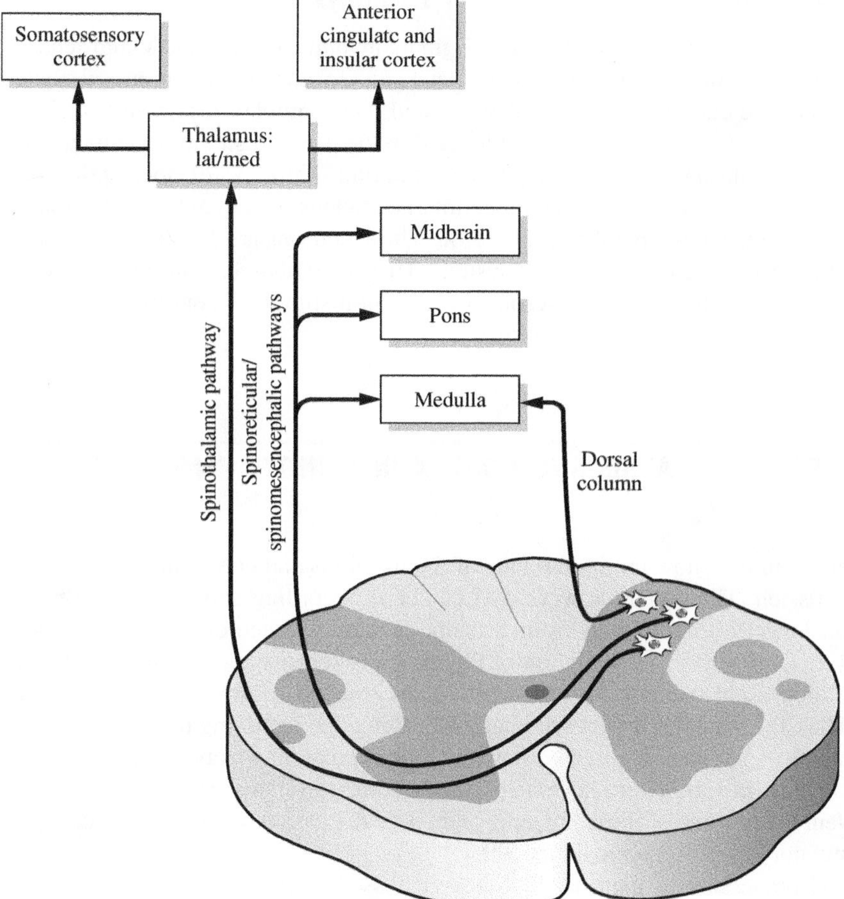

Figure 4.9. Illustration of the ascending pain pathways: spinothalamic, spinoreticular (to midbrain, pons, and medulla), and the postsynaptic dorsal column pathway to the medulla.

mechanical stimuli and may play an important role in thermal nociception (87). It has also been suggested that this pathway may be responsible for activating the body's control systems to limit pain (88–90). However, this model emphasizing the role of laminae I spinothalamic tract neurons has recently been questioned (91). Several investigators support a role for WDR spinothalamic tract cells; particularly those in laminae V (91).

Postsynaptic Dorsal Column Pathway

Postsynaptic dorsal column (PSDC) neurons are located in the dorsal horn of the spinal cord, are activated by innocuous and noxious stimuli, and send projections through the dorsal column to the brainstem (rostral ventromedial medulla, RVM), periaqueductal gray (PAG), and locus coeruleus (LC), in addition to the nucleus cuneatus and gracilis (92). Fifty percent of PSDC neurons, originating in laminae III and IV of the spinal cord, respond only to innocuous cutaneous stimuli, while another 50% are WDR neurons responding to both noxious and innocuous stimuli (93). In addition, PSDC neurons respond to noxious visceral stimuli (94). PSDC neurons do not transmit nociceptive information from cutaneous somatic tissue, but do from visceral tissue (94,95). Midline myelotomy, which removes the postsynaptic dorsal column pathway, selectively eliminates visceral pain in humans (96).

Spinomesencephalic and Spinorecticular Pathways

Cells of the spinomesencephalic pathway originate in laminae I, IV, and V and send projections to the midbrain, particularly the PG, the nucleus cuneiformis, and the pretectal nucleus (1,82). These neurons are classified as NS and WDR and have complex receptive fields. The cells of origin of the spinoreticular pathways are located in the deep dorsal horn, laminae VII and VIII, and project to brainstem areas involved in descending inhibition of nociception (see below). These nuclei include the nucleus gigantocellularis, nucleus paragigantocellularis lateralis, ventrolateral medulla, and the parabrachial region. These neurons are NS and are proposed to activate the human endogenous analgesia system. They may also activate brainstem centers that give rise to many of the autonomic responses to painful stimuli or conditions (e.g., increases in blood pressure, respiratory rate, sweating).

ROLES OF THE THALAMUS AND CORTEX IN PAIN TRANSMISSION AND PROCESSING

A number of studies show the importance of the thalamus and cortex in processing of nociceptive transmission. These include work by Lenz et al. recording and stimulating neurons in the human thalamus (97), recordings from thalamic and cortical neurons in animal models of pain (98), and imaging studies. Stimulation of the principle sensory nucleus in humans can produce pain sensations, and thalamic neurons in humans respond to noxious thermal or mechanical stimuli. Thus, the thalamus appears to integrate information regarding peripheral noxious stimuli. Recordings from neurons in animals show that nociceptive information is processed in the VPL of the thalamus, as well as in the somatosensory cortex, insular cortex, and anterior cingulated cortex. Neurons in some of these thalamic and cortical areas sensitize after tissue injury induced by inflammatory or neuropathic injury (99).

Central processing of pain has also been assessed with imaging techniques such as PET scans that look at cerebral blood flow changes after specific stimuli. It is thought that blood flow increases in an area with increased neuronal activity. Imaging studies of cerebral blood flow in humans reveal that cutaneous tactile/touch stimuli and painful stimuli activate separate regions of the cerebral cortex (100,101). These data show that the cortical regions most reliably activated by painful stimuli are SI and SII, the anterior cingulate cortex, and the anterior insular cortex. Innocuous tactile stimulation also activates the primary and secondary somatosensory cortexes in addition to the posterior cingulate cortex (100). Primary and secondary somatosensory cortexes may be involved in discrimination and localization of a painful stimulus, the sensory–discriminative component of pain (102). The motivational–affective component of pain is thought to involve the anterior cingulate and anterior insular cortexes.

ENDOGENOUS MECHANISMS OF PAIN INHIBITION

Over the past 40 years, substantial evidence has emerged demonstrating that nociceptive transmission throughout the central nervous system is subject to modulation at numerous locations. Experimental findings have demonstrated that the nervous system has the ability to both facilitate and inhibit nociceptive transmission. The focus of this section of the chapter is on how and where pain transmission can be inhibited, and on reviewing the evidence for the existence of endogenous pain-inhibiting processes.

Inhibition of Nociceptive Transmission Between Primary Afferent Nociceptors and Second-order Dorsal Horn Neurons

The foregoing discussion has demonstrated that nociceptive transmission, and hence pain perception can be significantly enhanced by processes that take place within the peripheral nervous system as well as in the central nervous system including the spinal cord dorsal horn is also where inhibition of nociceptive transmission may occur. The basic elements of mechanisms underlying inhibition of pain transmission within the dorsal horn of the spinal cord were first summarized with the publication of the *gate-control theory of pain* postulated by Melzack and Wall (10) in 1965. Melzack and Wall proposed that large diameter, non-nociceptive primary afferent fibers send input to the dorsal horn and interfere with the transmission of pain between nociceptors and dorsal horn neurons by inhibiting or "gating" activity in nociceptors. Their theory also suggested that this inhibitory spinal gating effect was under control descending from higher brain centers, and was activated by both cognitive and subconscious activity at these supraspinal centers. Extensive work has been performed over the last four decades to elucidate the anatomical pathways associated with gate control and the physiologic processes that mediate the inhibition of pain transmission at the spinal level.

Inhibition of Pain Transmission by Stimulation of Innocuous Sensory Afferents

Large-diameter primary afferent neurons can be activated by electrical stimulation of their peripheral terminals and axons or by stimulation of their central processes as they pass through the dorsal (posterior) columns of the spinal cord to the medulla. Peripheral sensory axons associated with nonpainful sensations (e.g., touch) are activated by electrical stimulation applied to the skin using relatively low-amplitude and short-duration electrical pulses. This procedure, brought to the medical community by Wall and Sweet (103), is called *transcutaneous electrical nerve stimulation*. The central processes of large-diameter primary afferents associated with the nonpainful senses can be activated using similar forms of electrical stimulation by placing electrodes over the dorsal (posterior) columns of the spinal cord (i.e., dorsal column stimulation). Using these and other techniques to activate non-nociceptive primary afferent fibers, several important findings have emerged that support the existence of a dorsal horn pain-gating mechanism activated by peripheral, nonpainful, sensory-level stimulation. Both peripheral nerve and dorsal column stimulation reduce the responses of dorsal horn neurons, including STT neurons, evoked by painful stimuli (104–108).

GABA, an inhibitory neurotransmitter in the dorsal horn of the spinal cord, produces both *presynaptic* and *postsynaptic inhibition* (Fig. 4.10). GABA is released in response to dorsal column stimulation, as well as in response to transcutaneous electrical nerve stimulation (TENS) at sensory intensity (109,110). Presynaptic inhibition is mediated by *axoaxononic synapses* between an interneuron that release the inhibitory neurotransmitter GABA and the terminal endings of Aδ and C fibers (Fig. 4.10A). The release of GABA produces presynaptic inhibition of primary afferent nociceptors by reducing the release of neurotransmitters from their central endings. This reduction in neurotransmitter release from the central terminals of primary afferents reduces excitatory input to second-order dorsal horn neurons. GABA also reduces excitability postsynaptically through $GABA_A$ and $GABA_B$ receptors located on spinothalamic neurons (Fig. 4.10B). GABA reduces the excitability of dorsal horn projection neurons, ultimately reducing the net output of signals transmitted to higher centers and thus reducing pain.

Adenosine is a neurotransmitter located in the dorsal horn of the spinal cord that exerts inhibitory actions through activation of the A1 receptor [for review, see Sawynok (111)]. The source of the adenosine and location of the receptors for adenosine have not yet been identified. However, spinal administration of adenosine, A1 receptor agonists, or drugs aimed at reducing

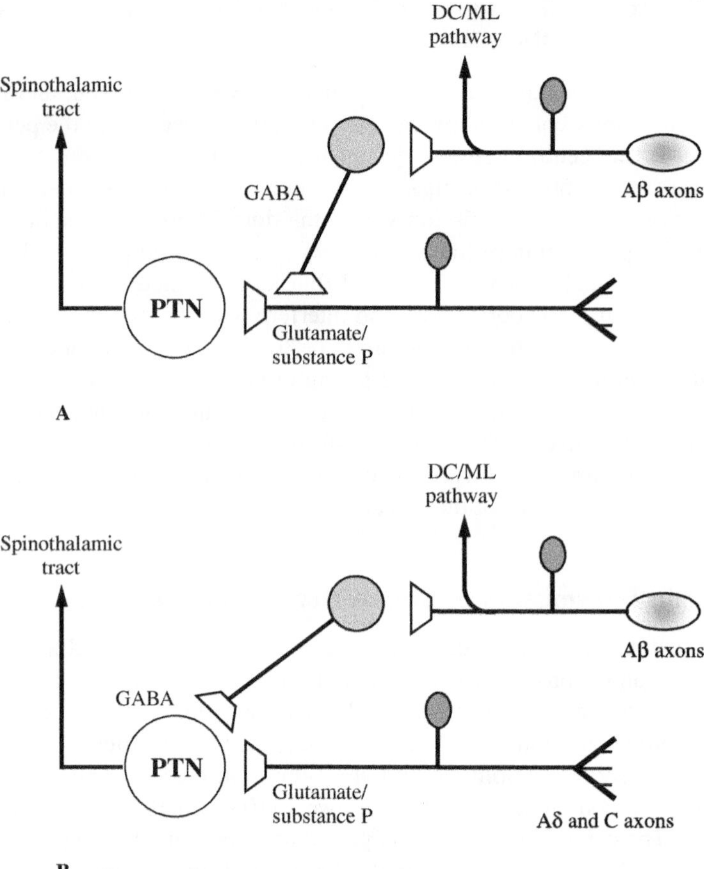

Figure 4.10. Spinal gating of pain transmission. **A:** Presynaptic inhibition of neurotransmitter release from nociceptors. **B:** Postsynaptic inhibition of pain transmission neurons (PTN). GABA, γ-aminobutyric acid; DC/ML, dorsal colum/medial lemniscus.

the degradation of adenosine are analgesic and reduce hyperalgesia in inflammatory and neuropathic pain conditions (112– 116). Recent studies have targeted adenosine modulation in humans as a method of reducing pain (117), and depletion of adenosine in human subjects with caffeine reduces the effectiveness of TENS (118).

Acetylcholine activates muscarinic receptors in the spinal cord. Cholinergic receptors are unique in that they mediate antinociception through interactions with most of the inhibitory receptors [i.e., 5-hydroxytryptamine (5-HT), adrenergic or opioid receptors] in the spinal cord (119–124). Both cholinergic nicotinic and cholinergic muscarinic receptors are localized to the dorsal horn, in Laminae I–IV (125–129). TENS produces part of its inhibitory effects through activation of muscarinic receptors.

Inhibition of Pain Transmission by Activation of Supraspinal Centers

Descending Inhibitory Pathways

Descending modulation of pain transmission can be produced by activation of many areas of the brain and brainstem, including the midbrain PAG, the RVM, and the lateral pontine tegmentum. These three sites were discovered early in the search for supraspinal centers that might give rise to the *descending pain inhibition* pathways originally proposed in the gate-control theory. Anatomically, the PAG sends projections to the RVM and the lateral pontine tegmentum, but not directly to the spinal cord. The RVM and lateral pontine tegmentum then project axons to the spinal cord and reduce dorsal horn pain neuron activity and ultimately the perception of pain.

DESCENDING INHIBITION ARISING FROM THE PAG-RVM

The central inhibitory control of pain was initially discovered by Reynolds (130), who found that electrical stimulation of the PAG in the midbrain produces analgesia in rats. This led to an explosion of work on so-called endogenous analgesia systems [for review, see Fields and Basbaum (131)]. The work focused primarily on two sites, the midbrain PAG and a site in the ventral medulla, the nucleus raphe magnus. Subsequent studies show that other nuclei in the rostral ventral medial medulla (RVM), including the nucleus raphe magnus, nucleus reticularis gigantocellularis pars alpha, and nucleus reticularis paragigantocellularis lateralis, are similarly involved in descending modulation of pain transmission at spinal cord levels (Fig. 4.11) [for review, see Fields and Basbaum (131) and Heinricher (132)]. The RVM projects to the spinal cord via fibers running in the dorsolateral funiculus.

Electrical stimulation of the PAG, which activates the RVM, and direct stimulation of the RVM cause analgesia in rats, cats, and humans (133–135). Electrical (136–138) or chemical (139,140)

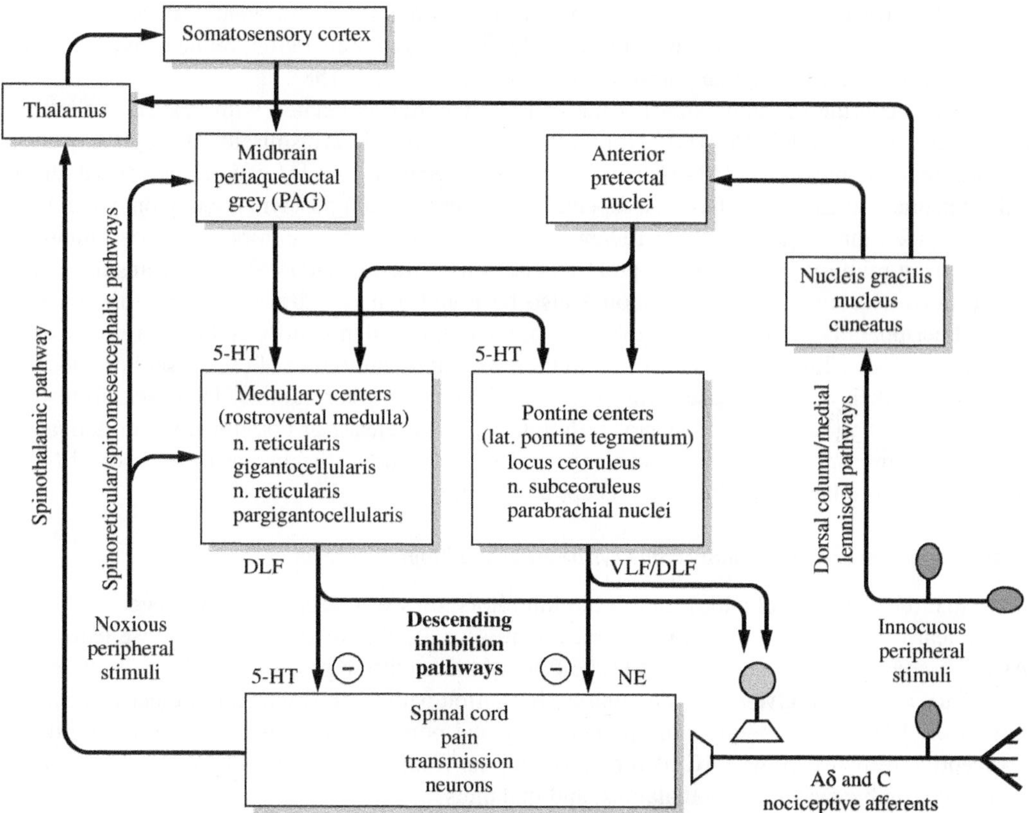

Figure 4.11. Pathways associated with descending inhibition arising from the pons and medulla. These descending inhibition pathways reduce the activity in spinal pain-transmission neurons by presynaptic inhibition of nociceptors and postsynaptic inhibition of pain-transmission neurons. 5-HT, serotonin; DLF, dorsolateral funiculus; VLF, ventrolateral funiculus; NE, norepinephrine.

stimulation of the RVM inhibits reflex and behavioral responses to noxious stimuli and also inhibits neurons in the spinal dorsal horn that receive nociceptive input (141).

Serotonin (5-HT) is a neurotransmitter in the RVM in neurons that send projections to the spinal cord and in PAG neurons that project to the RVM (142,143). Spinal blockade of serotonin receptors also prevents analgesia. In addition, application of serotonin to the spinal cord decreases the activity of dorsal horn neurons, producing analgesia through receptors located both postsynaptically on spinothalamic neurons and presynaptically on primary pain afferent endings (144).

In the spinal cord, three families of serotonin receptors are present: 5-HT1 (two subtypes, 5-HT1A and 5-HT1B), 5-HT2. and 5HT3 receptors (145,146). The role of individual serotonin receptors in nociceptive transmission is controversial. and serotonin receptors have been implicated in both inhibition and facilitation of nociception. 5-HT3 receptors are located on primary afferent pain fibers and dorsal horn pain projection neurons (145) and are involved in descending inhibition from stimulation of the RVM (147–149). 5-HT1A receptors, in contrast, are not found on primary afferent fibers (150) and mediate descending facilitation (147,151–153) as well as inhibition (152,153). 5-HT2 receptors include a number of subtypes that appear to be involved in inhibition of nociceptive responses (151).

DESCENDING INHIBITION ARISING FROM DORSOLATERAL PONS

A second pathway that mediates brainstem descending inhibition arises from neurons in the LC, nucleus subcaeruleus, and parabrachial nucleus of the pons (Fig. 4.11). The axons of these pontine nuclei project to the dorsal horn of the spinal cord through the ventrolateral funiculus. Chemical or electrical stimulation of these nuclei causes antinociception, reduces hyperalgesia, and decreases activity of spinal pain-transmission neurons (154–158).

Norepinephrine (noradrenaline) is the neurotransmitter associated with descending inhibition from pontine nuclei (159,160). Noradrenaline inhibits pain transmission through activation of α_2-adrenergic receptors (161–164). α_2-Adrenergic receptors are located on the central terminals of primary nociceptive afferents, especially nociceptors, and postsynaptically on dorsal horn neurons [see Stone et al. (165) for review]. Activation of these receptors decreases glutamate release from primary afferent nociceptors and decreases the excitatory synaptic transmission to dorsal horn neurons (166,167). It should also be noted that α_2-adrenergic receptors are also located peripherally on the terminal of nociceptors and on inflammatory cells [see references in King et al. (168)]. Taken together with a direct postsynaptic inhibition of the dorsal horn neuron, there would then be a decreased transmission of pain to higher centers. However, following sensory-level high- and low-frequency TENS, there is no release of noradrenaline or activation of spinal or supraspinal α_2-adrenergic receptor (168,169). Part of the analgesic effect of TENS is mediated by peripheral α_2-adrenergic receptors (168).

Activation of Descending Inhibitory Pathways by Brain and Brainstem Areas

Once that the existence of endogenous pain inhibitory sites was demonstrated, it became important to learn what areas of the brain or brainstem were capable of activating of these pathways. As discussed previously, the neurons in the PAG of the midbrain project to both the pontine and medullary nuclei that give rise to descending inhibition pathways. Chemical or electrical activation of the PAG excites neurons in the medullary and pontine nuclei that result in inhibition of nociceptive responses. The PAG also receives inputs from and may be activated by the frontal cortex, the limbic system, hypothalamus, and thalamus.

Another brainstem area that makes similar connections is the anterior pretectal nucleus. A number of lines of evidence suggest an important role for the anterior pretectal nucleus in the activation of descending inhibition pathways (170). First, stimulation of the anterior pretectal nucleus results in long-lasting antinociception without the additional aversive effects seen with stimulation of PAG (171,172). Second, lesions or local anesthetic blockade of the RVM partially reduces anterior pretectal nucleus antinociception (173,174). Blockade of opioid, adrenergic, and serotonergic receptors prevents the analgesia produced by electrical stimulation of the anterior pretectal nucleus (172,175). Of particular relevance to electrotherapy is the finding that the anterior pretectal nucleus receives input from the nucleus gracilis (170,176). The nucleus gracilis, a component of the dorsal column-medial lemniscal system, relays sensory input related to touch, proprioception, and kinesthesia to the somatosensory cortex. It is interesting that electrical stimulation of the dorsal columns, at an intensity that only activates large afferent fibers, excites cells in the anterior pretectal nucleus, and the analgesia produced by stimulation of the dorsal column is abolished by cutting the dorsal column axons rostral to the site of stimulation (177). The activation of descending inhibition pathways resulting from the stimulation of ascending sensory pathways with origins in nonpainful somatosensory systems supports the hypothesis that pain control achieved through innocuous sensory-level stimulation is in part mediated by these pathways.

Although innocuous stimulation may activate descending inhibitory pathways, the most reliable method of activating the PAG, RVM, or pontine cell groups is by noxious stimulation arising from input from spinal cord through the spinomesencephalic and spinoreticular pathways (178). Activation of these systems can also occur from the hypothalamus, cortex, and limbic system.

Descending Inhibition Arising from the Somatosensory Cortex via the Corticospinal Tract

In addition to receiving nociceptive input for discrimination of pain, the somatosensory cortex, also sends fibers that inhibit nociceptive transmission through the corticospinal tract directly to the spinal cord, or indirectly through thalamus or PAG. Electrical stimulation of somatosensory cortex inhibits STT neurons (179). In addition, stimulation of somatosensory cortex causes primary afferent depolarization, a measure of presynaptic inhibition (180). In contrast, lesioning the corticospinal tract eliminates primary afferent depolarization produced by stimulation of the somatosensory cortex (180). These findings demonstrate that inhibition of pain transmission at the spinal cord level from stimulation of the somatosensory cortex is mediated by both presynaptic inhibition of the central terminals of primary afferent nociceptors and postsynaptic inhibition of STT neurons. Thus, activation of the corticospinal tract (as with voluntary exercise) may reduce nociceptive input through the descending postsynaptic inhibition of spinal pain-transmission neurons or presynaptic inhibition primary-afferent pain fibers.

Endogenous Opioid System and Pain Inhibition

Substances derived from opium or opium like compounds have been used for hundreds of years to relieve pain. A resurgence in research investigating the mechanisms underlying "exogenous opioid" analgesia occurred in the early 1970s. At that time it was learned that receptors binding opioids are present in many areas of the central nervous system. Many of the sites containing opioid receptors are the same as associated with stimulation-produced analgesia described above. These areas include the PAG, RVM, and LC, which give rise to descending inhibition of pain, and the spinal cord dorsal horn, where pre- and postsynaptic inhibition of pain transmission occurs. The discovery of opioid receptors throughout the nervous system led to the hypothesis that the central nervous system contains "endogenous substances" with analgesic properties like those of natural or synthetic origin. The endogenous opioids include: β-endorphins, methionine- and leucine-enkephalin, endomorphin 1 and 2, and dynorphin A and B [for review, see Fields and Basbaum (131)]. Each compound has a distinct anatomical distribution and activates specific receptors.

β-Endorphins are found in hypothalamic neurons and in the anterior and intermediate lobes of the pituitary (131). Neurons located in the hypothalamus send β-endorphin projections to the

PAG and can "turn on" the descending inhibitory pathways (181). Release of β-endorphin from the pituitary also occurs with vigorous exercise and stress, and there is an increase in measurable levels in the bloodstream during these times (182–185). β-Endorphins do not readily cross the blood–brain barrier, and thus their role in stress-induced or exercise-induced analgesia is not known. However, removal of the pituitary decreases the effectiveness of stress-induced analgesia (178). As there is an increase in the number of opioid receptors on the peripheral terminals of primary afferent fibers following inflammation, the increased plasma concentrations of β-endorphin likely produce their pain-inhibiting effects peripherally.

Enkephalins, endomorphins, and dynorphins are found in neurons in the brain and dorsal horn in areas involved in analgesia such as the PAG, RVM, and dorsal horn of the spinal cord (131). Activation of opioid receptors with selective agonists, systemically or locally in the PAG, RVM, or spinal cord, produces analgesia and reduces hyperalgesia in a number of pain models, including inflammatory, acid-induced muscle pain, and neuropathic pain (186,187). Dorsal horn neurons containing the neurotransmitter enkephalin produce both presynaptic inhibition of primary afferent nociceptors and postsynaptic inhibition of dorsal horn neurons.

MECHANISMS OF ACTION OF TRANSCUTANEOUS ELECTRICAL NERVE STIMULATION FOR PAIN CONTROL

TENS has been used both experimentally and clinically for more than 40 years to control pain. TENS is noninvasive and employs surface electrodes of various sizes, shapes, and materials to activate peripheral terminals and axons. TENS interventions are characterized by the intensity of stimulation, which is determined by adjustment of the amplitude and duration of pulses, and by the frequency (rate) of the pulses. The intensity of stimulation controls the recruitment of peripheral axons, as discussed in Chapter 3. Frequencies of stimulation generally range from a few (<10) pulses per second (i.e., low) to up to 100 to 150 pulses per second (i.e., high). At the low end of the spectrum, intensity is adjusted to activate the larger diameter sensory afferents; this form of stimulation is referred to as sensory-level stimulation. As the amplitude of stimulation is increased, a muscle contraction may be induced; this form of stimulation is called motor-level stimulation. If the stimulation intensity is increased more, greater numbers of motor axons are activated, and the magnitude of the evoked contraction increases. Increasing intensity of stimulation to higher levels can activate primary afferent nociceptors producing the perception of pain; this is called noxious-level stimulation. At times, depending on the placement of the electrodes and the relative location of peripheral axons, noxious-level stimulation may be reached either before motor axon recruitment, or in the absence of muscle contraction. The point is that all TENS interventions are not the same. TENS interventions differ in terms of intensity and frequency of stimulation as well as in the overall duration (in minutes) of stimulation. These variables characterize the "dosage" of TENS as it is used in contemporary clinical practice. As important as the TENS dosage is the placement and size of the electrodes used during treatment, which should be described in detail in every clinical or experimental study designed to investigate the mechanisms underlying the intervention as well as the efficacy of the intervention.

Although clinically TENS is applied and described in an intensity-dependent and not a frequency-dependent manner, the basic science research to date suggests that the effects of TENS are frequency dependent once a strong sensory intensity (just below motor contraction) is achieved. Increasing intensity to twice the motor threshold has no increased analgesic effect and appears to use the same mechanisms (described below). Thus, this section is organized based on frequency of stimulation as either low (<10 Hz) or high (>50 Hz) and further suborganized by intensity, where applicable. A series of experiments in animals has shown that noxious-level stimulation is also analgesic, this is addressed in a separate section.

Several theories have been put forth to explain the mechanisms of action of TENS. The gate-control theory of pain is most commonly used to explain the inhibition of pain by TENS. According to the gate-control theory of pain, stimulation of large-diameter, primary afferent fibers inhibits nociceptor-evoked responses in the dorsal horn (10). In addition, the original theory suggested that descending inhibitory pathways might exist and that spinal nociceptive transmission may be inhibited by these descending influences. Specific neurotransmitters or their receptors were not suggested at that time because the pharmacology of the nervous system was not yet fully elucidated. There are now much more detailed data on mechanisms of actions of TENS that include anatomical pathways, neurotransmitters and their receptors, and the types of neurons involved in the inhibition of pain transmission at the spinal cord dorsal horn. Release of endogenous opioids has also been used to explain the actions of TENS, particularly low-frequency stimulation. Recent data support this theory for low-frequency as well as for high-frequency TENS stimulation (188).

Effect of Transcutaneous Electrical Nerve Stimulation on Acute Pain Measures and Hyperalgesia

Early studies on mechanisms of action of TENS were performed in normal, uninjured animals. These studies provided valuable information regarding potential mechanisms of action of TENS. More recent studies have translated and extended these data by examining mechanisms of action of TENS in animal models of pain. The animal models of pain that have been used to investigate the mechanisms underlying TENS interventions are outlined in Table 4.6. The studies in animal models of pain have revealed pharmacological and anatomical pathways that mediate the reduction in pain produced by TENS (189).

Effects of High-frequency, Sensory-Intensity Transcutaneous Electrical Nerve Stimulation

In human and animals subjects, recording from the median nerve, high-frequency (100 Hz), sensory-intensity (three times the sensory threshold) TENS activates only large-diameter, Aβ

Table 4.6. Animal Models Used to Study Pain Mechanisms and the Effects of Transcutaneous Electrical Nerve Stimulation Interventions to Control Pain

Type of Pain	*Intervention/Agent*	*Similar to*
Musculoskeletal pain	Ischemia	Peripheral vascular disease
	Repeated acid injections	Noninflammatory chronic pain
	Carrageenan	Inflammatory acute and chronic pain
	Freund adjuvant	Chronic inflammatory pain
	Capsaicin	Acute inflammatory pain
	Formalin	Acute inflammatory pain
Nerve pain	Sciatic nerve ligation	Neuropathic pain
	Spinal nerve ligation	Neuropathic pain
Cutaneous pain	Capsaicin	Acute cutaneous inflammatory pain
	Turpentine oil	Acute cutaneous inflammatory pain
	Formalin	Acute cutaneous inflammatory pain
	Noxious heat	Acute pain
	Noxious mechanical (e.g., pinch)	Acute pain
	Noxious electrical stimulation	Acute pain

Table 4.7. Summary of the Physiologic Mechanisms Underlying Transcutaneous Electrical Nerve Stimulation (TENS) Interventions for the Control of Pain

Type of TENS	*Spinal Cord Gating Mechanisms*	*Descending Inhibitory Mechanisms*	*Endogenous Opioid Mechanisms*	*Serotonin Receptors*	*Noradrenaline Receptors*	*Muscarinic Receptors*
HF/motor	+	+	+	+	+	?
HF/sensory	+	+	+	−	−	+
LF/motor	+	?	+	?	?	?
LF/sensory	+	+	+	+	−	+
HF/noxious	?	+	+	+	+	?
LF/noxious	?	+	+	+	+	?

HF, high frequency; LF, low frequency.
Key: (+), evidence for activation with the specified form of TENS; (−), tested and no effect with the specified form of TENS; (?), equivocal evidence for activation with the specified form of TENS or unknown.

fibers (190,191). Recording from STT cells, stimulation at an intensity activating Aβ fibers, three times the threshold, has no effect on the spontaneous firing rate (104). In contrast, inhibition of dorsal horn neurons and responses to pinch occur with high frequencies at intensities that would be within the sensory stimulation range (105,106). High-frequency TENS at an intensity two times the sensory threshold decreases the reflex ventral root activity produced by stimulation of C fibers (192). However, the studies by Garrison and Foreman (105,106) and by Sjolund (192) show that increasing intensity increases inhibition (see below).

In an animal model of joint inflammation, high-frequency, sensory-intensity TENS has long-lasting effects on both primary and secondary heat and mechanical hyperalgesia (193–195). In fact, these studies show that high-frequency, sensory-intensity TENS partially reverses the primary hyperalgesia and completely reverses the secondary hyperalgesia associated with carrageenan inflammation for 24 hours. Modulation of frequency (4 Hz vs. 100 Hz), intensity (sensory vs. motor), or pulse duration (100 μs vs. 250 μs) demonstrated a frequency-dependent, but not an intensity- or pulse-duration-dependent, effect on primary hyperalgesia to mechanical and heat stimuli in animals with carrageenan paw inflammation (194). The increased responsiveness of dorsal horn neurons to innocuous and noxious mechanical stimuli that occurs after inflammation is completely reduced after high-frequency, sensory-intensity TENS treatment applied to the inflamed paw (196). This reduction in sensitization of high threshold and WDR dorsal horn neurons parallels the effects of TENS on secondary hyperalgesia. Using the sciatic nerve ligation model of neuropathic pain, Somers and Clemente (197) demonstrated that high-frequency, sensory-intensity TENS stimulation over the paraspinal musculature reduced heat but not mechanical hyperalgesia that normally occurs in this model. This inhibition of heat hyperalgesia only occurs if the high-frequency, sensory-level TENS was started the first day after injury, but not if it was started three days after injury.

Several lines of evidence suggest a role for opioid peptides in mediating the effects of high-frequency, sensory-level TENS. Concentrations of β-endorphins increase in the bloodstream and cerebrospinal fluid of healthy subjects after administration of high-frequency, sensory-intensity TENS (198,199). Increased concentrations of methionine enkephalin, a δ-opioid agonist, are observed in the lumbar cerebrospinal fluid after treatment of patients with high-frequency, sensory-intensity TENS (200).

Blockade of δ-opioid receptors in the spinal cord or the RVM reverses the analgesic effect produced by high-frequency, sensory-intensity TENS in animals with carrageenan knee joint inflammation (193,201). A second neurotransmitter that appears to mediate high-frequency, sensory-level TENS effects is acetylcholine. Blockade of muscarinic receptors, which are activated by acetylcholine in the spinal cord, also partially reverses the antihyperalgesia produced by high-frequency, sensory-intensity TENS (202). Another potential neurotransmitter involved in high-frequency, sensory-intensity TENS is adenosine. If human subjects are given caffeine, which blocks adenosine receptors, before treatment with high-frequency, sensory-intensity TENS, the analgesia produced by TENS is significantly reduced compared to placebo treatment (118). In contrast, blockade of serotonin or noradrenergic receptors has no effect on the reversal of hyperalgesia produced by high-frequency, sensory-intensity TENS (202).

Effects of High-Frequency, Motor-Intensity Transcutaneous Electrical Nerve Stimulation

Early studies using acute pain tests show that high-frequency, motor-level TENS increases the tail flick latency to heat (i.e., analgesia) (203,204). Recordings from dorsal horn neurons similarly show that increasing intensity or frequency produces greater decreases in spontaneous activity and responses to noxious pinch (105,106). Thus, TENS at motor intensity is analgesic and reduces activity in neurons that transmit nociceptive information.

In animals that were spinalized to remove descending inhibitory pathways, inhibition of the tail flick by high-frequency, motor-intensity TENS still occurs but is reduced by about 50% (204). Thus, these studies suggest both spinal and descending inhibition are involved in the analgesia produced by high-frequency, motor-intensity TENS. Studies using carrageenan knee joint inflammation suggest that δ-opioid receptors are activated by high-frequency, motor-intensity TENS. Specifically, repeated application of high-frequency, motor-intensity TENS produces tolerance (reduced effectiveness) to the antihyperalgesic effects. This tolerance occurs at spinal opioid receptors because there is a reduced effect of SNC80 (a δ-opioid agonist) when given intrathecally (205). Pharmacologically, high-frequency, motor-intensity TENS is blocked by systemic blockade of opioid receptors with naloxone and systemic depletion of serotonin (203,204).

Effects of Low-Frequency, Sensory-Intensity Transcutaneous Electrical Stimulation

In primates without tissue injury, low-rate burst TENS (3 bursts per second and 7 pulses per burst with an internal frequency of 85 Hz) at an intensity that activates Aβ fibers (presumable sensory intensity, three times the sensory threshold) has no effect on either the spontaneous activity or responses to noxious stimuli of STT cells (104). Low-frequency TENS, regardless of intensity, has no effect on the primary mechanical or heat hyperalgesia produced by carrageenan inflammation (194). However, low-frequency, sensory-intensity TENS fully reverses secondary heat hyperalgesia and partially reverses secondary mechanical hyperalgesia (193,195). In these studies, increasing intensity to twice the motor threshold does not further reduce the secondary mechanical hyperalgesia (195). The increased responsiveness of dorsal horn neurons to innocuous and noxious mechanical stimuli that occurs after inflammation is equally reduced after low-frequency, sensory-intensity TENS treatment of the inflamed paw (201). This reduction in sensitization occurs for high threshold (nociceptive specific) and WDR dorsal horn neurons with a complete reversal of the sensitization.

Low-frequency, sensory-intensity TENS antihyperalgesia is prevented by blockade of μ-opioid receptors with naloxone delivered to the spinal cord or the RVM (193,201). Low-frequency, sensory-intensity TENS is also reduced by blockade of serotonin receptors 5-HT2A and 5-HT3 in the spinal cord. Muscarinic receptors are also implicated in the reversal of hyperalgesia produced by low-frequency, sensory-intensity TENS (202). Taken together, these studies suggest a role of opioid, serotonin, and muscarinic receptors in the spinal cord and supraspinal opioid mechanisms in the action of low-frequency, sensory-intensity TENS.

Effects of Low-Frequency, Motor-Intensity Transcutaneous Electrical Nerve Stimulation

Low-frequency TENS at motor intensity reduces sensitization of dorsal horn neurons and decreases hyperalgesia in animal models of pain. After spinal nerve ligation, Leem et al. (206) recorded responses of dorsal horn neurons before and after application of low-frequency, motor-intensity TENS and compared these effects to those from animals without tissue injury. TENS reduces the responsiveness to noxious mechanical stimulation of dorsal horn neurons in both normal and neuropathic animals. However, the responsiveness of spinal neurons to innocuous mechanical stimulation is only inhibited by TENS in neuropathic animals (206). In rats with nerve injury, low-frequency, motor-intensity TENS reduces mechanical hyperalgesia and cold allodynia (207).

Studies using carrageenan knee joint inflammation suggest that δ-opioid receptors are activated by low-frequency, motor-intensity TENS. Specifically, repeated application of motor-level TENS produces tolerance (reduced effectiveness) to the antihyperalgesic effects. This tolerance occurs at spinal δ-opioid receptors, as demonstrated by the reduced effect of morphine when given intrathecally (205).

The effect of low-frequency, motor-intensity TENS on cold allodynia, but not on mechanical hyperalgesia, is reduced by systemic phentolamine, which blocks α-adrenergic receptors, suggesting that activation of sympathetic noradrenergic receptors may mediate the effects of TENS (207). However, effects of phentolamine could block central receptors, and future studies should address this issue.

Effects of Noxious-Intensity Transcutaneous Electrical Stimulation

Noxious-intensity TENS is expected to activate Aδ nociceptors and would be considered painful. Animal studies show that increasing intensity of stimulation to motor threshold only activates Aα and Aβ fibers; increasing intensity to twice motor threshold activates Aδ nociceptors regardless of frequency (low or high) (191). Therefore, the activation of Aδ nociceptors occurs with motor intensities well above motor threshold and may utilize different mechanisms to reduce pain compared to activation of Aβ fibers alone.

Recordings from STT tract neurons show that both low- and high-frequency TENS at intensities that activate Aδ nociceptors, in addition to Aβ primary afferent fibers, reduces spontaneous activity and responses to noxious heat or pinch (104) and decreases the flexion reflex response to noxious stimuli (192).

Noxious-intensity TENS is typically applied for short durations (<1 minute) to produce pain relief. Various studies have extensively investigated the analgesic effects of brief noxious stimuli applied to the paws (3 minute). Brief noxious stimuli (60 Hz, continuous for 1.5 to 3 minutes) applied to the front paw or the hind paw produce analgesia outside the site of stimulation, in the tail (208–211). The analgesia produced by noxious stimulation involves multiple and distinct pathways. Short-duration foot shock applied to the front paw is reversed by naloxone in the spinal cord (211). In contrast, brief foot shock applied to the hind paw is not naloxone reversible, but longer duration (30 minutes) foot shock applied to the hind paw is naloxone reversible (208–211). Further, the foot shock applied to the forepaw (but not the hind paw) uses serotonin and noradrenaline in the spinal cord (212) and activates the RVM supraspinally (213). In contrast, noxious foot shock applied to the hind paw, but not the forepaw, uses muscarinic receptors supraspinally (214). Thus, short-duration noxious electrical stimuli of the forepaws (but not the hind paws) produces both opioid-mediated analgesia and nonopioid-mediated analgesia depending on the area stimulated. It should be noted that this type of foot shock induced noxious stimulation may be distinctly different from that applied to human subjects for pain relief and is likely a stress-induced analgesic effect. Further, all experiments were done in animals without tissue injury, and effectiveness and mechanisms may be distinctly different in animals with tissue injury.

Similarly, dorsal horn neurons in the spinal cord are strongly inhibited when a noxious stimulation is applied to any part of the body outside the receptive field, called *diffuse noxious inhibitory controls* (DNIC) [see LeBars et al. (215) for review]. DNIC is also thought to be nonopioid mediated and does not involve activation of classical pathways (i.e., PAG and RVM). Rather, the subnucleus reticularis dorsalis in the caudal medulla appears to mediate the inhibition caused by DNIC.

ELECTRODE PLACEMENT IN TRANSCUTANEOUS ELECTRICAL NERVE STIMULATION INTERVENTIONS

In one study, the effect of electrode placement was evaluated by placing electrodes within the receptive field for a STT neuron, outside the receptive field of the neuron but on the same limb, and at the mirror site (104). The greatest degree of inhibition of STT cell activity occurred with electrodes placed within the receptive field for the neuron, and only minimal inhibition occurred when the electrode was placed on the same hind limb but outside the receptive field. These data suggest that electrode placement is important and that the greatest effect will occur if the electrode is placed at the site of injury, where one would be expected to affect the receptive fields of sensitized neurons.

ACCOMMODATION DURING TRANSCUTANEOUS ELECTRICAL NERVE STIMULATION INTERVENTIONS

A common practice in the use of TENS for pain control is to increase the stimulus intensity once accommodation occurs so that the "same stimulus" is being given. Using microneurographic recordings, Janko and Trontelj (216) examined the effects of perceptual accommodation to TENS and the activation of primary afferent fibers in human subjects. Although accommodation to TENS occurred as measured by patient perception, the evoked action potential response did not change. Increasing intensity of the stimulation to give the same perception (as before accommodation) increases the amplitude of the neuronal response. This suggests that there is no need to increase intensity to regain perception of the TENS stimulation, and that increasing intensity to account for accommodation actually increases the initial intensity of stimulation.

AFFERENT FIBERS ACTIVATED BY TRANSCUTANEOUS ELECTRICAL NERVE STIMULATION

It is generally assumed that TENS reduces pain and hyperalgesia through activation of cutaneous afferent fibers because patients perceive the stimulus in the skin. A recent study provides evidence contradictory to this assertion. Using animals with knee joint inflammation, lidocaine was applied to the skin under the electrodes or into the knee joint before TENS (either low-frequency or high-frequency TENS at sensory intensities). TENS was equally effective, compared to placebo, in animals where cutaneous afferents were anesthetized with lidocaine cream, but effects of TENS were prevented when knee joint afferents were anesthetized with lidocaine (191).

COMBINED USE OF PHARMACOLOGICAL AGENTS AND TRANSCUTANEOUS ELECTRICAL NERVE STIMULATION

Clinicians who treat pain, particularly chronic pain, prescribe a combination of exercise and functional training. Chronic pain is also typically managed with pharmaceutical agents, and thus patients are probably treated with a combination of pharmaceutical and nonpharmaceutical agents. Understanding the mechanisms will better assist the clinician in the appropriate choice of pain control treatment. Parameters of stimulation can be based on basic knowledge, and a particular modality such as electrical stimulation can be used in a more educated manner. Specific examples are given below that address these issues.

If a patient is taking opioids (currently those available activate μ-opioid receptors), high-frequency TENS may be more appropriate. Repeated application of opioids produces tolerance to the opioid such that a higher dose is necessary to produce the same effect. This is based on the fact that low-frequency, sensory-intensity TENS, but not high-frequency, sensory-intensity TENS, is ineffective if given in animals tolerant to morphine (217). Furthermore, it follows that repeated treatment with the same frequency of TENS would produce tolerance to its analgesic effects. Indeed, daily treatment with either low-frequency or high-frequency TENS in animals with knee joint inflammation produces tolerance to TENS and a cross-tolerance to either spinally administered μ- or δ-opioid agonists, respectively (205). Thus, TENS is ineffective if morphine tolerance is present, and it produces opioid tolerance with repeated use.

It might be possible to enhance the effects of TENS clinically if given in combination with certain agonists or antagonists. High-frequency TENS only partially reduces primary hyperalgesia, and low-frequency TENS is ineffective on primary hyperalgesia (194). However, either high- or low-frequency TENS is more effective in reducing primary hyperalgesia if given in combination with acute administration of morphine (218) or clonidine (219). This is likely a result of synergism between endogenous opioid agonists released by TENS and the α_2 agonist clonidine. Use of TENS in combination with morphine or clonidine should reduce the dose of morphine or clonidine necessary to reduce hyperalgesia, and thus reduce side effects of morphine and increase analgesia.

SUMMARY

One objective of this chapter was to provide a more contemporary perspective on the sensory pathways associated with pain transmission and perception as a basis for understanding the multidimensional nature of pain and a number of clinical phenomena related to pain. A second objective was to discuss endogenous pain control systems and review evidence that illustrates how these systems influence components of the pain pathways to reduce pain. Finally, the chapter provided a review of the scientific evidence that illustrates how various TENS interventions activate endogenous analgesic systems to control pain. Issues related to the actual clinical efficacy of TENS for pain control are presented in Chapter 5.

The data summarized support the theory that low-frequency TENS (sensory and motor) activates descending inhibitory pathways from the RVM to the spinal cord to produce analgesia by activation of serotonin, acetylcholine, and μ-opioid receptors in the spinal cord. In contrast, high-frequency TENS (sensory and motor) activates descending inhibitory pathways from the RVM to the spinal cord to produce analgesia by activation of acetylcholine and δ-opioid receptors in the spinal cord. Noxious-intensity TENS has multiple mechanisms (opioid and nonopioid), but likely involves activation of descending inhibitory pathways from the brainstem, RVM, PAG, and subnucleus reticularis dorsalis to produce inhibition via opioid, serotonin, and/or noradrenergic receptors in the spinal cord. Low and high frequency, as well as sensory-, motor-, and noxious-intensity TENS all produce analgesia in animal models of pain and reduce responses of dorsal horn neurons to nociceptive stimuli.

SELF-STUDY QUESTIONS

For answers, see Appendix B.

1. Define the following terms: pain, hyperalgesia, allodynia, and referred pain.
2. Compare and contrast acute pain and chronic pain.
3. Diagram the simplified three-neuron pathway for pain transmission and identify the value and the limitations of this concept.
4. Describe the dimensions of pain and neuroanatomical pathways that appear to mediate each dimension.
5. Characterize primary pain afferents in terms of the type of neuron, the locations of their cell bodies, the sites of origin of their peripheral processes, and the destination of their central processes.
6. Identify the chemicals released at the site of tissue inflammation that activate primary nociceptors.
7. Discuss the difference in pain responses between primary afferent fibers innervating skin, muscle, and joint.
8. Name three excitatory neurotransmitters found in the central terminals of primary afferent nociceptors and their respective receptors on spinal cord pain transmission neurons.
9. Compare and contrast the types of spinal cord pain-transmission neurons.
10. Describe how the inputs from peripheral nociceptors to spinal cord pain-transmission neurons may provide an explanation for referred pain.
11. Characterize sensitization of primary nociceptive afferents and identify the substances that appear to produce this sensitization.
12. What are the three processes that give rise to sensitization of spinal cord pain-transmission neurons?
13. Describe the gate-control theory of pain.
14. What two processes appear to reduce pain transmission between primary pain afferents and spinal cord pain-transmission neurons?
15. Describe the ascending pain pathways from the spinal cord to supraspinal centers.
16. What pathways are involved in descending inhibition of pain transmission?
17. Describe the endogenous opioid system and its role in controlling pain transmission.
18. Describe potential mechanisms of action for high-frequency TENS, both sensory and motor intensity. Describe similarities and differences between these.
19. Describe the potential mechanisms of action for noxious-level TENS.

20. Based on the pharmacology of low-frequency TENS (sensory and/or motor intensity), what potential pharmaceutical therapies could be combined with TENS to enhance its effectiveness?

REFERENCES

1. Willis WD, Coggeshall RE. *Sensory Mechanisms of the Spinal Cord.* Kluwer Academic, New York; 2004.
2. McMahon SB, Koltzenberg M. *Textbook of Pain.* 5th ed. Edinburgh: Churchill Livingstone; 2006.
3. Loeser JD, Butler SHC, Chapman R, et al. *Bonica's Management of Pain.* Philadelphia: Lippincott Williams & Wilkins; 2001.
4. Merskey H, Bogduk N. *Classification of Chronic Pain: Description of Chronic Pain Syndromes and Definition of Pain Terms.* Seattle: IASP Press; 1994.
5. Melzack R, Casey KL. Sensory, motivational, and central control determinants of pain: a new conceptual model. In Kenshalo D, ed. *The Skin Senses* Springfield, IL: Charles C. Thomas; 1968:423–443.
6. Cervero F, Laird JM. Mechanisms of touch-evoked pain (allodynia): a new model. *Pain.* 1996; 68:13–23.
7. Head H. On disturbances of sensation with especial reference to the pain of visceral disease. *Brain.* 1893;16:1–132.
8. IASP Task Force on Taxonomy. Available at: http://www.iasp-pain.org/dict_toc.html. Accessed May 2007. [Adapted from Merskey H, Bogduk N. *Classification of Chronic Pain: Descriptions of Chronic Pain Syndromes and Definitions of Pain Terms.* 2nd ed. Seattle, Wash: IASP Press; 1994.]
9. Robinson AJ. Central nervous system pathways for pain transmission and pain control. *J. Hand Ther.* 1997;10:64–77.
10. Melzack R, Wall PD. Pain mechanisms: a new theory. *Science.* 1965;150:971–978.
11. Lloyd DPC, Chang HT. Afferent fibers in muscle nerves. *J Neurophysiol.* 1948;11:199–207.
12. Gasser HS, Grundfest H. Average diameters in relation to spike dimensions and conduction velocity in mammalian fibers. *Am J Physio.* 1939;127:393.
13. Schaible H-G, Schmidt RF. Effects of an experimental arthritis on the sensory properties of fine articular afferent units. *J Neurophysiol.* 1985;54:1109–1122.
14. Schaible H-G, Schmidt RF. Time course of mechanosensitivity changes in articular afferents during a developing experimental arthritis. *J Neurophysiol.* 1988;60:2180–2194.
15. Berberich P, Hoheisel U, Mense S. Effects of a carrageenan induced myositis on the discharge properties of group III and IV muscle receptors in the cat. *J Neurophysiol.* 1988;59:1395–1409.
16. Diehl B, Hoheisel U, Mense S. Histological and neurophysiological changes induced by carrageenan in skeletal muscle of cat and rat. *Agents Actions.* 1988;25:210–213.
17. Mense S, Stahnke M. Responses in muscle afferent fibres of slow conduction velocity to contraction and ischaemia in the cat. *J Physiol.* 1983;342:383–387.
18. Marchettini P. Muscle pain: animal and human experimental and clinical studies. *Muscle Nerve,* 1993;16:1033–1039.
19. Mense S. Nociception from skeletal muscle in relation to clinical muscle pain. *Pain.* 1993; 54:241–289.
20. Schaible H-G, Grubb BD. Afferent and spinal mechanisms of joint pain. *Pain.* 1993;55:5–54.
21. Kellgren JH. Observations on referred pain arising from muscle. *Clin Sci.* 1938;3:175–190.
22. Simone DA, Marchettini P, Caputi G, et al. Identification of muscle afferents subserving sensation of deep pain in humans. *J Neurophysiol.* 1994;72:883–889.
23. Marchettini P, Cline M, Ochoa J. Innervation territories for touch and pain afferents of single fascicles of the human ulnar nerve. *Brain.* 1990;113:1491–1500.

24. Svensson P, Beydoun A, Morrow TJ, et al. Human intramuscular and cutaneous pain: psychophysical comparisons. *Exp Brain Res.* 1997;114:390–392.

25. Witting N, Svensson P, Gottrup H, et al. Intramuscular and intradermal injection of capsaicin: a comparison of local and referred pain. *Pain.* 2000;84:407–412.

26. Schneider SP, Perl ER. Selective excitation of neurons in the mammalian spinal dorsal horn by aspartate and glutamate *in vitro*: correlation with location and synaptic input. *Brain Res.* 1985;360:339–343.

27. Schneider SP, Perl ER. Comparison of primary afferent and glutamate excitation of neurons in the mammalian spinal dorsal horn. *J Neurosci.* 1988;8:2062–2073.

28. Hollmann M, Hartley M, Heinemann S. Ca2+ permeability of KA-AMPA–gated glutamate receptor channels depends on subunit composition. *Science.* 1991;252:851–853.

29. Mao J, Price DD, Hayes RL, et al. Differential roles of NMDA and non-NMDA receptor activation in induction and maintenance of thermal hyperalgesia in rats with painful peripheral mononeuropathy. *Brain Res.* 1992;598:271–288.

30. Sorkin LS, Yaksh TL, Doom CM. Pain models display differential sensitivity to Ca2+-permeable non-NMDA glutamate receptor antagonists. *Anesthesiology.* 2001;95:965–973.

31. Zahn PK, Brennan TJ. Lack of effect of intrathecally administered N-methyl-D-aspartate receptor antagonists in a rat model for postoperative pain. *Anesthesiology.* 1998;88:143–156.

32. Zahn PK, Umali E, Brennan TJ. Intrathecal non-NMDA excitatory amino acid receptor antagonists inhibit pain behaviors in a rat model of postoperative pain. *Pain.* 1998;74:213–223.

33. Millan MJ. The induction of pain: an integrative review. *Prog Neurobiol.* 1999;57:1–164.

34. Zubrzycka M, Janecka A. Substance P: transmitter of nociception minireview). *Endocr Regul.* 2000;34:195–201.

35. Wilcox GL. Pharmacological studies of grooming and scratching behavior elicited by spinal substance P and excitatory amino acids. *Ann NY Acad Sci.* 1988;525:228–236.

36. Radhakrishnan V, Henry JL. Novel substance P antagonist, CP-96345, blocks responses of cat spinal dorsal horn neurons to noxious cutaneous stimulation and substance P. *Neurosci Lett.* 1991;132:39–43.

37. Sluka KA, Milton MA, Westlund KN, et al. Differential roles of neurokinin 1 and neurokinin 2 receptors in the development and maintenance of heat hyperalgesia induced by acute inflammation. *Br J Pharmacol.* 1997;120:1263–1273.

38. Fleetwood-Walker SM, Mitchell R, Hope PJ, et al. The involvement of neurokinin receptor subtypes in somatosensory processing in the superficial dorsal horn of the cat. *Brain Res.* 1990;519:169–182.

39. Yashpal K, Radhakrishnan V, Coderre TJ, et al. CP-96,345, but not its stereoisomer, CP,96,344, blocks the nociceptive responses to intrathecally administered substance P and to noxious thermal and chemical stimuli in the rat. *Neuroscience.* 1993;52:1039–1047.

40. Radhakrishnan V, Henry JL. Antagonism of nociceptive responses of cat spinal dorsal horn neurons *in vivo* by the NK-1 receptor antagonists CP-96,345 and CP-99,994, but not by CP-96,344. *Neuroscience.* 1995;64:943–958.

41. Neugebauer V, Weiretter F, Schaible H-G. Involvement of substance P and neurokinin-1 receptors in the hyperexcitability of dorsal horn neurons during development of acute arthritis in rat's knee joint. *JJ Neurophysiol.* 1995;73:1574–1583.

42. Suzuki R, Morcuende S, Webber M, et al. Superficial NK1-expressing neurons control spinal excitability through activation of descending pathways. *Nature Neurosci.* 2002;5:1319–1326.

43. Khasabov SG, Rogers SD, Ghilardi JR, et al. Spinal neurons that possess the substance P receptor are required for the development of central sensitization. *J Neurosci.* 2002;22:9086–9098.

44. Sun RQ, Tu YJ, Lawand NB, et al. Calcitonin gene-related peptide receptor activation produces PKA- and PKC-dependent mechanical hyperalgesia and central sensitization. *J. Neurophysiol.* 2004;92:2859–2866.

45. Neugebauer V, Ruemenapp P, Schaible, H-G. Calcitonin gene-related peptide is involved in the spinal processing of mechanosensory input from the rat's knee joint and in the generation and maintenance of hyperexcitability of dorsal horn neurons during development of acute inflammation. *Neuroscience.* 1996;71:1095–1109.

46. Sun RQ, Lawand NB, Willis WD. The role of calcitonin gene-related peptide (CGRP) in the generation and maintenance of mechanical allodynia and hyperalgesia in rats after intradermal injection of capsaicin. *Pain.* 2003;104:201–208.
47. Schaible H-G, Hope PJ, Lang CW, et al. Calcitonin gene-related peptide causes intraspinal spreading of substance P released by peripheral terminals. *Eur J Neurosci.* 1992;4:750–757.
48. Woolf CJ, Wiesenfeld-Hallin Z. Substance P and calcitonin gene-related peptide synergistically modulate the gain of the nociceptive flexor withdrawal reflex in the rat. *Neurosci Lett.* 1986;66:226–230.
49. Hylden JLK, Nahin RL, Traub RJ, Dubner R. Expansion of receptive fields of spinal lamina I projection neurons in rats with unilateral adjuvant-induced inflammation: the contribution of dorsal horn mechanisms. *Pain.* 1989;37:229–243.
50. Schaible H-G, Schmidt RF, Willis WD. Enhancement of the responses of ascending tract cells in the cat spinal cord by acute inflammation of the knee joint. *Exp Brain Res.* 1987;66:489–499.
51. Hoheisel U, Mense S, Simons DG, et al. Appearance of new receptive fields in rat dorsal horn neurons following noxious stimulation of skeletal muscle: a model for referral of muscle pain? *Neurosci Lett.* 1993;153:9–12.
52. Palecek J, Dougherty PM, Kim SH, et al. Responses of spinothalamic tract neurons to mechanical and thermal stimuli in an experimental model of peripheral neuropathy in primates. *JJ Neurophysiol.* 1992;68:1951–1965.
53. Davies SN, Lodge D. Evidence for involvement of N-methylaspartate receptors in 'wind- up' of class 2 neurons in the dorsal horn of the rat. *Brain Res.* 1987;424:402–406.
54. Dickenson AH, Sullivan AF. Subcutaneous formalin-induced activity of dorsal horn neurones in the rat: differential response to an intrathecal opiate administered pre or post formalin. *Pain.* 1987;30:349–360.
55. Woolf CJ, Thompson SW. The induction and maintenance of central sensitization is dependent on N-methyl-D-aspartic acid receptor activation; implications for the treatment of post injury pain hypersensitivity. *Pain.* 1991;44:293–299.
56. Sluka KA, Westlund KN. An experimental arthritis in rats: dorsal horn aspartate and glutamate increases. *Neurosci Lett.* 1992;145:141–144.
57. Malmberg AB,Yaksh TL. Hyperalgesia mediated by spinal glutamate or substance P receptor blocked by spinal cyclooxygenase inhibition. *Science.* 1992;257:1276–1279.
58. Skyba DA, Lisi TL, Sluka KA. Excitatory amino acid concentrations increase in the spinal cord dorsal horn after repeated intramuscular injection of acidic saline. *Pain.* 2005;119:142–149.
59. Dougherty PM, Palecek J, Paleckova V, et al. The role of NMDA and non-NMDA excitatory amino-acid receptors in the excitation of primate spinothalamic tract neurons by mechanical, chemical, thermal, and electrical stimuli. *J Neurosci.* 1992;12:3025–3041.
60. Chapman V, Dickenson AH. Time-related roles of excitatory amino acid receptors during persistent noxiously evoked responses of rat dorsal horn neurones. *Brain Res.* 1995;703:45–50.
61. Neugebauer V, Lucke T, Schaible HG. N-Methyl-D-aspartate NMDA) and non-NMDA receptor antagonists block the hyper excitability of dorsal horn neurons during development of acute arthritis in rats knee joint. *JJ Neurophysiol.* 1993;70:1365–1377.
62. Ren K, Hylden JL, Williams GM, et al. The effects of a non-competitive NMDA receptor antagonist, MK-801, on behavioral hyperalgesia and dorsal horn neuronal activity in rats with unilateral inflammation. *Pain.* 1992;50:331–344.
63. Sluka KA, Westlund KN. Centrally administered non-NMDA but not NMDA receptor antagonists block peripheral knee joint inflammation. *Pain.* 1993;55:217–225.
64. Skyba DA, King EW, Sluka KA. Effects of NMDA and non-NMDA inotropic glutamate receptor antagonists on the development and maintenance of hyperalgesia induced by repeated intramuscular injection of acidic saline. *Pain.* 2002;98:69–78.
65. Coderre TJ, Fisher K, Fundytus ME. The role of inotropic and metabotropic glutamate receptors in persistent nociception. In Jensen TJ, Turner JA, Wiesenfeld-Hallin Z, eds. *Proceedings of the 8th World Congress on Pain.* Seattle, Wash: IASP Press; 1997:259–275.

66. Calcutt NA, Chaplan SR. Spinal pharmacology of tactile allodynia in diabetic rats. *Br J Pharmacol.* 1997;122:1478–1482.

67. Mao J, Price DD, Hayes RL, et al. Differential roles of NMDA and non-NMDA receptor activation in induction and maintenance of thermal hyperalgesia in rats with painful peripheral mononeuropathy. *Brain Res.* 1992;598:271–288.

68. Moore KA, Kohno T, Karchewski LA, et al. Partial peripheral nerve injury promotes a selective loss of GABAergic inhibition in the superficial dorsal horn of the spinal cord. *J Neurosci.* 2002;22:6724–6731.

69. Ibuki T, Hama AT, Wang X-T, et al. Loss of GABA-immunoreactivity in the spinal dorsal horn of rats with peripheral nerve injury and promotion of recovery by adrenal medullary grafts. *Neuroscience.* 1997;76:845–858.

70. Eaton MJ, Plunkett JA, Karmally S, et al. Changes in GAD- and GABA-immunoreactivity in the spinal dorsal horn after peripheral nerve injury and promotion of recovery by lumbar transplants of immortalized serotonergic precursors. *J Chem Neuroanat.* 1998;16:57–72.

71. Ralston DD, Behbehani M, Sehlhorst SC, et al. Decreased GABA immunoreactivity in rat dorsal horn is correlated with pain behavior: a light and electron microscopic study. In: Jensen TS, Turner JA, Wiesenfeld-Hallin Z, eds. *Proceedings of the Eighth World Congress on Pain.* Seattle, Wash: IASP Press; 1997:547–560.

72. Somers DL, Clemente FR. Dorsal horn synaptosomal content of aspartate, glutamate, glycine and GABA are differentially altered following chronic constriction injury to the rat sciatic nerve. *Neurosci Lett.* 2002;323:171–174.

73. Satoh O, Omote K. Roles of monoaminergic, glycinergic and GABAergic inhibitory systems in the spinal cord in rats with peripheral mononeuropathy. *Brain Res.* 1996;728:27–36.

74. Polgar E, Hughes DI, Riddell JS, et al. Selective loss of spinal GABAergic or glycinergic neurons is not necessary for development of thermal hyperalgesia in the chronic constriction injury model of neuropathic pain. *Pain.* 2003;104:229–239.

75. Lin Q, Peng YB, Willis WD. Inhibition of primate spinothalamic tract neurons by spinal glycine and GABA is reduced during central sensitization. *JJ Neurophysiol.* 1996;76:1005–1014.

76. Garrison CJ, Dougherty PM, Kajander KC, et al. Staining of glial fibrillary acidic protein GFAP) in lumbar spinal cord increases following a sciatic nerve constriction injury. *Brain Res.* 1991;565:1–7.

77. Sweitzer SM, Colburn RW, Rutowski M, et al. Acute peripheral inflammation induces moderate glial activation and spinal IL-1 beta expression that correlates with pain behavior in the rat. *Brain Res.* 1999;829:209–221.

78. Fu Y, Light AR, Matsushma GK, et al. Microglial reactions after subcutaneous formalin injection into the rat hindpaw. *Brain Res.* 1999;825:59–67.

79. DeLeo JA, Colburn RW, Nichols M, et al. Interleukin IL)-6 mediated hyperalgesia/allodynia and increased spinal IL-6 in a rat mononeuropathy model. *J Interferon Cytokine Res.,* 1996;16, 695–700.

80. Reeve AJ, Patel S, Fox A, et al. Intrathecally administered endotoxin or cytokines produce allodynia, hyperalgesia and changes in spinal cord neuronal responses to nociceptive stimuli in the rat. *Eur J Pain.* 2000;4:247–257.

81. Watkins LR, Milligan ED, Maier SF. Glial activation: a driving force for pathological pain. *Trends Neurosci.* 2001;24:450–455.

82. Willis WD, Westlund KN. Neuroanatomy of the pain system and of the pathways that modulate pain. *J Clin Neurophysiol.* 1997;14:2–31.

83. Ralston HJ III, Ralston DD. Medial lemniscal and spinal projections to the macaque thalamus: an electron microscopic study of differing GABAergic circuitry serving thalamic somatosensory mechanisms. *J Neurosci.* 2001;14:2485–2502.

84. Jones SL, Light AR. Serotoninergic medullary raphespinal projection to the lumbar spinal cord in the rat: a retrograde immunohistochemical study. *J Comp Neurol.* 1992;322:599–610.

85. Kenshalo DR, Iwata K, Sholas M, et al. Response properties and organization of nociceptive neurons in area 1 of monkey primary somatosensory cortex. *JJ Neurophysiol.* 2000;84:719–729.

86. Garber JE, Hassenbusch SJ. Neurosurgical operations on the spinal cord. InLoeser JD, Butler SH, Chapman CR, Turk DC, eds. *Bonica's Management of Pain.* 3rd ed. – New York: Lippincott Williams & Wilkins; 1999:2023–2037.

87. Craig AD, Bushnell MC, Zhang ET, et al. A thalamic nucleus specific for pain and temperature sensation. *Nature.* 1994;372:770–773.

88. McMahon SB, Wall PD. Descending excitation and inhibition of spinal cord lamina I projection neurons. *JJ Neurophysiol.* 1988;59:1204–1219.

89. Wall PD. The biological function and dysfunction of different pain mechanisms. In: Sicuteri F, ed. *Advances in Pain Research and Therapy.* Vol 20. New York: Raven Press; 1992:19–28.

90. Rees H, Roberts MHT. The anterior pretectal nucleus: a proposed role in sensory processing. *Pain.* 1993;53:121–135.

91. Willis WD, Zhang X, Honda CN, et al. A critical review of the role of the proposed VMpo nucleus in pain . *J Pain.* 2002;3:79–94.

92. Wang CC, Willis WD, Westlund KN. Ascending projections from the area around the spinal cord central canal: a *Phaseolus vulgaris* leucoagglutinin study in rats. *J Comp Neurol.* 1999;415:341–367.

93. Lu GW, Bennett GJ, Nishikawa N, et al. Extra- and intracellular recordings from dorsal column postsynaptic spinomedullary neurons in the cat. *Exp Neurol.* 1983;82: 456–477.

94. Al Chaer ED, Westlund KN, Willis WD. Sensitization of postsynaptic dorsal column neuronal responses by colon inflammation. *Neuro Report.* 1997;8:3267–3273.

95. Cliffer KD, Giesler GJ Jr. Postsynaptic dorsal column pathway of the rat. III. Distribution of ascending afferent fibers. *J Neuorsci.* 1989;9:3146–3168.

96. Gildenberg PL, Hirshberg RM. Limited myelotomy for the treatment of intractable cancer pain. *J Neurol Neurosurg Psychiatry.* 1984;47:94–96.

97. Lenz FA, Lee JI, Garonzik IM, et al. Plasticity of pain-related neuronal activity in the human thalamus. *Prog Brain Res.* 2000;129:259–273.

98. Treede RD. Transduction and transmission properties of primary nociceptive afferents. *Ross Fiziol Zh Im I M Sechenova.* 1999;85; 205–211.

99. Guilbaud G. 15 Years of explorations in some supraspinal structures in rat inflammatory pain models, some information, but further questions. *Pain Forum.* 1994;3:168–179.

100. Coghill RC, Talbot JD, Evans AC, et al. Distributed processing of pain and vibration by the human brain. *J Neurosci.* 1994;14:4095–4108.

101. Jones BE, Holmes CJ, Rodrignez-Veiga E, et al. GABA-synthesizing neurons in the medulla: their relationship to serotonin-containing and spinally projecting neurons in the rat. *J Comp Neurol.* 1991;313:349–367.

102. Rainville P, Duncan GH, Price DD, et al. Pain affect encoded in human anterior cingulate but not somaotosensory cortex. *Science.* 1997;277:968–971.

103. Wall PD, Sweet WH. Temporary abolition of pain in man. *Science.* 1967;155:108–109.

104. Lee KH, Chung JM, Willis WD. Inhibition of primate spinothalamic tract cells by TENS. *J Neurosurg.* 1985;62:276–287.

105. Garrison DW, Foreman RD. Decreased activity of spontaneous and noxiously evoked dorsal horn cells during transcutaneous electrical nerve stimulation TENS *Pain.* 1994;58:309–315.

106. Garrison DW, Foreman RD. Effects of prolonged transcutaneous electrical nerve stimulation TENS) and variation of stimulation variables on dorsal horn cell activity. *Eur J Phys Med Rehab.* 1997;6:87–94.

107. Foreman RD, Applebaum AE, Beall JE, et al. Responses of primate spinothalamic tract neurons to electrical stimulation of hindlimb peripheral nerves. *JJ Neurophysiol.* 1975;38:132–145.

108. Foreman RD, Beall JE, Applebaum AE, et al. Effects of dorsal column stimulation on primate spinothalamic tract neurons. *JJ Neurophysiol.* 1976;39:534–546.

109. Linderoth B, Stiller CO, Gunasekera L, et al. Gamma-aminobutyric acid is released in the dorsal horn by electrical spinal cord stimulation: an in vivo microdialysis study in the rat. *Neurosurgery.* 1994;34:484–488 [discussion, 488–489].

110a. Maeda Y, Lisi TL, Vance CG, Sluka KA. Release of GABA and activation of GABA (A) in the spinal cord mediates effects of TENS in rats. *Brain Res.* 2007;1136:43–50.

110b. Sluka KA, Vance CG, Lisi TL. High frequency, but not low frequency, transcutaneous electrical nerve stimulation reduces aspartate and glutamate release in spinal cord dorsal horn. *J Neurochem.* 2005;95:1794–1801.

111. Sawynok J. Adenosine receptor activation and nociception. *Eur J Pharmacol.* 1998;317:1–11.

112. Sawynok J, Reid A, Nance D. Spinal antinociception by adenosine analogs and morphine after intrathecal administration of the neurotoxins capsaicin, 6-hydroxydopamine and 5,7-dihydroxytryptamine. *J Pharmacol Exp Ther.* 1991;258:370–380.

113. Sawynok J, Sweeney MI, White TD. Classification of adenosine receptors mediating antinociception in the rat spinal cord. *BrJ Pharmacol.* 1986;88:923–930.

114. Pan HL, Xu Z, Leung E, et al. Allosteric adenosine modulation to reduce allodynia. *Anesthesiology.* 2001;95:416–420.

115. Li X, Conklin D, Pan HL, et al. Allosteric adenosine receptor modulation reduces hypersensitivity following peripheral inflammation by a central mechanism. *J Pharmacol Exp Ther.* 2003; 305:950–955.

116. Jarvis MF, Mikusa J, Chu KL, et al. Comparison of the ability of adenosine kinase inhibitors and adenosine receptor agonists to attenuate thermal hyperalgesia and reduce motor performance in rats. *Pharmacol Biochem Behav.* 2002;73:573–581.

117. Eisenach JC, Curry R, Hood DD. Dose response of intrathecal adenosine in experimental pain and allodynia. *Anesthesiology.* 2002;97:938–942.

118. Marchand S, Li J, Charest J. Effects of caffeine on analgesia from transcutaneous electrical nerve stimulation. *N Engl J Med.* 1995;333:325–326.

119. Chiang CY, Zhuo M. Evidence for the involvement of a descending cholinergic pathway in systemic morphine analgesia. *Brain Res.* 1989;478:293–300.

120. Gordh T, Jansson I, Hartvig P, et al. Interactions between noradrenergic and cholinergic mechanisms involved in spinal nociceptive processing. *Acta Anaesthesiol Scand.* 1989;33:39–47.

121. Li YJ, Zhang ZH, Chen JY, et al. Effects of intrathecal naloxone and atropine on the nociceptive suppression induced by norepinephrine and serotonin at the spinal level in rats. *Brain Res.* 1994;666:113–116.

122. Obata H, Saito S, Sasaki M, et al. Possible involvement of a muscarinic receptor in the anti-allodynic action of a 5-HT2 receptor agonist in rats with nerve ligation injury. *Brain Res.* 2002;932:124–128.

123. Chen SR, Pan HL. Spinal endogenous acetylcholine contributes to the analgesic effect of systemic morphinein rats. *Anesthesiology.* 2001;95:525–530.

124. Honda K, Koga K, Moriyama T, et al. Intrathecal alpha2 adrenoceptor agonist clonidine inhibits mechanical transmission in mouse spinal cord via activation of muscarinic M1 receptors. *Neurosci. Lett.* 2002;322:161–164.

125. Arimatsu Y, Seto A, Amano T. An atlas of alpha-bungarotoxin binding sites and structures containing acetylcholinesterase in the mouse central nervous system. *J Comp Neurol.* 1981;198:603–631.

126. Ninkovic M, Hunt SP. Alpha-bungarotoxin binding sites on sensory neurons and their axonal transport in sensory afferents. *Brain Res.* 1983;272:57–69.

127. Kayaalp SO, Neff NH. Regional distribution of cholinergic muscarinic receptors in spinal cord. *Brain Res.* 1980;196:429–436.

128. Coggeshall RE, Carlton SM. Receptor localization in the mammalian dorsal horn and primary afferent neurons. *Brain Res Rev.* 1997;24:28–66.

129. Eisenach JC. Muscarinic-mediated analgesia. *Life Sci.* 1999;64:549–554.

130. Reynolds DV. Surgery in the rat during electrical analgesia induced by focal brain stimulation. *Science.* 1969;164:444–445.

131. Fields HL, Basbaum AI. Central nervous system mechanisms of pain modulation. In Wall PD, Melzack R, eds. *Textbook of Pain.* 3rd ed. New York: Churchill Livingstone; 1999:243–257.

132. Heinricher MM. Organizational characteristics of supraspinally mediated responses to nociceptive input. In Yaksh TL, ed. *Anesthesia: Biologic Foundations.* Philadelphia: Lippincott-Raven Publishers; 1998, 643–661.

133. Mayer DJ, Wolfe TL, Akil H, et al. Analgesia from electrical stimulation in the brainstem of the rat. *Science.* 1971;174:1351–1354.

134. Liebeskind JC, Guilbaud G, Besson JM, et al. Analgesia from electrical stimulation of periaqueductal grey matter in the cat: Behavioral observations and inhibitory effects on spinal cord interneurons. *Brain Res.* 1973;50:441–446.

135. Dubuisson D, Melzack R. Analgesic brain stimulation in the cat: effect of intraventricular serotonin, norepinephrine, and dopamine. *Exp Neurol.* 1977;57:1059–1066.

136. Zorman G, Belcher G, Adams JE, et al. Lumbar intrathecal naloxone blocks analgesia produced by microstimulation of the ventromedial medulla in the rat. *Brain Res.* 1982;236:77–84.

137. Aimone LD, Gebhart GF. Stimulation-produced spinal inhibition from the midbrain in the rat is mediated by an excitatory amino acid neurotransmitter in the medial medulla. *J Neurosci.* 1986;6:1803–1813.

138. Aimone LD, Jones SL, Gebhart GF. Stimulation-produced descending inhibition from the periaquaductal gray and nucleus raphe magnus in the rat: mediation by spinal monoamines but not opioids. *Pain.* 1987;31:123–136.

139. Dickenson AH, Oliveras JL, Besson JM. Role of the nucleus raphe magnus in opiate analgesia as studied by the microinjection technique in the rat. *Brain Res.* 1979;170:95–111.

140. Rossi GC, Pasternak GW, Bodnar RJ. Mu and delta opioid synergy between the periaqueductal gray and the rostro-ventral medulla. *Brain Res.* 1994;665:85–93.

141. Ness TJ, Gebhart GF. Quantitative comparison of inhibition of visceral and cutaneous spinal nociceptive transmission from the midbrain and medulla in the rat. *J Neurophysiol.* 1987; 58:850–865.

142. Bowker RM, Westlund KN, Coulter JD. Origins of serotonergic projections to the lumbar spinal cord in the monkey using a combined retrograde transport and immunocytochemical technique. *Brain Res Bull.* 1982;9:271–278.

143. Beitz AJ. The sites of origin of brainstem neurotensin and serotonin projections to the rodent nucleus raphe magnus. *J Neurosci.* 1982;2:829–842.

144. Headley PM, Duggan AW, Griersmith BT. Selective reduction of noradrenaline and 5-hydroxytryptamine of nociceptive responses of cat dorsal horn neurones. *Brain Res.* 1978;145:185–189.

145. Hamon M, Gallisot MC, Menard F, et al. 5-HT_3 receptor binding sites are on capsaicin-sensitive fibers in the rat spinal cord. *Eur J Pharmacology.* 1989;164:315–322.

146. Marlier L, Teilhac J-R, Cerruti C, et al. Autoradiographic mapping of 5-HT_1, 5-HT_{1A}, 5-HT_{1B} and 5-HT_2 receptors in the rat spinal cord. *Brain Res.* 1991;550:15–23.

147. Calejesan AA, Ch'ang, MHC Zhuo M. Spinal serotonergic receptors mediate facilitation of a nociceptive reflex by subcutaneous formalin injection into the hindpaw in rats. *Brain Res.* 1998;798:46–54.

148. Glaum SR, Proudfit HK, Anderson EG. 5-HT_3 receptors modulate spinal nociceptive reflexes. *Brain Res.* 1990;510,12–16.

149. Alhaider AA, Lei SZ, Wilcox GL. Spinal 5HT_3 receptor-mediated antinociception: possible release of GABA. *J Neurosci.* 1991;11:1881–1888.

150. Chen CC, England S, Akopian AN, et al. A sensory neuron-specific, proton-gated ion channel. *Proc Natl Acad Sci USA.* 1998;95:10240–10245.

151. Solomon RE, Gebhart GF. Mechanisms of effects of intrathecal serotonin on nociception and blood pressure in rats. *J Pharmacol Exp Ther.* 1988;245:905–912.

152. Alhaider AA, Wilcox GL. Differential roles of 5-hydroxytryptamine$_{1A}$ and 5- hydroxytryptamine$_{1B}$ receptor subtypes in modulating spinal nociceptive transmission in mice. *J Pharmacol Exp Ther.* 1993;265:378–385.

153. Eide PK, Joly NM, Hole K. The role of spinal cord5-HT_{1A} and 5-HT_{1B} receptors in the modulation of a spinal nociceptive reflex. *Brain Res.* 1990;536:195–200.

154. Holden JE, Schwartz EJ, Proudfit, HK. Microinjection of morphine in the A7 catecholamine cell group produces opposing effects on nociception that are mediated by al. *Neuroscience.* 1999;91:979–990.

155. Tsuruoka M, Willis WD. Descending modulation from the region of the locus coeruleus on nociceptive sensitivity in a rat model of inflammatory hyperalgesia. *Brain Res.* 1996;743:86–92.

156. Li W, Zhao ZQ. Yohimbine reduces inhibition of lamina X neurones by stimulation of the locus coeruleus. *Neuroreport.* 1993;4:751–753.

157. Zhao, Z-Q, Duggan AW. Idazoxan blocks the action of noradrenaline but not spinal inhibition from electrical stimulation of the locus coeruleus and nucleus Kolliker-fuse of the cat. *Neuroscience.* 1988;25:997–1005.

158. Jones SL, Gebhart GF. Spinal pathways mediating tonic, coeruleospinal, and raphe-spinal descending inhibition in the rat. *JJ Neurophysiol.* 1987;58:138–159.

159. Westlund KN, Bowker RM, Ziegler MG, et al. Descending noradrenergic projections and their spinal terminations. *Progress in Brain Res.* 1983;57:219–238.

160. Clark FM, Proudfit HK. The projection of locus coeruleus neurons to the spinal cord in the rat determined by anterograde tracing combined with immunocytochemistry. *Brain Res.* 1991;538:231–245.

161. Yaksh TL. Pharmacology of spinal adrenergic systems which modulate spinal nociceptive processing. *Pharmacol Biochem Behav.* 1985;22:845–858.

162. Proudfit HK. Pharmacologic evidence for the modulation of nociception by noradrenergic neurons. *Prog Brain Res.* 1988;77:357–370.

163. Kuraishi Y, Hirota N, Sato Y, et al. Noradrenergic inhibition of the release of substance P from primary afferents in the rabbit spinal cord dorsal horn. *Brain Res.* 1985;359:177–182.

164. Sato A, Sato YSRF. *Impact of Somatosensory Input on Autonomic Functions.* Heidelberg: Springer; 1997.

165. Stone LS, Fairbanks CA, Wilcox GL. Moxonidine, a mixed α_2-adrenergic and imidazoline receptor agonist, identifies a novel adrenergic target for spinal analgesia. *Ann N Y Acad Sci.* 2003;1009:1–8.

166. Li X, Eishenach JC. α_2A-adrenoreceptor stimulation reduces capsaicin-induced glutamate release from spinal cord synaptosomes. *J Pharmacol Exp Ther.* 2001;299:939–944.

167. Pan YZ, Li DP, Pan HL. Inhibition of glutamatergic synaptic input to spinal lamina II_0 neurons by presynaptic α_2 adrenergic receptors. *J Neurophysiol.* 2002;87:1938–1947.

168. King EW, Audette K, Athman GA, et al. Transcutaneous electrical nerve stimulation activates peripherally located alpha-2A adrenergic receptors. *Pain.* 2005;115:364–373.

169. Radhakrishnan R, King EW, Dickman J, et al. Blockade of spinal 5-HT receptor subtypes prevents low, but not high, frequency TENS-induced antihyperalgesia in rats. *Pain.* 2003;5:205–213.

170. Roberts MHT, Rees H. 1986 The antinociceptive effects of stimulating the pretectal nucleus of the rat. *Pain.* 25:83–93.

171. Prado WA, Roberts MHT. An assessment of the antinociceptive and aversive effects of stimulating identified sites in the rat brain. *Brain Res.* 1985;340:219–228.

172. Rees H, Roberts MHT. Anterior pretectal stimulation alters the responses of spinal dorsal horn neurones to cutaneous stimulation in the rat. *J Physiol.* 1987;385:415–436.

173. Terenzi MG, Rees H, Morgan SJ, et al. The antinociception evoked by anterior pretectal nucleus stimulation is partially dependent upon ventrolateral medullary neurones. *Pain.* 1991;47:231–239.

174. Chiang CY, Dostrovsky JO, Sessle BJ. Periaqueductal gray matter and nucleus raphe magnus involvement in anterior pretectal nucleus-induced inhibition of jaw-opening reflex in rats *Brain Res.* 1991;544:71–78.

175. Mamede Rosa ML, Prado WA. Antinociception induced by opioid or 5-HT agonists microinjected into the anterior pretectal nucleus of the rat. *Brain Res.* 1997;757:133–138.

176. Wiberg M, Blomqvist A. The spinomesencephalic tract in the cat: its cells of origin and termination pattern as demonstrated by the intra-axonal transport method. *Brain Res.* 1984;291:1–28.

177. Rees H, Roberts MHT. Antinociceptive effects of dorsal column stimulation in the rat: involvement of the anterior pretectal nucleus. *J Physiol.* 1989;417:375–388.

178. Basbaum AI, Fields HL. Endogenous pain control systems: Brainstem spinal pathways and endorphin circuitry. *Annu Rev Neurosci.* 1984;7:309–338.

179. Yezierski RP, Gerhard KD, Shrock BJ, et al. A further examination of effects of cortical stimulation on primate spinothalamic tract cells. *JJ Neurophysiol.* 1983;49:424–441.

180. Carpenter D, Lundberg A, Norrsell U. Primary afferent depolarization evoked from the sensorimotor cortex. *Acta Physiol Scand.* 1963;59:126–142.

181. Watson SJ, Akil H. Alpha-MSH in rat brain: occurrence within and outside of beta-endorphin neurons. *Brain Res.* 1980;182:217–223.

182. degli Uberti EC, Petraglia F, Bondanelli M, et al. Involvement of mu-opioid receptors in the modulation of pituitary- adrenal axis in normal and stressed rats. *J EndocrinolInvest.* 1995;18:1–7.

183. Harte JL, Eifert GH, Smith R. The effects of running and meditation on beta-endorphin, corticotropin- releasing hormone and cortisol in plasma, and on mood. *Biol Psychol.* 1995;40:251–265.

184. Schedlowski M, Fluge T, Richter S, et al. Beta-endorphin, but not substance-P, is increased by acute stress in humans. *Psychoneuroendocrinology* 1995;20:103–110.

185. Schwarz L, Kindermann W. Changes in beta-endorphin levels in response to aerobic and anaerobic exercise. *Sports Med.* 1992;13:25–36.

186. Yaksh TL. Central pharmacology of nociceptive transmission. In: Wall PD, Melzack R, eds. *Textbook of Pain.* 4th ed. New York: Churchill Livingstone; 1999:253–308.

187. Sluka KA, Rohlwing JJ, Bussey RA, et al. Chronic muscle pain induced by repeated acid injection is reversed by spinally administered μ and δ but not κ, opioid receptor agonists. *J Pharmacol Exp Ther.* 2002;302:1146–1150.

188. Sluka KA, Deacon M, Stibal A, et al. Spinal blockade of opioid receptors prevents the analgesia produced by TENS in arthritic rats. *J Pharmacol Exp Ther.* 1999;289:840–846.

189. Sluka KA, Walsh DM. TENS: basic science mechanisms and clinical effectiveness. *J Pain.* 2003;4:109–121.

190. Levin MF, Hui-Chan CW. Conventional and acupuncture-like transcutaneous electrical nerve stimulation excite similar afferent fibers. *Arch PhysMed Rehabil.* 1993;74:54–60.

191. Radhakrishnan R, Sluka KA. Deep tissue afferents, but not cutaneous afferents, mediate TENS-induced antihyperalgesia. *J Pain.* 2005;6:673–680.

192. Sjolund BH. Peripheral nerve stimulation suppression of C-fiber evoked flexion reflex in rats. Part 1: Parameters of continuous stimulation. *J Neurosurg.* 1985;63:612–616.

193. Sluka KA, Bailey K, Bogush J, et al. Treatment with either high or low frequency TENS reduces the secondary hyperalgesia observed after injection of kaolin and carrageenan into the knee joint. *Pain.* 1998;77:97–102.

194. Gopalkrishnan P, Sluka KA. Effect of varying frequency, intensity and pulse duration of TENS on primary hyperalgesia in inflamed rats. *Arch Phys Med Rehabil.* 2000;81:984–990.

195. King EW, Sluka KA. The effect of varying frequency and intensity of transcutaneous electrical nerve stimulation on secondary mechanical hyperalgesia in an animal model of inflammation. *J Pain.* 2001;2:128–133.

196. Ma YT, Sluka KA. Reduction in inflammation-induced sensitization of dorsal horn neurons by transcutaneous electrical nerve stimulation in anesthetized rats. *Exp Brain Res.* 2001;137:94–102.

197. Somers DL, Clemente FR. High-frequency transcutaneous electrical nerve stimulation alters thermal but not mechanical allodynia following chronic constriction injury of the rat sciatic nerve. *Arch Phys Med Rehabil.* 1998;79:1370–1376.

198. Hughes GS, Lichstein PR, Whitlock D, et al. Response of plasma beta-endorphins to transcutaneous electrical nerve stimulation in healthy subjects. *Phys Ther.* 1984;64:1062–1066.

199. Salar G, Job I, Mingrino S, et al. Effect of transcutaneous electrotherapy on CSF β-endorphin content in patients without pain problems. *Pain.* 1981;10:169–172.

200. Han JS, Chen XH, Sun SL, et al. Effect of low and high frequency TENS on met-enkephalin-arg-phe and dynorphin A immunoreactivity in human lumbar CSF. *Pain.* 1991;47:295–298.

201. Kalra A, Urban MO, Sluka KA. Blockade of opioid receptors in rostral ventral medulla prevents antihyperalgesia produced by transcutaneous electrical nerve stimulation TENS *J Pharmacol Exp Ther.* 2001;298:257–263.

202. Radhakrishnan R, Sluka KA. Blockade of knee joint but not cutaneous afferents prevents TENS-induced antihyperalgesia. *J Pain.* 2003;4:48.

203. Woolf CJ, Barrett GD, Mitchell D, et al. Naloxone-reversible peripheral electroanalgesia in intact and spinal rats. *Eur J Pharmacol.* 1977;45:311–314.

204. Woolf CJ, Mitchell D, Barrett GD. Antinociceptive effect of peripheral segmental electrical stimulation in the rat. *Pain.* 1980;8:237–252.

205. Chandran P, Sluka KA. Development of opioid tolerance with repeated TENS administration. *Pain.* 2003;102:195–201.

206. Leem JW, Park ES, Paik KS. Electrophysiological evidence for the antinociceptive effect of transcutaneous electrical nerve stimulation on mechanically evoked responsiveness of dorsal horn neurons in neuropathic rats. *Neurosci Lett.* 1995;192:197–200.

207. Nam TS, Choi Y, Yeon DS, et al. Differential antinociceptive effect of transcutaneous electrical stimulation on pain behavior sensitive or insensitive to phentolamine in neuropathic rats. *Neurosci Lett.* 2001;301:17–20.

208. Hayes RL, Price DD, Bennett GJ, et al. Differential effects of spinal cord lesions on narcotic and non-narcotic suppression of nociceptive reflexes: further evidence for the physiologic multiplicity of pain modulation. *Brain Res.* 1978;155:91–101.

209. Hayes RL, Bennett GJ, Newlon PG, et al. Behavioral and physiological studies on non-narcotic analgesia in the rat elicited by certain environmental stimuli. *Brain Res.* 1978;155:69–90.

210. Lewis JW, Cannon JT, Liebeskind JC. Opioid and nonopioid mechanisms of stress analgesia. *Science.* 1980;208:623–625.

211. Watkins LR, Cobelli DA, Faris P, et al. Opiate vs. Non-opiate footshock-induced analgesia: the body region shocked is a critical factor. *Brain Res.* 1982;242:299–308.

212. Watkins LR, Johannessen JN, Kinscheck IB, et al. The neurochemical basis of footshock analgesia: the role of spinal cord serotonin and norepinephrine. *Brain Res.* 1984;290:107–117.

213. Watkins LR, Cobelli DA, Mayer DJ. Opiate vs. non-opiate footshock induced analgesia FSIA): descending and intraspinal components. *Brain Res.* 1982;245:97–106.

214. Watkins LR, Katayama Y, Kinscheck IB, et al. Muscarinic cholinergic mediation of opiate and nonopiate environmentally induced analgesias. *Brain Res.* 1984;300:231–242.

215. LeBars D. The whole body receptive field of dorsal horn multireceptive neurones. *Brain Res Rev.* 2002;40:29–44.

216. Janko M, Trontelj JV. Transcutaneous electrical nerve stimulation a microneurographic and perceptual study. *Pain.* 1980;9:219–230.

217. Sluka KA, Judge MA, McColley MM, et al. Low frequency TENS is less effective than high frequency TENS at reducing inflammation induced hyperalgesia in morphine tolerant rats. *Eur J Pain.* 2000;4:185–193.

218. Sluka KA. Systemic morphine in combination with TENS produces an increased analgesia in rats with acute inflammation. *J Pain.* 2000;1:204–211.

219. Sluka KA, Chandran P. Systemic administration of clonidine in combination with TENS produces an increased antihyperalgesia in rats. *Pain.* 2002;100:183–190.

ACKNOWLEDGMENTS

I thank the Arthritis Foundation and the National Institutes of Health (grants K02 AR02201 and R01 NS39734) for financial support. I also thank all my colleagues (graduate students, postdoctoral fellows, and collaborators) who contributed much of the work presented in this chapter: Drs. Westlund, Willis, Ma, Radhakrishnan, Hoeger Bement, and Ms. Gopalkrishnan, Kalra, and Mr. Chandran.

CHAPTER 5

Electrical Stimulation for Pain Modulation

Tara Jo Manal and Lynn Snyder-Mackler

In *The Puzzle of Pain*, Ronald Melzack describes a patient with a congenital inability to sense pain. By the time of her premature death at age 29, she had suffered third-degree burns, broken bones, arthritis, and other problems (1). She had what we as clinicians seek for our patients, freedom from pain, and that is in essence what she died from. Although most of this chapter addresses the amelioration of pain, remember that pain serves a protective function, and that in all but a few number of conditions, electrical stimulation for pain modulation should be used adjunctively with treatments of the underlying pathology.

Electroanalgesia can be traced to the presentation of the gate-control theory of pain transmission by Melzack and Wall in 1965 (2). Its application in clinical practice in modern times began with Shealy's (3) and Long et al.'s (4) use of implanted dorsal column stimulators and their serendipitous discovery that transcutaneous stimulation appeared equally effective for control of pain. Subsequently, the therapeutic use of electrical stimulation for pain control has increased exponentially. The objectives of this chapter are to present (i) common methods used to assess and measure pain; (ii) ways in which electrical stimulation is used to modulate pain; (iii) a review of the literature with emphasis on prospective, randomized clinical trials; and (iv) representative case studies as illustrative examples.

CLINICAL ASSESSMENT OF PAIN

Most forms of pain assessment attempt to quantify and objectify the patient's response to the query, "tell me about your pain." The study of pain assessment is a discipline unto itself, and this section can only touch on its complexity. A brief discussion of pain assessment, however, is integral to the review of literature regarding pain control with electrical stimulation and to the evaluation of electrical stimulation as a therapeutic intervention for individuals with pain.

Pain perception has *sensory–discriminative* and *affective–motivational* components. That is, patients can describe pain intensity/location (sensory–discriminative) and unpleasantness (affective–motivational) (4). Pain is multidimensional, and pain assessment that focuses only on the sensory component, with the argument that it is the only physiologic or "real" pain, misses the boat clinically. The study of experimentally-induced pain focuses on the sensory dimension of pain and does not capture the entirety of clinical pain. Pain perception is colored by many factors, and accounting for those factors can be useful in assessing the effectiveness of therapeutic interventions.

When to Treat Pain

Acute pain is a response to current or impending tissue injury or damage and provides an inherent protective function. A patient who has recently sustained an ankle sprain will have pain with weight bearing, encouraging them to adopt a less stressful, non–weight-bearing posture during healing. If pain is prematurely abolished, it may allow the patient to perform activities that place the healing structures at risk for further injury or delayed healing. Pain reduction should not interfere with the beneficial protective response. When pain complaints persist even though tissue healing would benefit from progressive exposure to stress, the pain is now no longer protecting the structures but is inhibiting recovery. *Chronic pain* is not protective and outlasts tissue healing or can be out of proportion to tissue injury (components contributing to this persistent pain are outlined in Chapter 4). Once pain is no longer providing a protective response but instead contributing to the maintenance of abnormal function and therapeutic progression, pain must be managed to ensure a successful outcome. In an overuse syndrome, pain may result from prolonged, repetitive activity in the face of insufficient muscle strength or endurance. In this situation, muscular training may alleviate the deficit that led to the onset of the painful condition (e.g., tendonitis). However, if pain is present with resisted muscular contractions and cannot be controlled, muscle recovery is unlikely to occur. In this case, pain should be directly managed as a potential contributor to treatment failure.

Patient Interview and History

Pain can be evaluated in part by the interview process, where the clinician elicits the pain history with a series of questions, avoiding the use of leading questions or those that are too broad. A question like "Does your back pain radiate down the back of your leg?" is suggestive. "Tell me about your pain" does not help direct the examiner because it does not constrain the answer. Specific questions that are not leading and that help the examiner focus the problem include

What activities initiate or worsen your pain?
Was the onset of pain sudden or gradual?
How do you relieve your pain?
Where is your pain?
When did the pain start?
Has the pain changed since it began?

Although the reliability and validity of the pain interview are not clearly established, the interview provides a means for identifying, confirming, and disconfirming information about pain patterns. Other means of assessing pain include pain drawings, questionnaires, verbal rating scales, visual analog scales, and indirect measures such as the assessment of analgesic use or relative levels of activity.

Pain Drawings

Pain drawings are visual representations of the distribution and quality of a patient's pain (Fig. 5.1). Pain drawings can be completed by the clinician, the patient, or both. Evidence suggests that patient and clinician versions of pain drawings can be very different. When pain drawings extend beyond anatomical structures or describe pain that is shooting out of the body into the air, a clinician may

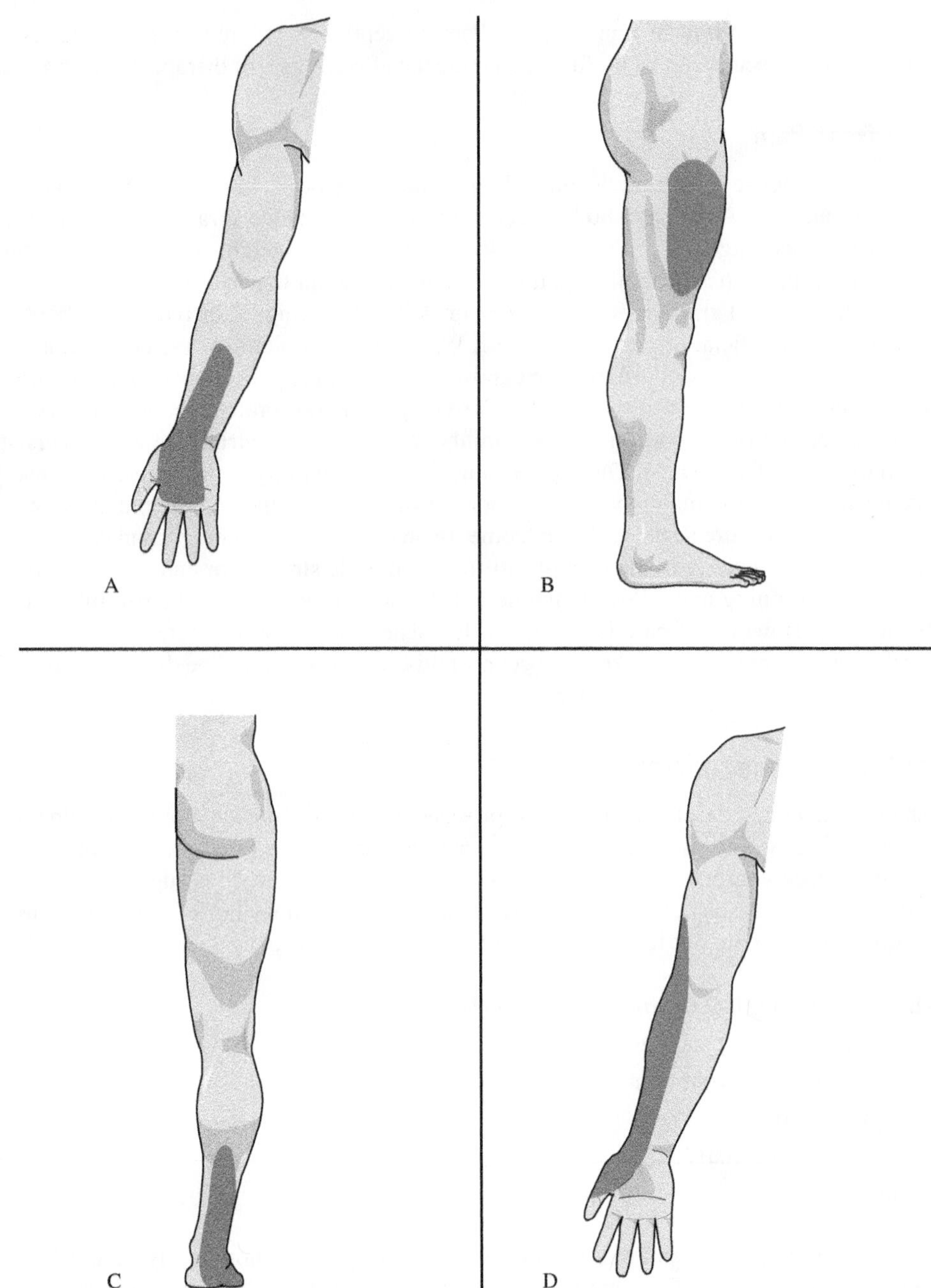

Figure 5.1. Sample pain drawings. **A:** Upper-extremity, aching pain in carpal tunnel syndrome. **B:** Anterolateral thigh pain in meraglia paresthetica. **C:** Lower-extremity pain of S1 nerve root compression. **D:** Upper-extremity pain with C6 nerve root compression.

need to consider if the affective–motivational component of pain is contributing significantly to the patient complaint (5). Less successful treatment outcomes should be anticipated when psychological services are not included in the management of pain with a strong affective component. The reliability and validity of these drawings have not been demonstrated (6). Pain drawings, however, can be clinically helpful in identifying locations of pain, prompting a therapist to further evaluate for pathology in an underlying structure. There are some pain patterns that are suggestive of underlying structural pathology. For example, subacromial impingement of the shoulder can refer down the middle deltoid area. If that pattern is identified on a pain drawing, it may initiate screening a patient for shoulder impingement. Pain patterns seen in drawings or described by patients can also indicate a cervical or lumbar peripheral nerve root radiculopathy (7), muscular trigger point distribution (8), cutaneous nerve entrapment, or even relate to pain of a visceral origin (e.g., jaw pain and arm pain associated with cardiac involvement). Comparison of the pain drawing, patient complaints, and the results of the evaluation can lead a therapist in the direction of effective patient care (9).

Pain Rating Scales

Pain rating scales are often used to record baseline pain levels and can be used to describe changes in pain over time. It is important in pain management to use many different measures to capture responses to therapeutic interventions. Pain rating scales are popular because they are easy to administer and can demonstrate even small changes in patient complaints. The scale can first be given to patients during their initial physical therapy evaluation and be repeated on subsequent visits or during periodic re-evaluations.

Visual analog scales (VAS) are lines conventionally 10 cm long and numbered from 1 to 10 (most common), 1 to 100, or not numbered. These scales vary from rather detailed to very sparse. A patient is usually asked to describe the pain intensity at the moment. A variation of the numerical VAS is the graphic rating scale (GRS), which has equally spaced descriptors on the line. These scales can be vertical or horizontal, and either the left (top) or right (bottom) margin may represent maximal pain intensity (Fig. 5.2). The VAS and GRS are reliable tools when a horizontal

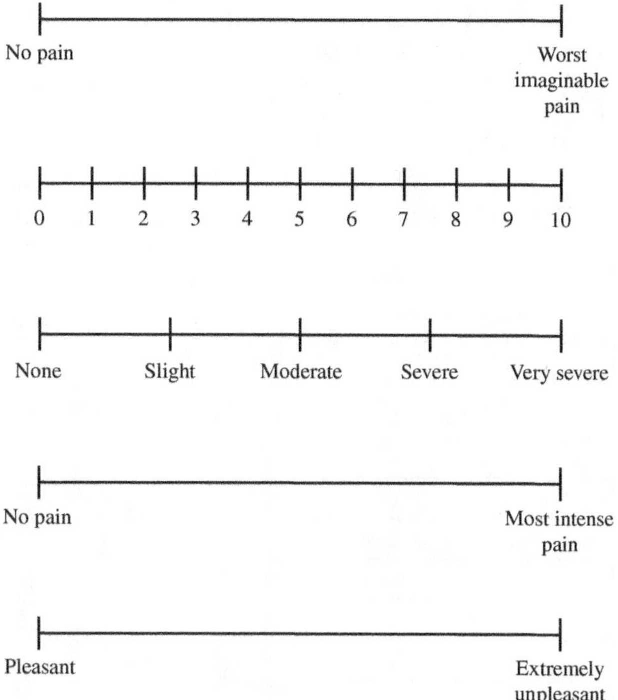

Figure 5.2. A sample of different types of visual analogue pain scales for assessment of the magnitude and unpleasantness of pain.

Table 5.1.

Identification Number										
O	O	O	0	O	O	0	O	O	O	O
O	O	O	1	O	O	1	O	O	O	O
O	O	O	2	O	O	2	O	O	O	O
O	O	O	3	O	O	3	O	O	O	O
O	O	O	4	O	O	4	O	O	O	O
O	O	O	5	O	O	5	O	O	O	O
O	O	O	6	O	O	6	O	O	O	O
O	O	O	7	O	O	7	O	O	O	O
O	O	O	8	O	O	8	O	O	O	O
O	O	O	9	O	O	9	O	O	O	O

OSWESTRY LOW BACK PAIN QUESTIONNAIRE

This questionnaire has been designed to give the physical therapist information as to how your pain has affected your ability to manage everyday life. Please answer all sections. Completely fill in only one circle in each section that applies to you. We realize that you may consider that two or more choices apply to you, but please fill the one circle that most clearly describes your problem.

Section 1—PAIN INTENSITY

O I have no pain.
O I have no pain except when I move a certain way.
O I have minimal pain most of the time.
O I have moderate pain most of the time.
O I have severe pain most of the time.
O I have intense/intolerable pain most of the time.

Section 2—PERSONAL CARE (washing, dressing, etc.)

O I can take care of myself normally without causing extra pain.
O I can take care of myself normally, but it causes extra pain.
O It is painful to take care of myself and I am slow and careful.
O I need some help, but manage most of my personal care.
O I need help every day in most aspects of self care.
O I do not get dressed, wash with difficulty, and stay in bed.

Section 6—STANDING

O I can stand as long as I want without pain.
O I can stand as long as I want, but it gives me extra pain.
O Pain prevents me from standing more than one hour.
O Pain prevents me from standing more than 30 minutes.
O Pain prevents me from standing more than 15 minutes.
O Pain prevents me from standing at all.

Section 7—SLEEPING

O Pain does not prevent me from sleeping well.
O I can sleep well only by taking medication.
O I have less than 6 hours sleep because of pain.
O I have less than 4 hours sleep because of pain.
O I have less than 2 hours sleep because of pain.
O Pain prevents me from sleeping at all.

Section 3—*LIFTING*

- O I can lift heavy weights without pain.
- O I can lift heavy weights, but it causes extra pain.
- O Pain prevents me from lifting heavy weights off the floor but I can manage if they are conveniently positioned on a table.
- O Pain prevents me from lifting heavy weights, but I can manage light to medium weights if conveniently positioned.
- O I can lift only very light weights.
- O I cannot lift or carry anything at all.

Section 4—*WALKING*

- O Pain does not prevent me from walking any distance.
- O Pain prevents me from walking more than one mile.
- O Pain prevents me from walking more than $^1/_2$ mile.
- O Pain prevents me from walking more than $^1/_4$ mile.
- O I can only walk using a cane or crutch.
- O I am in bed most of the time.

Section 5—*SITTING*

- O I can sit in a chair as long as I like.
- O I can only sit in my favorite chair as long as I like.
- O Pain prevents me from sitting more than one hour.
- O Pain prevents me from sitting more than 30 minutes.
- O Pain prevents me from sitting more than 10 minutes.
- O Pain prevents me from sitting at all.

Section 8—*SEX LIFE*

- O My sex life is normal and causes no extra pain.
- O My sex life is normal, but causes extra pain.
- O My sex life is nearly normal, but is very painful.
- O My sex life is severely restricted because of pain.
- O My sex life is nearly absent because of pain.
- O Pain prevents any sex life at all.

Section 9—*SOCIAL LIFE*

- O My social life is normal and gives me no extra pain.
- O My social life is normal, but gives me extra pain.
- O Pain has no effect on my social life other than limiting some energetic interests like dancing.
- O Pain has restricted my social life and I do not go out as often.
- O Pain has restricted my social life to my home.
- O I have no social life because of pain.

Section 10—*TRAVELING*

- O I can travel anywhere without extra pain.
- O I can travel anywhere, but it gives me extra pain.
- O Pain is bad, but I manage trips over 2 hours.
- O Pain restricts me to trips of less than one hour.
- O Pain restricts me to trips of less than 30 minutes.
- O Pain prevents me from traveling except to the doctor or hospital.

line is used (10). Because pain rating reflects individual differences in pain perception, a clinician needs to be cautious in attempting to draw meaning from pain rating data (validity). Those patients who score higher may or may not have greater underlying pathology; therefore individual changes in pain rating (i.e., initial pain rating minus current pain rating = pain relief) may be more clinically useful data (10).

Verbal rating scales (VRS) use descriptive words, with patients picking the words that best categorize their pain. A verbal rating scale that is used often clinically is to ask the patient to verbally rate pain on a scale of 1 to 10. The reliability of the VAS is superior to that of the VRS (11,12).

For both visual analog and verbal rating scales, the choice of descriptors or anchors for the scales is important. A scale that uses "no pain" and "worst pain imaginable" as anchors does not allow for discrimination of sensory and affective components of pain. The use of anchors such as "no pain," "most intense pain" or "pleasant," "extremely unpleasant" allows for differentiation that has important clinical and experimental implications (Fig. 5.2).

Pain Questionnaires

Pain questionnaires help patients describe pain in a reliable and reproducible way and often have subdivisions that assess different qualities of pain complaints. Many questionnaires attempt to separate out the affective–motivational component of the pain from the sensory–discriminative components, and many go a step further in attempting to capture the functional limitations induced by pain complaints. Functional-status questionnaires have been used to measure the pain and disability associated with chronic pain conditions. The Sickness Impact Profiles (SIP) and Oswestry Low Back Pain Questionnaire (Table 5.1) have been used both in research and in many clinical settings. These questionnaires address the issue of whether pain-associated dysfunction is affected. These questionnaires are useful to the clinician in determining the impact pain has on daily life, in identifying functional losses that can be the basis of therapeutic goals, and in monitoring within- and between-treatment changes in patient complaints.

Another commonly used questionnaire is the McGill Pain Questionnaire, which is available in both a short (15 items) and a long version (20 items) (14,15). The McGill questionnaire is a global assessment tool that uses variations of the tools mentioned above: line drawings, pain descriptors, items to assess changes in pain over time, and pain intensity. Both versions of the McGill questionnaire use grouped descriptors to quantify patients' pain characteristics. The reliability of these questionnaires, as demonstrated by Melzack and others, is acceptable, and the short form correlates highly with the pain rating indices of the long form (13–17). These types of questionnaires appear to also have high validity in the population of patients with chronic pain (18).

Alternative Methods of Pain Assessment

Investigators have monitored analgesic intake to assess the relative intensity of pain (19). It is assumed that patients take fewer pills (lower dosage of analgesic) if pain intensity is lower, but this becomes problematic with different types of drugs. Some researchers have developed means of converting analgesics to aspirin equivalents, but the validity of this is questionable. Recording the medication intake of patients is an essential component of a thorough evaluation, and changes in the frequency and amount of pain medications used by a patient may be helpful in reflecting changes in their condition. This information may be less useful when comparing that change to the changes seen in different patients taking different medications. The clinician should also gather information regarding pharmacological methods used to manage the patient's pain to ensure that considerations for cross-tolerance between stimulation-produced analgesia and pharmacological analgesia are made. This includes specific questions related to opioid medications that would favor the use of high-frequency transcutaneous electrical nerve stimulation (TENS) over low-frequency TENS. In cases of morphine tolerance, the use of TENS is contraindicated (see Chapter 4).

Evaluation of daily activity and levels of activity has also been used. The assumption is that patients are more active when pain is less intense, but evidence suggests that patients may not assess their activity level accurately (20). Clinically, therapists may find benefit from recording activity and pain onset and intensity. *Irritability* consists of information regarding ease of pain provocation combined with symptom severity and duration. A patient is more irritable if symptoms are easily provoked and if the symptoms last for a long time compared to a patient whose symptoms are easily provoked but the symptoms diminish quickly. Irritability data can be helpful in monitoring changes in these three entities, but also can be useful in determining how aggressive treatment intervention can be. For example, if a patient has pain in the knee that is provoked with running for longer than one hour, it is unlikely that a therapeutic exercise program will contribute to an increase in their pain or worsening of their condition. In this case, the pain is likely to resolve without direct treatment, and correction of the underlying causes of strength or flexibility should resolve the pain complaints. Conversely, if a patient has extreme pain (8 out of 10 on a 10 point scale) with any movement of the spine beyond the neutral position, a much slower and more pain-control–oriented approach may be necessary. In this case, immobilization with bracing and direct treatment for pain management may be necessary before a more movement-based treatment evaluation or program can be introduced. In this case the irritability of the patient's pain is high, and direct management of pain correspondingly ranks higher in the treatment order.

Magnitude estimation is a technique in which pain is measured (either the affective–motivational component, the sensory–discriminative component, or both) against a standard, representing the maximum value on a scale of intensity or unpleasantness. Delitto et al. (21) used a 20-mA DC stimulus as the reference for maximum intensity/unpleasantness in a study of discomfort with electrical stimulation. The subjects were informed that the 20-mA intensity was equal in value to a score of 100 for intensity or unpleasantness (22). When other levels of current were applied, the subjects were asked to relate those perceived factors in relation to the "100" reference current. Magnitude estimation yields ratio-scaled measurements with high reliability (22). This process may need to be considered and used when perceptions of current must be compared across subjects rather than within subjects.

Methods of pain rating described above have been used to assess the effectiveness of agents for modulation of experimentally-induced and clinical pain. The use of these agents in clinical practice has been largely in the chronic pain population. The predictive value of these measures is unknown, primarily because of unsystematic and sporadic use in daily clinical practice. The use of one or more of the reliable pain assessment measures, combined with thorough, accurate documentation of treatment procedures, could aid tremendously in the evaluation of pain control treatments.

MODES OF STIMULATION FOR PAIN CONTROL

Electrical stimulation has been used for pain modulation for more than a century. Refinements in equipment design have made this approach to pain management significantly easier over the years. Even with the new delivery systems, attempts to modulate pain by electrotherapy are characterized in one of four ways: *subsensory-level stimulation*, *sensory-level stimulation*, *motor-level stimulation*, and *noxious-level stimulation* (Fig. 5.3; Table 5.2). Many commercially available stimulators can produce each of these levels of stimulation, although the performance characteristics of some stimulators may be better suited to only one level of stimulation. Each

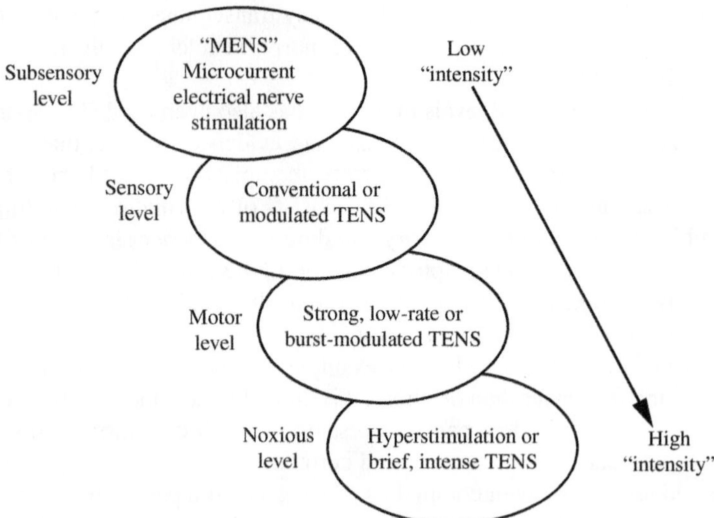

Figure 5.3. Clinical levels of electrical stimulation used for pain control correlated with the traditional designations for these interventions and the relative intensity of stimulation.

mode of stimulation has unique responses and requirements, as described below. *Transcutaneous electrical nerve stimulation* (TENS) is a term used to represent all the various forms of electrical stimulation for pain control that use surface electrodes applied to the skin.

Subsensory-level Stimulation

Stimulators have been marketed that do not produce phase charges sufficient to excite peripheral nerve fibers and reach sensory threshold. Such devices are called *microcurrent electrical nerve stimulators* (MENS). Because their peak current amplitudes are very low (below 1 mA) and

Table 5.2. Commonly Used Stimulation Parameters Associated with the Four Clinical Levels of Stimulation for Pain Control

Mode of Stimulation	*Amplitude Adjusted to Produce*	*Phase/Pulse Duration (μs)*	*Frequency (pps, bps)*	*Duration of Treatment*	*Duration of Analgesia*[a]
Subsensory level	No perception of stimulation	Not specified	<3	Not specified	Not known
Sensory level	Perceptible tingling ("pins and needles")	2–50 μs	50–100	20–60 min	Short: none to few minutes
Motor level	Strong visible muscle contraction	>150 μs	2–4	30–45 min	Long: hours
Noxious level	Painful sensation	≤1 ms	1–5 or <100	Seconds to few minutes	Long: hours

[a]Both the time to onset of anlagesia and the duration of analgesia have not been clearly established in the literature for the majority of commonly encountered pain syndromes that may be managed with TENS interventions.
pps: pulses per second, bps: bursts per second.

pulse durations are very short, these devices activate neither nerve nor muscle. Trade publications and clinical seminars have touted the effectiveness of MENS for a range of conditions but, to date, no studies of the clinical effectiveness of this mode of stimulation demonstrate a better effect than sham stimulation (23–25). Zizic et al. (26) evaluated the benefit of subsensory stimulation on patients with osteoarthritis of the knee. The authors compared 78 patients randomly assigned to a TENS and sham TENS group over an 8-week trial of 100 pulses per second (pps), low-voltage stimulation. The electrodes were placed around the knee, and the stimulation amplitude was increased until tingling was felt. The amplitude was turned down below sensory threshold for the TENS group, and the unit was turned off for the sham TENS group. Both groups used the unit on the painful knee for 6 to 10 hours per day for 4 weeks. There was a 2-week baseline period, followed by a post-testing evaluation in which more subjects (24%) in the active TENS group demonstrated improvement in VAS, self-rating of knee function, and physician global rating of knee evaluation compared to those in the sham TENS group (6%). The intensity of this stimulation was likely insufficient to create sensory nerve depolarization. The authors cite the influence of microcurrent on cellular activity as an explanation of their results; however, based on the mechanisms described in the Chapter 4, there is insufficient evidence for the efficacy of electrical stimulation below sensory threshold for pain management.

Sensory-level Stimulation

High-frequency sensory-level stimulation for pain modulation has been the best studied of any electrotherapeutic technique for pain control. Sensory-level stimulation is defined as stimulation at or above the sensory threshold and below the motor threshold. Sensory-level stimulation is most often accomplished by using a frequency in the 50- to 100-pps range, relatively short pulse or phase durations (2 to 50 μs), and relatively low intensities. Short pulse duration is used to minimize the chance of producing uncomfortable, tetanic muscular contraction. If longer pulse durations are applied, although sensory responses still occur, the therapeutic effect can be confounded by resulting muscular contractions. Muscular contractions may be undesirable as they can create apprehension, compress a joint, or even move a painful joint. Generally, when sensory TENS is being administered, muscular movement is unnecessary and often undesirable. This form of stimulation (Fig. 5.4A; Table 5.2) is also called *conventional TENS*.

Amplitudes are commonly adjusted in response to patient feedback based upon patient perception. In other words, current amplitude is increased until the patient perceives a comfortable *paresthesia* (buzzing, tingling, or "pins and needles," sensation) beneath the electrodes. The clinician should not be able to see or palpate muscle contraction. At this level of stimulation, the large-diameter, superficial cutaneous nerve fibers are preferentially activated. The likely mechanism of pain modulation is either a direct peripheral block of transmission (27) or activation of central inhibition mechanisms of pain transmission by large-diameter fiber stimulation (analogous to the original gate-control theory; see Chapter 4).

Sensory-level stimulation is usually perceived by the patient as very comfortable and is often the first choice in electrotherapeutic intervention for pain control. A patient may be frightened or nervous about the use of electricity, and sensory-level stimulation introduces electrotherapy gently. If this mode of stimulation is successful in improving pain or function, use of motor or noxious stimulation is unnecessary.

The patient response to sensory-level stimulation is often an immediate decrease in the perception of pain. However, pain reduction does not generally persist after the stimulation is stopped (28), although some longer lasting analgesia has been seen in animal models (see Chapter 4). Because the improvement in patient pain levels is expected only while the device is turned on, conventional TENS is used most often as needed throughout the day. If a patient has pain complaints while performing work or while sleeping, the unit is most effective if used during those behaviors.

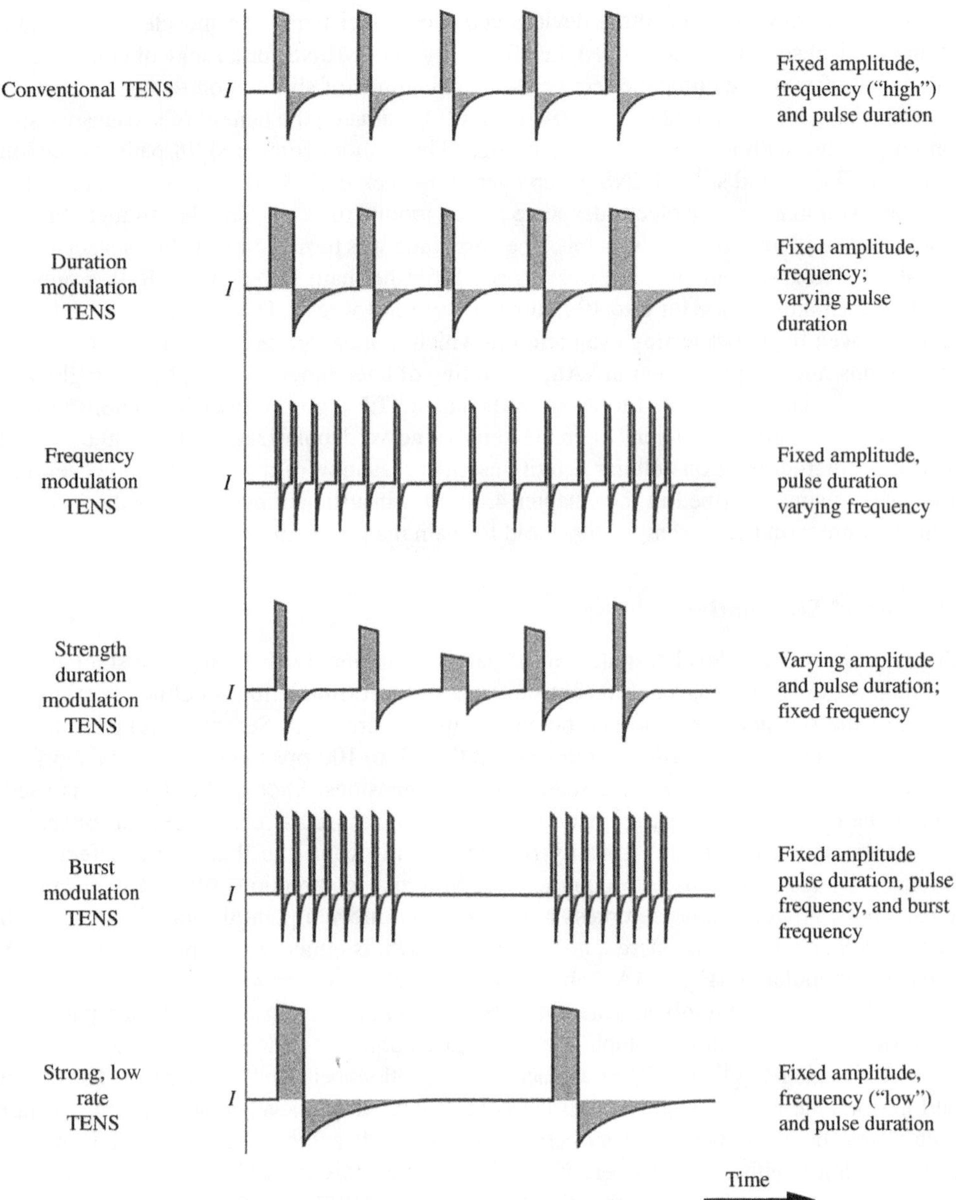

Figure 5.4. Illustration of examples of different types of pulse patterns produced by clinical and portable TENS units.

The key consideration in the use of pain-modulating current with activity is to be confident that the pain relief will not place the patient at risk of worsening their condition or furthering their injury. In cases where pain is inhibiting function, use of sensory-level TENS with activity can improve functional recovery. In a case of a secretary with neck pain during computer activity, if the addition of TENS can increase her time to pain onset, it may allow her to train her body to perform the work functions while the painful areas recover. If pain onset or intensity is alerting the patient that rest is required, sensory-level TENS may be more helpful if applied after the activity to promote rest and decreases in secondary hyperalgesia rather than during the activity.

The response to sensory-level TENS depends on the duration of the problem, the activity level, and pain level of the patient. Patients adapt readily to this type of stimulation, and perception of the stimulation can decline as the treatment progresses. Much as one becomes conditioned to external stimuli (e.g., night traffic noises in the city), one can adapt to a consistent stimulus. This is demonstrated in chronic problems where sensory-level stimulation is usually the first mode used but is rarely sufficient for full remediation. For this reason, modulations of conventional TENS (usually amplitude or duration modulations) (Fig. 5.4B–D) are used to diminish the adaptation and enhance the perceived effectiveness of the stimulation. The modulations are designed to prevent the patient from "ignoring" the stimulus provided. If the stimulus feels as though it has diminished over time, increasing intensity can quickly reverse this perception. As discussed in Chapter 4, even though the patient perceives the TENS intensity has diminished over time, the evoked action potential response remains stable; therefore, when the intensity is increased to return the patient's perception to "strong tingling." a net increase in evoked action potentials is produced. There are no negative implications to this practice, and intensity is routinely increased to restore the patient's perception; current modulation may be necessary to avoid the patient's perceived accommodation.

Stimulators are often designed with *current modulation* programs. In the continuous mode, the pulses are delivered without interruption or alteration based on the parameters chosen, providing a constant, unchanging pulse duration and frequency. Burst modes generally modulate the intensity temporally. The pulse amplitude is increased and decreased through a discrete time interval to provide a feeling of a wave or crescendo to a peak and then return to a baseline valley. In some individuals, burst modulation often has the sensation of a massage as the wave builds and degrades and can be relaxing for a patient. In other patients, burst modulation can be distracting or create apprehension as the peak amplitudes of stimulation approach. The clinician can decide on the modulation choice based on patient comfort and preference, as well as assessment of treatment effectiveness. If a patient's pain is not demonstrating a desired response, modulation to avoid adaptation can be considered and modified.

Many clinicians and investigators, most notably Mannheimer and Lampe (4), consider electrode placement to be critical to the success of this type of stimulation. Clinicians should examine electrode placement sites carefully for each patient. Electrode placements must be individually tailored to each patient's unique set of circumstances. There is not, for example, an optimal low-back pain placement, but rather a set of choices to be tried systematically and accepted or rejected based on patient response. No cookbook approach to electrode placement will replace a sound knowledge of anatomy, neuroanatomy, and pathology.

When sensory-level stimulation is chosen, electrodes are most commonly placed around or over the site of pain. There is some evidence that placement in remote areas (e.g., acupuncture points or trigger points) (8) may also result in the amelioration of pain, but the preponderance of evidence for effectiveness is placement directly over the pain site or over very closely related anatomical structures, bounding the pain source with electrodes, which allows for stimulation of the receptive field of the sensitized neurons responsible for the pain (see Chapter 4). Pads can be adjusted based on the patient's response to the stimulation provided. For direct stimulation, it is important that the pain generator (source) is bounded by the electrodes. Once the electrodes are applied, the amplitude is increased to ensure that the patient can feel the sensation covering the area where the pain occurs. If this does not occur, the stimulator should be turned off and the location of the pads adjusted before resuming the treatment. This process is repeated until a location is identified that surrounds the pain source, minimizes or avoids muscular response, and is identified by the patient as a strong tingling sensation.

A wide range of current amplitudes produces electroanalgesia via sensory-level stimulation. Sensory-level stimulation at higher frequencies (greater than 100 pps) and longer pulse durations (greater than 50 μs) than those described for conventional TENS can be used to allow some specific procedures to be performed. This form of stimulation, combined with relatively close electrode placement, causes instantaneous interelectrode analgesia (23,27). Using smaller electrodes in close approximation will increase the current density in the area. Current density is defined as the concentration (mA per cm^2) of current beneath stimulating electrodes. When the intensity is high and the area of electrodes are small, a higher current density can be achieved compared to large electrodes placed a great distance apart. When the goal of the stimulation application is to achieve a local analgesic response, the selected site is bound closely with the stimulating electrodes, and the intensity is raised to the highest level tolerated. The stimulation-induced analgesia allows the clinician to perform short-duration therapeutic procedures that might prove too painful for the patient otherwise. Examples of such procedures include transverse friction massage, wound debridement, suture removal, and joint mobilization. The duration of the electrical stimulation treatment depends on the length of the procedure because the response is only expected during and possibly shortly after cessation of the stimulation.

The clinical decision to use interelectrode analgesia as an adjunct to an otherwise painful procedure is challenging. This intervention is time consuming because the safety of stimulation application must be evaluated, the device must be set up, maximal analgesic response must be assessed before applying the painful procedure, and the electrical setup must be removed. Some treatments create discomfort, and patients are surprisingly tolerant of these iatrogenic effects. In some situations, the pain tolerance of the patient interferes with his or her ability to permit a necessary procedure or allow for the appropriate intensity of a procedure to ensure its effectiveness. Under these circumstances, the additive benefit of electrically-induced analgesia may outweigh the time commitment. The clinician should evaluate the added benefit of the procedure to determine if the outcome justifies the use of therapeutic time. The need to perform the procedure in conjunction with wound debridement or suture removal is an easy variable to measure. In other situations, outcome measures can assist a therapist in determining if the stimulation is useful. When applied with joint mobilizations, range-of-motion gains after the treatment application can be compared to gains when stimulation was not provided. If the addition of the stimulation results in range gains beyond those achieved when no stimulation was applied, the treatment should continue. Once the additive benefit of the electrically-induced analgesia is no longer discernable, the treatment should be discontinued.

Motor-level Stimulation

Motor-level stimulation for pain modulation is used primarily for control of chronic pain. By definition, motor-level stimulation produces a visible muscle contraction. The efficacy of this stimulation is maximal when it is applied to a site anatomically or physiologically related to the site of pain (27). Motor-level stimulation for pain control most often involves continuous stimulation at a frequency in the 2- to 4-pps or bursts per second (bps) range, with relatively long phase durations (>150 μs), and amplitudes high enough to produce a strong, visible muscle contraction. This form of stimulation is also called *strong, low-rate (frequency) motor TENS* (Fig. 5.4F; Table 5.2). A continuous mode of higher frequencies and shorter pulse durations (*high-frequency motor TENS*) has been used. The common factor is the production of a rhythmic muscle contraction. In addition, brief bursts of pulses have been applied for pain control at levels that elicit muscle contraction. This form of stimulation (Fig. 5.4E) has been called *burst-modulated TENS*.

The magnitude of the induced muscle contraction varies from barely perceptible to extremely strong. Evidence supports the contention that stronger contractions produce better analgesia (23,24). It is reasonable to assume that pain fibers are not activated at the lower levels of motor stimulation. A nonpainful contraction is induced, and stimulation may simply effect pain relief in much the same way as sensory-level stimulation (peripheral block or activation of central inhibition).

The response of patients to motor-level stimulation is usually not immediate but is often long lasting (29,30). There is evidence for control of secondary mechanical hyperalgesia and improvements in blood flow (see Chapter 4). The motor-level TENS that produces rhythmic contraction may also activate the endogenous opiate mechanisms of analgesia (31). Muscular contraction produced in response to stimulation indicates to the health care provider that motor level of stimulation has been reached. Patients receiving motor-level TENS are informed that muscular activation is an expected response to this stimulation, preparing them for the involuntary contraction produced by motor level stimulation. It can be disconcerting for patients to see and feel their muscles respond in a manner not under their active control. Explaining the anticipated action and rationale is generally sufficient to allay any fears. The clinician should also prepare the patient's body for uncontrolled movement. In large muscle groups such as the lumbar spine or quadriceps, twitching may be visible but does not create significant motion; however, stimulation to muscles of the forearm or even the deltoid can generate distal motion. The patient should be positioned in a resting position and supported (i.e., with pillows) to minimize aberrant motion. If the target muscle is placed in a shortened position, less motion will occur compared to contraction in a stretched position. For example, if the target muscle is the gastrocnemius, placing the patient in supported slight knee flexion and ankle plantar flexion can allow for strong muscle contractions with little movement, compared to the same application in knee extension with ankle dorsiflexion. Because stronger contractions are more desirable (23,24), patient positioning will assist the clinician in achieving the maximal desired results from this procedure.

Motor-level stimulation has been shown to be effective in the modulation of experimentally-induced and clinical pain. It is most often used clinically with patients who complain of deep, throbbing, or chronic pain. This mode of stimulation has been called *noninvasive electroacupuncture* and *acupuncturelike TENS* (32) because it is often applied to remote areas that may correspond to acupuncture points. Motor-level stimulation evokes a visible muscle contraction. Patients can be intolerant of this, especially with strong muscle contractions in the painful area. For this reason, electrodes are most commonly placed in an area remote from the pain site. Although acupuncture points have been used, it is advisable to apply electrodes to sites that are anatomically or physiologically related to the pain site, such as the related myotome; for example, for C5 irritation the placement can be over the deltoid muscle. Reliance on motor point or acupuncture point charts for electrode placement is not advised because each patient has anatomical variations and specific problems. The charts are normative, and as such fit everyone to a certain extent but no one well. Again, a sound anatomical and neuroanatomical base is necessary and sufficient for good electrode placement. Here, a knowledge of not just dermatomal and myotomal distributions, but also scleratomal (segmental innervation of bone) distributions is helpful.

Often, point stimulators are used to deliver this type of stimulation via small-probe electrodes. Point stimulators generally have small-diameter applicators coupled with a larger (dispersive) electrode. This configuration creates a large current density under the smaller applicator and a lower, often imperceptible, density at the larger electrode. Clinically, this application is generally reserved for small target areas such as trigger points (8,33) or acupuncture-related sites. Palpation of an active trigger point in a patient can induce pain in a specific distribution. When the pain created recreates the complaints causing the patient to seek treatment, the trigger point is likely a contributor to the patient's problem. The clinician can expect that direct stimulation to the trigger point may reproduce the patient's complaints at the time of the treatment. Recordings of pain provocation or a decreased irritability of the patient's complaints between treatments are indicators of treatment success. Patient response is the best determinant of usefulness of motor stimulation in painful areas.

Induction of analgesia is usually not immediate with motor-level stimulation. For this reason, treatment times are longer than with sensory-level stimulation (45 minutes or longer versus

20 to 30 minutes). This allows the induction of analgesia before treatment is terminated. When treatment is performed at home, it is usually done 2 to 3 times per day. This type of treatment is also performed several times per week in clinical settings.

Noxious-level Stimulation

Noxious-level stimulation for pain amelioration is the application of electrotherapeutic currents to produce a painful stimulus in or remote from the pain site. Noxious-level stimulation is produced using either low-frequency 1 to 5 pps) or high-frequency (80 to 100 pps) stimuli with long pulse durations of up to 1 second and amplitudes that produce pain beneath the electrodes with or without muscle contraction. Although activation of motor nerves routinely occurs before activation of pain fibers, noxious-level stimulation is often applied to areas with no motor nerve fibers, minimizing the potential for producing muscle contraction. The pulse duration and frequency characteristics described above are those in common use, but the only requirement is that the patient perceives the stimulus as painful.

Noxious-level stimulation is believed to effect pain amelioration by an endorphin-mediated mechanism. Pain production in a related or unrelated area is thought to result in a systemic release of endogenous opiates, which increases the patient's pain threshold. Noxious-level stimulation may also cause a quick-onset pain modulation called *hyperstimulation analgesia*, which has been hypothesized to interfere with the patterned-reverberation pain circuitry described by Nabe (34). Noxious-level stimulation can be effective in the relief of clinical and experimentally-induced pain. Because of its inherent discomfort, it is rarely used clinically as a first approach. It is most often used after adaptation to sensory-level stimulation or in cases where sensory-level or motor-level stimulation has not been effective.

Electrode placement for noxious-level stimulation is the most varied and arbitrary of all the stimulation modes used for electroanalgesia. Electrodes are most often placed over the pain site, perhaps to reintroduce a noxious, regional stimulation into the homeostasis developed in the chronic pain situation. Direct stimulation of the receptive field to the sensitized neurons is likely to generate the best response. Associated acupuncture points, motor points, trigger points, and unrelated sites are also used and have similar efficacy. Noxious-level stimulation applied anywhere in the body may be as effective as stimulation applied to a site anatomically or physiologically related to the pain site in the amelioration of that pain (35,36).

Neuraxial Implants for Pain Control

In some cases, pain unresponsive to TENS, from a widespread area, or pain resulting from injury to the nervous system can be a candidate for a neuraxis (spinal cord and deep brain) stimulator. In these cases, controlled stimulation of the spinal cord is achieved through the use of implanted electrodes to activate axons in the dorsal (posterior) columns and intracerebral areas such as periaqueductal and periventricular gray matter (37–45). Spinal cord stimulators are more successful for the treatment of neuropathic pain than nociceptive pain and have been used for multiple conditions such as arachnoiditis, failed cervical and low back syndrome, complex regional pain syndrome, peripheral nerve injury, postamputation pain syndrome, postherpetic neuralgia, and other types of chronic, intractable pain (46–49). Once a pain syndrome with a cause such as those listed above is identified and psychopathology is excluded, if the topography of the patient's pain will be covered by stimulation paresthesia, a trial of implanted stimulation can be considered (44,46,47). Electrodes can be either percutaneous or plate-type, which requires implantation under direct vision. Multipolar systems seem to outperform monopolor designs (37,40). The stimulator can be an "all-inside" approach which means the electrodes and the pulse generator are placed beneath the skin and are programmed transdermally via remote computer. These stimulators require battery replacement on average every 3 to 5 years, but the stimulator runs without patient management and is only turned on or off via an external magnet. In a partially implanted system, the implanted electrode is connected to a radio frequency receiver, and an external radio frequency transmitter generates stimulation in the implanted receiver when the two contact one another (44,45). This system does not require internal battery adjustment, but the parameters are easily within patient control for modification. The parameters are usually a patient-selected modification of 40- to 120-pps, 100- to 250-μs pulse duration and amplitude to pleasant tingling sensation. Parameters are adjusted based on patient response and clinician experience, but when necessary, the radio frequency device is capable of 1400 Hz. On/off times vary.

Much of the data available on the efficacy of spinal stimulation for pain control are presented in retrospective series and reviews. More rigorous methodology is needed to clearly identify the success rate of this intervention. Studies demonstrate a 25% to 50% success rate with spinal cord stimulators in patients with failed low back syndrome. "Success" is characterized by at least a 50% reduction in the patient's pain level even up to 2 years after implantation (50,51). Similar findings are seen in studies with patients with complex regional pain syndrome, peripheral vascular disease, and intractable angina (52–55).

Peripheral nerve stimulators with implanted electrodes are also used when a local peripheral anesthetic block provides relief from pain. Patients with complex regional pain syndrome, plexus injury, neuromas, and neuropathies may be appropriate candidates for this procedure. Surgical exposure of the nerve of interest is required, and the electrode is secured with a graph to the connective tissue surrounding the nerve (44). After a trial period, if a 50% reduction in pain is achieved, a pulse generator is implanted. Pain relief of 50% or greater has been seen in patients with peripheral nerve injury and chronic pain syndromes (56,57).

Motor cortex stimulation for pain control was introduced in the 1950s (58) but has not been fully developed. The early work has demonstrated some success in patients with central pain and trigeminal neuropathy, although the optimal stimulation parameters are unknown (59–61). The technical demands of implantation aided with computerized tomography or magnetic resonance visualization of the target tissue are no less difficult than the complex cases motor cortex stimulation may be best suited to help. Continued exploration of this form of stimulation is likely (43).

The benchmark for success with stimulation via implanted electrodes is high. Although clinicians and patients may be willing to accept lower than 50% reduction in pain levels as a successful outcome for the intervention, the treatment is not without risk. Many medical conditions, such as bleeding disorders, implanted cardiac demand-type pacemakers or defibrillators, or the inability of the patient to use or understand the device are contraindications to use of this form of pain management. Risks also exist during and after the implantation procedure. The most significant risk is neurological damage during the surgical procedure or cord compression from an intraspinal clot (45). Other risks include infection, leakage of cerebrospinal fluid, equipment migration, and hardware failure (44). There are concerns for the functional integrity of the microcircuitry if the patient is exposed to therapeutic radiation or MRIs; therefore, significant functional improvement in patient behaviors will likely be a continued benchmark for treatment efficacy (46).

LITERATURE ON EFFECTIVENESS OF ELECTRICAL STIMULATION FOR PAIN CONTROL

In this review of the literature on electrical stimulation and treatment of pain, we attempt to correlate stimulation characteristics with the various theories of pain transmission and control to provide a rational basis for their use. The preponderance of the literature reports on the use of portable TENS devices. Only one randomized, controlled clinical trial of the use of interferential current for pain control has demonstrated no effect of electrical stimulation over placebo (62). There are no similar studies of the effects of high-voltage pulsed current on pain control in the peer-reviewed literature.

In a recent review of the use of electrical stimulation for pain control, Long (64, p. 16) stated, "There are no comparative studies of TENS with other modalities in the treatment of acute pain." Nevertheless, electrical stimulation is generally assumed to be the most effective treatment for acute and postoperative pain (64,65).

Transcutaneous Electrical Nerve Stimulation and Chronic Pain Control

TENS effectiveness studies can be most easily divided into low-frequency (LFTENS) and high-frequency (HFTENS) categories. In 2002 the *Cochrane Review on TENS for Chronic Pain* determined that too few studies with sufficient rigor for subject randomization, objective outcome variables, and explanation of relevant TENS parameters exist to make definitive conclusions on the benefits of TENS for chronic pain (66). The chronic pain conditions included rheumatoid arthritis, osteoarthritis, pancreatitis, myofascial pain, diabetic neuropathy, and low back pain, and used pain scales including visual and verbal rating scales.

High-frequency Transcutaneous Electrical Nerve Stimulation for Chronic Pain Control

In the review, eight studies were identified with sufficient rigor to be examined for the analgesic efficacy of HFTENS compared to sham TENS. Five of the eight studies cited demonstrated an immediately positive response for analgesia, contrasted with two that found no positive effects on pain (67–73). In the Ableson et al. study (67), 32 patients with rheumatoid arthritis of the wrist were randomized to HFTENS (70 pps) and sham TENS applied directly over the painful site for 3 weekly doses with a treatment duration of 15 minutes. The treatment had a positive effect on VAS during rest and on gripping activity immediately after the treatment for those receiving HFTENS; however, no long-term follow-up was performed. Vinterberg et al. (71) had similar response in their study of 14 patients with HFTENS (70 to 100 pps) over the site of pain on the wrists of patients with rheumatoid arthritis. They demonstrated an improvement in VAS at rest during pre- and postcomparisons following one 60-minute session of stimulation, but found no statistically significant impact on pain with gripping.

Moystad et al. (69) used a cross-over design in which each of the 19 patients with rheumatoid arthritis of the temporomandibular joint received HFTENS (100 pps) and sham TENS over the site of pain on two separate trials. Immediately and 24 hours after one 30-minute treatment, the HFTENS outperformed the sham TENS on VAS scores for movement. In the study by Hseuh et al. (68), 60 patients with mild and moderate pain from trigger points in the upper trapezius muscle were treated with HFTENS (60 pps) for one 20-minute treatment applied directly to the trigger point. Immediate improvement was seen on a VAS for pain intensity in the HFTENS group compared to sham TENS and LFTENS (10 pps) groups; however, no long-term data were collected and the variable pretesting pain levels in the patients make comparisons difficult.

Smith et al. (70) evaluated the benefits of HFTENS (50 Hz) versus sham TENS on 32 randomized patients with knee osteoarthritis treated twice a week for 20-minute sessions over 4 weeks. Treatments varied between local tender points and acupuncture sites. The patients treated with HFTENS and those with sham TENS had 50% pain improvement or greater on a seven-point pain scale immediately after the treatment, and those with HFTENS outperformed those in the sham TENS group, with greater than 50% improvements in pain response at 4 weeks

(67% vs. 27%) and 8 weeks (46% vs. 27%); the number of patients who benefited long term declined over the 2-month follow-up, and more than one-fourth of those receiving sham TENS demonstrated both short- and long-term benefits from treatment with electrodes not connected to an active TENS unit.

In another study of acupuncture site stimulation in patients with knee osteoarthritis, Lewis et al. (74) randomized 29 patients into a crossover design of HFTENS (70 pps) and sham TENS. The patients had three daily sessions of 30 to 60 minutes for 3 weeks. After 3 weeks, 46% of those in the HFTENS group and 43% of those in the sham TENS group reported greater than 50% reduction in their pain levels. Forty-three percent of the HFTENS group compared to 14% in the sham TENS group intended to continue with TENS use after the study. Grimmer et al. (72) did not see an improvement with HFTENS (80 pps) after one 30-minute treatment to an acupuncture site in 60 patients with knee osteoarthritis randomized to HFTENS, LFTENS (80 pps, 3 bursts per second), and sham TENS groups. There was no immediate response in either active TENS group, and a short-term response at 24 hours only for the LFTENS group. In another study by Lewis et al. (75), subjects with knee osteoarthritis were given HFTENS (70 pps, 100 μs) to acupuncture points of the spleen and stomach for 30 to 60 minutes, three times daily for 3 weeks, and this was compared to nonsteroidal anti-inflammatory medications and sham TENS. There was no significant impact of TENS on the patients pain levels; however, when asked whether the treatment they were currently using was effective on their pain, 54% felt the HFTENS was effective, compared to 36% when the TENS was sham. Twenty-four percent of the patients said they would continue to use the HFTENS after the study concluded, and 14% expressed a desire to continue the sham TENS treatment. A placebo effect is evident, and the authors believe that this effect was responsible for the inability to achieve statistically significant changes in the pain measures they recorded. In a study by Moore et al. (73) in 28 patients with low back pain treated in a crossover design comparing HFTENS (100 pps) and sham TENS, after two sessions of 5 hours of stimulation each, there was no statistically significant post-treatment response in mean pain levels in the active stimulation group, yet 8% of the patients in both the stimulation and sham stimulation groups planned to continue with the treatment after the study.

Comparisons among these studies are challenging. The parameters the studies cite are highly variable, including treatment frequency, duration, locations, and sessions. Some of these studies administered treatment at the site of pain, and others used acupuncture-related or trigger points, and the ranges in treatment dosage were highly erratic. There are simply insufficient data to generate direct clinical conclusions.

Low-frequency Transcutaneous Electrical Nerve Stimulation for Chronic Pain Control

Early studies of motor-level electrical stimulation for the relief of chronic pain had positive results similar to those obtained in early studies of the effectiveness of sensory-level stimulation for pain control. Here, too, the preponderance of literature involved case reports, retrospective chart reviews, and, at best, crossover designs. Few prospective randomized clinical trials have been performed. Melzack et al. (76) compared motor-level electrical stimulation (4 to 8 Hz with electrodes placed over the low back) with suction-cup massage in the treatment of patients with chronic low back pain. Forty-one patients were randomly assigned in this double-blind prospective study. The McGill Pain Questionnaire pain rating index and present pain index plus straight leg raise measurements were used to assess outcome. The electrical stimulation group was statistically better than the massage group in all measures (4,76).

In the 2002 *Cochrane Review on TENS for Chronic Pain*, five studies of sufficient rigor were evaluated for analgesic efficacy after LFTENS compared to sham TENS. The overall conclusion was that three studies demonstrated a positive response and two did not (68,69,72,77). As previously noted in the Grimmer study (72), LFTENS (80 pps, 3 bursts per second) outperformed HFTENS and sham TENS on 24-hour after-treatment pain reports in patients with osteoarthritis of the knee, although no immediate post-treatment improvements were seen compared to sham TENS. In the Hseuh et al. study (68) of patients with trigger point of the upper trapezius muscle, LFTENS (10 pps) and HFTENS (60 pps) directly over the trigger point outperformed sham stimulation on immediate after-treatment VAS measures of pain intensity. Kumar et al. (77) studied LFTENS (70 pps in 2 bursts per second) in 31 patients with pain resulting from diabetic neuropathy. Thirty-minute daily home treatment sessions over 4 weeks were performed over four areas of the leg. No immediate after-treatment assessments were performed, but improvements in VAS were seen in the LFTENS group at the end of the 4-week treatment duration compared with the group receiving sham TENS. Moystad et al. (69) compared a single 30-minute dose of LFTENS (2 pps) to sham TENS on patients with rheumatoid arthritis of the temporomandibular joint after finding a benefit with HFTENS (100 pps). There was no immediate response to the LFTENS treatment, and no further assessment was made.

When HFTENS and LFTENS were compared to one another, four studies did not detect a difference between these two types of stimulation, one reported a difference in favor of HFTENS, and two reported a difference in favor of LFTENS (68,72,78–82). Jensen et al. (78) randomized 20 patients with knee osteoarthritis into LFTENS (2 pps) or HFTENS (80 pps) groups. Five treatment sessions each 30 minutes long yielded a positive response for pain improvement for both HFTENS and LFTENS at the end of the treatment week and at a 3-week follow-up. Neither HFTENS nor LFTENS outperformed the other, and no sham TENS group was included in this protocol. Nash et al. (79) evaluated 200 patients with a variety of chronic pain conditions and compared four variations of TENS for durations of up to 2 years. This study compared continuous and pulsed HFTENS (100 pps) with continuous and pulsed LFTENS (10 pps). Although the information provided to allow a clinician to reproduce the procedures on specific patients was sparse, all stimulation forms demonstrated a positive effect on pain. At one year of treatment, between 24% and 47% of the subjects reported a 50% reduction in their pain ratings, although no one type of stimulation was deemed most effective and comparisons to sham treatment were not made.

Grimmer et al. (72) saw no immediate response to HFTENS (80 pps) or LFTENS (80 pps at 3 bursts per second) compared to sham in patients with knee osteoarthritis. A delayed improvement was seen in only the LFTENS burst group a day after the single 30-minute treatment administration. This response favored LFTENS in this study, but no long-term follow-up was performed. Mannheimer and Carlsson (80) evaluated three forms of stimulation on 20 patients with rheumatoid arthritis of the wrist in a crossover design. A 10-minute single treatment of HFTENS (70 pps), LFTENS (3 pps), or frequency-modulated TENS (70 pps at 3 bursts per second) was performed over the wrist. Improvement was noted as a change from baseline of at least two grades on a 1 to 5 scale. In general, the LFTENS was less effective than the other two stimulation types, although some patients demonstrated improvement from this form of stimulation.

Tulgar et al. (81,82) evaluated variations of HFTENS and LFTENS on patients with a variety of chronic painful conditions. The number of treatment sessions ranged from 20 to 30 per stimulation pattern, and the form of stimulation deemed most successful by the patient was used for a subsequent 3-month trial. Three modes of electrical stimulation were applied: constant frequency sensory-level stimulation (70 pps); burst-modulated sensory-level stimulation (90 ms trains of 100 pps; 10 trains at 2 Hz); and frequency-modulated sensory-level stimulation (continuous pulses ranging from 90 to 55 Hz over 90 ms). In general, burst-modulated and HFTENS were more effective than continuous, frequency-modulated TENS. In 8 of 14 patients who continued with their preferred choice of stimulation for 3 months, 2 subjects had 50% reduction in pain long term. In general, if a theoretical rationale for stimulation parameters can be made, the response is positive. If one form of stimulation is not generating the desired response, a change to other forms may be considered.

Transcutaneous Electrical Nerve Stimulation and Control of Chronic Low-back Pain

The Deyo et al. study (83) randomly assigned 145 patients with chronic low back pain to a trial of electrical stimulation [HFTENS (80 to 100 pps) for 2 weeks followed by LFTENS (2 to 4 pps), with the third 2-week trial at the self-selected favorite], sham electrical stimulation, electrical stimulation and exercise, or sham electrical stimulation and exercise. The HFTENS was administered for 2 weeks as 45-minute sessions three times daily or more. Then LFTENS was introduced as a trial for 2 weeks and patients were allowed to choose the mode they preferred for the remaining 2 weeks. Electrodes were located over the area of pain. All subjects improved over the study period, although they returned to baseline at the 3-month follow-up. A modified SIP, a VAS, and an activity rating scale were used to determine effect of treatment. Exercise was more effective than electrical stimulation, and electrical stimulation was no more effective than placebo. No statistically significant differences were found in any outcome between the subjects with true or sham TENS after 2 weeks, 4 weeks, and at 3 months, although 68% of those using active TENS and 56% of those using sham TENS wished to continue TENS therapy after completion of the study.

The authors admitted that in chronic pain this form of counterstimulation may be inadequate for some people with low back pain (83). The patients averaged 4.1 years of low back pain, and it is unlikely that HFTENS would have profound effects on this population because the literature points instead to active therapy, occupational factors, and even fear-avoidance beliefs as factors affecting recovery following back pain (84,85). HFTENS would only have been theorized to provide pain relief while the stimulation was ongoing; three daily sessions of 45 minutes is not expected to have lasting relief over a day, and even less of a response would be expected weeks after discontinuation. This study had a profound effect on reimbursement for TENS for patients with low back pain and prompted much discussion in the literature. Criticism ranged from the inclusion of patients who were not in active treatment and an apparent failure of the randomization with respect to previous surgery, to disagreement regarding the current characteristics and timing of the stimulation. Many suggestions were made to correct the identified flaws with this study (83).

In 1997 the Moore and Shurman study (73) also demonstrated no change in chronic back pain after two 5-hour sessions of HFTENS. Herman et al. (86) designed a study to evaluate a new use of TENS on patients with acute, occupational, low back pain. Their TENS unit switched between HFTENS and LFTENS among six predetermined body sites regardless of pain source or location. The stimulation was performed 30 minutes before exercise and was compared to a sham TENS plus exercise group. A variety of outcome measures including disability questionnaires, VAS three times daily, and return to work rate were collected. In this study, however, there was a statistically significant drop in patient's pain in the treatment group (almost 50%) compared with less than 10% in the sham group. No data on typical TENS can be extrapolated from this report, and this novel approach to multisite stimulation requires further testing.

Marchand et al. (87) used a pseudo-randomization technique (controlling for sex, weight, diagnosis, and pain severity) to HFTENS, sham TENS, or control group. A preassessment of pain severity was performed using a VAS. During preparation for use of the real and sham stimulators, the authors noted that all patients reported a sensation, including those with sham treatment. Patients recorded pain complaints for both intensity and unpleasantness on a VAS every 2 hours for 10 weeks. The subjects followed up with ratings for 3-day periods at 11 weeks, 22 weeks, and 34 weeks after treatment. The HFTENS group demonstrated a statistically significant reduction in pain ratings before and after treatment of greater than 40% compared to 17% in the sham TENS group. Over the 10-week treatment period of two 30-minute treatments weekly, the pretreatment pain complaints were reduced in the HFTENS group only. The effectiveness of TENS treatment continued into the 11th week after cessation of the actual TENS treatment. Both the TENS and sham TENS groups demonstrated greater pain relief than the control group at 22 and 34 weeks. The authors cite both the placebo effect and a potential increase in activity in both TENS conditions as a result of the decrease in pain as explanations for their findings. The study needs to be replicated with true randomization and measurement of activity levels and medications to assist in interpreting these results.

A retrospective analysis was performed on 376 patients owning TENS units (most commonly patients with herniated discs, sciatica, and lumbar surgery) and using the units for 6 months or longer (88). Although the authors relied on patient reports of pre-TENS condition and post-TENS success, they reported significant improvement in pain interference with activity, decreased use of therapies, and decreased use of pain and anti-inflammatory medications. The authors note issues related to the possible sources of error with this type of reporting but consider that, even if overestimated, the results may provide insight into not only short-term but also long-term benefits of TENS for the control of chronic pain with continued use.

Johnson et al. (28), studied long-term users of portable TENS devices. Approximately 50% of the patients reported that TENS relieved their pain by more than half. Electroanalgesia had a rapid onset and was not long lasting after the device was turned off. One-third of the patients used TENS for more than 61 hours per week. Approximately half of the patients reported pain reduction from a burst modulation, and most used stimulation frequencies between 1 and 70 pps. It is interesting that two-thirds of those who reported no electroanalgesia nevertheless used the stimulators on a daily basis.

Transcutaneous Electrical Nerve Stimulation and Acute Pain Control

All studies included in this section have examined the efficacy of high-frequency TENS in the management of acute pain. The stimulation parameters are in the range of conventional TENS settings. In many cases, descriptions of the parameters used are inadequate. Some studies have demonstrated the effectiveness of electrical stimulation for control of acute pain.

Early reports, case studies, and retrospective reviews suggested that electrical stimulation was quite effective for the treatment of postoperative and acute pain (89–91). In problems as varied as low back pain (89), pancreatitis (90), and postherpetic neuralgia (91), sensory-level stimulation had been shown to be an effective modulator of acute pain. The effectiveness of TENS for pain control in more recent studies has been less than that found in earlier studies. Reported benefits of postoperative electroanalgesia have included decreased length of stay, reduced pulmonary complications, and less narcotic usage.

Schomburg and Carter-Baker (92) reported on a retrospective chart review of 150 patients who had undergone laparotomy, 75 of whom received sensory-level stimulation paraincisionally after surgery. The 75 patients in the comparison group were operated on before the institution of the postoperative electrical stimulation program. Length of stay and medication usage were the only comparisons made between groups, but pain intensity and unpleasantness were measured using VAS in the electrical stimulation group. The authors found a statistically lower medication usage in the electrical stimulation group than in the comparison group, but no difference in length of stay. Issenman et al. (93) compared 20 patients after spinal fusion with Harrington rods. Ten patients received sensory-level stimulation paraincisionally after surgery. Ten age-matched control patients were also studied. Length of stay and medication usage were lower in the electrical stimulation group. Results were presented descriptively without statistical analysis.

Hargreaves and Lander (94) randomly assigned 75 abdominal surgery patients to electrical stimulation (100 pps, 0.4 ms), sham electrical stimulation, and control groups. The conventional TENS was applied 15 minutes before and during the dressing change that occurred on the second day after surgery. A VAS for pain intensity was used. There was significantly greater pain relief in the electrical stimulation group, and no difference between the sham electrical stimulation and control groups. Benedetti et al. (95) randomly assigned 324 patients after thoracic surgery procedures to one of three groups: HFTENS (100 pps, 200-μs pulse duration), placebo-TENS, and standard postoperative medications. TENS had no effect on the management of severe pain, provided an additive effect to typical pain medications for moderate pain, and was successful in replacing medications in mild pain conditions.

These studies are in the minority in demonstrating effectiveness. Caroll et al. (96) performed a review of the impact of nonrandomization on estimating the benefits of TENS on postoperative pain. The overall conclusion based on the evidence that met the author's inclusion criteria was that the benefits of TENS in the postoperative period are overestimated. Postoperative pain management with the use of TENS has been evaluated under many conditions, including abdominal surgery, coronary artery bypass, gastric bypass, and thoracotomy (97–101).

The results of randomized prospective studies of the effectiveness of electrical stimulation on acute and postoperative pain have not been as positive as one might have expected from conventional wisdom. Reuss et al. (102) randomly assigned 64 patients who were undergoing elective cholecystectomy to one of two groups: electrical stimulation (50 pps, 170-ms pulse duration) and no electrical stimulation. A commercially available TENS device was set to deliver sensory-level stimulation, and electrodes were placed within 2 cm of the surgical incision. There was no statistically significant difference in length of stay, narcotic usage, or pulmonary complications between groups (102).

Carman and Roach (103) studied children 11 to 21 years of age who were undergoing spinal surgery. Patients were randomly assigned to one of three groups (15 in each group): analgesics and electrical stimulation, analgesics and sham electrical stimulation, and analgesics alone. Duration-modulated sensory-level stimulation at 60 pps was delivered. There was no difference in narcotic usage or length of stay between groups (103). Smedley et al. (104) randomly assigned 62 men scheduled for hernia repair into two groups: electrical stimulation (70 pps) or sham electrical stimulation. Sensory-level stimulation was used. There was no significant difference between groups in postoperative opiate usage, pulmonary function, or visual analog pain ratings (104).

Walker et al. (105) performed a sequential trial in the treatment of 30 patients after unilateral total knee arthroplasty. Sensory-level stimulation (70 pps, 100 μs) applied to the knee along with constant passive motion was compared to constant passive motion without electrical stimulation. There was no difference between treatments for length of stay, knee flexion range of motion, and analgesic use (105). All these studies suggest that even in the cases where electrical stimulation is theoretically most likely to be effective, when subjected to the rigor of prospective randomized design, effectiveness is not readily demonstrated.

Studies on postoperative TENS generally agree that TENS is not effective in the face of severe pain, and in many studies no change on measured outcomes is demonstrated (96). Short-term improvements such as decreased 24-hour analgesic use or shorter lengths of stay in the recovery room have been seen, yet they can be deemed insignificant when pain management is the clinical goal (106,107). In general, the role of TENS on postoperative pain can benefit from larger clinical trials with variables to include the ability to customize the TENS settings, evaluations of pain, medication usage, functional recovery (ability to walk or cough sooner), and inclusion of both sham TENS and control groups to manage the placebo effect. As VanderArk and McGrath said in 1975 (109, p. 340), "although TENS obviously is not a panacea as a future analgesic, its role should be assessed critically and not denied."

Dawood and Ramos (109) used a randomized crossover design to compare the effectiveness of electrical stimulation (sensory level, 100 pps, 100 μs) to that of sham electrical stimulation and ibuprofen in the treatment of acute pain in primary dysmenorrhea. During the cycles of treatment with electrical stimulation, the women studied required less rescue medication than during the placebo electrical stimulation cycles, and had pain relief comparable to that during the ibuprofen cycles (109). Milsom et al. (110) found a similar response comparing HFTENS to oral naproxen in women with primary dysmenorrhea in a 2-day crossover design. HFTENS (70 to 100 pps) 0.2-ms constant pulses were administered through electrodes located on either side of the umbilicus, suprapubic area, and sacroiliac region on one day, and the strong stimulation (40 to 50 mA) was compared to an oral dose of 500 mg of naproxen, given the alternate day. Naproxen demonstrated improvement in intrauterine pressures and pain ratings after the 90-minute postadministration time that continued until 240 minutes, although the benefits waned over time. HFTENS did not affect intrauterine pressure measurements but resulted in a significant reduction in pain after the first 15-minute recording interval and before the second 30-minute interval that lasted throughout the 240-minute time period. Although both methods were effective, TENS was quicker and no less effective than the oral nonsteriodal and as long lasting. This supports a growing body of work suggesting that TENS may be effective for primary dysmenorrheal pain, especially when typical pharmacological agents are not tolerated or desired.

Transcutaneous Electrical Stimulation Research Shortcomings

The Cochrane Report (67, p. 2) on the effectiveness of TENS on chronic pain concluded that "the published trials do not provide information on the stimulation parameters which are most likely to provide optimum pain relief, nor do they answer questions about long-term effectiveness." Clinicians must rely on a theoretical approach based on the available evidence and understanding of the biology of pain when choosing parameters likely to accomplish the clinical goal.

Published TENS research is riddled with shortcomings in experimental design. In general, reporting of the methods used and numbers of subjects recruited are inadequate. Rarely do parameters include electrical stimulation unit, electrode number, size and location, current intensity, and clear descriptions of stimulation frequency or modulation. The measurement methods and data for different analgesic outcomes are often absent or ill-defined. Response time frames are also variable. Most studies have some immediate measure of pain relief, but few extend the testing time frame to 24 hours and beyond, which is necessary for the determination of treatment efficacy. Some studies evaluate a single dose response and others assess the response of a myriad of multiple dose combinations. Of 109 studies identified in the population of patients with chronic pain, the Cochrane study could only evaluate 19 studies due to inadequate methodology (66). The poor methodology cited in the 19 included trials made meta-analysis impossible and led to inconclusive results on the effectiveness of TENS of any type in this population.

Research projects need to be randomized and reflect clinical practice. In the chronic pain population, TENS can be used for long periods of time, in excess of 6 to 8 hours per day, and single-dose trials may simply be misguided in design (28). Stimulation parameters can be idiosyncratic, and in the majority of the studies available to date, the subjects were not permitted to adjust parameters to optimize their response. Long-term follow-up including evaluations and pain diaries have been suggested by the Cochrane Report and reflect clinically relevant changes in complaints. In short, clinicians cannot rely on the evidence to provide definitive characteristics for TENS treatment by treatment condition or stimulation type. The artful management of the devices coupled with the consistent and long-term evaluation of patient response may be the best tools currently available to determine individual treatment effectiveness.

Dose–Response Issues in Electrical Stimulation for Pain Control

One of the major criticisms of studies of electrical stimulation where effectiveness has not been demonstrated is that the investigators did not use the "right" stimulation characteristics (111). Some studies have been undertaken that compared the relative effectiveness of different stimulation characteristics. Johnson et al. (112) examined control of cold-induced pain by different frequencies of electrical stimulation. They found that the greatest analgesia occurred at frequencies between 20 and 80 pps for sensory-level stimulation. Frequencies above and below this range were less effective (112). Tulgar et al. (81) examined patterns of stimulation in two studies on chronic pain cited above. In the first study, three delivery modes were tested: constant-frequency sensory-level stimulation (70 pps), burst-modulated sensory-level stimulation (90 ms trains of 100 pps; 10 trains at 2 Hz), and frequency-modulated sensory-level stimulation (continuous pulses ranging from 90–55 Hz over 90 msec). The patients, all of whom had chronic pain, preferred the modulated modes to the constant-frequency mode (80). In the second study, constant-frequency high-rate frequency-modulated (55 to 90 pps), low-rate frequency-modulated (20 to 60 pps), and burst-modulated sensory-level stimulation were tested for relief of chronic pain in 14 patients with a variety of pain conditions as measured by a VAS of pain intensity (81). Six of the 14 patients did not report any effect of the stimulation on their pain. Among the remaining patients, there was a preference for the high-rate, frequency-modulated and burst-modulated modes. These studies are beginning to address the dose–response issues regarding frequency and frequency modulation, but other characteristics (current intensity, pulse duration) have yet to be systematically examined.

Placebo Effects of Electrical Stimulation for Pain

Electrical stimulation has a profound placebo effect that has been underscored in many studies and throughout this chapter. Petrie and Hazleman (113) demonstrated that sham electrical stimulation can be a strong placebo. Langley et al. (114), in a randomized, double-blind study of patients with chronic pain, demonstrated a clear placebo effect of sensory-level electrical stimulation. Although effectiveness has been reported in some studies, any clear benefit of TENS other than that which can be explained by the placebo effect has not been shown convincingly in randomized, prospective studies.

PRECAUTIONS, CONTRAINDICATIONS, AND ADVERSE EFFECTS OF TRANSCUTANEOUS ELECTRICAL STIMULATION FOR PAIN CONTROL

Table 5.3 lists the contraindications and or precautions/warnings for the use of electrical stimulation for pain control. Some literature actually calls the rationale for certain of the listed precautions into question. For example, demand-inhibited (synchronous) pacemakers are sensitive to electromagnetic interference. Most pacemakers in use today are of this type. An electrical signal within the pacemaker's range can inhibit pacing by indicating a normal heart rhythm when none occurs. Performing an electrocardiogram during a trial of TENS has been suggested to ensure normal pacemaker function. Chen et al. (115) reported on two patients with synchronous pacemakers who were using TENS for control of chronic pain. Electrocardiogram tracings showed no interference, but extended cardiac monitoring (Holter) showed inhibition of pacemaker function by the TENS devices. One patient used the stimulator with electrodes on the back and legs, the other with electrodes on the neck and shoulder. In both cases, the pacemakers were reprogrammed to change their sensitivities, and no further inhibition of pacing occurred. This study's recommendation for extended cardiac monitoring for patients with synchronous pacemakers appears to be a prudent one.

Table 5.3. Contraindications, Precautions, Warnings, and Adverse Reactions for TENS Applications

Contraindications	TENS should not be used: Over or near medical stimulators, monitors, or their leads; e.g., demand-type cardiac pacemakers; sleep apnea monitors; cardioverter difibillators; phrenic nerve stimulators; bladder stimulators; ECG monitors In confused or uncooperative patients TENS should not be applied over: Damaged skin or subcutaneous tissues Skin with impaired sensation Malignancies Arterial or venous thrombus (e.g., thrombophlebitis) Anterior neck to avoid stimulation of the carotid Sinus, laryngeal, or pharyngeal muscles Phrenic nerve or vagus nerve
Precautions/warnings	Safety of TENS use during pregnancy has not been established; TENS use in a woman who is pregnant should only be performed following consultation with and approval from the woman's obstetrician Patients should be closely monitored when TENS use may pass current across the head (transcranial) or through the chest (transthoracic) Monitoring of vital signs (e.g., blood pressure) should be performed in patients with disorders such as heart disease, hypertension, or hypotension Caution should be exercised in patients with diagnosed or suspected epilepsy TENS should be used only under the continued, regular supervision of a qualified health professional Use only for the specific pain problem identified by the health professional Keep TENS devices out of the reach of children TENS should be used with caution while operating machinery or vehicles Turn the stimulator off prior to applying, adjusting, or removing surface electrodes Long-term stimulation at the same electrode site may cause skin irritation Response of the skin under the electrodes should be monitored after treatment
Potential adverse reactions to TENS therapy	Allergic reaction to tape, electrodes, or gel Skin irritation or burn beneath the electrodes Dizziness, syncope (fainting) Nausea and vomiting Increased pain

The evidence underlying the rationale behind a number of other contraindications commonly cited for the use of TENS is lacking. Manufacturers of TENS devices list the use of TENS over metal implants as a contraindication for the use of TENS. This fails to take into account the low electrical conductivity of certain metals such as titanium. The Food and Drug Administration suggests that electrical stimulation should not be used over the abdomen of women who are pregnant, but there are many reports of the use of electrical stimulation during labor and delivery, and no adverse effects have been demonstrated (116,117). Interference with fetal monitoring has been reported (118). The safety for the fetus of prolonged or repetitive stimulation over the abdomen or back has not been determined.

Electrical stimulation for pain control should be used cautiously, if at all, when the patient's pain is serving a protective or useful function. For example, if pain is to be used as a limitation for progression of weight bearing or range of motion, it would be inappropriate to use electrical stimulation to reduce the pain.

Users of electrical stimulation for pain control and other applications of electrical stimulation should refer regularly to the instruction manuals that are provided by manufacturers of stimulators in order to refresh or update their understanding of the contraindications and precautions/warnings associated with the use of these devices.

The most common complication from portable stimulator use is skin irritation, primarily near or under the electrodes (18). In general, the adverse effects reported with the use of TENS are not serious. The complaints range from skin rash, to burning sensations and skin irritation (67,70,77,79). This complication is most likely a function of the electrode interface (26). The use of self-adhesive electrodes that are composed of synthetic materials should mitigate this response.

CLINICAL CASE STUDIES

The case studies that follow are examples of the types of patient pain problems that may be amenable to remediation by electrical stimulation. Regardless of the other treatment goals, pain modulation is common to all, and electrical stimulation for pain modulation is a component of each treatment plan. For brevity, only essential additional treatment is included (e.g., ultrasound in a combination treatment, or the therapeutic procedure being performed under electroanalgesia). The reader should remember that electrotherapy for pain is primarily adjunctive to other treatments crucial for a successful outcome. Cases 5 and 6 demonstrate some special circumstances in which patients whose problems are not traditionally within the scope of physical therapy may be helped by electrotherapeutic intervention.

Case 1

A 36-year-old longshoreman injured his low back 2 days ago while lifting a heavy object at work. Medical history is noncontributory; x-rays of the spine are negative.

Objective

Examination reveals marked limitation in all lumbar motions with pain rated as 10/10 on a verbal rating scale for all motions. Test maneuvers produce no peripheralization or centralization of symptoms, but complete testing was precluded by pain. There is significant lumbar muscle guarding and diffuse low back pain. Neurological signs are negative.

Assessment

Significant resultant pain and muscle tenderness precludes complete examination. Muscle guarding and pain need to be diminished in order for examination to be completed.

Plan

Thermal agents
Electrical stimulation for pain control
Activity of daily living instruction and modification
Complete examination when pain is diminished sufficiently to allow for movement testing.

Detailed Electrotherapeutic Plan

Mode of stimulation: sensory-level stimulation
Type of stimulator: portable; two available circuits
Electrodes and placement: four large electrodes placed to surround pain area (Fig. 5.5)
Duration of treatment: 20 to 30 minutes

Rationale

High-frequency sensory-level stimulation is an appropriate starting point for the management of acute pain because the patient should tolerate it well and it should be effective. HFTENS is expected to help manage primary and secondary hyperalgesia (see Chapter 4). A portable stimulator was chosen to attempt to assist the patient in managing the pain with activities of daily living until the acuteness of the situation is resolved. Because the painful area is rather large,

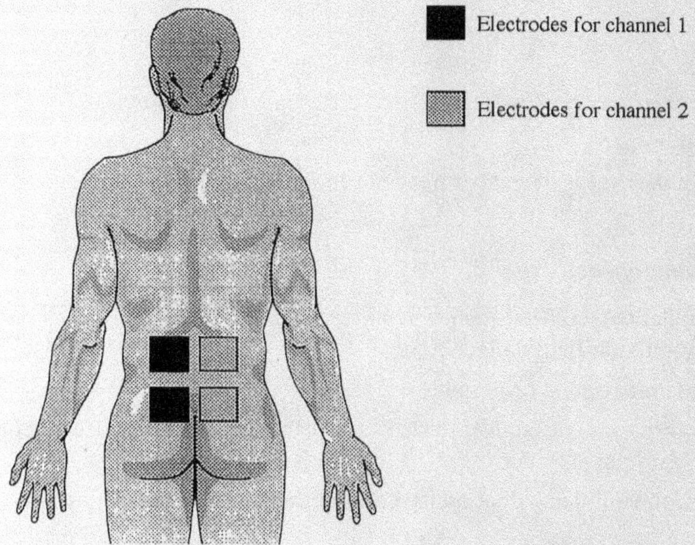

Figure 5.5. Illustration of electrode placement for case 1.

larger electrodes are chosen, and four electrodes from either one or two circuits are used. If the target area is too tender to allow placement over the site, electrodes may be placed over lower lumbar myotomes. The duration of treatment should be sufficient to produce electroanalgesia with sensory-level stimulation to the strongest yet comfortable sensation. As described in Chapter 4, the greater the intensity, the greater the inhibition that can result due to the acute inflammatory response of this condition. This patient has pain with all activity and will benefit from any relief from this discomfort; however, the patient must be educated on avoiding aggravating positions. The TENS treatment is expected to provide relief from some level of the pain reported, but it may give the patient a false perception of activity ability. This patient would benefit from advice on activity control, movement limitations, and beneficial posturing to complement the TENS treatment.

Case 2

A 62-year-old woman sustained a Colles fracture of the left wrist 8 weeks ago. X-rays showed excellent healing and her cast was removed this morning.

Objective

Examination reveals marked, equal limitation in wrist extension and flexion with empty end feels and slightly limited supination with a muscular end feel. The wrist and fingers are mildly edematous. She has at least "fair" grade distal upper-extremity musculature, but she is unable to accept any resistance secondary to pain. She is extremely tender to palpation and will not allow any passive motion to be performed.

Assessment

Joint restriction at the midcarpal and radiocarpal joints and probable muscle weakness secondary to immobilization. Pain inhibits full evaluation and treatment.

Plan

Whirlpool

Mobilization to radiocarpal, midcarpal, and distal radioulnar joints

Remedial exercise

Electrical stimulation for the performance of mobilization and exercise

Detailed Electrotherapeutic Plan

Mode of stimulation: high-frequency sensory-level stimulation to allow passive and active ROM and joint mobilization techniques

Type of stimulator: clinical or portable

Electrodes and placement: small, placed on volar and dorsal surface surrounding (but not over) the wrist joint (Fig. 5.6)

Duration of treatment: dependent on duration of therapeutic procedures

Rationale

Restricted joint motion after immobilization can cause significant pain. If the joint cannot be moved secondary to this pain, it will continue. This cycle can be broken by electrical stimulation. High-frequency with high-intensity sensory-level stimulation causes an instantaneous interelectrode analgesia that allows mobilization and exercise. Either clinical or portable stimulators of almost all types could be used. Small electrodes are necessary because the wrist area is small. Placement is around rather than over the joint so as not to interfere with movement. Stimulation should be applied throughout the procedures and may be left on for a short time afterward to minimize postmobilization soreness.

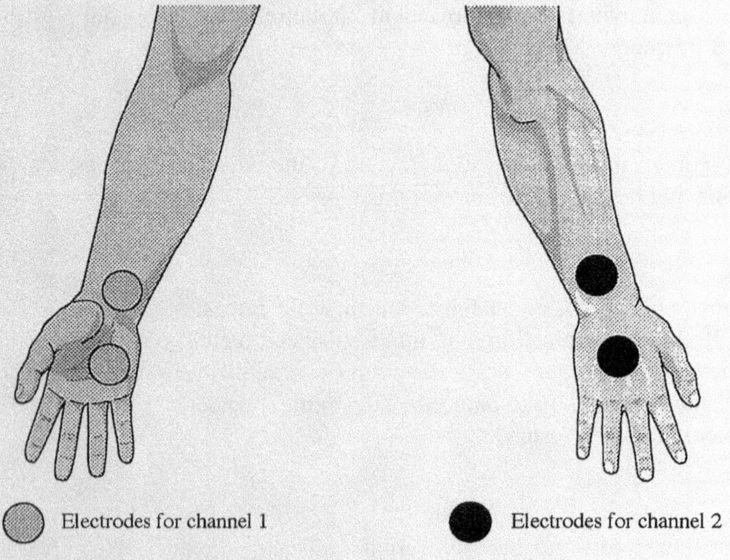

Figure 5.6. Illustration of electrode placement for case 2.

Case 3

A 45-year-old man presents with complaints of longstanding, constant, left-sided low-back pain with some radiation into the left buttock and posterior thigh 2 years after left L4-5 laminectomy and discectomy.

Objective

Examination reveals a slight loss of the lumbar lordosis and lateral shift to the right. There is a 25% loss of lumbosacral flexion, a 50% loss of extension, and 50% loss of lateral bending to the left and rotation to the right with "stretching" pain at the end of these ranges. Movement tests reproduce these "stretching" symptoms but do not produce peripheralization or centralization of the patient's symptoms. Patient has less motion in extension coupled with left side-bending (reproducing the stretching pain) compared to extension with right side bending. Straight leg raise and sitting root tests are negative bilaterally. Deep tendon reflexes and sensation testing are normal. Motor function of the L2-S1 myotomes is normal. Sacroiliac torsion, compression, and distraction tests are negative. Oswestry score is 54/100.

Assessment

Mechanical lumbar dysfunction accompanied by chronic low back pain.

Plan

Manipulation

Remedial exercise

Thermal agents

Electrical stimulation for pain modulation

Detailed Electrotherapeutic Plan

Mode of stimulation: motor-level stimulation

Type of stimulator: portable and/or clinical

Electrodes and placement: two electrodes paraspinally at L4-5 and two at distal extent of pain or electrodes on the motor points of the hamstrings and gluteal muscles (Fig. 5.7)

Duration of treatment: at least 30 to 45 minutes

Rationale

This patient has a chronic problem, and sensory-level stimulation will likely be insufficient to fully remediate it. Motor-level stimulation gives longer lasting analgesia. A portable stimulator is preferable because the unrelenting nature of the patient's pain will probably require more than intermittent, clinic-based treatment. This treatment can be combined with the use of a clinical stimulator for in-clinic treatments. Electrodes can be placed directly over the target area or, if that is not well tolerated, over associated myotomes. The duration of treatment must be sufficient to allow induction of analgesia by endorphin-mediated mechanisms.

Case 4

A 35-year-old college professor presents with periodic complaints of severe headaches unaccompanied by any somatic complaints. The headaches are primarily concentrated in the suboccipital areas bilaterally but eventually involve the entire head. He states that they are accompanied by a

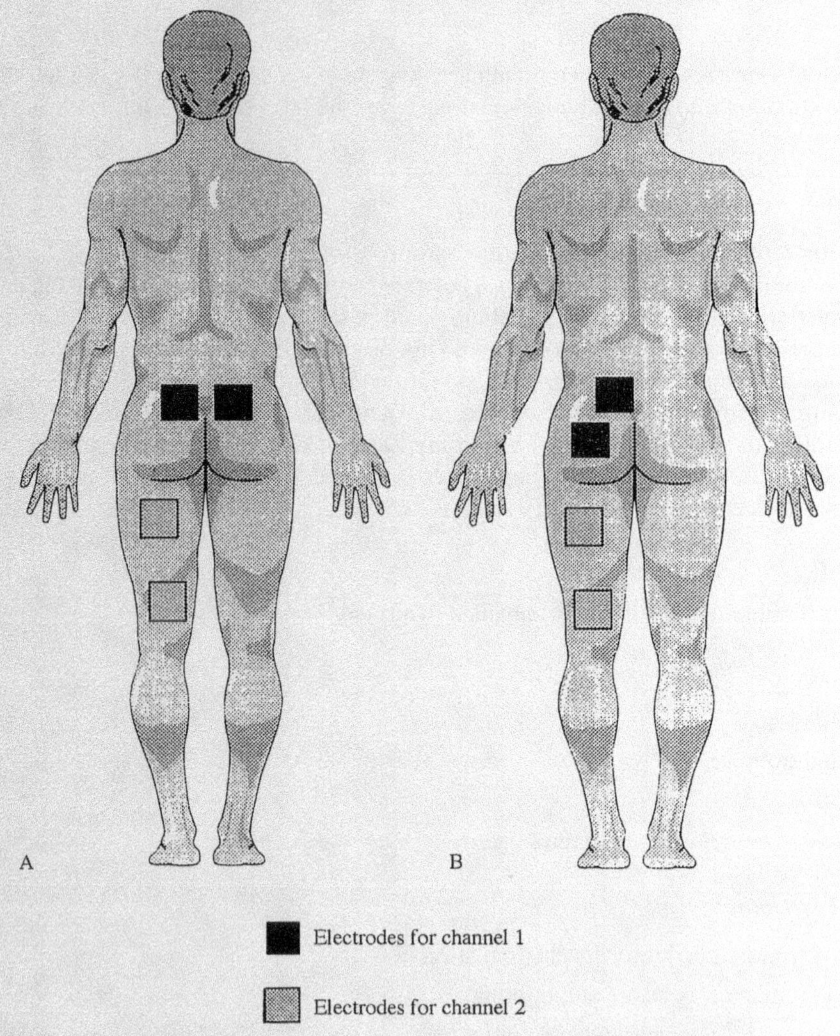

Figure 5.7. Illustration of electrode placement for case 3.

"tight" feeling in his neck and shoulders and are brought on by "stress." Medical evaluation has been negative.

Objective

Musculoskeletal evaluation is negative, with the exception of some muscle spasm and tenderness to palpation in both upper trapezei. He rates his pain as 10/10 when it occurs.

Assessment

Muscle-contraction headache.

Plan

Relaxation training

Electrical stimulation for pain modulation

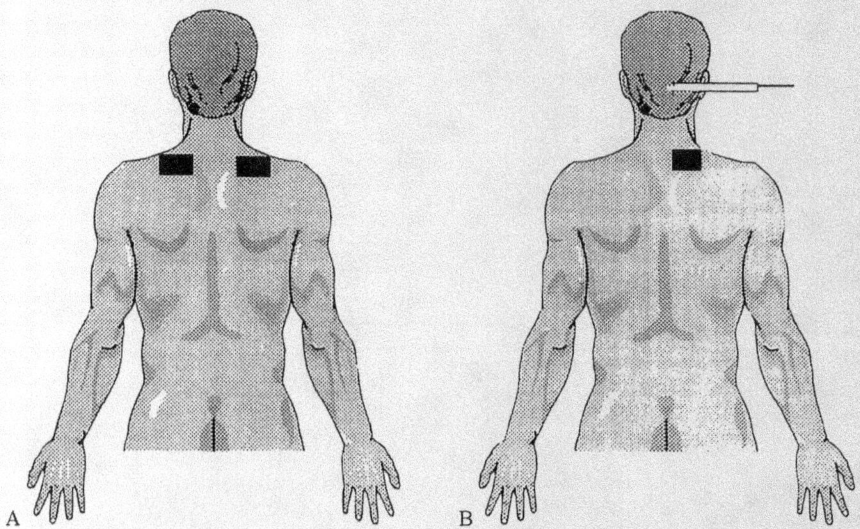

Figure 5.8. Illustration of electrode placement for case 4.

Detailed Electrotherapeutic Plan

Mode of stimulation: noxious- and motor-level stimulation

Type of stimulator: clinical for noxious level; portable for motor level

Electrodes and placement: probe electrode to stimulate bilaterally over occipital protuberances for noxious level, bilaterally over motor points of the upper trapezei for motor level (Fig. 5.8)

Duration of stimulation: 30 to 60 seconds per stimulation site for noxious level, at least 30 to 45 minutes for motor level

Rationale

Both motor-level and noxious-level stimulation provide long-lasting pain relief and are indicated for this type of problem. This patient may be amenable to clinic-based treatment, but if his complaints are only manifested when he has a headache, the electrotherapeutic treatment may need to be performed at home. A probe electrode is chosen for the noxious-level stimulation because the occipital protuberances are not accessible to traditional electrodes. The duration for noxious-level stimulation is brief, as patient tolerance for this mode of stimulation is low.

Case 5

A 40-year-old woman, 12 weeks after rotator cuff repair, presents with unrelenting posterior shoulder pain with shoulder movement and the physician cannot explain the continued symptoms. Evaluation reveals pain in the posterior shoulder with radicular symptoms in the upper extremity that mimic C8 distribution. The pain is increased with horizontal adduction, and palpation reveals a palpable trigger point in the teres minor with reproduction of the patient's complaint.

Plan

Motor, "acupuncture TENS" for pain control of the trigger point.

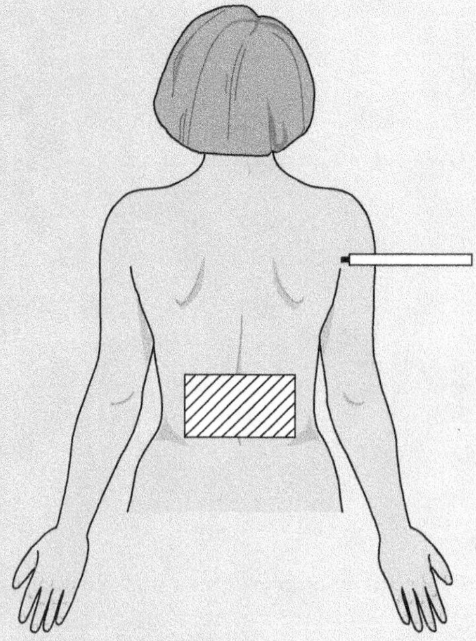

Figure 5.9. Illustration of electrode placement for case 5.

Detailed Electrotherapeutic Plan

Mode of stimulation: low-frequency TENS to trigger point

Type of stimulator: line powered

Electrodes and placement: large, dispersive on the back, use of small point stimulator for point application of the stimulation to trigger point of the teres minor (Fig. 5.9)

Duration of treatment: 10 minutes with rest as necessary

Rationale

TENS may provide some relief from local trigger points via direct motor stimulation. The stimulation is the maximal tolerable, and the patient will be positioned for comfort considering that motion of the affected limb is expected.

Case 6

A 44-year-old mildly obese woman with a 2-week history of right upper-quadrant pain is referred for instruction in the use of TENS for postoperative pain management. She is scheduled for a cholecystectomy tomorrow. She has a noncontributory past medical history and no history of narcotic use.

Plan

Electrical stimulation for postoperative pain.

Detailed Electrotherapeutic Plan

Mode of stimulation: sensory-level stimulation

Type of stimulator: portable

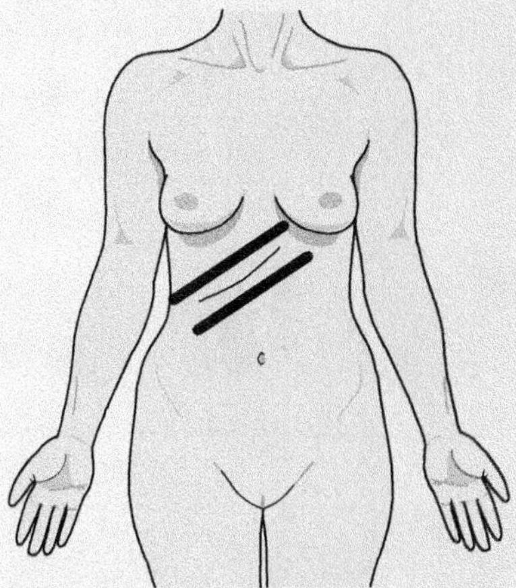

Figure 5.10. Illustration of electrode placement for case 6.

Electrode placement: paraincisional sterile postoperative electrodes placed in operating room by surgical team (Fig. 5.10)

Duration of treatment: as needed for incisional pain

Rationale

Sensory-level stimulation is used because stimulation above the motor threshold will interfere with the incision. Portable stimulators are used because the patient is moved from the operating room to the recovery area to her room, all areas with little extra space. Electrodes are placed paraincisionally and are removed when the bandage is removed. Treatment is controlled by the patient but may be continuous throughout her hospital stay.

Case 7

A 21-year-old woman presents with chronic bilateral patellar tendonitis after participating in a cross-country bicycle tour 6 months ago. Her patellar tendons are thickened and red. She cannot tolerate deep palpation of the tendons. She has pain with knee flexion past 90 degrees, resisted knee flexion, and inferior patellar glide. She rates her pain as 7/10 at rest and 10/10 with activity.

Plan

Electrical stimulation to allow for increased weight-bearing activity and transverse friction massage.

Detailed Electrotherapeutic Plan

Mode of stimulation: sensory-level stimulation, high-intensity

Type of stimulator: clinical

Electrode placement: small (1 inch × 1 inch), on either side of the patellar tendon (Fig. 5.11)

Duration of treatment: 10 minutes at the beginning of each treatment

Rationale

High-intensity sensory-level stimulation is used to cause analgesia of the patellar tendons to allow them to be manipulated and to allow for weight-bearing activity. Clinical stimulator is used

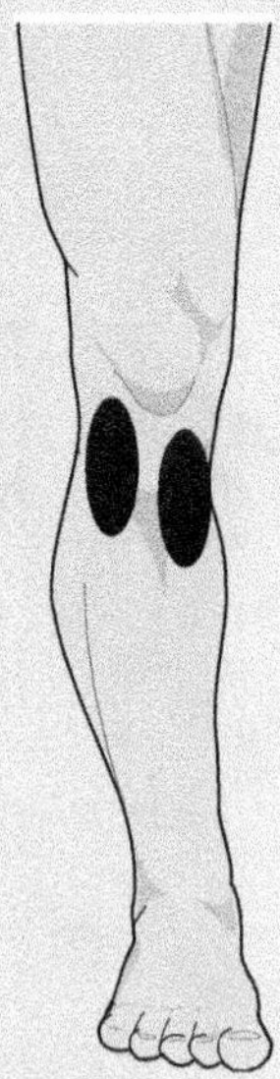

Figure 5.11. Illustration of electrode placement for case 7.

to provide very high-intensity stimulation, and because short-duration, in-clinic treatment is planned. Electrodes are placed to focus the current on the tendons. The therapist will control the intensity to the highest tolerable level.

Case 8

A 12-year-old girl sustained a first-degree ankle sprain 1 month ago. Over the month she has developed severe reflex sympathetic dystrophy. She displays hyperesthesia and dystonia. She is unable to bear any weight at all on her left lower extremity. Her left foot and ankle are shiny, swollen, and red. She has had a sympathetic ganglion block, which resulted in a short-term decrease in her symptoms. Her pain level is rated as 90/100 using a visual analog pain rating scale.

Plan

Sensory-level stimulation to facilitate progressive weight-bearing activity on the left ankle and foot.

Detailed Electrotherapeutic Plan

Mode of stimulation: sensory-level stimulation

Type of stimulator: portable

Electrode placement: over the peripheral sensory nerves that innervate the ankle and foot (Fig. 5.12)

Duration of treatment: in the clinic and at home during weight-bearing activities (initially, begin with the patient seated, and have her attempt to bear a small amount of weight with her foot on a pillow)

Rationale

Sensory-level stimulation is used because of the patient's hypersensitivity and the fact that motor-level stimulation could interfere with the activities. A portable stimulator is used because

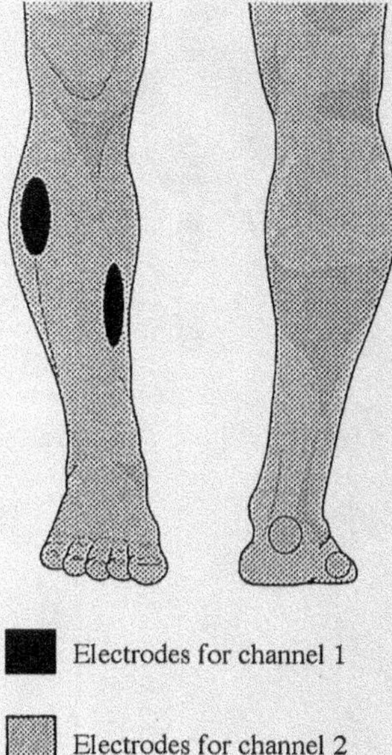

Figure 5.12. Illustration of electrode placement for case 8.

the patient will be progressing to more vigorous activities that could not be performed if she were tethered. The patient will control the stimulation intensity.

Case 9

A 55-year-old businesswoman was driving 2 weeks ago and was hit from the rear while stopped at an intersection. She was wearing a seat belt. She was taken to the emergency room where x-rays were taken of the cervical spine and were reported as negative. She was given a soft cervical collar and a prescription for analgesics and was told to go home and rest. She has had continued neck pain and went to see her family physician yesterday, who referred her for physical therapy.

Examination

The patient states that she has pain in the back of her neck and between her shoulder blades. It is exacerbated with weight bearing and activity and relieved with rest. There is no radiation into the upper extremities and no complaints of paresthesia or numbness.

Postural evaluation reveals a forward head, decreased cervical lordosis, and increased thoracic kyphosis. Passive range of motion (ROM) is full and pain-free with the exception of "stretching" pain with full flexion. Resisted isometrics and active ROM reveal pain with extension. Compression is negative; traction produces the same "stretching" pain. Deep tendon reflexes are 2+ and equal bilaterally. Sensory testing reveals no abnormality. Upper-extremity myotomal screening is negative. Patient is tender to palpation paraspinally from the occiput to approximately T5. There is no evidence of muscle guarding or trigger points.

Assessment

Subacute strain of the cervical and thoracic extensors.

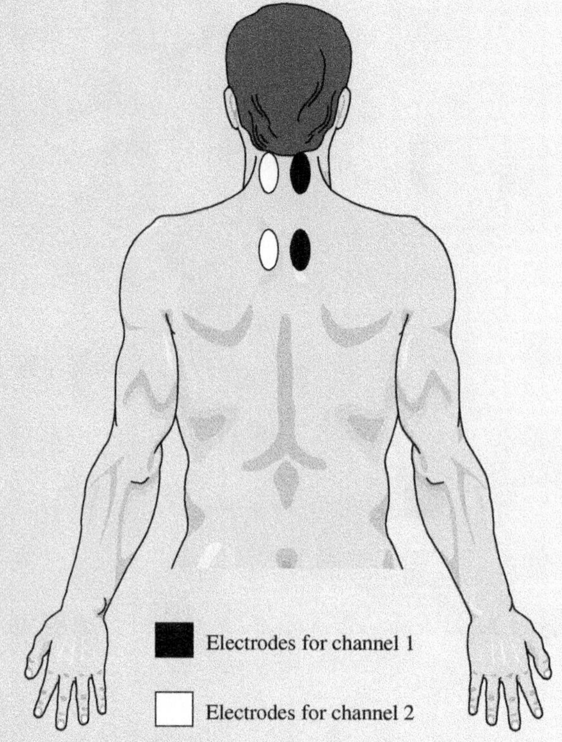

Figure 5.13. Illustration of electrode placement for case 9.

Plan

Remedial exercise

Electrotherapy for pain modulation

Detailed Electrotherapeutic Plan

Mode of stimulation: sensory-level

Type of stimulator: clinical

Electrodes and placement: four electrodes placed paraspinally from C2 to T5 (Fig. 5.13)

Duration of stimulation: 20 to 30 minutes

Rationale

See case 1. After approximately 10 minutes, the patient reports that there has been no change in her symptoms.

Action

Change electrode placement so that the circuits cross (currents intersect).

Rationale

Before drastically changing treatment modes or stimulator type, it is advisable to attempt electrode configuration changes, as this often results in an improved outcome.

The patient responds well to this treatment and makes marked improvement over a 2-week period. She decides that she is ready to return to work, but you are concerned both that the increased activity may limit availability for treatment and necessitate stronger pain modulation. You determine that her clinic-based time should be spent on exercise.

Action

Change to a portable stimulator and instruct her in its use to provide sensory-level and motor-level stimulation. Instruct her in appropriate electrode placement for motor-level stimulation.

Rationale

The use of a portable stimulator at home and work will permit the clinic time to be used for exercise and may facilitate the patient's return to work. The introduction of motor-level stimulation to the regimen will allow her to get longer-lasting analgesia from a brief treatment.

The patient gradually returns to her premorbid mobility level and is weaned from both treatment and stimulator over the next 2 months.

SUMMARY

This chapter has addressed the approaches used in electrical stimulation to modulate pain. There remains much to be investigated in this area of clinical practice. In the words of Lewis Thomas, "In real life, every field of science I can think of is incomplete, and most of them are still in the earliest stage of their starting point. The next week's issue of any scientific journal can turn a whole field upside down"(from *Late Night Thoughts on Listening to Mahler's Ninth Symphony p. 148*). Regard this chapter as a beginning, a clinical guide to the ways in which various stimulators, modes of stimulation, and electrode placements can be used to effect electroanalgesia. Take this information and use it to expand the scope of your practice and enhance patient care.

SELF-STUDY QUESTIONS

For answers, see Appendix B.

1. Under what circumstances should the clinician choose to use electrical stimulation as an intervention to reduce or relieve a patient's pain?
2. State the types of questions a clinician should pose to a patient in pain that would assist in establishing the underlying causes and determining the type of electrical stimulation that would be most suitable for pain management.
3. Identify tools used to assess patients' perception of pain.
4. Compare and contrast the parameters of stimulation for sensory-level (conventional TENS), motor-level (strong low rate), and noxious level (acupuncturelike) electrical stimulation for pain control.
5. What is the purpose of modulation of stimulation parameters in sensory-level stimulation, and what parameters of stimulation may be modulated?
6. What are the reasons that sensory-level stimulation for pain control is generally the type of TENS chosen for initial use in a patient with pain?
7. Where are electrodes usually placed for sensory-level electrical stimulation for pain control, and what is the rationale for this electrode placement?
8. Identify six conditions for which neuraxial implants have been used for pain control.
9. Identify conditions or situations that would contraindicate the use of electrical stimulation for pain control.
10. Identify potential adverse reactions to electrical stimulation for pain control.
11. When one form of TENS does not appear to be adequate for pain control, what alternatives are available to the clinician?
12. What does the literature suggest regarding the effectiveness of subsensory microcurrent electrical nerve stimulation?
13. What are the important conclusions of the 2002 Cochrane Study on the effectiveness of TENS in the management of chronic pain?
14. Identify several chronic painful conditions for which the literature suggests that high-frequency sensory-level stimulation may be effective for pain control.

15. Identify several chronic painful conditions for which the literature suggests that low-frequency motor-level stimulation may be effective for pain control.

16. What is the placebo effect, and is this effect relevant to electrical stimulation for pain control?

17. What were the treatments used and what was the reported outcome of the Deyo et al. (84) study on the use of electrical stimulation for chronic low back pain?

18. What were the treatments used and what was the reported outcome of the Marchand et al. (88) study on the use of electrical stimulation for chronic low back pain?

19. What are the shortcomings of much of the research that has been reported on the efficacy of TENS for pain control?

20. What has research shown regarding the control of pain in primary dysmenorrhea?

REFERENCES

1. Melzack R. *The Puzzle of Pain*. New York: Basic Books; 1973.
2. Melzack R, Wall PD. Pain mechanisms: a new theory. *Science*. 1965;150:971–976.
3. Shealy CN. Six years experience with electrical stimulation for control of pain. *Congr Neurol Surg*. 1974;4:775–782.
4. Mannheimer J, Lampe G, Long DM, et al. Transcutaneous electrical stimulation for relief of chronic pain. *Clinical transcutaneous electrical nerve stimulation*. Philadelphia: FA Davis 1983.
5. Robinson J, Turk D, Loeser J. Pain evaluation: fifth edition approaches. *The Guides* [newsletter of the American Medical Association]. 2002;Jan/Feb.: 1–5, 9–11.
6. Cummings GS, Routan JL. Validity of unassisted pain drawings by patients with chronic pain [abstract]. *Phys Ther.* 1985;65:668.
7. Rothstein J, Roy S, Wolf S. *The Rehabilitation Specialist's Handbook*. Philadelphia: FA Davis; 1991:207–210.
8. Travell JG, Simons DG. Myofascial pain and dysfunction. *The Trigger Point Manual*. Vols 1 and 2. Baltimore, Md: Williams and Wilkins; 1983.
9. Lo Y, Pavanni R. Electrophysiological features in the management of meraligia paraesthetica. *Anna Acta Med Singapore*. 1998;27:530–532.
10. Scott J, Huskisson EC. Graphic representation of pain. *Pain*. 1976;2:175–185.
11. Agnew B, Mersky H. Words of chronic pain. *Pain*. 1976;2:43–81.
12. Ohnhaus EE, Adler R. Methodological problems in the measurement of pain: a comparison between the VRS and the VAS. *Pain*. 1975;1:379–384.
13. Melzack R. The short-form McGill pain questionnaire. *Pain*. 1987;30:191–197.
14. Melzack R. The McGill pain questionnaire: major properties and scoring methods. *Pain*. 1975;1: 277–299.
15. Graham C, Bond SS, Gerkovich MM, et al. Use of the MPQ in the assessment of cancer pain: replicability and consistency. *Pain*. 1982;8:377–387.
16. Melzack R. The McGill pain questionnaire: from description to measurement. *Anesthesiology*. 2005;103:199–202.
17. Mystakidou K, Parpa E, Tsilika E, et al. Greek McGill pain questionnaire: validation and utility in cancer patients. *J Pain Symptom Manage*. 2002;24:379–387.
18. Deyo RA, Diehl AK. Measuring physical and psychosocial function in patients with low-back pain. *Spine*. 1983;8:635–642.
19. Elton D, Burrows GD, Stanley GV. A multidimensional approach to the assessment of pain. *Aust J Physiother*. 1979;25:33–37.

20. Kremer EF, Block A, Gaylor M. Behavioral approaches to treatment of chronic pain: the inaccuracy of patient self-report measure. *Arch Phys Med Rehabil.* 1981;62:188–191.
21. Delitto A, Strube MJ, Shulman AD, et al. A study of discomfort with electrical stimulation. *Phys Ther.* 1992;72:410–412.
22. Lodge M. Magnitude scaling: quantitative measurement of opinion. In: Sullivan JL, ed. *Quantitative Applications in the Social Sciences.* Beverly Hills, Calif: Sage Publications; 1981:24–41.
23. Picker RI. Current trends: low-volt pulsed microamp stimulation, part I. *Clin Manage Phys Ther.* 1988;9:10–14.
24. Picker RI. Current trends: low-volt pulsed microamp stimulation, part II. *Clin Manage Phys Ther.* 1989;9:28–33.
25. Becker RO, Selden G. *The Body Electric: Electromagnetism and the Foundation of Life.* New York: William Morrow; 1985.
26. Zizic TM, Hoffman KC, Holt PA, et al. The treatment of osteoarthritis of the knee with pulsed electrical stimulation. *J Rheumatol.* 1995;22:1757–1761.
27. Ignelzi R, Nyquist J. Direct effect of electrical stimulation on peripheral nerve evoked stimulation on peripheral nerve evoked activity: implications in pain relief. *J Neurosurg.* 1976;45:159–165.
28. Johnson MI, Ashton CH, Thompson JW. An in-depth study of long-term users of transcutaneous electrical nerve stimulation: implications for clinical use or TENS. *Pain.* 1991;44:221–229.
29. Sjolund B, Ternis L, Eriksson M. Increased CSF of endorphins after electro-acupuncture *Acta Physiol Scand.* 1977;100:382–384.
30. Duranti R, Pantealeo T, Bellini F. Increase in muscular pain threshold following low frequency-high intensity peripheral conditioning stimulation in humans. *Brain Res.* 1988;452:66–72.
31. Sjolund B, Eriksson M. The influence of naloxone on analgesia produced by peripheral conditioning stimulation. *Brain Res.* 1979;173:295–301.
32. Johnson MI. The analgesic effects and clinical use of acupuncture-like TENS. *Phys Ther Rev.* 1998;3:73–93.
33. Travell J, Rinzler S. The myofascial genesis of pain. *Postgrad Med.* 1952;11:425–434.
34. Nabe JB. A quantitative theory of feeling. *J Gen Psychol.* 1929;2:199–204.
35. Chapman CR, Wilson ME, Gehrig JD. Comparative effects of acupuncture and TCS on the perception of painful dental stimuli. *Pain.* 1976;2:265–291.
36. Chapman CR, Chen AC, Bonica JJ. Effects of intrasymental electrical acupuncture on central pain: evaluation of threshold estimation and sensory decision theory. *Pain.* 1977;3:213–224.
37. Rushton D. Electrical stimulation and the treatment of pain. *Disability Rehabil.* 2002;24:407–415.
38. Long DM. The current status of electrical stimulation of the nervous system for the relief of chronic pain. *Pain.* 1998;49:142–144.
39. Kay AD, Mcintyre MD, Macrae WA, et al. Spinal cord stimulation—a long term evaluation in patients with chronic pain. *Br J Neurosurg.* 2001;15:335–341.
40. Holsheimer J. Effectiveness of spinal cord stimulation in the management of chronic pain: analysis of technical drawbacks and solutions. *Neurosugery.* 1997;40:990–999.
41. Tseng SH. Treatment of chronic pain by spinal cord stimulation. *J Formos Med Assoc.* 2000;99:267–271.
42. Stanton-Hicks M, Salamon J. Stimulation of the central and peripheral nervous system for the control of pain. *J Clin Neurophysiol.* 1997;14:46–62.
43. Myerson BA. Neurosurgical approaches to pain treatment. *Acta Anaesthesiol Scand.* 2001;45: 1108–1113.
44. Day M. Neuromodulation: spinal cord and peripheral nerve stimulation. *Curr Rev Pain.* 2000; 4:374–382.
45. Barolat G. Spinal cord stimulation for chronic pain management. *Arch Med Res.* 2000;31:258–262.
46. May R, Volder S. Chronic pain management and spinal cord stimulation; patient-screening guidelines to improve outcome. *Pain Digest.* 1999;9:353–363.

47. Segal R, Stacey B, Rudy T. Spinal cord stimulation revisited. *Neurol Res.* 1998;20:391–396.
48. Kumar K, Toth C, Nath R. Spinal cord stimulation for chronic pain in peripheral neuropathy. *Surg Neurol.* 1996;46:363–369.
49. Turner J, Loeser J, Bell K. Spinal cord stimulator for chronic low back pain; a systematic literature synthesis. *Neurosugery.* 1995;37:1088–1095.
50. De LaPorte C, Van de Kelft E. Spinal cord stimulation in failed low back syndrome. *Pain.* 1993;52:55–61.
51. Burchiel K, Anderson V, Brown E, et al. Prospective, multicenter study of spinal cord stimulation for relief of chronic low back and extremity pain. *Spine.* 1993;18:191–194.
52. Calvillo O, Racz G, Dedie J, et al. Neuroaugmentation in the treatment of complex regional pain syndrome of the upper extremity. *Acta Orthop Belg.* 1998;64:57–63.
53. Kemler M, Barendse G, Van Kleef M, et al. Electrical spinal cord stimulation in reflex sympathetic dystrophy: retrospective analysis of 23 patients. *J Neurosurg.* 1999;90:79–83.
54. Broseta J, Barbera j, De Vera J, et al. Spinal cord stimulation in peripheral arterial disease. *J Neurosurg.* 1986;64:71–80.
55. Eliasson T, Augustinsson I, Mannheimer C. Spinal cord stimulation in severe angina pectoris—presentation of current studies, indications and clinical experience. *Pain.* 1996;65:169–179.
56. Law J, Swett J, Kirsch W. Retrospective analysis of 22 patients with chronic pain treated by peripheral nerve stimulation. *J Neurosurg.* 1980;52:482–485.
57. Nashold B, Goldner J, Mullen J, et al. Long-term pain control by direct peripheral nerve stimulation. *J Bone J Surg.* 1982;64A:1–10.
58. Tsubokawa T, Katayama Y, Yamamoto T. Chronic motor cortex stimulation in patients with thalamic pain. *J Neurosurg.* 1993;78:393–401.
59. Nguyen JP, Lefaucherur JP, Decq P, et al. Chronic motor cortex stimulation in the treatment of central and neuropathic pain. Correlations between clinical, electrophysiological and anatomical data. *Pain.* 1999;82:245–251.
60. Meyerson BA, Lindblom U, Linderoth B, et al. Motor cortex stimulation as treatment of trigeminal neuropathic pain. Acta Neurochir Suppl(Wien) Vol 58. Wien: Springer-Verlag; 1993:150–153.
61. Katayama Y, Fukaya C, Yamamoto T. Poststroke pain control by chronic motor cortex stimulation: neurological characteristics predicting a favorable response. *J Neurosurg.* 1998;89:585–591.
62. Taylor K, Newton RA, Personius WJ, et al. Effects of interferential current stimulation for treatments of subjects with recurrent jaw pain. *Phys Ther.* 1987;67:346–349.
63. Long D. Fifteen years of transcutaneous electrical stimulation for pain control. *Stereotact Funct Neurosurg.* 1991;56:2–19.
64. Schomburg FL, Carter-Baker SA. Transcutaneous electrical nerve stimulation for post laparotomy pain. In: *Electrical Stimulation: Management of Pain.* Vol 2. Alexandria: APTA (American Physical Therapy Assoc); 1983:191–196.
65. Issenman J, Nolan MF, Rowley J, et al. Transcutaneous electrical nerve stimulation for pain control after spinal fusion with Harrington rods. In: *Electrical Stimulation: Management of Pain.* Vol 2. Alexandria: APTA (American Physical Therapy Assoc); 1983:197–200..
66. Carroll D, Moore RA, McQuay HJ, et al. Trancutaneous electrical stimulation (TENS) for chronic pain (Cochrane Review). In: *The Cochrane Library*, Issue 3. New York: Wiley Interscience; 2002:1–58.
67. Abelson K, Langley GB, Sheppeard H, et al. Transcutaneous electrical nerve stimulation in rheumatoid arthritis. *N Z Med J.* 1983;96:156–158.
68. Hseuh T, Cheng P, Kuan T, et al. The immediate effectiveness of electrical nerve stimulation and electrical muscle stimulation on myofascial trigger points. *Am J Phys Med Rehabil.* 1997; 76:471–476.
69. Moystad A, Drogstad BS, Larheim TA. Transcutaneous nerve stimulation in a group of patients with rheumatic disease involving the temporomandibular joint. *J Prosthet Dent.* 1990;64:596–600.

70. Smith CR, Lewith GT, Machin D. Preliminary study to establish a controlled method of assessing transcutaneous nerve stimulation as treatment for the pain caused by osteo-arthritis of the knee. *Physiotherapy.* 1983;69:266–268..

71. Vinterberg H, Donde R, Andersen RB. Transcutaneous nerve stimulation for relief of pain in patients with rheumatoid arthritis. *Ugeskr Laeger.* 1978;140:1149–1150..

72. Grimmer K. A controlled double blind study comparing the effects of strong burst mode TENS and high rate TENS on painful osteoarthritic knees. *Austral J Physiother.* 1992;48:49–56..

73. Moore SR, Shurman J. Combined neuromuscular electrical nerve stimulation and transcutaneous electrical nerve stimulation for treatment of chronic back pain: a double blind, repeated measures comparison. *Arch Phys Med Rehabil.* 1997;78:55–60.

74. Lewis D, Lewis B, Sturrock RD. Transcutaneous electrical stimulation in osteoarthrosis: a therapeutic alternative? *Ann Rheum Dis.* 1984;43:47–49.

75. Lewis B, Lewis D, Cumming G. The comparative analgesic efficacy of transcutaneous electrical nerve stimulation and a non-steroidal anti-inflammatory drug for painful osteoarthritis. *Br J Rheumatol.* 1994;33:455–460.

76. Melzack R, Vetere P, Finch L. Transcutaneous electrical nerve stimulation for low back pain: a comparison of TENS and massage for pain and range of motion. *Phys Ther.* 1983;63:489–492.

77. Kumar D, Marshall HJ. Diabetic peripheral neuropathy: amelioration of pain with transcutaneous electrostimulation. *Diabetes Care.* 1997;20:1702–1705.

78. Jensen H, Zesler R, Christensen T. Transcutaneous electrical nerve stimulation (TNS) for painful osteoarthritis of the knee. *Intl J Rehabil Res.* 1991;14:356–358.

79. Nash TP, Williams JD, Machin D. TENS: does the type of stimulus really matter? *Pain Clinic.* 1990;3:161–168.

80. Tulgar M, McGlone F, Bowsher D, et al. Comparative effectiveness of different stimulation modes in relieving pain. Part 1, a pilot study. *Pain.* 1991;47:151–155.

81. Tulgar M, McGlone F, Bowsher D, et al. Comparative effectiveness of different stimulation modes in relieving pain. Part 2, a double-blind controlled long-term clinical trial. *Pain.* 1991;47:157–162.

82. Mannheimer C, Carlsson C. The analgesic effect of transcutaneous electrical nerve stimulation (TNS) in patients with rheumatoid arthritis. A comparative study of different pulse patterns. *Pain.* 1979;6:329–334.

83. Deyo R, Walsh NE, Martin DC, et al. A controlled trial of transcutaneous electrical nerve stimulation and exercise for chronic low back pain. *N Engl J Med.* 1990;322:1627–1634.

84. George SZ, Fritz JM, Erhard RE. A comparison of fear avoidance beliefs in patients with lumbar spine and cervical spine pain. *Spine.* 2001;26:2139–2145.

85. Fritz JM, Wainner R, Hicks G. The use of nonorganic signs and symptoms as a screening tool for return to work in patients with acute low back pain. *Spine.* 2000;25:1925–1932.

86. Herman E, Williams R, Stratford P, et al. A randomized controlled trial of TENS (Codetron) to determine its benefits in a rehabilitation program for acute occupational low back pain. *Spine.* 1994;19:561–568.

87. Marchand S, Charest J, Li J, et al. Is TENS purely a placebo effect? A controlled study on low back pain. *Pain.* 1993;54:99–106.

88. Fishbain DA, Chabal C, Abbott A, et al. TENS treatment outcome in long-term users. *Clin J Pain.* 1996;12:201–214.

89. Ersek RA. LBP: prompt relief with transcut neurostimulation. A report of 35 consecutive pts. *Orthoped Rev.* 1976;5:27–31.

90. Roberts HJ. TENS in the management of pancreatitis pain. *South Med J.* 1978;71:396–399.

91. Nathan PW, Wall PD. Treatment of post-herpetic neuralgia by prolonged electrical stimulation. *Br Med J.* 1974;3:645–647.

92. Schomburg FL, Carter-Baker SA. Transcutaneous electrical nerve stimulation for postlaparotomy pain. In: *Electrical Stimulation: Management of Pain.* Vol 2. Alexandria: American Physical Therapy Assoc; 1983;191–196.

93. Issenman J, Nolan MF, Rowley J, et al. Transcutaneous electrical nerve stimulation for pain control after spinal fusion with Harrington rods. In: Electrical Stimulation: Management of Pain. Vol. 2. CITY: PUBLISHER; 1983:197–200.

94. Hargreaves A, Lander J. Use of transcutaneous electrical nerve stimulation for postoperative pain. *Nursing Res.* 1989;38:159–161.

95. Benedetti F, Amanzio M, Casadio C, et al. Control of postoperative pain by TENS after thoracic operations. *Ann Thorac Surg.* 1997;63:773–776.

96. Caroll D, Tramer M, McQuay H, et al. Randomization is important in studies with pain outcomes: systematic review of TENS in acute postoperative pain. *Br J Anesthes.* 1996;77:798–803.

97. Cooperman AM, Hall B, Mikalacki K, et al. Use of TENS in the control of postoperative pain: Reults of a prospective, randiomized, control study. *Am J Surg.* 1977;133:185–187.

98. Forster EL, Kramer JF, Lucy D, et al. Effect of TENS on pain, medications and pulmonary function following coronary artery bypass graft surgery. *Chest.* 1994;106:1343–1348.

99. Klin B, Uretzky G, Magora F. TENS after open heart surgery. *J Cardiovasc Surg.* 1984;25:445–448.

100. Strayhorn G. TENS and postoperative use of narcotic analgesics. *J Natl Med Assoc.* 1983;75:811–816.

101. Rooney S-M, Jain S, Goldiner PL. Effect of TENS on postoperative pain after thoracotomy. *Anesth Analg.* 1983;62:1010–1012.

102. Reuss R, Cronen P, Abplanalp L. Transcutaneous electrical nerve stimulation for pain control after cholecystectomy: lack of expected benefits. *South Med J.* 1988;81:1361–1363.

103. Carman D, Roach JW. Transcutaneous electrical nerve stimulation for the relief of postoperative pain in children. *Spine.* 1988;13:109–110.

104. Smedley F, Taube M, Wastell C. Transcutaneous electrical nerve stimulation for pain relief following inguinal hernia repair: a controlled trial. *Eur Surg Res.* 1988;20:233–237.

105. Walker RH, Morris BA, Angulo DL, et al. Postoperative use of continuous passive motion, transcutaneous electrical nerve stimulation, and continuous cooling pad following total knee arthroplasty. *J Arthroplasty.* 1991;6:151–156.

106. Conn IG, Marshall AH, Yadav S, Daly JC, Jaffer M: TENS following appendectomy: the placebo effect. *Ann R Coll Surg.* 1986;68:191–192.

107. Warfield CA, Stein JM, Frank HA. The effect of TENS on pain after thoracotomy. *Ann Thorac Surg.* 1985;39:462–465.

108. VanderArk GD, McGrath KA. TENS in treatment of postoperative pain. *Am J Surg.* 1975; 130:338–340.

109. Dawood MY, Ramos J. Transcutaneous electrical nerve stimulation for the treatment of primary dysmenorrhea: a randomized crossover comparison with placebo TENS and ibuprofen. *Obstet Gynecol.* 1990;75:656–660.

110. Milsom I, Hedner N, Mannheimer C. A comparative study of the effects of high-intensity TENS and oral naproxen on intrauterine pressure and mestrural pain in patients with primary dymenorrhea. *Am J Obstet Gynecol.* 1994;170:125–132.

111. Barr JO, Winter A, Conwill DE, et al. Letter to the editor. *N Engl J Med.* 1990;323:1423–1425.

112. Johnson MI, Ashton CH, Bousfield DR, et al. Analgesic effects of different frequencies of transcutaneous electrical nerve stimulation on cold-induced pain in normal subjects. *Pain.* 1989;39:231–236.

113. Petrie I, Hazleman B. Credibility of placebo transcutaneous nerve stimulation and acupuncture. *Clin Exp Rheumatol.* 1985;6:936–939.

114. Langley BG, Sheppard H, Johnson M, et al. The analgesic effects of transcutaneous electrical nerve stimulation and placebo in chronic pain patients: a double-blind non-crossover comparison. *Rheumatol Intl.* 1984;4:119–123.

115. Chen D, Philip M, Philip PA, et al. Cardiac pacemaker inhibition by transcutaneous electrical nerve stimulation. *Arch Phys Med Rehabil.* 1990;7:27–30.

116. Van der Ploeg J, Vervest H, Liem A. Transcutaneous nerve stimulation (TENS) during the first stage of labour: a randomized clinical trial. *Clin Exp Obstet Gynaecol.* 1996;9:95–97.

117. Harrison R, Woods T, Shore M, et al. Pain relief in labour using transcutaneous electrical nerve stimulation (TENS). *Br J Obstet Gynaecol.* 1986;93:739–746.

118. Grim LC, Morey SH. Transcutaneous electrical nerve stimulation for relief of parturition pain. *Phys Ther.* 1985;65:337–340.

SUGGESTED READING

Mannheimer J, Lampe G. Clinical transcutaneous electrical nerve stimulation. Philadelphia: FA Davis; 1983.

Melzack R, Wall PD. Pain mechanisms: a new theory. *Science.* 1965;150:971–976.

Nolan, MF. A chronological indexing of the clinical and basic science literature concerning TENS, 1967–1987. Alexandria, Va: American Physical Therapy Association; 1987.

Section on Clinical Electrophysiology. Electrotherapeutic terminology in physical therapy. Alexandria, Va: Section on Clinical Electrophysiology of the American Physical Therapy Association; 1990.

Thomas, L. *Late Night Thoughts on Listening to Mahler's Ninth Symphony, penguin, New York; 1983.*

Wolf SL, Gersh MR, Rao VR. Examination of electrode placement and stimulating parameters in treating chronic pain with conventional electrical nerve stimulation (TENS). *Pain.* 1981;11:37–47.

CHAPTER 6

Electrical Stimulation of Muscle: Techniques and Applications

Sara J. Farquhar and Lynn Snyder-Mackler

Electrical stimulation of muscle is commonly used as a therapeutic intervention for muscle strengthening. *Neuromuscular electrical stimulation* (NMES) has been made more readily available by the development of new, versatile stimulators. A renewed interest in NMES for strengthening began with reports in the 1970s of the effectiveness of NMES training programs to promote strength development in elite athletes and healthy individuals. Yakov Kots, a Russian scientist, advocated a stimulus regimen for increasing muscle force that he claimed was able to increase the maximum voluntary contraction in elite athletes by more than 50% [see Ward and Shkuratova (1)]. Kots investigated the optimal protocols to maximize NMES strengthening while keeping fatigue at a minimum.

Contemporary work on the effects of NMES on skeletal muscle focuses primarily on its usefulness as a strengthening tool in the management of weak muscles, and also on its effects on healthy muscle. The purposes of this chapter are to (i) describe general adaptations of skeletal muscle to changes in patterns of activation; (ii) describe procedures used to assess muscle strength, activation, and endurance using NMES; (iii) review studies examining the effectiveness of NMES for strengthening healthy and weak muscle; (iv) outline the current evidence for the clinical use of NMES; (v) outline the general clinical considerations and procedures for NMES for strengthening muscle; (vi) describe common features and parameters for the use of NMES devices; and (vii) outline conditions considered to be precautions or contraindications to the use of NMES. In addition, case studies are presented at the end of this chapter to illustrate how NMES for strengthening can be integrated into a comprehensive treatment plan for clients with muscle weakness.

SKELETAL MUSCLE CHANGES IN RESPONSE TO ELECTRICAL STIMULATION

Skeletal muscle characteristics are not immutable (2). In response to changes in muscle use, the structural, biochemical, and physiological characteristics of muscle adapt to meet the imposed demands more appropriately.

Adaptations to Prolonged, Low-force-level Activity

Muscles that are required to perform at relatively low-force levels for prolonged periods of time in day-to-day activities develop an enhanced capability to provide ATP from energy stores to fuel repetitive muscle contraction. This so-called endurance muscle has an enhanced capability to oxidatively metabolize muscle fats, carbohydrates, and protein. Frequent low-level use of skeletal muscle increases the activity of *oxidative metabolic enzymes* within muscle and is associated with an increase in the number of mitochondria where these enzymes are located. The increase in a muscle's oxidative enzymes in response to use is accompanied by an increase in the content of *myoglobin,* the oxygen transport protein, and a rise in the number of capillaries bringing oxygen to the muscle fibers. These changes characterize the adaptive muscle response not only to voluntary endurance training programs, but also to the changes in use brought about by chronic low-level electrical stimulation of muscle (3).

Adaptations to Intermittent, High-force-level Activity

When muscle is activated so that the majority of muscle fibers are recruited, high forces are generated. The strength of these contractions requires high energy. As a result, the energy stores used to fuel these contractions are rapidly depleted. Consequently, this form of contraction can be sustained for only short periods of time before fatigue begins to set in. In spite of the rapid onset of fatigue, this pattern of muscle contraction is associated with changes in the muscle that lead to increases in muscle strength.

Histochemical, biochemical, and physiological studies reveal that the major adaptation of muscle to high force level contractions is an increase in the content of *actin* and *myosin,* the muscle's contractile proteins. As the amount of contractile protein in muscle fibers is increased, the number of cross-bridges that may be formed increases. The force produced by the muscle contraction is directly proportional to the number of cross-bridges that form, which accounts for the marked increase in the muscle's ability to generate tension in response to high-level activation. Both volitional activation and electrical stimulation can induce a rise in the amount of muscle fiber contractile protein.

ASSESSMENT OF VOLUNTARY MUSCLE STRENGTH, ACTIVATION, AND ENDURANCE

NMES can be used to augment the strength of either injured or healthy muscle. *Strength* is defined as the maximal force or *torque* a muscle or muscle group can generate at a specified velocity (4). *Muscle fatigue* has been defined as a decrease in the force-generating capacity of a muscle after recent activation (5,6). *Muscle endurance* has an inverse relationship with muscle fatigue. In this section we review electrical tests that assess muscle strength, activation, and endurance, and the results of experimental studies on (i) levels of torque produced in muscle in response to NMES; (ii) the levels of activation of a muscle; (iii) comfort; (iv) the strengthening effect of NMES training in healthy individuals and patient populations; and (v) muscle fatigue in response to NMES.

Determining Muscle Strength and Activation

Muscle strength is typically assessed as a *maximal voluntary-contraction* (MVC) force or torque. Isometric, isotonic, isokinetic, eccentric, or concentric contractions can be measured. Determination of MVC is best done by providing the subject a visual target representing their force (Fig. 6.1A and B). Targeting is combined with a superimposed electrical stimulus, producing the subject's best attempt. A superimposed pulse or a burst of supramaximal electrical stimulation to evaluate the force-generating capacity of a muscle has been used as a research tool for many years. The patient contracts volitionally and a supramaximal stimulus [100 pulses per second (pps), 600 μs duration] is superimposed on the contraction. If the patient is not activating the muscle completely, an increase in force as a result of the stimulus is recorded (Fig. 6.2). If the patient is contracting fully, no augmentation of force is noted in response to stimulation, or a slight decrease in force is seen (7) (Fig. 6.2). This technique has been used to evaluate muscles with weaknesses attributed to a significant central nervous system component, such as a failure of voluntary activation, or *reflex inhibition* (8–10). The amount of reflex inhibition, or *activation failure*, is determined by a simple ratio where the MVC force divided by the force produced with the burst augmentation equals the muscle activation of the subject, or the *central activation ratio* (CAR). Activation >95% is considered full activation; <95% is considered activation failure. This technique has been shown to provide useful clinical information. In fact, the failure to use

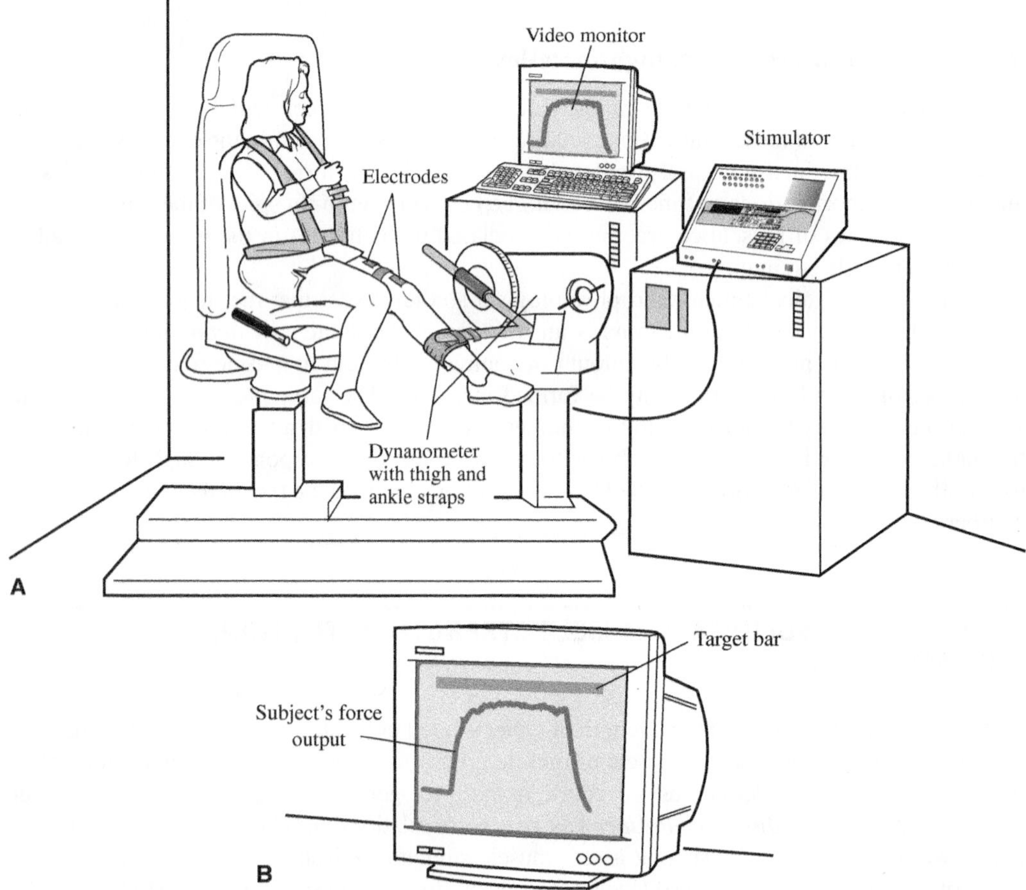

Figure 6.1. A: A person seated in the Kin-Com Dynamometer. **B:** Image shows a different view of the target screen.

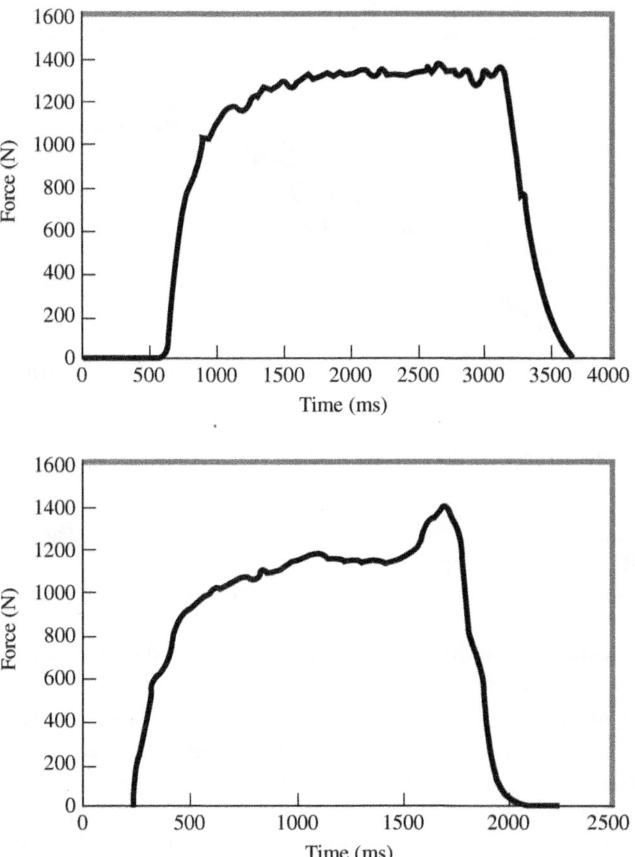

Figure 6.2. Top trace shows complete activation with no augmentation in the volitional force by the burst of electricity. **Bottom trace** shows an augmentation in force when the burst of electricity is applied to the quadriceps muscle. (Reprinted with permission from Chmielewski TL, et al. A prospective analysis of incidence and severity of quadriceps inhibition in a consecutive sample of 100 patients with complete actue anterior cruciate ligament rupture. *J Orthop Res.* 2004;22:925–930.)

this technique may result in a gross underestimation of the torque-generating capability of a muscle (11,12).

A mathematical model demonstrated that the relationship between force of the MVC and the level of activation of the quadriceps muscle is curvilinear, based on a second-order polynomial (12) (Fig. 6.3). This model has been evaluated in healthy subjects (12), older adults (13), and in subjects following anterior cruciate ligament rupture (14,15). In subjects with low levels of activation (<70%), this model is shown to be more accurate than the results of the *burst superimposition* testing, which underestimates muscle activation at this level. However, at high levels of activation (>70%) use of the model is not needed, as the results of burst superimposition testing are accurate. Errors in clinical judgment can result from failure to accurately measure strength. If the level of activation is not tested, the force output may be misinterpreted. If a patient has activation failure, volitional exercise alone will not allow for complete recovery.

The uninvolved limb may also show activation deficits (14–17). When rehabilitating a patient with quadriceps muscle weakness, side-to-side strength comparisons are made, often with the assumption that the uninvolved limb is of normal strength. If the level of muscle activation is not tested, however, the strength of the uninvolved limb and the side-to-side ratio may be underestimated. The wrong clinical strategy may be implemented as a result of such erroneous information.

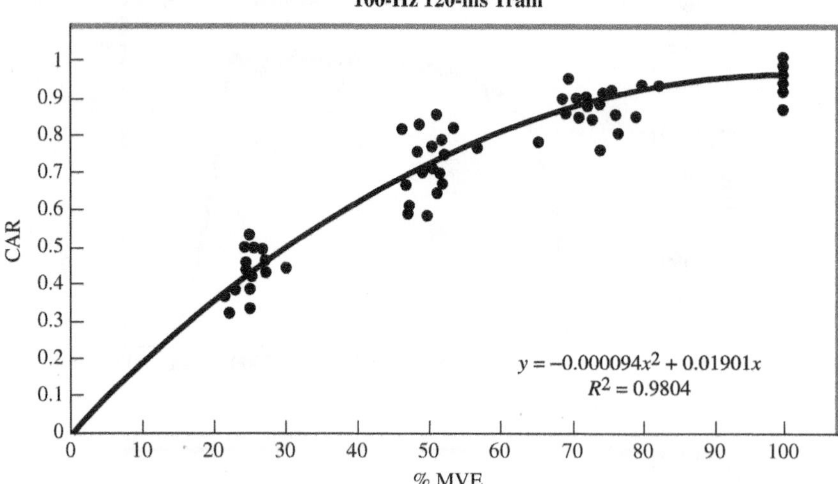

Figure 6.3. The relationship between the percent maximum voluntary effort (%MVE) and the central activation ratio (CAR) is curvilinear. (Reprinted with permission from Stackhouse SK, et al. Measurement of central activation failure of the quadriceps femoris in healthy adults. *Muscle Nerve.* 2000;23:1706–1712.)

Volitional strength testing alone does not determine whether the measurement reflects muscle atrophy, motivational factors, or an inability to activate all motor units (the reflex inhibition). The appropriate clinical strategies to treat each of these causes of low-force output differ substantially (Table 6.1). For atrophy, a program of volitional strengthening exercise is most common. Motivation requires only training in fully activating the muscle, as there is no true weakness or inhibition. It has been shown that with practice and training, patients can improve their performance and increase their quadriceps activation during a burst superimposition testing session. In the case of reflex inhibition, volitional exercise alone will not help; another strategy, such as the use of electromyographic (EMG) biofeedback, or NMES, is more appropriate.

Snyder-Mackler et al. have investigated the use of the burst superimposition technique to evaluate the presence of reflex inhibition in patients with anterior cruciate ligament (ACL) rupture (8), osteoarthritis (18), and after total knee arthroplasty (TKA) (19). The burst superimposition technique resulted in a higher torque value in each of these groups. Training patients to produce an MVC was not difficult, and in all studies, all patients were trained within a single test session. No patient required more than four trials; most required only two to learn to maximally activate the quadriceps. Snyder-Mackler et al. demonstrated that some patients do have a failure of voluntary activation after ACL rupture, with osteoarthritis (18), and after surgery [ACL reconstruction or TKA (8,20)]. If the burst superimposition technique had not been used, the

Table 6.1. Causes and Management of Muscle Weakness

Cause of Muscle Weakness	*Strategy to Manage*
Muscle Atrophy	Volitional exercise alone will be effective if activation is complete
Incomplete Neural Activation of the Muscle	Training to fully activate the muscle using NMES or biofeedback
Reduced Motivation	Exercise training of the ability to volitionally activate the muscle completely

weakness may erroneously have been attributed to atrophy rather than incomplete activation. Patients with incomplete activation will not respond well to the typical treatment prescribed for weakness, a volitional exercise program.

Older adults have been shown to have a reduced ability to activate their biceps brachii when tested using a twitch-interpolation technique (20). Fourteen younger (30.6 ± 4.3 years old) and 14 older (71 ± 6.1 years old) adults participated. Testing was done at 100 pps, 160 V, 0.1 to 0.3 μs pulse duration, and activation was determined by the force produced at each pulse duration on a by-subject basis. The younger group generated significantly higher forces than the older group. The mean activation level for the older group was 93.7% ± 2.9%, which was significantly lower than the activation level of the younger group (96.8% ± 3.7%). A decline in the number of neurons and in myelin of axons occurs with aging. The authors suggest that the loss of voluntary strength is a result of a reduced ability to activate the muscle and of muscle atrophy (20).

Assessing Muscle Fatigue and Endurance

Volitionally and electrically-elicited fatigue tests have been used to quantify muscle endurance. A potential disadvantage of tests in which volitional contraction forces are used to assess the amount of fatigue is that it may not be possible to isolate the site of fatigue. If subjects are not well-motivated or have a disorder that affects central drive (e.g., following a cerebral vascular accident), measured losses in force generation may not reflect actual failure of the contraction within muscle. However, clinically, volitional effort may be most representative of the clinical entity being evaluated.

Many investigators have attempted to use electrically-elicited fatigue tests as a clinical tool to sustain force output through repeated contraction (21,22). Before reviewing the specifics of this literature, it is important to point out the limitations of clinical fatigue tests and the clinical decisions that can be made based on the results of these tests. Operationally defining fatigue and endurance is an elusive task, whether using electrically-elicited or volitional contractions. Physiologically, fatigue has a very strict definition related to the oxidative capacity of a muscle, an increase in the aerobic capacity (VO_2). Clinicians may use volitional or electrical tests to evaluate changes in endurance capabilities in response to treatments; however, they may be attempting to quantify something other than physiological fatigue. Does the clinical observation that muscles appear to fatigue more quickly indicate that the involved muscles are truly less enduring, or are the observed phenomena due solely to muscle weakness? Because the involved muscles are weaker, they must be contracting at a higher percentage of their capacity to perform typical functional tasks, such as ambulation. Thus, even if both involved and uninvolved muscles fatigue at the same rate, the weaker muscles will be able to maintain functional force levels for shorter periods of time and will appear to the clinician to fatigue sooner.

Electrically-elicited fatigue tests have provided new insights into muscle physiology. These tests are attractive for two reasons: the physiological differences between electrical and volitional activation, and the fact that the stimulus to the muscle can be standardized and is not affected by central factors such as motivation or effort. Binder-Mcleod and Snyder-Mackler (21) used a modification of a fatigue test, originally described by Burke et al. (23) to characterize fatigue in cat single motor units, to assess muscle endurance in patients after surgical repair of their ACL. A 600-μs monophasic pulse is delivered at a train frequency of 100 pps for one-third of a second each second for 3 minutes (21). Binder-Mcleod and Snyder-Mackler found that the rate of fatigue during the application of electrical stimulation is greater than is seen with volitional contractions.

McDonnell et al. (22) investigated the use of electrical stimulation to assess the fatigue characteristics of muscle using a commonly available electrical stimulator. Using a 2500-Hz alternating current interrupted at 50 bursts per second (bps) with a 5 seconds on:2 seconds off duty cycle, these researchers recorded the torque decrement over 50 electrically-elicited contractions of the quadriceps femoris of healthy subjects. From an initial value of 60% of maximal voluntary isometric torque, declines of 65% were noted. This measure of electrically-elicited fatigue was reproducible in repeated testing of healthy subjects. These studies provide physiological insights, such as contractile characteristics and muscle fiber composition. Clinically, they provide information about the rate of fatigue, potentially providing a means of measuring muscle fatigue.

The literature shows different results for activation levels in older adults. One reason for this may be the techniques used to test muscle strength and activation. Stevens et al. (13) found small differences in strength and activation using the burst superimposition technique. When the mathematical model of Stackhouse et al. (12) was applied to the data, the same older adults showed much less activation. The CAR from the burst superimposition testing was significantly lower than the CAR calculated by the mathematical model. The activation deficits found in older adults again highlights the need to augment volitional strengthening programs with NMES.

STRENGTH OF CONTRACTIONS PRODUCED BY NEUROMUSCULAR ELECTRICAL STIMULATION

Voluntary exercise to augment strength is based on the *overload principle.* Strengthening may be achieved if training is conducted at high contraction levels (>75% of maximum) for a low number of repetitions (usually fewer than 10). In an effort to establish analogous paradigms for NMES strength training, investigators have compared maximal electrically-elicited torque and the *maximal voluntary isometric torque* (MVIT).

Kramer et al. (24) compared the torque-generating capabilities of three different forms of stimulation on the quadriceps muscle (Table 6.2) and found volitional force did not exceed the force produced with electrical stimulation. They also found that superimposition of NMES onto voluntary isometric contractions (MVIC) produced no appreciable increase in torque. More than 75% MVIC can be reached, but not necessarily by all NMES stimulation programs.

Walmsley et al. (25) performed a similar study comparing the torque-generating capabilities of four different stimulators on the quadriceps muscle (Table 6.2). Superimposition of voluntary contraction on NMES contraction increased torque levels for all stimulators but in no instance exceeded MVIT. Snyder-Mackler et al. (26) compared the isometric torque-generating capabilities of three stimulators on the quadriceps muscle (Table 6.2). These investigators also noted tremendous intersubject variation.

Locicero (27) studied the isotonic torque-generating ability of a 2500-Hz alternating current modulated at 50 bps at three different velocities (0, 60, and 240 degrees per second). The stimulator was able to generate an average of 93% to 104% of the MVC of the quadriceps femoris muscles of 20 women and 10 men (27).

Delitto et al. (28) evaluated the torque-producing capability of 2500-Hz current interrupted at 75 bps in healthy college students while studying discomfort with stimulation (28). Similar to Snyder-Mackler et al. (26), they found that subjects who participated were able to generate an average of 70% of their MVIT.

From the levels of contraction evoked in these and other studies, one can conclude that many forms of NMES are capable of producing torque comparable to those volitional contraction levels that induce strengthening on repeated application. But can muscles be activated at levels greater than MVC? Delitto et al. (29) reported average training contraction intensities of 112% of the quadriceps MVIT in a single-subject study of an elite weight lifter, the only study to date where training contraction intensities in excess of 100% of MVIT have been demonstrated. It should be noted, however, that this subject is precisely the type of subject described by Kots. Kots reported at a conference in 1977 that he was able to increase the MVC of elite athletes by up to 40%; however, the brief conference notes do not contain the details [see Ward and Shkuratova (1)].

Table 6.2. Comparison of Maximal Electrically Elicited Torques and Maximal Volitional Isometric Torques

Study	Parameters of Electrical Stimulation		Percent = Electrical Torque / Volitional Torque
Kramer et al.	ES1	1-μs PD asymmetrical AC at 100Hz	93%
	ES2	200-μs PD asymmetrical AC at 100Hz	67%
	ES3	2-μs PD monophasic pulsed at 100 Hz	53%
Walmsley et al.	ES1	2500 Hz AC interrupted at 10-ms intervals to produce 50 bursts/s	87%
	ES2	250-μs PD 4000-Hz AC at 75 beats/min	46%
	ES3	400-μs PD asymmetrical, biphasic pulsed current at 50 pps	84%
	ES4	200-μs PD monophasic pulsed current at 60 pps	68%
Snyder-Mackler et al.	ES1	AC 2500-Hz interrupted at 10-ms intervals to produce 50 bursts/s	68%
	ES2	250-μs PD AC 4000-Hz modulated at 50 beats/min	45%
	ES3	400-μs PD symmetrical, biphasic pulsed current at 50 pps	61%

Enoka et al. (30,31) have made the argument that the MVC does not represent the maximal force that a muscle can exert. Rather, the MVC represents a relative maximum, one that can be achieved under the constrained conditions of the test. Most studies that have examined motor unit discharge during high-force contraction have reported that neither the instantaneous nor the average discharge rate approaches the frequencies necessary to electrically elicit the maximal force (30,31). This argument supports the possibility of the kind of activation found by Kots (1) and Delitto et al. (29).

In summary, there are many options available clinically that will produce high levels of electrically-elicited contractions (Table 6.2). In using electrical stimulation, the parameters can be modified to produce the maximal force desired. Modifications to the parameters can also affect the patient's perceived comfort of the stimulation (see below).

STIMULATION CONTRACTION REQUIRED TO STRENGTHEN SKELETAL MUSCLE

One assumption implicit in the studies of torque-generating capability is that stronger stimulation will result in greater strengthening effects. In a recent study of 52 patients after ACL reconstruction, Snyder-Mackler et al. (32) described a dose–response relationship for NMES. They found that the greater the electrically-elicited training contraction force, the greater the quadriceps femoris muscle recovery after ACL reconstruction. Training contraction intensity was linearly related to quadriceps femoris muscle strength only for training contraction intensities >10% of the uninvolved MVC force. This suggests that there is a threshold training contraction intensity for strengthening of the quadriceps femoris muscle group using this technique.

FACTORS DETERMINING PATIENT COMFORT DURING NEUROMUSCULAR ELECTRICAL STIMULATION FOR STRENGTHENING

One classic approach to studying experimental pain methodologies is to use electrical stimulation. Patient discomfort is often the limiting factor in using electrical stimulation in clinical settings, especially when high contractile forces are sought for strength-training regimens. Numerous studies have investigated discomfort associated with electrical stimulation administered clinically (28,33–37). The methodologies used in these studies were visual analog scales, categorical scales, forced-choice techniques, and magnitude estimation.

Most studies have focused on subject preference for various current characteristics, studying electrical stimulation as though discomfort was solely a function of current form (e.g., waveform, pulse duration, frequency). Delitto and Rose (34) evaluated the relative comfort of three different waveforms (triangular, sinusoidal, and square), delivered at 2500 Hz and interrupted at 10-ms intervals to produce 50 bps, and found that individual preferences existed for each current form. Bowman and Baker (33) reached a similar conclusion when comparing 2500-Hz sinusoidal current delivered in 10-ms bursts at 50 bps to "single pulsed" current (symmetrical biphasic current, 300-μs pulse duration) when using a forced-choice paradigm. In a study comparing identical current forms with either low- or high-frequency sine waves, Grimby and Wigerstad-Lossing (35) found no difference in the torque produced with the current forms. They also reported no qualitative or quantitative difference between the stimulators in perceived discomfort.

Two limitations are apparent in the previous studies. First, the contractile force elicited differed substantially, with Delitto and Rose (34) eliciting contractile forces in excess of 60% of MVC, and Bowman and Baker (33) eliciting contractile forces of as little as 20 foot-pounds, the latter most likely less than 10% of MVC. Second and more important, the discomfort associated with electrical stimulation is studied as though it is a sole function of current form, as if one particular current will stimulate the maximal number of motor neurons and the minimal number of nociceptors. This is not consistent with most pain theories, which make it clear that discomfort and pain are not solely a function of nociceptor input, and instead are moderated by an individual's cognitive and behavioral factors.

Delitto et al. (28) attempted to address these limitations by studying cognitive behavioral influences of subject tolerances to electrically-elicited contractions at contractile forces that are reported to have training (e.g., strengthening) effects, as well as electrical stimulation in which there were no contractile forces (nociceptive input only). The results of this study suggested that three variables are important when considering discomfort associated with electrical stimulation: the subject's preferred coping style, whether the stimulus causes a muscle contraction, and whether the subject is judging the intensity or the unpleasantness of the stimulation. Therefore, Delitto et al. suggest that clinicians be aware that individual differences exist in preferred coping styles when a patient is faced with an aversive event (e.g., electrical stimulation), which may include monitoring (information-seeking) or blunting (information-avoiding) behaviors. The clinician should attempt to match the environment to the patient's coping style. For example, if a patient prefers a blunting strategy, providing a quiet environment with some type of distraction (e.g., music via headphones) may improve his or her tolerance to electrical stimulation. If a patient prefers a monitoring strategy, education about electrical stimulation and its effectiveness may improve the patient's tolerance to electrical stimulation. The clinician should also be aware that in addition to the nociceptive input, the electrically-elicited contractile force contributes uniquely to the discomfort associated with electrical stimulation; that is, the greater the force, the more intense the discomfort, regardless of current intensity.

Miller et al. (37) investigated two stimulation parameters and the effectiveness of the stimulation coupled with the subject's report of comfort. In one part of the experiment, subjects received four submaximal MVC contractions at 100 Hz, 150 V, 50-ms pulse trains, with monophasic rectangular waves of 0.2-ms pulse duration, and four contractions at 100 HZ, 150 V, 100-ms pulse trains, with monophasic rectangular waves of 0.2-ms pulse duration. In the second part of the study, subjects received four pulse train stimuli at 100 Hz, 150 V, and 100 ms, with 0.1-ms pulse duration, then four with 0.2-ms pulse duration. Subjects evaluated pain levels on a visual analogue scale after each trial. The authors found that the 100-ms pulse duration produced higher torque than the 50-ms pulse duration; however, the discomfort reported was higher with the 100-ms pulse duration than with the 50-ms pulse duration. Subjects reported significantly less discomfort with 0.1-ms pulse duration than with the 0.2-ms pulse duration; this parameter change did not influence torque increment size (37).

Pulsed electromagnetic field (PEMF) therapy, when combined with NMES, is more comfortable that NMES alone; however, it is more cumbersome to set up and use (36). There is little in the literature regarding the use of PEMF for muscle strengthening. Currier et al. (36) compared NMES and NMES combined with PEMF superimposed on volitional quadriceps/hamstring contraction with the knee in full extension. Patients reported that NMES alone was twice as painful as NMES combined with PEMF. Currently, research is underway to confirm the findings of Currier et al.

EVIDENCE SUPPORTING NEUROMUSCULAR ELECTRICAL STIMULATION FOR STRENGTHENING

Two issues must be kept in mind when reviewing the literature related to the strengthening effect of NMES: subject selection (patients or healthy college students) and the type of stimulator used (battery powered or line-current driven). There are numerous studies in which the general purpose was to compare electrical stimulation to volitional exercise. Taken as a whole, the results of these studies vary with regard to which is more effective. The picture becomes more distinct when the studies are separated according to the characteristics of the populations from which each study obtained samples.

Neuromuscular Electrical Stimulation-induced Strengthening in Healthy Subjects

Massey et al. (38) examined the strengthening effect of NMES in four groups of United States Marine Corps recruits: group A (electrical stimulation alone), group B (progressive resistive exercise), group C (isometric exercise), and group D (unexercised control). A monophasic, pulsed current of unspecified pulse duration was delivered at 1000 pps. The middle deltoid, pectoralis major, trapezius, biceps, triceps, wrist flexor, and wrist extensor muscles were stimulated bilaterally in group A at the *maximally tolerated contraction* (MTC) level. All groups trained three times per week for 9 weeks. Isometric shoulder, elbow, and grip strengths were used as dependent measures. Training with NMES produced strength gains equivalent to those of volitional exercise (groups B and C). All three experimental groups demonstrated increased strength versus unexercised controls. This study is one of the few that has shown similar increases in strength for both NMES and volitional exercise programs.

Halbach and Straus (39) compared NMES to isokinetic exercise for muscle strengthening in six subjects. A monophasic pulsed current of 500 μs duration was delivered at 50 pps to the quadriceps femoris to elicit *maximally tolerated isometric contractions* (MTICs) in training. The voluntary exercise group was trained isokinetically. Training occurred five times per week for 3 weeks. NMES was found to be inferior to isokinetic exercise for increasing strength. However, the voluntary exercise group was trained in the same fashion as all groups were tested, whereas the NMES group trained isometrically, which may have affected the validity of the dependent measure.

Eriksson et al. (40) compared quadriceps NMES (using a 500 μs monophasic pulse delivered at 200 pps at 15 seconds on and 15 seconds off) to isometric exercise in eight subjects. MTICs and isometric exercise training occurred three to four times per week for 4 weeks. Increases in isometric strength were equivalent for both groups. Using several t-tests, the researchers reported biochemical changes after stimulation similar to those seen in intense voluntary exercise.

NMES using a 2500-Hz, sinusoidal alternating current interrupted for 10 ms at 10-ms intervals (resulting in 50 10-ms bps) became the focus of a great deal of attention beginning in 1977. These current characteristics were described by Soviet researcher Yakov Kots during a symposium on NMES (1,41) and were purported to produce intense muscle contractions (110% to 130% of MVIC) with no discomfort in elite athletes. Training for 3 to 4 weeks reportedly produced 30% to 40% strength gains as well as functional gains (in vertical jump and other measures). Endurance was reported to be increased after 6 to 8 weeks of training. No data were presented [see Kramer and Mendryk (42)].

Spurred by these reports, Kramer and Semple (43) examined the effects of isometric exercise and muscle stimulation of the quadriceps femoris. Due to the unavailability of a machine capable of producing the current characteristics described above, these investigators used a symmetrical, rectangular alternating current of unspecified pulse duration and frequency to stimulate the muscle to MTIC. Using similar training regimens, subjects treated with NMES alone, NMES plus isometric exercise, and isometric exercise alone were compared to unexercised controls. All experimental groups produced significant gains in isometric strength when compared with the control group, but there was no difference among the experimental groups.

In the late 1970s, a stimulator was developed that produced the current characteristics described by Kots. This device was used to provide training sessions of 10-second contractions followed by 50 seconds of rest for 10-minute sessions (1). Using this device, Currier and Mann (44) compared the quadriceps femoris of subjects treated with isometric exercise, NMES, and simultaneous NMES with that of an unexercised control group. These authors were the first to report the amplitude of the stimulated contraction as a percentage of the MVIT, producing a standard that was analogous to that used in the voluntary exercise and strengthening literature. In this study, current amplitude was increased to 60% of pretest MVIT. Training occurred three times per week for 5 weeks. Stimulation produced significant gains in isometric strength in quadriceps when compared to controls, but not when compared to the isometric exercise group. No additional benefit was noted with simultaneous NMES and isometric exercise. In addition, no increase in isokinetic torque-producing capability was found in any of the groups.

Selkowitz (45) compared NMES to unexercised controls and continuously-monitored training intensity, which averaged 91% of pretest MVIT. Training occurred seven days per week for 4 weeks. The NMES group increased quadriceps MVIT by 18%, suggesting that the pretest MVITs may have been artificially low. Training intensities and strength gains in the experimental group were positively and significantly correlated.

Mohr et al. (46) compared subjects treated to NMES and isometric exercise with unexercised controls using a 20-μs pulse duration, monophasic pulsed current at 50 pps. Subjects trained five times per week for 3 weeks. No significant increase in MVIT was noted in the quadriceps femoris of the NMES group when compared with unexercised controls. This type of current may not produce contractions of sufficient magnitude to elicit a strengthening effect because of its extremely short pulse duration.

Stefanovska and Vodovnik (47) compared subjects treated to a 2500-Hz alternating current burst-modulated 25 times per second to a 300-μs, monophasic pulsed current delivered at 25 pps with an unexercised control group. Quadriceps training intensities were only 5% of MVIT. Subjects trained five times per week for 3 weeks. Their training paradigm included MVIT measurements for the NMES groups before and after each training session. Although MVIT increases were noted for both NMES groups when compared to unexercised controls, the relatively low NMES training intensities compared to the high amplitude of multiple daily MVICs might indicate that the MVIT increases in the NMES groups were attributable to the voluntary exercise of the MVIT measurements.

Wolf et al. (48) compared an exercise group, a simultaneous NMES and exercise group, and an unexercised control group. The stimulator used in this study delivered a 300-μs, monophasic pulse at 75 pps. Intensity was set at MTIC of the quadriceps, bilaterally. A full body squat was the training exercise. Dependent measures included force measurements from a computerized squat machine and two functional measures, 25-yard dash time and vertical jump. Again, NMES and exercise was comparable to exercise alone for quadriceps strengthening. Of particular interest in this study is the carryover to functional tasks of the increase in strength. In both experimental groups there was an increase in vertical jump and decrease in 25-yard dash time.

Alon et al. (49) examined the effect of NMES alone or combined with volitional exercise on the strength of the abdominal musculature. Subjects participated in NMES or voluntary training three times per week for 4 consecutive weeks. Measurements of abdominal strength were taken at 1-week intervals over the course of the study. NMES to the abdominal musculature was provided with symmetrical biphasic waveforms at maximal tolerable intensities with 5 seconds on time and 5 seconds off time initially. Contract/relax cycles were increased to 7.5, 10, and 12.5 seconds over the remaining weeks of training. The number of contraction repetitions was increased by 20% weekly from baseline voluntary repetition levels determined in pretest measures. NMES combined with stimulation produced the greatest increases in muscle strength, followed by stimulation alone.

Evidence for Neuromuscular Electrical Stimulation-induced Strengthening in Patient Populations

Quadriceps Strengthening

The literature is replete with studies investigating the effects of NMES on strengthening of the quadriceps. A variety of stimulation parameters are used, as well as a variety of treatment times and frequency and electrode number and placement. The information presented here is a sampling of the literature. It is important to note strength gains that occur in the groups receiving NMES and the groups receiving exercise, and the specifics of the NMES parameters and the exercise protocols. Although most studies found NMES to be more effective than exercise alone (32,41,42,49–53), not all did (24,54,55).

William and Street (56), in a study of 20 patients with quadriceps femoris atrophy, used 20 minutes of NMES per session for 13 sessions and found recovery of normal quadriceps function in the majority of cases. The current characteristics were not described, and no control group was used. Johnson et al. (57) studied the effects of electrical stimulation on quadriceps MVIT in 40 patients with chondromalacia patellae. NMES of unspecified current characteristics was delivered at 65 Hz, three times per week for 6 weeks. Each session consisted of 10 to 15 minutes of NMES. A 36% increase in MVIT was noted. No control group was used.

Eriksson and Haggmark (54), in their study on healthy subjects cited earlier, used an identical regimen to compare NMES and isometric exercise in eight patients who had undergone knee ligament surgery. They reported less observable atrophy of the thigh, marked functional improvement (using an ordered rating scale), and an increase in oxidative activity in the NMES group as compared to the isometric exercise group.

Godfrey et al. (51) compared isometric exercise to NMES in 35 patients referred for strengthening who had recently either undergone knee surgery or sustained a knee injury. A 60-Hz alternating current was used to produce MTICs of the quadriceps femoris. The isometric exercise group trained at 75% of MVIT. Patients trained 5 days per week for 3 weeks, 10 to 15 minutes per day. The dependent measure was peak isokinetic torque measured at several velocities. Increase in peak torque at the slowest isokinetic speed (3 rpm) was significantly higher in the NMES group than in the exercise group. An aggregate score developed from the isokinetic measures at the three tested speeds (3, 10, and 25 rpm) was also significantly higher in the NMES group than in the exercise group.

Gould et al. (52) compared NMES to isometric exercise in 20 patients who had undergone open joint meniscectomy. A 100-μs, monophasic pulsed current delivered at 35 pps was used to produce MTICs of the involved quadriceps femoris. Training occurred daily for 2 weeks. The percentage of MVIT (compared to the unoperated limb) was significantly greater for the NMES group.

Morrissey et al. (58) compared patients receiving NMES to unexercised patients after ACL reconstruction. The portable stimulator used in this study produced a 350-μs, monophasic pulsed current delivered at 50 pps at an on time:off time of 10 seconds:50 seconds. Training consisted of 6 hours of cycled maximally tolerated muscle stimulation per day. The results showed a less pronounced decrease in quadriceps MVIT and in thigh circumference in the muscle stimulation group at the end of a 6-week immobilization period when compared to unexercised controls. Six weeks later (12 weeks postsurgery, 6 weeks after immobilization and NMES had ceased), all differences between the groups had disappeared.

Singer et al. (59) examined the effect of three different stimulators on patients with long-term knee pathology and quadriceps atrophy. The stimulators delivered pulsed current with pulse durations ranging from 75 to 350 μs and frequencies of 50 and 100 pps. Patients were stimulated to MTIC 15 minutes per day, 7 days per week for 4 weeks. An aggregate increase in MVIT for the 15 subjects was 22% over pretest values.

Delitto et al. (60) compared high-intensity electrical stimulation to volitional exercise in the early postoperative period of patients undergoing ACL surgery. Twenty patients were randomly and independently assigned to an NMES and to a volitional exercise group. All quadriceps activity was accompanied by simultaneous hamstring contraction to counter anterior translation forces at the knee. Their post-test design used a dependent measure of isometric strength measured at 65 degrees of flexion within the 4-to 6-week period after surgery. The results of this study clearly show a better response to high-intensity electrical stimulation than volitional training in the early postoperative period (Fig. 6.4).

Snyder-Mackler et al. (53) conducted a similar study, in that the postoperative ACL reconstruction patients were randomly assigned to an exercise or an electrical stimulation group, and a post-test design was used. A 2500-Hz alternating current, burst-modulated at 75 bps, was used to deliver 15 contractions per session, three times per week. Their dependent measures were isokinetic strength (90 and 270 degrees per second), as well as a more functional quadriceps strength measure that they operationalized as knee excursion during stance. The isokinetic results for the quadriceps femoris musculature are illustrated in Figure 6.5. Again, high-intensity stimulation showed a clear benefit over volitional training when co-contractions were used. In addition, the study showed that patients receiving high-intensity NMES had significantly better temporal gait measures. Finally, this study showed a significant correlation between quadriceps strength and the amount of knee flexion excursion during stance phase.

Snyder-Mackler et al. (61) randomly assigned 110 subjects immediately following ACL reconstruction to one of four groups: (i) high-level electrical stimulation, (ii) high-level volitional exercise, (iii) low-level electrical stimulation (portable stimulator), and (iv) combined high- and low-level electrical stimulation. After 4 weeks, quadriceps femoris muscle strength and stance phase knee kinematics were assessed. Quadriceps strengths averaged >70% of the uninvolved quadriceps for the two high-level electrical stimulation groups (high-level electrical stimulation and combined), 57% for the high-level volitional exercise, and 51% for the low-level

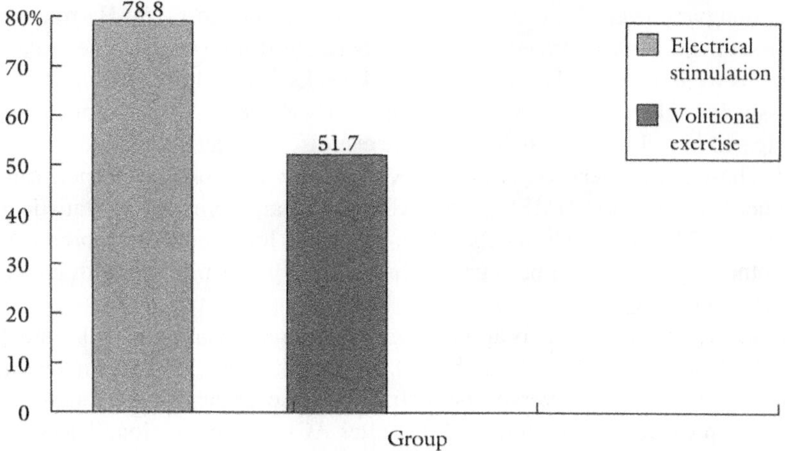

Figure 6.4. A comparison of isometric quadriceps femoris muscle torque expressed as a percentage of the maximal voluntary isometric contraction of the uninvolved quadriceps for electrical stimulation and volitional exercise groups.

electrical stimulation group. Knee joint kinematics were again directly and significantly correlated with quadriceps strength.

Lieber et al. (62) investigated NMES compared to volitional exercise alone in patients after ACL reconstruction (n = 40; 15 to 44 years old). Each contraction cycle, either stimulated or volitional, was for 10 seconds, followed by 20 seconds rest, for 30 minutes. For the NMES

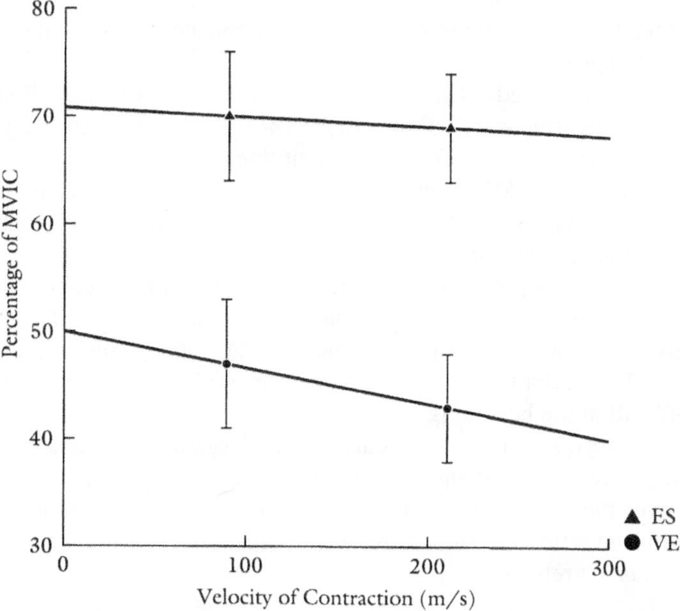

Figure 6.5. Isokinetic torque of the quadriceps femoris as a function of contraction velocity. ES, electrical stimulation group; VE, volitional exercise group. (Reprinted with permission from Snyder-Mackler L et al. Electrical stimulation of the thigh muscles after reconstruction of the anterior cruciate ligament. Effects of electrically elicited contractions of the quadriceps femoris and hamstring muscles on gait and strength of the thigh muscles. *J Bone Joint Surg Am.* 1991;73:1025–1036.)

group, stimulation parameters were asymmetrical, biphasic waveform, 50-Hz frequency, 250-μs pulse duration, at maximally tolerated intensity. A portable stimulator was used in a clinical setting. Both groups were treated 5 days per week for 4 weeks. The volitional contraction group was given progressively higher force targets based on MVIC of the first session of each week. Both groups participated in a clinician-monitored home exercise program as an adjunct to the contraction protocol. These researchers found that the volitional contraction group performed at a significantly higher level than the NMES group. After one year, there was no statistical difference among the groups. This study shows that both methods, long term, may produce equivalent results. The authors speculate that both groups had similar protocols, and with increasing intensities, both techniques may be equally effective.

There are studies where NMES is applied for long treatment durations of several hours, such as the studies by Sisk et al. (55) and Lamb et al. (63). Sisk et al. (55) investigated the effect of NMES plus isometric exercise versus isometric exercise alone on the quadriceps femoris strength of a group of 22 patients immobilized after ACL reconstruction. The stimulator produced a 300-μs pulse duration, balanced, symmetrical, biphasic pulsed current at 40 pps and a timing cycle of 10 seconds on:30 seconds off. Training was at MTIC, 8 hours per day, 7 days per week, for 6 weeks. No difference in MVIT was noted between the groups.

Lamb et al. (63) investigated NMES of the quadriceps after hip fracture in 24 elderly subjects (83.9 ± 2.9 years old). The patients were randomized in to two groups: one receiving patterned neuromuscular strengthening (PNMS) or a placebo stimulation. The portable stimulator PNMS parameters were a balanced, asymmetric biphasic pulsed current with 300-μs pulse duration, 30 seconds:15 seconds on:off timing cycle, set at the minimum required for a visible muscle contraction. The stimulators were used 3 hours per day, every day, for 6 weeks. Both groups received physical therapy as inpatients, and at discharge were given a home exercise program to follow. Their results showed significant improvements in walking speed and in postural stability in the PNMS group after treatment. These results show that low levels of stimulation are effective in this patient population; by strengthening the uninjured leg, they placed less reliance on the uninvolved limb and improved walking speed.

Currier et al. (36) compared NMES and NMES combined with PEMF superimposed on volitional quadriceps/hamstring contraction with the knee in full extension. They compared thigh girth before surgery to that after 6 weeks of treatment three times per week with 10 contractions per session. Although using PEMF is an intriguing approach to strength training, the study by Currier et al. is the only study done on patients using this technique. The cumbersome procedure makes this option less attractive than electrical stimulation.

Karmel-Ross et al. (64) reported a case series of patients with spina bifida. The quadriceps femoris muscles were stimulated during standing or walking for 30 minutes each day. Stimulation intensity was adjusted to patient tolerance. A battery-powered stimulator using a pulse duration of 347 μs and a frequency of 35 pps was used. On:off times ranged from 8 seconds on:24 seconds off at the beginning of the study, to 8 seconds on:8 seconds off at the completion of the study. Dependent measures included quadriceps torque and timed functional tasks (level walking, stair ascending, and stair descending). Four of the five subjects improved at the functional tasks over the treatment period, and only two (the oldest subjects) had improved quadriceps torque production. Karmel-Ross et al. suggested that the muscle testing in the youngest subjects was not reliable.

Lumbar Paraspinal Strengthening with Neuromuscular Electrical Stimulation

Starring et al. (65) published a case report of a patient with persistent low back pain. A 2500-Hz alternating current with a burst frequency of 75 bps and a 15 seconds:50 seconds on:off ratio was used. Electrodes were placed bilaterally over the erector spinae in the lumbar region. After

6 weeks of treatment the patient was asymptomatic. No measures of lumbar extensor muscle strength were taken, but the author notes that substantial electrically-elicited contractions were achieved, necessitating stabilization with straps over the pelvis to prevent anterior pelvic tilt.

Kahanovitz et al. (66) compared NMES to an exercised and an unexercised control group in a study of the erector spinae muscles in patients with low back pain. The stimulator produced a 425-μs pulse duration symmetrical, biphasic pulsed current. Training consisted of daily 20-min sessions of either exercise or maximally tolerated electrical contraction for 4 weeks. The increase in isokinetic strength was significantly greater in the NMES group than in either the exercise or control group.

Neuromuscular Electrical Stimulation Strengthening in Other Populations

Low-intensity therapeutic electrical stimulation to the deltoid and biceps muscles was evaluated in a series of 13 children with spinal muscular atrophy (9.9 ± 3.36 years old) over a period of 6 months (67). The stimulation parameters were 300-μs pulse width, pulse frequency 35–45 Hz, peak intensity no more than 10 mA, and a 1:1 on:off cycle for 15-minute sessions. This protocol did not effectively improve muscle strength. This result is unusual for NMES; however, the low-intensity current may not have been sufficient to overcome the primary abnormality of fewer motor units.

A randomized, controlled clinical trial was conducted on the effects of NMES in patients with chronic obstructive pulmonary disease (68). Fifteen patients with moderate ventilatory impairment and incapacitating breathlessness without concomitant neurologic conditions were included. Stimulation was applied to the quadriceps femoris muscles of both legs. Patients were randomized into group 1, which initially received 6 weeks of NMES treatments ($n = 9$), or group 2, which received the same NMES treatment after a 6-week control period. NMES parameters were symmetrical biphasic square pulsed current at 50 Hz, 300 to 400 μs, using the highest tolerable amplitude (patients were started at 10 mA, increasing to 100 mA), and a duty cycle that started at 2 seconds on:18 seconds off and increased to 10 seconds on:30 seconds off. Treatment sessions were 15 minutes in the first week and 30 minutes thereafter. Following NMES protocol, the patients show statistically significant improvement in VO_2 max, endurance, muscle strength, and muscle fatigue index. Patients also reported decreased dyspnea. The use of NMES offers the potential for muscle strengthening via an essentially passive exercise protocol, without fatigue or ventilatory distress, to patients with a condition that manifests itself as breathlessness and that results in exercise intolerance.

Limitations to the Use of Neuromuscular Electrical Stimulation for Strengthening

NMES for strengthening is generally used on the superficial muscles of the arms and shoulder girdle, the legs, and low back. An isolated injury with specific muscular strength deficits, such as quadriceps weakness or lumbar paraspinal weakness, is the most common impairment that is treated with NMES for strengthening. NMES for strengthening is appropriate when weakness is limited to a few weakened muscles. In the presence of generalized weakness, NMES for strengthening may benefit if the appropriate muscle groups are targeted, or combined with the use of functional electrical stimulation (see Chapter 7). However, generalized weakness will probably require other interventions.

Summary of Neuromuscular Electrical Stimulation for Strengthening

The focus of the research on NMES for strengthening is primarily on the quadriceps femoris muscles There are few studies of NMES for strengthening other muscle groups. However, application procedures used on the quadriceps femoris can theoretically be used effectively in an analogous fashion on other muscles groups. The studies of NMES for strengthening do not include NMES for restoring strength to denervated muscles, and this information is presented below. The literature is replete with studies on the use of functional electrical stimulation in patients following central damage, such as stroke or spinal cord injury. This literature and the evidence for the use of FES is presented in Chapter 7.

EFFECTIVENESS OF PORTABLE VERSUS CLINICAL STIMULATORS FOR STRENGTHENING

Until recently, studies have suggested that portable stimulators were not as effective as clinical stimulators (32,50,55,58,69,70) in generating torques required in rehabilitation. Recent work (71,72) indicates that portable stimulators are capable of producing adequate quadriceps muscle contractions.

Laufer et al. (71) investigated force generation produced with the use of different waveforms and muscle fatigue caused by repeated contractions with these waveforms. They examined differences in fatigue and muscle force production between men and women with these waveforms. They used two portable stimulators and one clinical stimulator. Fifteen subjects (mean, 28.2 years old; range, 22 to 35 years) participated in three test sessions to test each of the three stimulators (Table 6.3). The fatiguing test had a 7 seconds:2 seconds on:off time cycle until 48 contractions were produced, or until zero torque was generated. Laufer et al. found that the

Table 6.3. Stimulation Parameters Used in Comparing Portable and Clinical Stimulators

	Lyons et al. (2005)		***Laufer et al. (2001)***		
	Clinical Stimulator	***Portable Stimulator***	***Portable Stimulator***	***Portable Stimulator***	***Clinical Stimulator***
Pulse rate	2500-HZ carrier frequency at 75 bps	75 pps	50 Hz	50 Hz	50 Hz bursts
Pulse duration	400 μs	250 μs	200 μs	200 μs	200 μs
Burst duration	6.7 ms	N/A			10 ms bursts, 10 ms burst intervals, with 25 alternating pulses per burst
On time	10 s (2 s ramp up, with 8 s at dose intensity)	10 s (2 s ramp up, 6 s at dose intensity, 2 s ramp down)	3 s	3 s	3 s
Off time	50 s	50 s	57 s	57 s	57 s
Amplitude	Subject tolerance	Subject tolerance	150 mA maximum	150 mA maximum	100 mA maximum
Waveform	Symmetrical, biphasic, triangular	Symmetrical, biphasic, square	Monophasic	Biphasic	Polyphasic

maximally tolerated muscle contraction produced by the line-powered stimulator was weaker than the portable stimulators with the biphasic or monophasic waveforms. They also found that the 2500-Hz AC waveform produced the greatest fatigue. There was no difference in the rate of fatigue between men and women. These results indicate that battery-operated stimulators may be effective tools with patient rehabilitation at home and in the clinic.

Lyons et al. (72) investigated the force generation produced with use of a portable stimulator and a clinical stimulator, as well as self-reported pain during NMES with the two types of stimulators. Subjects had no history of knee injury. Subjects were seated on dynamometers with the knee stabilized at 60 degrees of flexion. Subjects' MVIC was determined, then a dosing phase was completed to determine the maximal amplitude each subject could tolerate using the parameters chosen (Table 6.3), up to 25% to 50% of their MVIC. After a rest period, the testing phase began, with 10 isometric contractions at the testing intensity. A second test session was performed within 1 week, repeating the testing procedures with the second stimulator. There were no differences in peak torque or pain ratings between the clinical and portable stimulator. The portable stimulator produced a greater average torque integral compared to the clinical stimulator during the course of the testing phase (Fig. 6.6). Testing of the current capacity of each instrument revealed that the portable stimulator used a greater percentage of its capacity as compared to the clinical stimulator, indicating that, although the two are comparable at producing torque, the portable stimulator may not have the reserve current capacity to maintain adequate torque as muscle torque increases with training.

Several studies suggest that the use of portable (battery-driven) electrical stimulators may not be as effective in producing strength gains in muscle as are clinical (60-Hz, AC-driven) stimulators. Sisk et al. (55) found no difference between NMES plus exercise and exercise alone in strengthening the quadriceps after reconstructive knee surgery. Morrissey et al. (58) found NMES using a portable stimulator better than nothing (unexercised controls) for quadriceps strengthening during immobilization, but this apparent effect was only temporary.

Draper et al. (69) compared EMG biofeedback and portable NMES used in conjunction with quadriceps setting and straight-leg-raise exercises, three times per day for 30 minutes per session, for 4 weeks. There was no control group or comparison group in which volitional exercise alone was used. All subjects had a recent ACL reconstruction. The biofeedback group recovered to 46% of the contralateral quadriceps MVIC, whereas the portable electrical stimulation group recovered to 38%. A comparison of these results with those of Delitto et al. (50) and Snyder-Mackler et al. (53), who used line-powered NMES, is illustrated in Figure 6.7. As can be

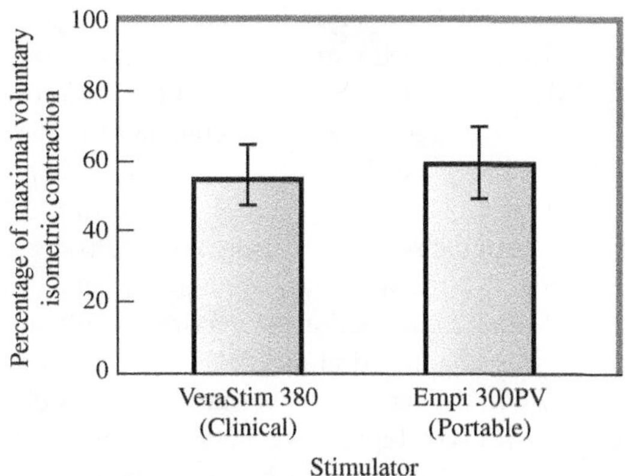

Figure 6.6. Mean torques between clinical versastim 380 and portable stimulator (Empi 300PV). (Reprinted with permission from Lyons CL, Robb JB, Irrgang JJ, Fitzgerald JI. Differences in quadricpes femoris muscle torque when using a clinical electrical stimulator versus a portable electrical stimulator. *Phys Ther* 2005;85:44–51.)

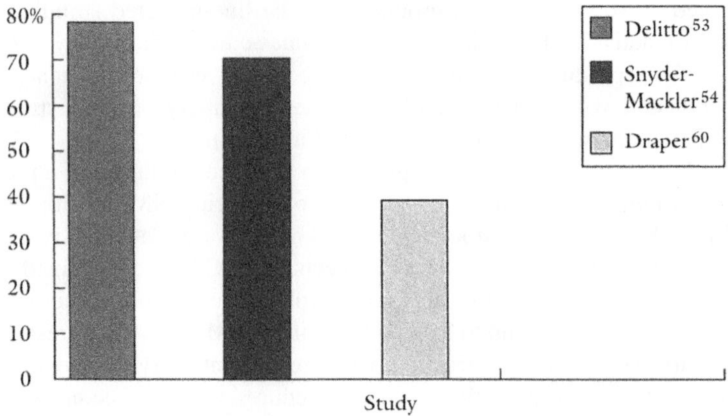

Figure 6.7. A comparison of quadriceps femoris muscle torque expressed as a percentage of the maximal voluntary isometric contraction of the uninvolved quadriceps for electrical stimulation groups in the three cited studies: Delitto et al. (50), Snyder-Mackler et al. (53), and Draper and Ballard (69).

seen in the graph, the magnitude of the experimental effect of the studies using line-powered NMES is much greater than that of those using the portable stimulation.

Snyder-Mackler et al. (32) established a dose-response curve for electrical stimulation regimens designed to improve quadriceps femoris muscle recovery in patients after ACL reconstruction. They analyzed data from a subsample (n = 52) of patients receiving electrical stimulation who were involved in a large (n = 110), multicenter, randomized clinical trial investigating treatment strategies designed to enhance quadriceps femoris recovery. Training contraction forces were monitored by logging the electrically-elicited knee-extension torque and expressing this as a percentage of the uninvolved quadriceps maximal voluntary-contraction force. After 4 weeks of training, isometric muscle performance was assessed, and a dose-response curve was generated. A significant linear correlation was found between training contraction force and quadriceps recovery. Subjects training with console-type clinical generators trained at higher contraction forces than those with portable, battery-operated generators; such training resulted in higher quadriceps femoris recovery and improved gait. The dose-response curve is illustrated in Figure 6.8. These results support the use of clinical, high-output electrical stimulation and do not support the use of low-output or battery-powered stimulators when the goal is quadriceps femoris recovery in the early phases of rehabilitation after ACL surgery.

Paternostro-Sluga et al. (73) conducted a randomized, double blind, controlled trial to evaluated the effectiveness of NMES after ACL reconstruction (n = 25) or repair (n = 25). NMES was given in addition to an exercise regimen and was compared to the exercise regimen alone. Subjects were randomly assigned to group 1 (NMES and exercise therapy), group 2 (TENS and exercise therapy), or group 3 (exercise therapy alone). Those in the NMES group (n = 16) received stimulation daily on a portable stimulator, using six-electrodes over the quadriceps muscles. A rectangular, monophasic, 0.2-ms wave was applied for set 1, using a 30 Hz, 5 seconds on:15 seconds off timing cycle, for 12 contractions at maximally tolerated amperage. A 6 minute rest was provided, then set 2 was conducted at a 50 Hz, 10 seconds on:50 seconds off timing cycle, for 12 contractions. Those in the sensory-level transcutaneous electrical nerve stimulation (TENS) group (n = 14) received 100-Hz, biphasic rectangular waveform with 220-μs pulse duration, for 30-minute treatment sessions, with intensity set at a perception threshold. The subjects could feel the TENS, but no muscle contraction was elicited. Subjects' quadriceps and hamstring torque was tested at 6 weeks, 12 weeks, and 1 year after the start of treatment. No statistically significant difference was found between the three treatment groups. The authors proposed that

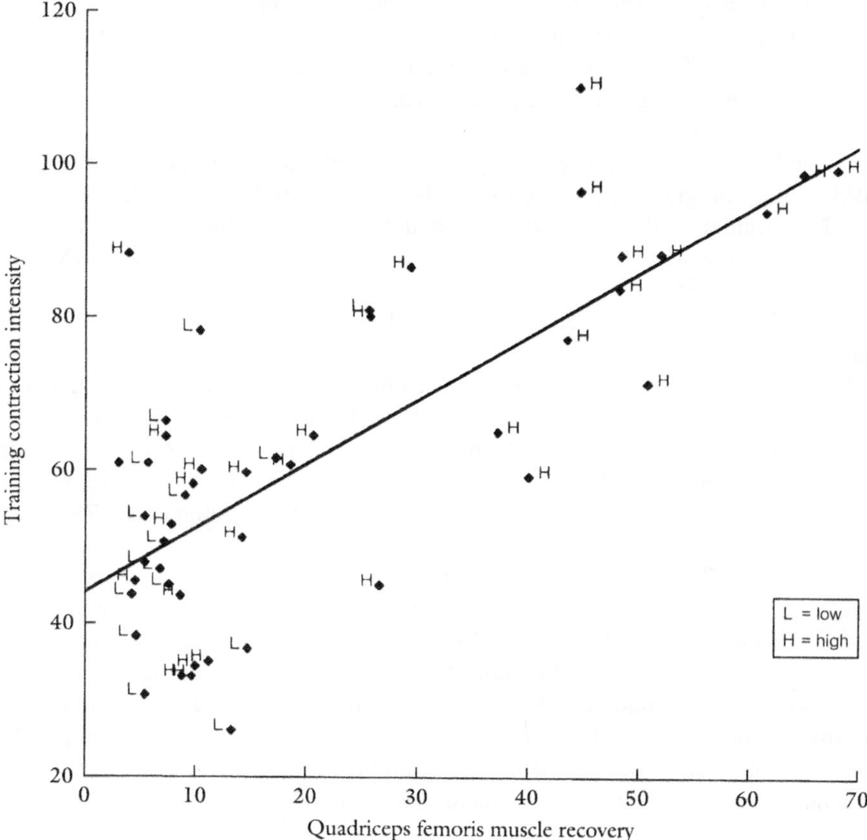

Figure 6.8. Training contraction intensity (electrically induced quadriceps force) versus quadriceps femoris muscle torque expressed as a percentage of the maximal voluntary isometric contraction of the uninvolved quadriceps.

their stimulation protocol and their exercise protocol were less aggressive than has been reported in other studies (36,53,70).

The results of Laufer et al. (71) and Lyons et al. (72) show that portable stimulators may be able to produce output of similar torque-generating power as clinical stimulators using the current generation of portable stimulators. This conflicts with earlier work of Snyder-Mackler (32). New advances in technology are making portable, battery-operated stimulators a more appropriate option in NMES applications for muscle strengthening.

EFFECT OF NEUROMUSCULAR ELECTRICAL STIMULATION FOR STRENGTHENING ON MUSCLE ENDURANCE AND FATIGUE

Few studies have been performed to date to investigate the effects of NMES training on the ability of muscle to sustain force over time with either repeated or sustained voluntary contractions. Alon et al. (49) found that abdominal musculature stimulation training designed to enhance muscle strength did not significantly influence the endurance characteristics of these muscles.

Hartsell (74) examined the effect of NMES training on the volitional endurance characteristics of the quadriceps in normal subjects. NMES training consisted of 10 daily MTCs (10-second contraction with 50 seconds rest each), 5 days per week for 6 weeks. Square waves with a pulse duration of 2 ms were applied at a frequency of 65 pps. Quadriceps endurance increased after the stimulation program, but the small increases were not significantly greater than those achieved through exercise alone. This finding is not surprising, in that the NMES training program used was based on volitional strength training programs and not on any feature analogous to voluntary endurance training programs.

One of the key problems in determining the effects of NMES on muscle fatigue is the fact that NMES training programs examined to date have been based on volitional strength training programs. No clinical studies are available that have applied the principles of volitional endurance training (low-amplitude contractions, high number of repetitions) to NMES training for improving muscle endurance.

That NMES can induce muscle fatigue is well known. The precise relationship between fatigue and stimulated contraction duration and rest has not been clearly established for most muscles. Packman-Braun (75) performed a study examining the effects of 1:2, 1:4, and 1:6 (timing cycles of 5 seconds on:5 seconds off, 5 seconds on:15 seconds off, 5 seconds on:25 seconds off, respectively) duty cycles on the development of fatigue in the wrist extensor musculature of hemiparetic patients. She found that 1:2, 1:4, and 1:6 timing cycles were progressively less fatiguing. These findings are in general agreement with those of Benton et al. (76) presented in the early 1980s.

Binder-Macleod (77) demonstrated that both contraction force and frequency directly affect fatigue, but their effects are independent of one another. To achieve the high force levels necessary for strengthening, frequencies higher than critical fusion frequency (tetany) are required. The higher the frequency, the more fatiguing the contraction. High contraction intensities also provoke fatigue. The manipulation of these variables to minimize fatigue is critical for functional electrical stimulation. The use of electrical stimulation to augment muscle strength, however, allows for much more flexibility in manipulating on:off times to minimize fatigue while using high frequencies and contractile forces to maximize strength gains.

EFFECTIVENESS OF ELECTRICAL STIMULATION IN RESTORING STRENGTH TO DENERVATED MUSCLES

Denervation of skeletal muscle, the disruption of peripheral motor nerve supply to the muscle, results in lost volitional control and produces profound structural and physiologic changes (78). Treatment of denervated muscle with electrical stimulation is controversial. The variety of stimulation characteristics used, targeted musculature in humans, and treatment protocols has made comparison difficult.

Researchers in this area have hypothesized that these morphological and functional changes in denervated muscle result from the inactivity of involved muscles, the loss of the influence of neurotrophic substances provided by the nerve fibers that normally innervate the muscle, or some combination of these two factors (Table 6.4). Because many believe that the degenerative changes in denervated muscle result from cessation of the normal patterns of muscle use, *electrical muscle stimulation* (EMS) to the denervated muscle in an effort to increase muscle activity has been examined in laboratory and clinical studies.

In 1841, Reid (79) first suggested that electrical stimulation of denervated muscle could offset the structural changes that accompany loss of motor innervation. Since that time, interest in and support of this therapeutic procedure has waxed and waned. Gutmann's text (80) on the use of EMS for denervated muscles provides a review and synthesis of the experimental findings through the 1950s. For every report that suggests that EMS prevents or retards the effects of denervation (80–92), another can be found that indicates that EMS is either ineffective (91,92) or, in fact, detrimental (93–96) to the maintenance or recovery of denervated muscle.

Table 6.4. Morphological and Physiological Changes in Denervated Skeletal Muscle

Muscle atrophy (red > pale muscle atrophy)
Decrease in muscle weight
Decrease in muscle contractile protein (myofibril)
Decrease in muscle sarcoplasm
Decrease in number of muscle fibers
Replacement of muscle by fibrous and adipose tissue
Changes in muscle excitability
Oscillations in resting membrane potential
Fibrillation potentials
Dispersion of acetylcholine receptors
Increase in chronaxie and rheobase

After a nerve has been severed, both the proximal and distal sections undergo changes. The distal portion shows degeneration of axon terminals and degradation of the axon and the myelin sheath of the nerve (*Wallerian degeneration*). With regeneration, growth cones form at the axonal tips and send out sprouts. These sprouts play a role in pathfinding and target recognition. Elongation of the axon proceeds by forward movement of the sprouts. If contact is made with a denervated muscle fiber, synaptogenesis begins, followed by recovery of muscle function. The rate of regeneration slows with distance from the motor nerve cell body, at approximately 1 to 2 mm per day. Studies have shown that electrical stimulation can reduce or inhibit sprouting (97,98).

Generally, EMS should be used if there is a likelihood of reinnervation. However, it can take months for a denervated muscle to re-establish innervation with a motor axon. Given the slow growth rate, it can take a year or more for a muscle to reinnervate if it is far from the lesion site (78). The optimal time to start stimulation is soon after the onset of denervation. A study in rats began stimulation 1 day after nerve section and prevented atrophy (99). Studies that began EMS at much later time frames have also been effective (82,88,100).

Reviews of the literature indicate that the controversy over the efficacy of EMS persists (101,102). Evidence from animal studies indicates that EMS of denervated muscles can preserve or restore properties of the muscles. Direct current was the conventional treatment for EMS; however, it has been recently replaced by alternating current. Use of direct current has declined after controversy over the effects on nerve growth and muscle reinnervation (78), and over the lack of therapeutic benefits (82). There are few studies of the use of EMS as a rehabilitation tool (82,84,88,89,100,103,104), and they have studied different musculature and therefore used different parameters (Table 6.5) to achieve their goal.

Stimulation protocols that retard the effects of denervation appear to have several features in common. Important considerations for obtaining positive therapeutic results with EMS include:

1. Use of supramaximal stimulus intensities: all of the denervated muscle fibers must be activated. EMS may be less successful in larger muscles because the stimulation intensities required to activate all muscle fibers may not be tolerated by the patient. Some authors (95) believe that stimulation of all muscle fibers can be attained only by use of implanted electrodes.
2. Isometric contraction in response to stimulation: isotonic contraction of denervated muscle during stimulation sessions has not been shown to be effective.
3. Initiation of sessions of stimulation as soon as possible after denervation, but not so soon as to inhibit axonal sprouting.

Table 6.5. Electrical Stimulation of Denervated Muscles: Comparison of Parameters

Study	Denervated Muscle(s)	Parameters	Outcome Measures
Schmitt et al.	Flexor pollicus longus	AC 1.5 KHz 75 bps sine wave	Muscle force production
Woodcock et al.	Variety of muscles	Range reported in the study: 0.05–200 Hz range 40 μs-16s PD	None reported
Kern et al.	Quadriceps femoris	AC 20 Hz 40 ms pulses	Cross sectional area, muscle force production
Valecic et al.	Tibialis anterior	20 ms square waves at 25 Hz for 20 minutes, 2x day 5 days/wk	Active dorsiflexion range of motion
Boonstra et al.	Variety of muscles	1 KHz square wave to elicit twitch contraction	
Modlin et al.	Quadriceps femoris`	AC 2 Hz 5 s on:2 s off duty	Cross sectional area, biopsies, muscle force production

4. Use of bipolar electrode placement: higher-magnitude evoked contractions have been obtained with this technique than with placement of one electrode of the stimulation circuit over the denervated muscle. A potential disadvantage of bipolar placement may be spread of current to adjacent innervated muscle or sensory structures, causing pain or discomfort.
5. Biphasic current pulses with long pulse-durations: the stimulation patterns now believed to be most optimal are those that resemble the normal activity of the motor neuron (78).

Optimal values for other important parameters of EMS protocols have not been established. Researchers do not agree about the most effective EMS parameters, how often to receive EMS, or total time to receive EMS. The efficacy of the stimulation depends on the stimulus parameters. Because the mechanism by which stimulation affects the course of denervation atrophy is not known, choice of parameters varies. Research in EMS to date has not clearly established optimal values for numerous treatment parameters, including:

1. Number of contractions in a single stimulation session.
2. Number of stimulation sessions per day or week.
3. Frequency of stimulation (pps or Hz).
4. On time:off time of stimulation in denervation training.

In spite of numerous studies, electrical stimulation of denervated muscle in humans is an area of electrotherapy where fundamental questions remain unresolved. EMS can be effective in preserving or restoring muscle strength in denervated muscles. Studies have shown that the best results are obtained if the stimulation pattern is similar to the activity of a normal motor neuron. The optimum time to start EMS is as soon as possible following injury; however, initiation of EMS months after injury will likely reverse the degenerative process as well. EMS does not hinder axon regeneration or muscle reinnervation. However, much of the work on EMS has been done in animal studies, and questions remain as to the appropriate stimulation parameters for use in humans.

CONCLUSIONS ABOUT THE USE OF NEUROMUSCULAR ELECTRICAL STIMULATION FOR STRENGTHENING

The basic question in the muscle stimulation literature is how does NMES of muscle compare to voluntary exercise or voluntary exercise in combination with NMES in the ability to alter muscle performance? After reviewing the literature on the use of NMES in healthy subjects with no apparent muscle weakness, and in subjects with muscle weakness, the following conclusions can be drawn:

1. Increase in strength usually occurs in the NMES group compared to a control group that does not receive NMES.
2. NMES has been found to be more effective than volitional exercise alone in strengthening the quadriceps muscles and in patients with knee injury, such as ACL rupture. The reason for this is that all muscle fibers are recruited with the external stimulus of NMES, whereas with volitional activation, not all muscle fibers are recruited.
3. Activation of <95% of the quadriceps femoris muscle fibers is an indicator of voluntary activation failure, commonly seen with knee injury. Burst superimposition provides information as to whether weakness is attributable to atrophy or incomplete activation.
4. In healthy individuals, no added benefit is attributed to simultaneous NMES and voluntary exercise over either alone.
5. In healthy individuals, electrically-elicited contractions of the quadriceps femoris muscle in the range of 80% to 100% of MVIT are possible; in some cases those in excess of 100% MVIT are also possible.
6. Evidence exists that certain muscle stimulation regimens produce greater strength gains than voluntary exercise in studies of patient populations with demonstrable weakness.
7. A positive correlation exists between training contraction intensity and strength gains in people with muscle weakness. This indicates that NMES for strengthening should be performed using the highest possible NMES-evoked contraction.
8. A positive correlation exists between phase charge and torque-generating capability in patients. The phase charge can be altered in an effort to generate as high of a force output as possible when using NMES for strengthening.
9. NMES activates motor units a subject is not able to activate volitionally, thus improving muscle activation and strength.
10. The focus of NMES research is primarily on the quadriceps femoris muscles. Evidence for strengthening effects of NMES in other muscle groups is minimal. However, application procedures used on the quadriceps femoris can likely be used in an analogous fashion on other muscles.

METHODOLOGICAL CONCERNS WITH STUDIES OF NEUROMUSCULAR ELECTRICAL STIMULATION FOR STRENGTHENING

Caution should be exercised in reading and interpreting studies comparing NMES and voluntary exercise for strengthening. Many studies lack sophistication in design, data sampling, analysis, and/or documentation. Some major flaws to be aware of when reviewing articles on NMES for strengthening include:

1. Use of change scores: pre- minus post-measurements (change scores) may lack reliability (105).
2. Failure to accurately describe methods: many studies do not completely report important experimental details, such as training parameters and current characteristics.

3. Inappropriate statistical analysis: use of multiple t-tests within one study without appropriate adjustment in the α-level. For example, one of the studies reviewed above used up to 20 independent t-tests. With an α-level of 0.05, 1 of the 20 t-tests will be significant by chance alone.
4. Generalizability of results: improvements in functional status cannot be inferred from improvements in isometric or isokinetic strength.
5. Specificity of results: results in one population cannot be extended to another group (e.g., healthy subjects vs. patients, young vs. old). In addition, results obtained from NMES experimentation on one muscle (e.g., quadriceps femoris) may not be valid for other muscles.

The results of a study exhibiting any of these flaws should not be automatically dismissed. Clinical research is difficult to perform without breaking some methodological rules. An awareness of possible methodological shortcomings should facilitate more discriminating review.

CLINICAL GUIDELINES FOR NEUROMUSCULAR ELECTRICAL STIMULATION FOR STRENGTHENING

A review of the literature concerning NMES strengthening and torque generation yields a number of general guidelines for clinical applications (Table 6.5). NMES strengthening procedures are based on several analogous volitional exercise programs for strengthening. In voluntary exercise programs, tetanic muscle contractions are produced at a relatively high percentage of the maximum voluntary torque levels (overload principle). In NMES for strengthening, stimulated contractions should be tetanic and at the highest tolerated torque level. The peak contraction torque ranges used for the quadriceps commonly exceed 60% of MVIT. Maximum torque levels for other lower extremity musculature may be comparable, and maximum torque levels for upper extremity and trunk musculature remain to be established.

Snyder-Mackler et al. have demonstrated a threshold contraction intensity for quadriceps strengthening (32). Although thresholds have not been described for other muscles, it is essential that the clinician consider two factors related to this when choosing a stimulator. The stimulator must be able to cause a contraction of sufficient intensity to strengthen the muscle. This necessitates measurement of electrically-elicited contraction intensity, not current amplitude or pulse charge. Additionally, the stimulator must have sufficient reserve current amplitude to continue to present a training stimulus to the muscle as it gets stronger.

Recommended Stimulator Features and Controls

A stimulator for NMES for strengthening should be designed to allow a high degree of freedom in adjusting current characteristics. Preset parameters or programs for stimulation may be somewhat limiting and do not allow the adjustment of current characteristics for each individual. A stimulator with considerable flexibility may be a better investment in the long run as more is learned about optimal stimulation characteristics for strengthening. Flexibility in stimulus adjustment places additional responsibilities on users who need to know the consequences of changing each stimulator setting to provide safe and effective treatment. Recommendations on the design and performance characteristics of stimulators intended for NMES applications are available from the Association for the Advancement of Medical Instrumentation (AAMI).

Output Channels and Amplitude Controls

A stimulator for NMES applications generally has at least two channels for stimulation. In a stimulator with two or more channels, controls are often provided to set either simultaneous stimulation from two channels, or alternating stimulation with both channels active at the same time. This is important, for example, during synchronous activation of two synergistic muscle groups to produce two-joint movement, or synchronous activation of two antagonistic muscle groups (co-contraction) to minimize joint movement by producing an isometric contraction. In contrast, alternating or reciprocal stimulation between channels is useful in providing alternating patterns of active movement (e.g., flexion followed by extension) across a joint.

Each channel on NMES devices should have independent amplitude controls. Controls should also be present to adjust stimulus pulse or phase duration, frequency of stimulation, ramp modulations, and on time:off time. Analog design of amplitude controls allows the user to carefully adjust stimulation to evoke maximal contraction.

Pulse Amplitude and Pulse/Phase Duration Controls

The pulse amplitude control and the phase (or pulse) duration control regulate the charge of each pulse and so determine the number of peripheral nerve fibers recruited with each stimulus. Analog amplitude controls, those that allow continuous amplitude adjustment over the available range, are preferable to incremental amplitude controls for NMES applications. Analog amplitude controls allow the user to make very small adjustments and thus provide fine control over the level of evoked muscle contraction.

Phase duration or pulse duration controls may or may not be provided on commercially available stimulators designed for NMES applications. Optimal pulse durations for NMES have not been definitively established. Investigators have suggested that the optimal pulse duration likely lies between 50 and 1,000 μs. Because the question of optimal pulse duration is unresolved, the contemporary "ideal" stimulator should provide pulse duration control in the 20- to 1,000-μs range. Each output channel of NMES units should have channel output indicators that allow the user to know when stimulation is being applied through the channel.

Frequency Controls

Continuous adjustment of rate from 1 pulse (or burst) per second to about 80 to 100 pps allows a user to closely regulate the rate at which muscle is activated. Smooth tetanic muscular contractions will be ensured in normally-activated muscle when the stimulation frequency is set at more than 50 pps. Stimulation at this frequency is rapid enough to elicit smooth contraction in even the most rapidly contracting motor units. Although 50-pps stimulation ensures a smooth tetanic contraction, some clinicians use stimulation at lower frequencies (e.g., 30 to 35 pps) and have reported positive results.

Theoretically, as the frequency of stimulation is increased, the opposition to current flow (impedance) by the tissue falls. This has led to the development of stimulators using bursts of stimulation with carrier frequencies in the 2,000- to 4,000-Hz range. Such devices were expected to be able to produce higher levels of muscle contraction with less patient discomfort than more traditionally available stimulators producing 1 to 100 pps stimulation. To date, experimental findings have not substantiated claims that 2,000 to 4,000-Hz burst-modulated (e.g., 50 bps) AC is superior to low-frequency (e.g., 50 pps) pulses in NMES applications.

On Time:Off Time Controls

On time:off time controls of NMES stimulators are necessary because continuous or uninterrupted stimulated skeletal muscle contraction leads to very rapid muscle fatigue or force failure. On times of muscle stimulation for many applications are usually set to 10 or 15 seconds. Off times are generally adjustable up to about 1 or 2, minutes and have been most thoroughly examined at about 60 seconds.

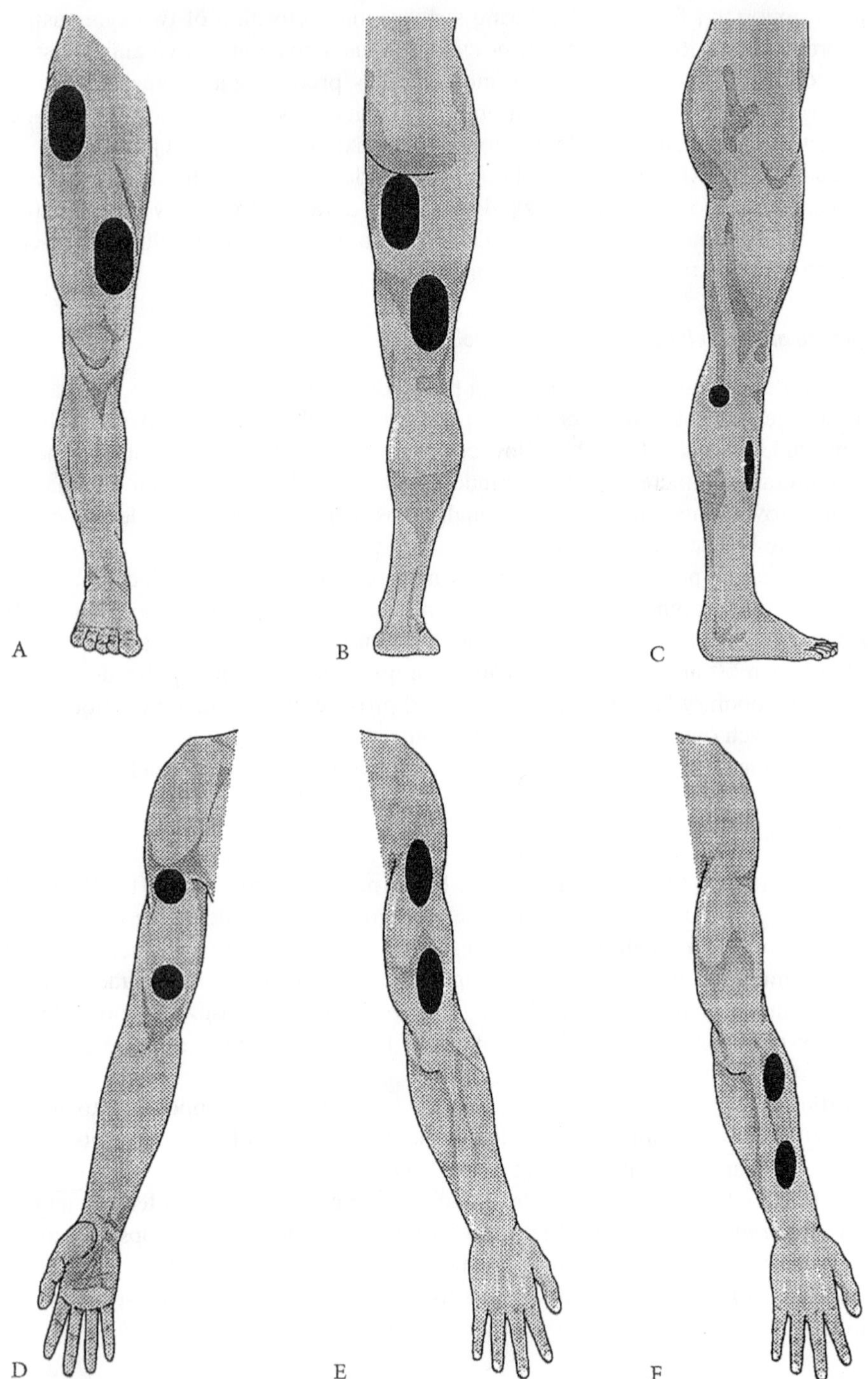

Figure 6.9. Common electrode placement sites for NMES of the quadriceps **(A),** the hamstrings **(B),** the tibialis anterior and peroneals **(C),** the biceps brachii **(D),** triceps brachii **(E),** wrist extensors **(F),** and lower back extensors **(G).**

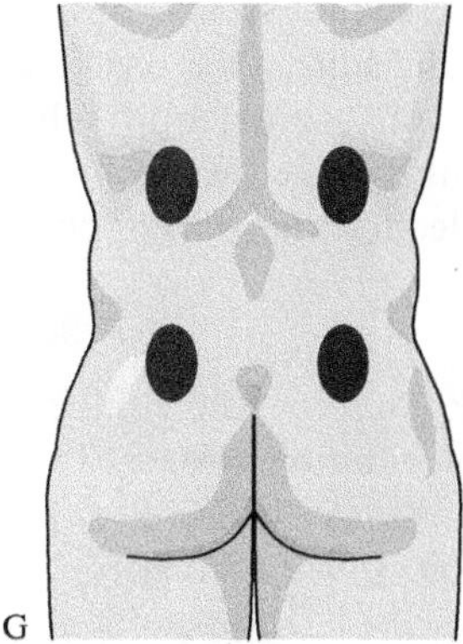

Figure 6.9. *Continued.*

Ramp Modulation Controls

Ramp modulation controls are included in neuromuscular electrical stimulators so that the phase or pulse charge of each stimulus can be gradually increased or decreased over 2 to 3 seconds. The gradual rise in stimulus charge over several seconds allows the gradual recruitment of nerve fibers and a more comfortable initiation of contraction for the subject. This type of modulation also allows more effective use of NMES in neurologically impaired patients. A declining ramp at the end of a contraction allows a smooth, gradual drop in the force produced by muscle.

Treatment Duration Controls

A treatment duration timer is usually included in NMES devices to provide control of the total duration of stimulation and automatic shutoff of the unit at the desired time. In general, treatment durations are adjustable up to 60 minutes. Many stimulators have a safety switch that can be used by the patient to shut off the stimulation if it becomes uncomfortable. Such safety switches override the treatment timer.

To achieve tetanic contractions, pulsatile or burst-modulated alternating currents are the most common forms of current successfully used at frequencies ranging from 30 to 80 pulses or bursts per second. Lower stimulation frequencies may not provide smooth tetanic contraction in all muscles. Stimulators must provide a range of available on and off times to mitigate the effects of fatigue.

Electrode Considerations

The selection and application of electrodes may influence the level of contraction evoked in response to NMES. Electrode sizes should suit the muscles to be activated. If electrodes are too large, current may spread to antagonistic muscle groups. If electrodes are too small, current density may be so high that subject tolerance is exceeded before sufficient levels of contraction are reached for strengthening. No available evidence suggests that one type of commercially available electrode or coupling agent is superior to others for strengthening applications.

Proper electrode placement is of paramount importance in NMES. Illustrations of common electrode placements are shown in Figure 6.9. In general, both electrodes from a single stimulator circuit are placed over the muscles to be activated. In some cases, four electrodes from two separate stimulator channels may be required to produce contraction levels sufficient to strengthen muscle. Commonly, motor points of the muscle to be activated are first located. The focus of NMES for strengthening is the quadriceps femoris muscle. Electrode placement on the quadriceps femoris (Fig. 6.9A) is proximally over the vastus lateralis and distally over the vastus medialis muscle bellies (53). The clinician should position electrodes over the belly of the muscle to be strengthened and carefully adjust their position as motor threshold level stimulation is applied to determine the site of optimal stimulation. When electrode position has been established, all electrodes should be firmly secured with elastic wraps to ensure uniform electrical contact with the skin and minimal electrode movement during stimulation.

Application Principles

Before beginning the first stimulation session, the clinician should explain clearly what sensations patients are likely to experience during NMES. The patient should experience a strong muscle contraction, with the electrical sensation between the two electrodes. The patient should not feel a single pin-prick sensation. If the patient reports this type of sensation, electrode integrity and contact should be evaluated. The patient should also be provided with a cutoff safety switch to stop stimulation if tolerance is exceeded. In addition, firm and proper patient stabilization should be provided. Minimal motion should occur in body segments proximal and distal to the region stimulated and in the joint influenced by the stimulated contraction. Many commercially available dynamometers and their attachments afford excellent positioning and stabilization for NMES applications.

Once the majority of stimulation parameters have been selected, the electrodes secured, and the subject stabilized, the initial stimulation session begins. The objective for muscle strengthening applications is to achieve the maximum tolerable level of muscle contraction. As treatment is initiated, the amplitude of stimulation should be increased gradually until motor threshold is reached and exceeded. In the first stimulation session, the amplitude of stimulation should be increased from contraction to contraction according to the patient's tolerance.

During early treatment sessions, some patients will not tolerate stimulation at amplitudes sufficient to produce muscle strengthening. In such patients, a 5- to 7-day program of stimulation designed to increase tolerance should be implemented. In these sessions, low amplitudes of stimulation are administered to produce threshold (just visible) contraction for periods of less than 10 seconds. This allows the patient to adapt to the feeling of the electrical current. After a rest period of 10 to 20 seconds, another 10-second contraction is attempted at a higher stimulus amplitude. In this fashion, the current amplitude is slowly increased until the desired level of contraction is obtained. Throughout this process, the ongoing encouragement and reassurance of the clinician is essential to achieve levels of stimulation sufficient to produce muscle strengthening. If adequate torque levels are not produced in response to NMES using a particular set of current parameters, other combinations of stimulation parameters can be tried by the clinician in attempts to improve the torque response to NMES.

PRECAUTIONS AND CONTRAINDICATIONS FOR NEUROMUSCULAR ELECTRICAL STIMULATION

The precautions for use of NMES for strengthening and endurance training include the following:

1. In hypertensive or hypotensive patients, autonomic responses to NMES may adversely affect control of blood pressure. With careful patient monitoring during the procedure, NMES can be used for strengthening. However, if the hypertension levels are not being controlled medically or monitored regularly by a physician, NMES should not be used.
2. In areas of excessive adipose tissue, as in obese patients, levels of stimulation required to activate muscle may produce adverse autonomic reactions. With careful patient monitoring during the procedure, NMES can be used for strengthening. The goal of an isometric contraction ≥60% of MVIC may not be safely achievable.

The contraindications for NMES strengthening and endurance training include the following:

1. Over the thoracic region NMES current may interfere with the function of vital internal organs, including the heart.
2. In the thoracic region of patients with demand cardiac pacemakers NMES current may interfere with pacemaker activity and may lead to asystole or ventricular fibrillation.
3. In regions of phrenic nerve or urinary bladder stimulators NMES current may interfere with the normal operation of these devices.
4. Over the carotid bodies NMES current may interfere with the normal regulation of blood pressure and cardiac contractility and may produce bradycardia or cardiac arrhythmia.
5. In areas of peripheral vascular disorders, such as venous thrombosis or thrombophlebitis, NMES may increase the risk of releasing emboli.
6. In regions of neoplasm or infection the effects of NMES on muscles and circulation may aggravate these conditions.
7. On the trunk of pregnant females there is a risk of NMES inducing uterine contractions that may influence the developing fetus. However, if the patient requires strengthening of distal limb musculature, being pregnant is a precaution, as long as the site receiving NMES is not over or adjacent to the fetus. NMES to the multifidi of the lumbar spine is a contraindication, but NMES to the wrist flexors, for example, is not a contraindication.
8. In close proximity to diathermy devices there is a potential for loss of control of NMES stimulation parameters.
9. In patients who are unable to provide clear feedback regarding the level of stimulation, such as infants, senile subjects, or individuals with mental disorders, NMES should not be used.
10. Electrodes should never be placed over the eyes.
11. In patients with skin injury, such as cuts or scratches, or frail skin that will break open easily, NMES should not be used, as a burn may result.

Careful observation by the clinician is required in all applications of electrical stimulation. Detrimental responses to stimulation often occur rapidly and require quick reaction to avoid serious injury. Patients should not be allowed to use NMES independently until the clinician is confident that they have been trained adequately in the safe use of the device and are aware of the signs and symptoms of adverse reactions.

Patients That May not be Appropriate for Neuromuscular Electrical Stimulation for Strengthening

Patients who are not able to provide clear feedback regarding the intensity and the sensation of electrical stimulation, such as infants, senile patients, or patients unable to follow commands or understand the process should not be subjected to NMES. Patients that are extremely obese should not receive NMES, as the intensity needed to elicit a muscle contraction through the excessive soft tissue may result in a skin burn. A woman who is pregnant should not receive NMES for strengthening in the vicinity of the fetus; however, NMES can be done at a distal location.

Conditions in the Area of Proposed Neuromuscular Electrical Stimulation That Preclude its Use

NMES should not be used over the site of a skin injury, such as cuts or scratches, or frail skin that will break open easily. NMES should not be used in areas of peripheral vascular disorders, such as venous thrombosis or thrombophlebitis, because of the risk of releasing emboli. NMES should not be used in regions of neoplasm or infection, because muscular and circulatory effects may aggravate these conditions.

Adverse Reactions to Neuromuscular Electrical Stimulation for Strengthening

SKIN BURNS

Skin burns may occur occasionally in NMES applications. The cause of skin burns may be related to faulty electrodes or nonuniform contact of electrodes during treatment. To reduce the potential for burns, disposable electrodes should be frequently replaced. Reusable electrodes (e.g., carbon rubber) should also be periodically replaced. Often the first indication of faulty electrodes is the perception on the part of the patient of a small area of intense and/or uncomfortable stimulation beneath the electrodes. As stated above, NMES for strengthening should not be done if the skin in the area of desired electrode placement is frail or broken. A local area of skin damage has a lower resistance to current, and the current will preferentially flow through this path of least resistance. Concentration of current in an area of low resistance may result in skin burn.

AUTONOMIC DYSREFLEXIA

Autonomic dysreflexia is characterized by an abrupt onset of excessively high blood pressure, increased spasticity, bradycardia, and often profuse sweating, caused by an uncontrolled sympathetic nervous system. It is most often seen in patients with spinal cord injuries, with injury levels above the sixth thoracic vertebrae. It is potentially life threatening and considered a medical emergency. A noxious stimulus below the level of the lesion can precipitate this syndrome. For more information on the use of electrical stimulation in patients with spinal cord injuries, see Chapter 7.

CLINICAL CASE STUDIES

The following case studies serve as examples of the ways NMES can be used to strengthen muscle. The electrotherapeutic treatment plan is described in detail, but additional treatment is only outlined.

Case 1

A 24-year-old female is referred to physical therapy 1 week after surgery for reconstruction of her left anterior cruciate ligament.

Examination

The patient is wearing a postoperative knee orthosis on the left and ambulates with the orthotic locked in full extension. Examination of the knee reveals no overt signs of inflammation and well-healed surgical incisions. Left thigh girth is 6 cm less than the right. Comparison of MVIT of left and right knee extensors and flexors shows significant weakness on the left using a burst superimposition technique.

Assessment

Well-healed postsurgical knee with demonstrable atrophy and weakness as compared to contralateral extremity.

Plan

Therapy will include volitional isometric exercise and NMES to augment strength of the thigh musculature by either co-contraction of both hamstrings and quadriceps, monitoring knee-extension torque, or NMES of the quadriceps with the patient stabilized in knee flexion greater than 45 degrees.

Detailed Electrotherapeutic Plan

Mode of stimulation: cycled NMES

Type of stimulator: clinical (line powered)

Electrodes and electrode placements: two equal-sized electrodes placed on the quadriceps (Figure 6.9A); knee extension must be blocked at 45 to 65 degrees.

Duration and frequency of treatment: three times per week, 10 contractions at >60% MVIC per session. Current amplitude is increased with each contraction to maximally tolerated contraction magnitude >60% of the quadriceps femoris MVIC.

Rationale

It is generally recognized that ligament protection must be observed by the clinician while exercising or electrically stimulating the quadriceps femoris muscle in patients with ACL pathology. Forceful knee extension through the range from 45 degrees of flexion to full extension may be accompanied by anterior translational forces that are deleterious to the reconstructed ACL and secondary supportive structures of the knee. The clinician can safely stimulate the quadriceps femoris in the way listed above. NMES can be used at any time during the rehabilitation phase after ACL surgery, but it is superior to voluntary exercise in increasing isometric strength of knee extensors. Electrode placement is designed to minimize compressive forces on the patellofemoral joint and decrease the likelihood of other lower extremity musculature being stimulated simultaneously.

A clinical stimulator is recommended because portable stimulators have not been shown to be effective for this type of NMES. The effectiveness of the program should be assessed weekly. Isometric knee extension and flexion torques should be measured, before stimulation, with the knee in 60 degrees of flexion.

Case 2

A 45-year-old man with a recent history of lumbar instability and pain in the right leg is referred for physical therapy.

Examination

Examination reveals a slight loss of the lumbar lordosis and no lateral shift. Movement tests into extension and right pelvic translocation produce centralization of the patient's symptoms; flexion peripheralizes them. Returning from a flexed position, he uses his hands to climb up his thighs in order to extend. Sacroiliac torsion, compression, and distraction tests are negative. The Oswestry score is 45/100. The patient states that his symptoms are easily evoked with changes in position. Sometimes sitting evokes his leg pain and sometimes standing and walking. This is borne out over several days of examination and treatment when he presents with lateral shifts alternating from left to right.

Assessment

This patient has symptoms that are consistent with those in the immobilization principle category described by Delitto et al. (106).

Plan

1. Stabilization exercise to strengthen the multifidi muscles.
2. Brace immobilization.
3. NMES to strengthen the multifidi muscles.

Detailed Electrotherapeutic Plan

Patient positioning: patient is placed prone on a treatment table and stabilized across the pelvis with a belt. This is the exception to isometric contraction and measuring contraction force principles because of the difficulty in stabilizing the patient in a dynamometer to measure back-muscle strength.

Electrode placement: electrodes are placed as in Figure 6.9G, bilaterally over the area of the multifidus muscle.

Type of stimulator, burst frequency, on and off times: clinical NMES, burst-modulated 2500-Hz AC; burst frequency, 50 to 75 bps; on time, 10 seconds; off time, 50 seconds.

Muscle contraction force: to tolerance, but at least sufficient to cause an anterior pelvic tilt.

Treatment duration: 10 to 15 contractions per session; 2 to 3 times per week.

Rationale

Intermittent, high-force, electrically-elicited contractions have been shown to augment muscle strength. Use of small electrodes (2 × 2 inch square) over the deep back extensors should permit more isolated strengthening of these muscles.

SUMMARY

This chapter has reviewed the essential features of neuromuscular electrical stimulators, the clinical application of NMES to augment muscle strength, the stimulation parameters and techniques used in NMES, and precautions and contraindications for NMES applications. Advances in NMES applications and techniques are occurring at a faster pace than ever before. Clinicians using NMES and other electrical techniques should strive to stay abreast of new developments in the field. Active clinicians are encouraged to add to the knowledge base in NMES through the careful design and implementation of clinical research studies. Through the coordinated efforts of laboratory and clinical researchers, both the breadth and depth of understanding and applications will increase. The patients we serve will benefit most from these efforts.

SELF-STUDY QUESTIONS

For answers, see Appendix B.

1. Given a patient with weakened right knee extension secondary to prolonged cast immobilization and a neuromuscular stimulator that produces rectangular, symmetric, biphasic pulsed current, describe the parameters of stimulation and a training program that may strengthen knee extension.

   Stimulation characteristics:
   - Amplitude:
   - Pulse/phase duration:
   - Frequency of stimulation:
   - On:off times of stimulation:

   NMES training program characteristics:
   - Number of contractions per training session:
   - Number of training sessions per week:

2. What are the major adaptations in skeletal muscle in response to:
   (a) high-amplitude (>30% MVIC), low-repetition (10-15 contractions) daily NMES?
   (b) low-amplitude (<30% MVIC), high-repetition (5 sets of 10 contractions each) daily NMES?

3. One pattern of NMES, developed by the Soviet researcher Kots, has been extensively studied with respect to NMES for strengthening. Completely describe the parameters of stimulation developed by Kots and outline the training regimen he used to improve strength in elite athletes.
   - Carrier frequency:
   - Burst frequency:
   - On:off times of stimulation:

4. What range of stimulation frequencies is used for electrical stimulation to augment muscle strength?

5. Why are the frequencies in question 4 used, as opposed to higher or lower frequencies?

6. Lengthening the off cycle of NMES is a good strategy for decreasing _________ during NMES for strengthening.

7. How can NMES be used to test the strength and activation of a muscle?

8. What are the essential characteristics of an electrical stimulator used for NMES?

   Pulse duration:
   Frequency:
   Amplitude:

9. Electrically-elicited training contraction force is __________ to strength augmentation.

10. The phase charge is __________ electrically-elicited muscle contraction force.

11. Identify several sites where NMES should not be applied, and describe the rationale for each contraindication.

12. Describe the autonomic dysreflexia response that may occur in a patient with spinal cord injury.

13. Identify potential adverse effects of NMES.

14. Identify patient considerations that may preclude the use of NMES.

15. Burst superimposition testing can be used to identify what useful information in the development of patient rehabilitation program?

16. Why is volitional activation an important consideration in determining the true force-producing capabilities of the muscle?

17. A patient is receiving NMES for muscle strengthening, and they find the NMES intolerable. What parameter changes can be made to improve patient comfort?

18. Is a portable stimulator as effective as a clinical stimulator in producing adequate levels of torque for rehabilitation?

19. Given a patient with muscle denervation, what stimulation parameters should be used?

   Amplitude:
   Frequency:
   Pulse/phase duration:
   On:off times of stimulation:

20. Why are the stimulation parameters in question 19 effective in patients with muscle denervation?

21. What are the benefits of NMES for muscle denervation?

22. What is one way to prevent fatigue with NMES, while continuing to deliver adequate intensities of stimulation to the muscle?

23. List the precautions for use of NMES.

24. (a) In preparing a patient to receive NMES, what should they experience and what should they be told? (b) What should they not experience that would require modification?

25. What are some stimulator control features that should be considered in purchasing an NMES device?

REFERENCES

1. Ward AR, Shkuratova N. Russian electrical stimulation: the early experiments. *Phys Ther.* 2002;82:1019–1030.
2. Rose SJ, Rothstein JM. Muscle mutability. Part 1. General concepts and adaptations to altered patterns of use. *Phys Ther.* 1982;62:1751–1830.
3. Salmons SJ, Henriksson J. The adaptive response of skeletal muscle to increased use. *Muscle Nerve.* 1981;4(2):94–105.
4. Knuttgen HG, Kraemer KW. Terminology and measurement in exercise performance. *J Appl Sport Sci Res.* 1987;1:1–10.
5. Bigland-Ritchie B, Woods JJ. Changes in muscle contractile properties and neural control during human muscular fatigue. *Muscle Nerve.* 1984;7:691–699.
6. Vollstad NK, Segersted SO. Biochemical correlates of fatigue. A brief review. *Eur J Appl Physiol.* 1988;57:336–347.
7. Snyder-Mackler L, Binder-Macleod SA, Williams PR. Fatigability of human quadriceps femoris muscle following anterior cruciate ligament reconstruction. *Med Sci Sports Exerc.* 1993;25: 783–789.
8. Snyder-Mackler L, Deluca PF, Williams PR, et al. Reflex inhibition of the quadriceps femoris muscle after injury or reconstruction of the anterior cruciate ligament. *J Bone Joint Surg Am.* 1994;764:555–560.
9. Newham DJ, Hurley HM, Jones DJ. Ligamentous knee injury and muscle inhibition. *J Orthop Rheumatol.* 1989;2:163–173.
10. Jones DW, Jones DA, Newham DJ. Chronic knee effusion and aspiration: the effect on quadriceps inhibition. *Br J Rheumatol.* 1987;26:370–374.
11. Shih Y-F. *Can Burst Superinposition Predict Maximal Voluntary Force?* [Masters Thesys]. University of Pittsburgh; 1994.
12. Stackhouse SK, Dean JC, Lee SCK, et al. Measurement of central activation failure of the quadriceps femoris in healthy adults. *Muscle Nerve.* 2000;2311:1706–1712.
13. Stevens JE, Stackhouse SK, Binder-Macleod SA, et al. Are voluntary muscle activation deficits in older adults meaningful? *Muscle Nerve.* 2003;27:99–101.
14. Chmielewski TL, Stackhouse SK, Axe MJ, et al. A prospective analysis of incidence and severity of quadriceps inhibition in a consecutive sample of 100 patients with complete acute anterior cruciate ligament rupture. *J Orthop Res.* 2004;22:925–930.
15. Farquhar SJ, Chmielewski T, Snyder-Mackler L. Accuracy of predicting maximal quadriceps force from submaximal effort contractions after anterior cruciate ligament surgery. *Muscle Nerve,* 2005;32:500–505.
16. Urbach D, Awiszus F. Impaired ability of voluntary quadriceps activation bilaterally interferes with function testing after knee injuries. A twitch interpolation study. *Int J Sports Med.* 2002;23:231–236.
17. Konishi Y, Konishi H, Fukubayashi T. Gamma loop dysfunction in quadriceps on the contralateral side in patients with ruptured ACL. *Med Sci Sports Exerc.* 2003;35:897–900.
18. Lewek MD, Rudolph KS, Snyder-Mackler L. Quadriceps femoris muscle weakness and activation failure in patients with symptomatic knee osteoarthritis. *J Orthop Res.* 2004;22:110–115.
19. Stevens, JE, Mizner RL, Snyder-Mackler L. Quadriceps strength and volitional activation before and after total knee arthroplasty for osteoarthritis. *J Orthop Res.* 2003;21:775–779.
20. Yue GH, Ranganathan VK, Siemionow V, et al. Older adults exhibit a reduced ability to fully activate their biceps brachii muscle. *J Gerontol A Biol Sci Med Sci.* 1999;54:M249–253.
21. Binder-Macleod SA, Snyder-Mackler L. Muscle fatigue: clinical implications for fatigue assessment and neuromuscular electrical stimulation. *Phys Ther.* 1993;73:902–910.
22. McDonnell MK, Delitto A, Sinacore DR, et al. Electrically elicited fatigue test of the quadriceps femoris muscle. Description and reliability. *Phys Ther.* 1987;67:941–945.

23. Burke RE, Levine DN, Tsairis P, et al. Physiological types and histochemical profiles in motor units of the cat gastrocnemius. *J Physiol.* 1973;234:723–748.

24. Kramer J, Lindsay D, Magee D, et al. Comparison of voluntary and electrical stimulation contraction torques. *J Orthop Sports Phys Ther.* 1984;5:324–331.

25. Walmsley RP, Letts G, Vooys J. A comparison of torque generated by knee extension with a maximal voluntary muscle contraction vis-a-vis electrical stimulation. *J Orthop Sports Phys Ther.* 1984;6:10–17.

26. Snyder-Mackler L, Garrett M, Roberts M. A comparison of torque generating capabilities of three different electrical stimulating currents. *J Orthop Sports Phys Ther.* 1989;11:297–301.

27. Locicero R. The effect of electrical stimulation on isometric and isokinetic knee extension torque: interaction of the Kinestim electrical stimulator and the Cybex II+. *J Orthop Sports Phys Ther.* 1991;13:143–148.

28. Delitto A, Strube MJ, Shulman AD, et al. A study of discomfort with electrical stimulation. *Phys Ther.* 1992;72:410–421 [discussion, 421–424].

29. Delitto A, Brown M, Strube MJ, et al. Electrical stimulation of quadriceps femoris in an elite weight lifter: a single subject experiment. *Int J Sports Med.* 1989;10:187–191.

30. Enoka RM, Fuglevand AJ. Neuromuscular basis of the maximum force capacity of a muscle. In: Grabiner M, ed. *Current Issues in Biomechanics.* Champaign, IL: Human Kinetics;1993:215–235.

31. Enoka RM, Stuart DG. Neurobiology of muscle fatigue. *J Appl Physiol.* 1992;72:1637–1648.

32. Snyder-Mackler L, Delitto A, Stralka SW, et al. Use of electrical stimulation to enhance recovery of quadriceps femoris muscle force production in patients following anterior cruciate ligament reconstruction. *Phys Ther.* 1994;74:901–907.

33. Bowman BR, Baker LL. Effects of waveform parameters on comfort during transcutaneous neuromuscular electrical stimulation. *Ann Biomed Eng.* 1985;13:59–74.

34. Delitto A. Rose SJ. Comparative comfort of three waveforms used in electrically eliciting quadriceps femoris muscle contractions. *Phys Ther.* 1986;66:1704–1707.

35. Grimby G, Wigerstad-Lossing I. Comparison of high- and low-frequency muscle stimulators. *Arch Phys Med Rehabil.* 1989;70:835–838.

36. Currier DP, Ray JM, Nyland J. Effects of electrical and electromagnetic stimulation after anterior cruciate ligament reconstruction. *J Orthop Sports Phys Ther.* 1993;17:177–184.

37. Miller M, Downham D, Lexell J. Effects of superimposed electrical stimulation on perceived discomfort and torque increment size and variability. *Muscle Nerve.* 2003;27:90–98.

38. Massey BH, Nelson RC, Sharkey BC, et al. Effects of high frequency electrical stimulation on the size and strength of skeletal muscle. *J Sports Med Phys Fitness.* 1965;5:136–144.

39. Halbach JW, Strauss D. Comparison of electro-myo stimulation to isokinetic power of the knee extensor mechanism. *J Orthop Sports Phys Ther.* 1980;2:20–24.

40. Eriksson E, Haggmark T, Kiessling KH, et al. Effect of electrical stimulation on human skeletal muscle. *Int J Sports Med.* 1981;2:18–22.

41. Kots Y. 1977. [as referenced in Ward AR, Shkuratova N. Russian Electrical stimulation: the early experiments. *Phys Ther.* 2002;82:1019–1030]

42. Kramer JF, Mendryk SW. Electrical stimulation as a strength improvement technique: a review. *J Orthop Sports Phys Ther.* 1982;4:91–98.

43. Kramer JF, Semple JE. Comparison of selected strengthening techniques for normal quadriceps. *Physiother Can.* 1983;35:300–304.

44. Currier DP, Mann R. Muscular strength development by electrical stimulation in healthy individuals. *Phys Ther.* 1983;63:915–921.

45. Selkowitz DM. Improvement in isometric strength of the quadriceps femoris muscle after training with electrical stimulation. *Phys Ther.* 1985;65:186–196.

46. Mohr T, Carlson B, Sulentic C, et al. Comparison of isometric exercise and high volt galvanic stimulation on quadriceps femoris muscle strength. *Phys Ther.* 1985;65:606–612.

47. Stefanovska A. Vodovnik L. Change in muscle force following electrical stimulation. Dependence on stimulation waveform and frequency. *Scand J Rehabil Med.* 1985;17:141–146.

48. Wolf SL, Ariel GB, Saar D, et al. The effect of muscle stimulation during resistive training on performance parameters. *Am J Sports Med.* 1986;14:18–23.

49. Alon G, McCombe SA, Koutsantonis S, et al. Comparison of the effects of electrical stimulation and exercise on abdominal musculature. *J Orthop Sports Phys Ther.* 1987;8:567–573.

50. Delitto A, Rose SJ, McKowen JM, et al. Electrical stimulation versus voluntary exercise in strengthening thigh musculature after anterior cruciate ligament surgery. *Phys Ther.* 1988;68(5):660–663.

51. Godfrey CM, Jayawardena H, Quance TA, et al. Comparison of electrostimulation and isometric exercise in strengthening the quadriceps muscle. *Physiother Can.* 1979;31:265–267.

52. Gould N, Donnermeyer D, Gammon GG, et al. Transcutaneous muscle stimulation to retard disuse atrophy after open meniscectomy. *Clin Orthop.* 1983;178:190–197.

53. Snyder-Mackler L, Ladin Z, Schepsis AA, et al. Electrical stimulation of the thigh muscles after reconstruction of the anterior cruciate ligament. Effects of electrically elicited contraction of the quadriceps femoris and hamstring muscles on gait and on strength of the thigh muscles. *J Bone Joint Surg Am.* 1991; 73:1025–1036.

54. Eriksson E, Haggmark T. Comparison of isometric muscle training and electrical stimulation supplementing isometric muscle training in the recovery after major knee ligament surgery. A preliminary report. *Am J Sports Med.* 1979;7:169–71.

55. Sisk TD, Stralka SW, Deering MB, et al. Effect of electrical stimulation on quadriceps strength after reconstructive surgery of the anterior cruciate ligament. *Am J Sports Med.* 1987;15:215–220.

56. William JC, Street PM. Sequential faradism in quadriceps rehabilitation. *Physiotherapy.* 1976; 62:252–254.

57. Johnson DH, Thurston P, Ashcroft P. The Russian technique of faradism in the treatment of chondromalacia patellae. *Physiother Can.* 1977;29:169–171.

58. Morrissey MC, Brewster CE, Shields CL, Jr., et al. The effects of electrical stimulation on the quadriceps during postoperative knee immobilization. *Am J Sports Med.* 1985;13:40–45.

59. Singer KP, Gow PJ, Otway WF, et al. A comparison of electrical muscle stimulation isometric, isotonic, and isokinetic strength training programmes. *N Z J Sports Med.* 1983;11:61–63.

60. Delitto A, McKowen JM, McCarthy JA, et al. Electrically elicited co-contraction of thigh musculature after anterior cruciate ligament surgery. A description and single-case experiment. *Phys Ther.* 1988;68:45–50.

61. Snyder-Mackler L, Delitto A, Bailey SL, et al. Strength of the quadriceps femoris muscle and functional recovery after reconstruction of the anterior cruciate ligament. A prospective, randomized clinical trial of electrical stimulation. *J Bone Joint Surg Am.* 1995;77:1166–1173.

62. Lieber RL, Silva PD, Daniel DM. Equal effectiveness of electrical and volitional strength training for quadriceps femoris muscles after anterior cruciate ligament surgery. J Orthop Res. 1996; 14:131–138.

63. Lamb SE, Oldham JA, Morse RE, et al. Neuromuscular stimulation of the quadriceps muscle after hip fracture: a randomized controlled trial. *Arch Phys Med Rehabil.* 2002;83:1087–1092.

64. Karmel-Ross K, Cooperman DR, Van Doren CL. The effect of electrical stimulation on quadriceps femoris muscle torque in children with spina bifida. *Phys Ther.* 1992;72:723–730.

65. Starring DT, Gossman MR, Nicholson GG, Jr., et al. Comparison of cyclic and sustained passive stretching using a mechanical device to increase resting length of hamstring muscles. *Phys Ther.* 1988;68:314–320.

66. Kahanovitz N, Nordin M, Verderame R, et al. Normal trunk muscle strength and endurance in women and the effect of exercises and electrical stimulation. Part 2: Comparative analysis of electrical stimulation and exercises to increase trunk muscle strength and endurance. *Spine.* 1987;12:112–118.

67. Fehlings DL, Kirsch S, McComas A, et al. Evaluation of therapeutic electrical stimulation to improve muscle strength and function in children with types II/III spinal muscular atrophy. *Dev Med Child Neurol.* 2002; 44:741–744.

68. Neder JA, Sword D, Ward SA, et al. Home based neuromuscular electrical stimulation as a new rehabilitative strategy for severely disabled patients with chronic obstructive pulmonary disease (COPD). *Thorax.* 2002; 57:333–337.

69. Draper V. Ballard L. Electrical stimulation versus electromyographic biofeedback in the recovery of quadriceps femoris muscle function following anterior cruciate ligament surgery. *Phys Ther.* 1991;71:455–461 [discussion, 461–464].

70. Wigerstad-Lossing I, Grimby G, Jonsson T, et al. Effects of electrical muscle stimulation combined with voluntary contractions after knee ligament surgery. *Med Sci Sports Exerc.* 1988;20:93–98.

71. Laufer Y, Ries JD, Leininger DM, et al. Quadriceps femoris muscle torques and fatigue generated by neuromuscular electrical stimulation with three different waveforms. *Phys Ther.* 2001;81:1307–1316.

72. Lyons CL, Robb JB, Irrgang JJ, et al. Differences in quadriceps femoris muscle torque when using a clinical electrical stimulator versus a portable electrical stimulator. *Phys Ther.* 2005;85:44–51.

73. Paternostro-Sluga T, Fialka C, Alacamliogliu Y, et al. Neuromuscular electrical stimulation after anterior cruciate ligament surgery. *Clin Orthop.* 1999;368:166–75.

74. Hartsell WF, Sarin P, Recine DC, et al. Long-term results of curative irradiation in pathologically staged IA and IIA Hodgkin disease. *Radiology.* 1993;186:565–568.

75. Packman-Braun R. Relationship between functional electrical stimulation duty cycle and fatigue in wrist extensor muscles of patients with hemiparesis. *Phys Ther.* 1988;68:51–56.

76. Benton LA, Baker LL, Bowman B, et al. Functional electrical stimulation: a practical clinical guide. Downey, CA: Professional Staff Association of the Rancho Los Amigos Hospital; 1981:65–71.

77. Binder-Macleod SA, Halden EE, Jungles KA. Effects of stimulation intensity on the physiological responses of human motor units. *Med Sci Sports Exerc.* 1995;274:556–565.

78. Eberstein A, Eberstein S. Electrical stimulation of denervated muscle: is it worthwhile? *Med Sci Sports Exerc.* 1996;28(12):1463–1469.

79. Reid J. On the relation between muscular contractility and the nervous system. *Lond Edinb Month J Med Sci.* 1841;1:320–329.

80. Gutmann E, ed. *The Denervated Muscle.* Prague: Publishing House of the Czechoslovak Academy of Sciences; 1962.

81. Al-Amood WS, Lewis DM. The role of frequency in the effects of long-term intermittent stimulation of denervated slow-twitch muscle in the rat. *J Physiol.* 1987;392:377–395.

82. Boonstra AM, Van Weerden JW, Eisma WH, et al. The effect of low-frequency electrical stimulation on denervation atrophy in man. *Scand J Rehabil Med.* 1987;19:127–134.

83. Carraro U, Catani C, Saggin L, et al. Isomyosin changes after functional electrostimulation of denervated sheep muscle. *Muscle Nerve.* 1988;11:1016–1028.

84. Kern H, Salmons S, Mayr W, et al. Recovery of long-term denervated human muscles induced by electrical stimulation. *Muscle Nerve.* 2005;31:98–101.

85. Nemeth PM. Electrical stimulation of denervated muscle prevents decreases in oxidative enzymes. *Muscle Nerve.* 1982;5:134–139.

86. Nemoto K, Williams HB, Nemoto K, et al. The effects of electrical stimulation on denervated muscle using implantable electrodes. *J Reconstr Microsurg.* 1988;4:251–255, 257.

87. Pachnter B, Eberstein A, Goodgold J. Electrical stimulation effect on denervated skeletal myofibers in rats: a light and electron microscopic study. *Arch Phys Med Rehabil.* 1982;63:427–430.

88. Schmitt LC, Schmitt LA, Rudolph KS. Management of a patient with a forearm fracture and median nerve injury. *J Orthop Sports Phys Ther.* 2004;34:47–56.

89. Valencic V, Vodovnik L, Stefancic M, et al. Improved motor response due to chronic electrical stimulation of denervated tibialis anterior muscle in humans. *Muscle Nerve.* 1986; 9:612–617.

90. Yanai A, Harii K, Okabe K. Preventing denervation atrophy of a grafted muscle. *J Reconstr Microsurg.* 1991;7:85–92.

91. Herbison GJ, Teng CS, Gordon EE. Electrical stimulation of reinnervating rat muscle. *Arch Phys Med Rehabil.* 1973;54:156–160.

92. Nix WA. Effects of intermittent high frequency electrical stimulation on denervated EDL muscle of rabbit. *Muscle Nerve.* 1990;13:580–585.
93. Girlanda P, Dattola R, Vita G, et al. Effect of electrotherapy on denervated muscles in rabbits: an electrophysiological and morphological study. *Exp Neurol.* 1982;77:483–491.
94. Merletti R. Pinelli P. A critical appraisal of neuromuscular stimulation and electrotherapy in neurorehabilitation. *Eur Neurol.* 1980;19:30–32.
95. Nix WA, Dahm M. The effect of isometric short-term electrical stimulation on denervated muscle. *Muscle Nerve.* 1987;10:136–143.
96. Schmirigk K, McLaughlin J, Gruninger W. The effect of electrical stimuation on the experimentally denervated rat muscle. *Scand J Rehabil Med.* 1977;9:55–60.
97. Hennig R. Late reinnervation of the rat soleus muscle is differentially suppressed by chronic stimulation and by ectopic innervation. *Acta Physiol Scand.* 1987;130(1):153–160.
98. Hennig R, Lomo T. Effects of chronic stimulation on the size and speed of long-term denervated and innervated rat fast and slow skeletal muscles. *Acta Physiol Scand.* 1987;130:115–131.
99. Westgaard RH, Lomo T. Control of contractile properties within adaptive ranges by patterns of impulse activity in the rat. *J Neurosci.* 1988;8:4415–4426.
100. Woodcock AH, Taylor PN, Ewins DJ. Long pulse biphasic electrical stimulation of denervated muscle. *Artif Organs.* 1999;23:457–459.
101. Davis H. Is electrostimulation beneficial to denervated muscle? A review of results from basic research. *Physiother Can.* 1983;35:306–310.
102. Hayes K. Electrical stimulation and denervation: proposed program and equipment limitations. *Top Acute Care Trauma Rehabil.* 1988;3:27–37.
103. Kern H, Boncompagni S, Rossini K, et al. Long-term denervation in humans causes degeneration of both contractile and excitation-contraction coupling apparatus, which is reversible by functional electrical stimulation (FES): a role for myofiber regeneration? *J Neuropathol Exp Neurol.* 2004;63:919–931.
104. Kern H, Hofer C, Modlin M, et al. Denervated muscles in humans: limitations and problems of currently used functional electrical stimulation training protocols. *Artif Organs.* 2002;26:216–218.
105. Cohen J, Cohen P. *Applied Multiple Regression Correlation for the Behavioral Sciences.* 2nd ed., Hillsdale, NJ: Lawrence Erlbaum Associates; 1983:72–73, 413–423.
106. Delitto A, Erhard RE, Bowling RW. A treatment based classification approach to low-back syndrome: identifying and staging patients for conservative treatment. *Phys Ther.* 1995;95:470–485.

CHAPTER 7

Electrical Stimulation of Muscle for Control of Movement and Posture

Scott Stackhouse

Electrical stimulation of muscle for the control of movement involves the application of either transcutaneous or percutaneous electrical stimulation to activate skeletal muscle to assist or control the movement or posture of the limbs or trunk. Electrical stimulation to control movement has been used and studied as a therapeutic intervention since the early 1960s. In 1961, Liberson et al. (1) coined the phrase *functional electrical stimulation* (FES) in which electrically elicited muscle contractions produce a functional movement. This first report on FES was a series of case studies in which portable, single-channel stimulators were used to activate the ankle dorsiflexors during the swing phase of gait in individuals with hemiplegia. Unfortunately, it has taken clinical researchers more than 30 years to systematically study the effects and efficacy of FES for dorsiflexion in people with hemiplegia. Over the past 10 years, however, technological advances and the need to demonstrate a positive outcome for FES applications has led to renewed interest in studying FES as an intervention in people with central nervous system dysfunction.

The original theoretical foundation for the application of electrical stimulation of muscle to control movement or posture was that electrical stimulation could replace lost nervous system control of muscle contractions—in effect, using electrical stimulation like an orthosis. In some of the initial cases reported by Liberson et al. (1), however, there was an unexpected improvement in the ability to clear the foot during swing phase of gait, even after the electrical stimulation was removed, in people with hemiplegia. Thus, from its beginnings, FES demonstrated the potential to do more than just act like an orthotic device; it had an actual therapeutic effect. The improved foot clearance without stimulation in some subjects with hemiplegia was perhaps the result of direct peripheral effects in the muscle (i.e., strengthening due to hypertrophy), improved activation of spared corticospinal pathways, improved activation of redundant pathways, or improved activation of indirect pathways.

Over the past 10 to 20 years, scientists have begun to study the plasticity of the central nervous system (CNS). Animal studies have shown that active repetitive training can influence the functional reorganization of the cortex (2,3). In humans, there is some evidence that forced-use and repetitive-task practice paradigms can improve motor recovery after stroke (4,5). Evidence has also been mounting for the existence of spinal networks (central pattern generators) that produce coordinated stepping in both quadruped mammals (6) and humans (7), and studies have shown that locomotor retraining using a bodyweight supported treadmill system has the potential to enhance locomotor ability after CNS disruption (7a). Using electrical stimulation in a functional context for retraining the CNS can be integrated into current motor control theory. Sensorimotor integration theory certainly would embrace the use of electrical stimulation to enhance the movement of a person with CNS dysfunction for retraining motor function. Perhaps combining motor-control theories such as sensorimotor integration and dynamical systems (interlimb coordination) with the use of electrical stimulation in functional contexts will lead to more robust motor recovery (8).

Electrical stimulation of muscle for the control of movement and posture has been used in an attempt to improve function after CNS disruption resulting from spinal cord injury (SCI), cerebral vascular accident (CVA), cerebral palsy (CP), multiple sclerosis (MS), and traumatic brain injury (TBI). Recently, the late actor and director Christopher Reeve brought media attention to FES-cycle training as one of the treatments he received several times per week to prevent muscle atrophy, prevent formation of deep vein thrombosis, improve cardiovascular fitness, and improve bone-mineral density in his femurs after his SCI. Great strides have been made in examining the clinical efficacy of FES since the last edition of this book was published. In an effort to reflect current perspectives in rehabilitation science, this chapter will help guide the clinician in choosing the appropriate stimulation devices and selecting appropriate candidates. The chapter provides an updated review of evidence that supports the use of electrical stimulation of muscle for the control of movement and posture in clinical populations. The learning objectives for this chapter are

1. The clinician will be able to identify attributes of electric stimulation devices necessary for use in control of movement and posture.
2. The clinician will be able to identify characteristics of patients that make them appropriate candidates for electrical stimulation of muscle for the control of movement and posture.
3. The clinician will be familiar with the evidence that supports the use of electrical stimulation of muscle for the control of movement and posture for a variety of medical conditions.

APPLICATION PRINCIPLES OF ELECTRICAL STIMULATION FOR CONTROL OF MOVEMENT AND POSTURE

To use neuromuscular electrical stimulation (NMES) for the control of movement, you must first have an appropriate stimulator available in the clinic. Clinicians have many choices when purchasing stimulators, and they need to be able to sift through the marketing jargon to find a device that is most suitable to their needs. Using NMES for the control of movement requires a stimulator that allows you to adjust stimulation parameters such as waveform, pulse duration, and pulse frequency. In addition, stimulation amplitude control should preferably allow amplitudes up to 100 mA. Aside from the control parameters of the stimulator, you may also have to consider if triggering systems such as manual trigger switches or footswitches can be integrated with the stimulator.

Table 7.1. Precautions to Take When Using Neuromuscular Electrical Stimulation (NMES) for Movement Control

- NMES should be avoided in regions of peripheral vascular disorders such as venous thrombosis or thrombophlebitis because of the risk of releasing the emboli.
- NMES should be avoided in people who are cognitively not able to provide clear feedback regarding the level of the stimulation.
- NMES in people with decreased or absent sensation can be performed, but careful inspection of skin integrity needs to be performed before and after stimulation.
- Stimulation over the thoracic region should be avoided because the current may interfere with the function of the electrical conduction system of the heart.
- Stimulation in the thoracic region in people with demand-type cardiac pacemakers should be avoided because the current may interfere with the function of the pacemaker.
- Stimulation over the carotid sinus should be avoided because the current may interfere with the normal regulation of blood pressure and cardiac contractility.
- Stimulation in the region of phrenic, bladder, or spinal cord stimulators should be avoided because the current may interfere with the function of the devices.
- NMES in people with uncontrolled hypertension or hypotension should be avoided because autonomic responses may adversely affect control of blood pressure.
- NMES in the area of neoplasms or infection should be avoided because muscular and circulatory effects may aggravate these conditions.
- NMES on the trunk of pregnant females should be avoided because of the risk of inducing uterine contractions that may influence the developing fetus.
- NMES in the area of excessive adipose tissue should be avoided because levels of stimulation required to activate muscle through excessive tissue may produce adverse autonomic reactions.
- NMES in people with spinal cord injury can be performed, but the clinician must be may vigilant for signs of autonomic dysreflexia.

Robinson AJ. Neuromuscular electrical stimulation for control of posture and movement. In: Robinson AJ Snyder-Mackler L (eds) *Clinical Electrophysiology Electrotherapy and Electrophysiologic Testing.* 2nd ed. Baltimore, Williams Wilkins; 1995

Next, you will need to be able to identify appropriate clinical problems and patients for the application of electrical stimulation. Most stimulators only offer simultaneous use of two channels, and thus will limit most clinicians to stimulating two muscle groups when using NMES for the control of movement. Additionally, the number of available support staff may also affect the selection of patients. For example, if a patient is going to need multiple support staff to assist during gait-retraining with FES, you will need to decide if this is feasible in your practice facility.

Perhaps the information most likely to affect your choice to use NMES is the patient's current health status. The application of NMES for the control of movement is a form of exercise, and the client will need to be able to withstand the cardiopulmonary demands of the treatment. Thus, adequate health screening will need to be a necessary part of an evaluation before NMES is used. Some commonly cited precautions for the use of NMES are given in Table 7.1.

A patient's specific impairments in strength and range of motion will also affect the ability to use NMES for the control of movement. Logically, if the patient has insufficient electrically-elicited strength or lacks range of motion to perform the movement, these impairments will need to be addressed before starting NMES for the control of movement.

Other patient-specific considerations may include motivation, home environment, family/caregiver support, and insurance coverage to pay for the intervention.

EVIDENCE THAT SUPPORTS THE USE OF ELECTRICAL STIMULATION FOR CONTROL OF MOVEMENT

This section of the chapter illustrates how successful interventions using electrical stimulation of muscle for the control of movement and posture were applied to the upper and lower extremities for a variety of dysfunctions.

Neuromuscular Electrical Stimulation for Scoliosis Management

Idiopathic scoliosis is a lateral curvature of the spine of unknown etiology. This condition is commonly found in children and, if untreated, produces severe postural deformities that may lead to impaired cardiopulmonary function, joint disease of the spine, back pain, and limitation in daily functional activities. In the previous edition of this book, NMES was discussed as a potential alternative to bracing for the management of idiopathic scoliosis. In large, multicenter studies conducted in the early 1980s, Brown et al. (9) and McCullough (10) found that NMES was able to halt the progression of idiopathic scoliotic curves in approximately 70% to 90% of patients. Brown et al. (9) treated curves between 20 degrees and 45 degrees, and McCullough (10) treated curves less than 30 degrees. The NMES was applied laterally over the midaxillary line of the thorax on the convex side of the curve. Brown et al. (9) used rectangular constant-current pulses of 220 μs duration and a frequency of 25 pulses per second (pps). The on:off times were 6 seconds on and 6 seconds off, and the amplitude was adjusted to produce spinal movement in the "straightening" direction. The duration of each NMES application was gradually increased to 8 hours, and the patients used the NMES each night until they reached skeletal maturity.

In recent studies, the effectiveness of NMES at stopping or reversing spinal curve progression has been compared to that of full-time and part-time orthotic bracing as well as to observation (no treatment). These comparative studies have shown NMES to be no better than observation (11,12). In fact, both of these studies provide evidence that bracing with an orthosis either full-time (23 hours per day) or part-time (16 hours per day) was superior to NMES treatment. Furthermore, there are no clear differences in methodology between the studies that show positive and negative treatment outcomes. The results summarized above coupled with the results of other studies (13–18) provide substantial evidence that NMES treatment for idiopathic scoliosis is not an effective treatment, especially when compared to orthotic intervention.

Upper Extremity Applications

Neuromuscular Electrical Stimulation for Prevention or Reduction of Shoulder Subluxation

Inferior subluxation of the glenohumeral joint is a frequent consequence of hemiplegia secondary to stroke. Immediately after stroke, muscles in the involved extremities become flaccid in approximately 90% of patients (19). The subsequent development of an inferior subluxation of the shoulder has been reported to occur with a widely varying incidence that ranges from 17% to 81% (20–23). The glenohumeral joint relies on muscular support for stabilization, and Basmajian (24,25) demonstrated that the supraspinatus and posterior deltoid muscles provide the active support to prevent inferior glenohumeral subluxation. When the upper limb is flaccid during the early stages after stroke, the force of gravity on the affected arm can potentially stretch the ligamentous and capsular passive support systems about the shoulder and lead to the development of an inferior subluxation. A common treatment for inferior shoulder subluxation is the application of a sling to mitigate the pull of gravity on the affected shoulder. There are two major drawbacks to slings: first, most slings are not effective at preventing or reducing the subluxation (26), and second, the slings that are effective cause patients not to use the affected arm and to hold the elbow in a flexed posture that may increase the risk of contracture development.

Electrical stimulation of the supraspinatus and posterior deltoid muscles has the potential, when used appropriately, to reduce and prevent the development of inferior subluxations of the glenohumeral joint. In 1986, Baker and Parker (27) conducted a study that compared the effectiveness of conventional slings to that of electrical stimulation of the supraspinatus and posterior deltoid on 63 people with hemiplegia with ≥5 mm of inferior subluxation as compared to their uninvolved side (Fig. 7.1). Pulse duration was not reported, but the stimulation pulse frequency

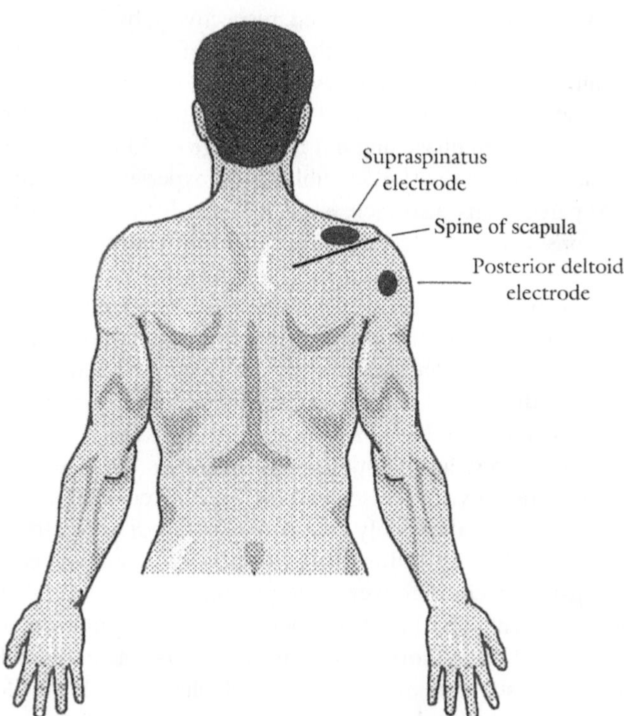

Figure 7.1. Electrode placement over the suprapinatus and posterior deltoid muscles for electrical stimulation for shoulder subluxation.

was set to produce a tetanic contraction and ranged from 12 to 25 pps. The length of each stimulation session was gradually progressed from three 30-minute sessions per day to a single 6- to 7-hour session, and the on:off time was increased from 1:3 seconds to 24:2 seconds as permitted by the ability to maintain subluxation reduction. This procedure was performed 5 days per week for 6 weeks. The participants that received electrical stimulation reduced their subluxation from 14.8 mm to 8.6 mm, whereas the unstimulated control group demonstrated no change (13.3 mm). At a 3-month follow-up assessment on a subset of participants from each group, the control group demonstrated no change in subluxation, and the group that received electrical stimulation had only a 1–2 mm increase in subluxation, thus demonstrating some maintenance of the reduction from the training period.

Baker and Parker (27) studied participants who already had an inferior shoulder subluxation (≥5 mm) before enrollment in the study, and who were being treated in a rehabilitation setting and were therefore past the acute, flaccid stage of recovery after stroke (~45 to 50 days after stroke). Faghri et al. (28) conducted a randomized study that assessed the effects of electrical stimulation on the reduction of shoulder subluxation, arm function recovery, and shoulder pain in participants 16 to 17 days after stroke, on average. The 26 participants with flaccid paralysis of one upper extremity were randomized into either control or electrical stimulation groups. Both groups received physical therapy (interventions not described), and the participants in the electrical stimulation group additionally received stimulation to the supraspinatus and posterior deltoid muscles. Stimulation pulse frequency was set at 35 pps, but the pulse duration was not reported. Electrical stimulation was performed 7 days per week for 6 weeks. The duration of the stimulation sessions and the on:off times were progressively increased based on whether full reduction of the subluxation could be attained at the end of each session. The duration of the sessions started at 1.5 hours and progressed to 6 hours, and the on:off times were initiated at 10:12 seconds and gradually progressed to 30:2 seconds. Once 6 hours of stimulation was attained, the on time and off times were increased and decreased, respectively, by 2 seconds, as tolerated. In the electrical stimulation group, the difference in the amount of side-to-side subluxation decreased from 6.0 mm to 2.46 mm after the 6-week intervention and increased slightly to 3.46 mm after a 6-week withdrawal phase. In the control group the subluxation increased from 4.0 mm to 9.85 mm over the 6-week intervention phase and did not change (9.35 mm) during the 6-week withdrawal phase. In addition to the reduction in subluxation experienced by the electrical stimulation group, stimulated participants also increased their arm function, passive shoulder external rotation prior to pain onset, and posterior deltoid electromyographic activity more than the control group.

The earlier treatment with electrical stimulation of the supraspinatus and posterior deltoid by Faghri et al. (28) led to smaller initial and post-intervention subluxations than those reported by Baker and Parker (27). It therefore appears that early treatment with electrical stimulation while the affected upper extremity is acutely flaccid is important in preventing and ultimately reducing the amount of glenohumeral joint subluxation. Chantraine et al. (29) conducted a large trial of electrical stimulation to reduce shoulder subluxation as the result of acute hemiparesis, with the intervention starting between the second and fourth weeks after stroke. This study followed 120 participants who were alternately assigned to a control or electrical stimulation group and followed through a 5-week intervention phase and periodically followed for up to 24 months after stroke. All participants received conventional rehabilitation therapy that followed the concepts of Bobath (29). Electrical stimulation was performed using pulse durations of 350 μs and with an on:off time of 1:5 but the authors did not specify if this was in seconds or if it represents a ratio. Additionally, the investigators did not specify the placement of the electrodes. The stimulation program was performed with three sequences: the first sequence was 90 minutes in duration with a stimulation pulse frequency of 8 pps, the second sequence was 30 minutes in duration with a pulse frequency of 40 pps, and the third sequence was 10 minutes in duration with a pulse frequency of 1 pps. No rationale was given for the selection of these stimulation parameters. Stimulation was performed for 5 weeks with increases to the length of stimulation by 5 minutes to sequences 1 and 2 during the second and fourth weeks. Unfortunately, both the number of days per week and the number of sessions per day that the electrical stimulation was performed were omitted from this report. The results of Chantraine et al. support the results of Baker and Parker (27) and Faghri and et al. (28) by demonstrating that participants in the electrical stimulation group had a greater reduction of shoulder subluxation and maintained it at 6, 12, and 24 months after stroke. Additionally, participants in the electrical stimulation group demonstrated less pain with range of motion and had increased amounts of active range of motion in shoulder forward flexion and abduction than the control group at each measurement period.

Another study has been conducted recently that further examined electrical stimulation for preventing subluxation. Linn et al. (30) reported on the efficacy of electrical stimulation at preventing the development of shoulder subluxation in a single-blind, randomized, and controlled study. Initial assessments and treatment started within 48 hours of admission to an acute stroke unit of a hospital, and participants were assessed after a 4-week intervention and after an 8-week withdrawal phase. Electrical stimulation was applied to the supraspinatus and posterior deltoid muscles during four sessions every day (2 to 4 hours total duration) with a 30-pps pulse frequency, a 300-μs pulse duration, and a 15:15 second on:off time. The results showed less subluxation in the electrical stimulation group after the intervention period; however, this difference was not maintained after the 8-week withdrawal phase. Explanations for the difference between this result and those of Baker and Parker (27) and Faghri et al. (28) may include both the longer daily time of stimulation sessions (4 vs. 6 to 7 hours) and the longer treatment period (4 vs. 6 weeks). In the Linn et al. (30) study, the shorter duration of the treatment period coupled with initiation of the treatment within 48 hours of admission to the hospital may have contributed to the lack of maintaining reductions in subluxation because the treatment may have ended before patients regained some functional control over the supraspinatus, and deltoid and before the time that adaptations in muscle start to occur. This idea may have some merit because Linn et al. (30) did find a significant correlation between reduction in subluxation and scores on the Motor Assessment Scale. Finally, this study also demonstrated that no participant who scored a grade of ≥2 on the Motor Assessment Scale developed a subluxation. This type of information is important for researchers to explore because it could allow clinicians to select appropriate candidates for this type of treatment intervention.

Kobayashi et al. (31) explored the use of electrical stimulation to reduce subluxation in people with chronic hemiplegia (≥1 year) using two electrical stimulation groups and a control group. One electrical stimulation group activated only the supraspinatus muscle, and the other group activated only the middle portion of the deltoid. The electrical stimulation was applied for two 15-minute sessions per day (5 days per week) for 6 weeks with a pulse frequency of 20 pps, a pulse duration of 300 μs and a 15:15 second on:off cycle time. After the 6-week intervention, no changes in subluxation were noted without stress, but when the affected arm was stressed by attaching a 3.5-kg weight, a significant reduction in subluxation was noted for the group receiving stimulation to the deltoid. Additionally, both electrical stimulation groups were able to generate a greater amount of shoulder abduction force than before treatment.

Wang et al. (32) compared the ability of electrical stimulation to reduce subluxation in people with acute (<21 days) versus chronic (>365 days) hemiplegia. Electrical stimulation was applied to the supraspinatus and posterior deltoid muscles 5 days per week for 6 weeks. The duration of daily treatment time was progressed during the first week from three 30-minute sessions to a single 6-hour session with a 1:3 on:off ratio (no exact on or off times given). Over the next 5 weeks, the stimulation on time was increased by 2 seconds every 1 to 2 days until 24 seconds was reached. When the on time reached 24 seconds, the off time was progressively decreased every 1 to 2 days until a time of 2 seconds was reached. Electrical stimulation pulse frequency was set to achieve a fused tetanic contraction (10 to 24 pps). Participants that had acute hemiplegia and received electrical stimulation had a reduction in the amount of shoulder subluxation after 6 weeks and had a slight increase in subluxation, although not back to baseline, after a 6-week withdrawal. Participants that had chronic hemiplegia did not show significant reductions in shoulder subluxation.

The results of Wang et al. (32) are in line with those of Kobayashi et al. (31) for nonstressed (by weight) radiographs. Kobayashi et al. had reduced stressed subluxation measurements, and this may be important for protecting the joint and surrounding structures if the person with hemiplegia is carrying an object. Using treatments longer than 6 weeks in duration may be necessary to shorten shoulder joint structures and rehabilitate musculature, and therefore reduce shoulder subluxation in people with chronic hemiplegia. Further research investigating the efficacy of electrical stimulation in reducing shoulder subluxation in people with chronic hemiplegia is warranted.

Literature-based Guidelines for Treating People with Glenohumeral Joint Subluxation Resulting from Hemiplegia

1. Treatment should be initiated early, while in the acute flaccid stage of recovery, in an attempt to prevent the development of glenohumeral joint subluxation.
2. Treatment should be at least 6 weeks in duration.
3. Electrical stimulation should involve the supraspinatus, posterior deltoid, and possibly the middle deltoid muscles.
4. Electrical stimulation should be performed at a high enough amplitude and frequency to attain tetany in order to produce a strong contraction to reduce subluxation at the time of treatment.
5. Electrical stimulation should be applied for relatively long sessions each day that total 4 to 7 hours in duration.

Neuromuscular Electrical Stimulation for Improving Wrist and Hand Movement

HEMIPLEGIA AFTER STROKE

The use of electrical stimulation to improve wrist extensor function and wrist range of motion has been fairly well studied. There are a few reports in the literature dating back to the early 1960s and mid-1970s; however, these studies (33–35) mainly focus on device development and feasibility. It was not until the late 1970s that a research group from the Rancho Los Amigos Hospital started to study the effects of electrical stimulation on the wrist extensors and identify which patients would benefit from this treatment. In their first study in people with hemiplegia, NMES was applied "passively" to produce wrist extension (36). In their second study, people with hemiplegia were "actively" trained in wrist extension using electromyographically (EMG) triggered NMES (37). In this section, both passive and active applications of electrical stimulation to the wrist extensors are discussed.

Passive Applications. Baker et al. (36) applied electrical stimulation to the wrist extensors in 16 people with hemiplegia (nine subacute, seven chronic) to examine the effects of electrical stimulation on sensation, spasticity, passive range of motion of wrist and fingers, and strength of wrist extensors. NMES of the wrist extensors was performed to produce the maximum comfortable extensor contraction using a pulsed current with pulse duration of 200 μs delivered at a frequency of 33 pps. The stimulation cycle was 7 seconds of stimulation, including a 3-second ramp-up time, followed by 10 seconds of rest time. Treatment sessions were performed initially for 15 minutes twice daily, and progressed to three 30-minute sessions per day over a 4-week treatment program. The stimulation program effectively prevented wrist and metacarpalphalangeal (MP) joint contracture development in the subacute stroke group, and dramatically increased the amount of passive range of motion in the same joints of the chronic stroke group. The chronic group averaged a 36-degree increase in wrist extension, and the average gain in extension at the MP joints was 27 degrees. An interesting finding from this study was the increase in wrist extensor strength from 1.55 to 2.46 Nm in participants who initially had some voluntary control at the wrist. On the premise of the increase in wrist extensor strength in subjects with some voluntary control at the wrist, Baker et al. designed a study that examined the effects of EMG-triggered electrical stimulation training (see next section below).

Since the early study by Baker et al. (36), two randomized, controlled studies have been reported for NMES of the wrist extensors in people with hemiplegia (38,39). Both studies reported gains in motor function after the treatment period with electrical stimulation. Chae et al. (38) treated study participants in an inpatient rehabilitation setting, and those in the NMES group received 1 hour of stimulation per day for a total of 15 sessions. The parameters for electrical stimulation were 300-μs pulse duration, frequency of 20 to 50 pps, amplitude sufficient to produce full wrist and finger extension, with a 10:10 seconds on:off cycle time. They calculated each participant's Fugl–Meyer Motor Assessment score, which measures motor recovery, and calculated the self-care component of the Functional Independence Measure (FIM), which measures upper extremity-related disability. After the 15 treatment sessions, they observed significant increases in Fugl–Meyer scores, but this increase in motor function did not translate into a decrease in upper-extremity-related disability. Perhaps the intervention period with the stimulation was too short (~2 weeks) for carryover of motor recovery into functional use.

Powell et al. (39) studied the effects of a protracted electrical stimulation program on isometric wrist extensor strength and upper extremity disability using the Action Research Arm Test (ARAT). Participants randomized into the electrical stimulation group performed three 30-minute electrical stimulation sessions per day for 8 weeks. The electrical stimulation parameters were 300-μs pulse duration, 20 pps frequency, and an amplitude that achieved full wrist extension. The stimulation cycled at 5:20 seconds on:off time, and was progressively decreased over the study to a 5:5 seconds on:off time. Isometric wrist extension strength at 0 degrees of extension increased over the 8-week intervention period and was maintained at the end of a 24-week withdrawal period. Two components of the ARAT (grasp and grip subscores) improved over the intervention phase; however, these gains were not maintained at the end of the 24-weeks of withdrawal. In a subgroup of participants who could produce wrist torque at the start of the study, the participants who received electrical stimulation had a increase in the total ARAT as compared to those in the control group after the 8-week intervention. Again, this difference was not maintained after 24 weeks of withdrawal.

Active Applications. Baker et al. (36), Chae et al. (38), and Powell et al. (39) demonstrated that electrical stimulation of the wrist extensors improved aspects of stroke recovery such as passive and active range of motion, strength, and motor function. The above studies, however, were less successful in decreasing upper-extremity disability. The lack of carryover into function might be from the lack of active patient participation during electrical stimulation. The next series of research reports used either joint position or muscle activation feedback to enhance the movement experience in people with hemiplegia. This type of application is theoretically based within the *sensorimotor integration theory*. In this theory, sensory input from the joint and limb movement are thought to directly affect subsequent motor output (40).

Bowman et al. (37) reported using positional feedback in combination with electrical stimulation of the wrist extensors of participants who had some residual voluntary control at the wrist. After stroke, 30 people were randomized into two groups (positional feedback coupled to electrical stimulation and unstimulated control) and treated 5 days per week for 4 weeks. Each group received standard rehabilitation of the wrist/hand of passive range of motion, active resistive exercise, neuromuscular facilitation, and activities of daily living training 5 days per week. The group that received positional feedback coupled to electrical stimulation performed 20 to 100 resisted repetitions for two 30-minute sessions each day. Electrical stimulation was performed using a 200-μs pulse duration delivered at 35 pps with a 6 to 8:20 second on:off cycle time. The electrical stimulation was initiated by the participant when they volitionally achieved a threshold level of wrist extension. This threshold was set daily for each individual. The positional feedback display gave instantaneous information about wrist-joint position using visual and auditory cues. Participants were also able to keep track of the number of successful repetitions in which they met the threshold level set for initiation of the electrical stimulation. Participants in the feedback plus electrical stimulation group increased their wrist extension torque measured at 0 degrees of extension from 0.43 Nm to more than 1.6 Nm (a 280% increase), whereas participants in the control group increased by about 25%. Similar gains were made for active range of motion in and out of synergy patterns, with the feedback-plus-electrical-stimulation group increasing their wrist extension motion by more than 30 degrees, and the control group increasing their motion by approximately 8 degrees. Unfortunately, this study does not report on any gains in functional ability with activities of daily living and subsequent reduction in disability.

A more recent pilot study reported outcomes related to function and disability by using the FIM. Francisco et al. (41) performed a pilot study on nine people with acute hemiplegia, with approximately 18 days between stroke onset and admission to the study. Four participants were randomly assigned to an EMG-triggered NMES group, and five participants to an unstimulated control group. The EMG-triggered NMES group performed two 30-minute intervention sessions per day, 5 days a week for the duration of the rehabilitation stay. EMG threshold was set daily, and triggered NMES of the extensor carpi radialis was applied with a pulse duration of 200 μs and a frequency that was set between 20 and 100 pps based on subject comfort. The duty cycle for the exercise was 5:5 seconds on:off. In addition, both groups received standard rehabilitation interventions such as neuromuscular re-education, range of motion exercises, strengthening, neuromuscular facilitation, and functional training. The EMG-NMES group made greater gains in both the Fugl–Meyer and FIM scores than the control group. After controlling for the length of stay, however, the Fugl–Meyer remained significantly higher for the EMG-NMES group, and the FIM results were reduced to a trend. This is the first study, however, that demonstrated a functional carryover of the EMG-triggered NMES training.

EMG-triggered NMES also has been demonstrated to increase motor function of the wrist in people with chronic hemiplegia (≥1 year). In their first study, Cauraugh et al. (8) trained seven participants with EMG-NMES, trained four participants with volitional wrist and finger extension. All participants had some residual wrist function and performed two treatment sessions of 30 wrist/finger extension movements three times per week for 2 weeks. Participants in the control group performed volitional contractions, and the experimental group initiated volitional wrist/finger extension to an EMG threshold and then completed the motion with NMES. Electrical stimulation was delivered at 50 pps with a 7:25 second on:off time that included 1 second each for ramp up and ramp down. After the short intervention period (2 weeks totaling 360 contractions), patients in the EMG-NMES group increased their ability to sustain the force during an isometric wrist extension contraction as compared to patients in the control group. In addition, the EMG-NMES group demonstrated carryover to a functional task by being able to move a greater number of blocks (9) during a Box and Block test.

Cauraugh and Kim (42) conducted a follow-up experiment in which they coupled EMG-triggered NMES of the involved wrist/finger extensors with the simultaneous performance of volitional wrist/finger extension of the uninvolved side. These training protocols are based on two motor control theories: *sensorimotor integration* and *dynamical systems theory*. The purpose of this study was to determine if integrating these two rehabilitation protocols would enhance recovery of motor function in the wrist/finger extensors. Twenty-five study participants were randomly assigned to one of three groups with the restriction that 20 people were assigned to the two intervention groups. The control group performed volitional wrist/finger extensions, the unilateral group performed EMG-triggered NMES, and the bilateral group performed volitional wrist/ finger extension of the uninvolved side and simultaneous EMG-triggered NMES to the involved side. EMG-triggered NMES was performed as described above, with the exception that three sessions were performed two times per week for 2 weeks. Both the unilateral and bilateral groups that performed EMG-triggered NMES improved their motor recovery; however, the bilateral group improved to a greater extent with more blocks moved on the Box and Block test, decreased reaction time, and an improved sustained force.

Mechanistically, the improvement in wrist and finger motor ability that is seen after NMES is poorly understood. Recently, Han et al. (43) demonstrated that NMES of the wrist extensor musculature produced bilateral cortical activation in the primary sensory cortex, primary motor cortex, and supplementary motor cortex activation, as demonstrated by functional magnetic resonance imaging. Cortical activation resulting from NMES may facilitate cortical plasticity that leads to increased motor function, but the relationship between cortical activation and plasticity has yet to be elucidated. Electrical stimulation of the wrist/finger extensors has also been applied to children with cerebral palsy (44,45). Both of the studies reported improvement in active wrist and finger motion, but neither study was a randomized-controlled trial. The studies do provide a basis from which to design and perform such investigations.

LITERATURE-BASED GUIDELINES FOR USING ELECTRICAL STIMULATION TO IMPROVE WRIST/FINGER EXTENSION IN PEOPLE WITH HEMIPLEGIA AFTER STROKE

1. Cyclic NMES and EMG-triggered NMES of the wrist extensors can improve motor recovery of subacute and chronic poststroke hemiplegia.
2. Active participation using EMG-triggered NMES of the wrist extensors also improves the functional use of the wrist and fingers in people with subacute and chronic poststroke hemiplegia.
3. Pulse durations ranged from 200 to 300 μs, and pulse frequencies ranged from 20 to 100 pps (with all but one study at ≤50 pps). Amplitudes of stimulation produced movement through the full available range of motion.
4. On times ranged from 5 to 10 seconds and off times from 5 to 25 seconds.
5. The goal of the stimulation was to achieve full wrist and finger extension.
6. Functional carryover was seen with as few as 360 EMG-triggered NMES contractions performed over a 2-week period; therefore, this treatment could feasibly be performed in most rehabilitation settings (inpatient rehabilitation, outpatient rehabilitation, or as part of a home exercise program if patient and caregiver are given proper training).

Neuromuscular Electrical Stimulation for Improved Hand Function in Spinal Cord Injury

Hanson and Franklin (46) surveyed men with quadriplegia and had them rank-order their functional losses due to SCI. This study revealed that 76% of the men rated the loss of arm and hand function as the greatest loss compared to bowel and bladder, leg, and sexual function. The use of electrical stimulation to improve wrist and hand function after SCI has focused on achieving functional grips to allow better object manipulation in individuals with motor level lesions of C5 and C6. People with C5 and C6 motor level SCI will have some control of shoulder flexion, elbow flexion, and wrist extension (C6 only), but will be unable to volitionally control the fingers, and therefore will have limited functional use of the hand. Improving upper-extremity function in people with SCI has been attempted with both implantable and surface electrical stimulation devices, and some of the studies that have been reported are reviewed below.

Use of Implanted Devices

In the early 1980s, rehabilitation researchers started to develop and test an implantable electrical stimulation system (*neuroprosthesis*) that would provide functional grasps to people with C5 and C6 motor level lesions. This neuroprosthesis has both external and implanted components (Fig. 7.2). The external controller communicates with the implanted stimulator via a radiofrequency coil. The stimulator has up to eight channels, which connect to the desired elbow, forearm, and hand musculature via electrodes placed on the epimysium of the desired muscles. These electrodes are surgically placed to produce the correct movement. The type of hand grasp that is produced is controlled by movements of the contralateral shoulder. Shoulder elevation–depression and protraction–retraction are detected using a shoulder position sensor, and shoulder movement is used to select different hand grasps and to grade the position and amount of grasp force (47). This neuroprosthesis provides two different hand grasps: the lateral pinch and palmar grasp. The lateral pinch grasp occurs when the thumb flexes against the lateral aspect of the index finger, and the palmar grasp occurs when the fingers are flexed to meet an opposed thumb.

Peckham et al. (47) performed a mulitcenter trial in which each participant's hand-grasp function was measured before and after neuroprosthesis implantation, and with and without the neuroprosthesis activated. They followed 51 patients for at least 3 years after implantation (median, 5.4 years), and collected data on lateral pinch force, palmar grasp force, grasp function, independence during activities of daily living, and satisfaction with the neuroprosthesis. The neuroprosthesis was able to increase lateral pinch and palmar force in almost all tested subjects.

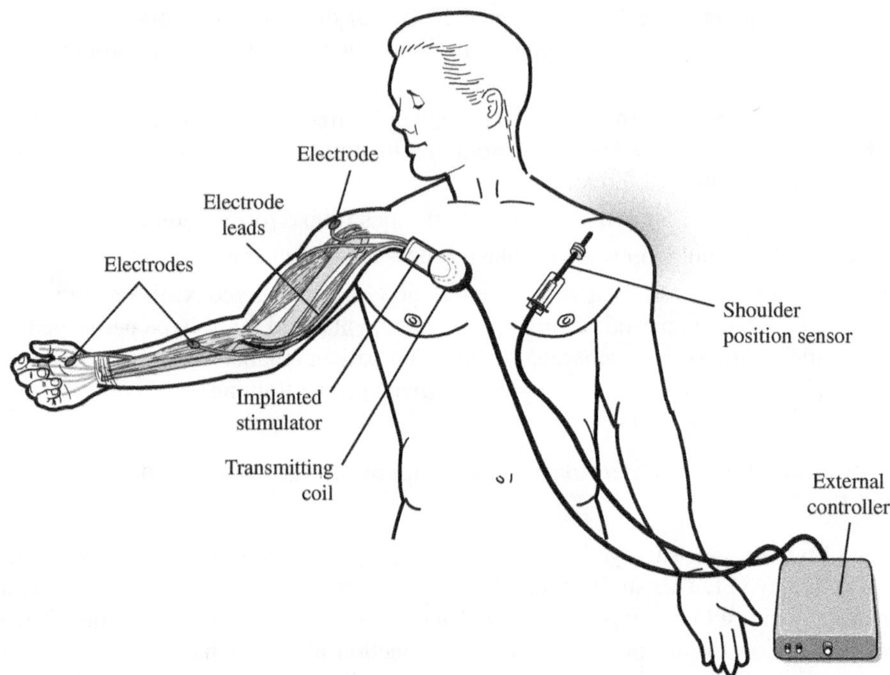

Figure 7.2. Schematic of the upper extremity implantable neuroprosthesis that provides palmar grasp and lateral pinch grip to people with C5 to C6 motor level spinal cord injury.

All but one subject improved his or her performance on a grasp function test, and all subjects were more independent with at least one activity of daily living. The subjects also rated their satisfaction with the neuroprosthesis highly, with >90% of participants stating that the neuroprosthesis improved their quality of life and that they would recommend the device to others. In a related study by this same research group (48), the economic consequences of implanting the neuroprosthesis were examined. Creasey et al. (48) determined that the cost of implementing the upper extremity neuroprosthesis would be recovered over the lifetime of the user if their attendant care time would be reduced by only 2 hours per day; however, this analysis did not consider other benefits, such as return to work, and therefore it may underestimate some of the economic advantages of the device.

One downside to the implanted neuroprosthesis is that the surgery, the device, and associated rehabilitation are initially costly. To combat the initial costs, several external (surface) neuroprosthesis systems have been developed to assist grasping function in people with C5 through C7 SCI. One system, the Bionic Glove, uses three channels of stimulation to activate the finger flexors and extensors, and thumb flexors, with the control signal coming from a wrist position transducer (49). The device is housed within a custom-fitted forearm/hand sleeve that needs to be positioned appropriately to stimulate the correct motor points for palmar grasp. Popovic et al. (49) reported on the functional outcomes of 12 people with cervical SCI. When subjects were excluded that had nearly normal scores on the quadriplegia index of function and functional independence measure tests ($n = 3$) or Brown-Séquard syndrome ($n = 1$), six of the remaining eight subjects demonstrated functional improvements on both functional scales after 6 months of use of the Bionic Glove. The subjects in the study, however, complained of difficulties in donning and doffing the system, and reported that small shifts in the position of the electrodes produced dramatic changes in function; that good control of the wrist was necessary to make the device most functionally useful (C6 or lower motor level); and that the rigidity of the hand portion of the glove interfered with small-object manipulation.

Another surface grasp–release system, the Handmaster (now NESS H200, Neuromuscular Electrical Stimulation Systems, Ltd.; see Fig. 7.3), combines wrist stabilization and electrical stimulation to produce lateral pinch, palmar grasp, and a static hand-open posture. The device connects with a small control unit, which has three exercise and three functional modes that can be activated by the user. Similar to the Bionic Glove, the Handmaster is custom fit to the user, and electrode placement and size are determined for the extensor digitorum communis, extensor

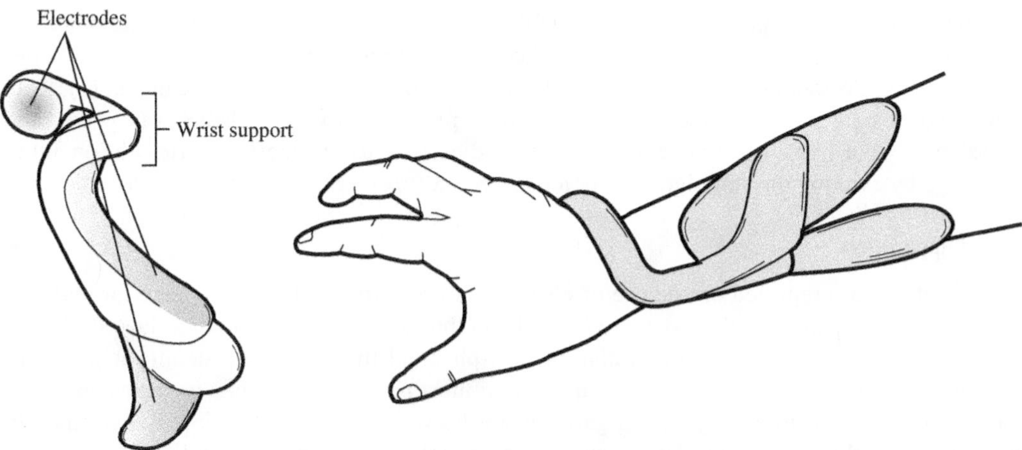

Figure 7.3. The Handmaster (now NESS H200; Neuromuscular Electrical Stimulation Systems, Ltd.; Ra'anana, Israel) combines wrist stabilization with electrical stimulation for hand grip and opening.

pollicis brevis, flexor digitorum superficialis, flexor pollicis longus, and the thenar muscles. Alon and McBride (50) studied five people with C5 and two people with C6 motor level injury over a 3-week training period. Over this short training period, improvements were demonstrated while using the neuroprosthesis during the activities of daily living/grasp-and-release tests. Without the neuroprosthesis, subjects were successful in only 3 of 14 attempts of the tasks on the activities of daily living/grasp-and-release tests; whereas with the neuroprosthesis activated, they improved to a 100% success rate after 3 weeks of training. In addition, grip strength improved from 0.57 N without the neuroprosthesis, to 16.5 N with the neuroprosthesis (50). Alon and McBride (50) suggested that compared to implanted systems that may require 6 to 8 months to develop complete control of the system, the subjects in their study only needed 1 to 2 weeks. They also speculated that the Handmaster neuroprosthesis could be a low-cost alternative or an early intervention that would enhance decision-making for people considering implantation of an upper-extremity neuroprosthesis.

Literature-based Guidelines for Using Electrical Stimulation to Improve Hand Grasp and Release Function in Patients after Spinal Cord Injury

This section of the chapter has focused on research-based and commercially available systems for improving hand function in C5 through C7 motor-level SCI, and it would not be expected that every clinician could devise such a system for their patients. It would be expected, however, that clinicians could do the following:

1. Perform an evaluation to see if the appropriate wrist and hand muscles can be electrically activated.
2. Determine if the person being treated might be an appropriate candidate for a neuroprosthetic system.
3. Discuss the different neuroprosthetic systems with the patient and be able to explain the differences and advantages and disadvantages of each system.
4. Serve as an advocate for the patient by appropriate referral to the distributor of the neuroprosthesis or to a research laboratory if the patient meets criteria to be a candidate and wants to pursue a neuroprosthetic system.

Neuromuscular Electrical Stimulation for Control of Lower Extremity Movement

Electrical stimulation to produce movement of the lower extremity in people with hemiplegia has been used in a similar manner as described for the upper extremity. Aside from the early case series report of using electrical stimulation for dorsiflexion assist during the swing phase of gait (1), there were studies that examined the recovery of force production when NMES was performed "passively" in a nonfunctional context, and studies that used electrical stimulation more "actively" by evoking the stimulation after a targeted motion or EMG level had been achieved.

Passive Applications

Merletti et al. (51) reported on the use of electrical stimulation to the tibialis anterior and peroneal muscles in people with poststroke hemiplegia that were in a rehabilitation hospital. They placed 49 patients into either a stimulation-plus-physical therapy group or into a physical-therapy-only group. The stimulation was applied in most patients while they were seated, while some used the stimulation only during gait. Electrodes were placed either directly over the tibialis anterior and peroneal muscles, or over the peroneal nerve in the popliteal fossa and at the fibular head. The stimulation parameters were a pulse duration of 300 μs and a pulse frequency of 30 pps. The elicited contractions were 1.5 seconds in duration with a 3-second rest time, and were performed for 20 minutes per day, 6 days per week for approximately 4 weeks. Isometric dorsiflexion force production was measured with a custom leg brace–strain gauge device. The subjects who received the electrical stimulation demonstrated a significantly greater recovery of force (as a percentage of their less-involved side; 17.00%) as compared to the physical-therapy-only treatment group (6.29%).

Active Applications

Winchester and colleagues (52) were one of the first group of researchers to use positional feedback training with electrical stimulation of the lower extremity. They recruited 40 patients in a rehabilitation hospital who had minimal knee extension as a result of poststroke hemiplegia. These subjects were divided into either a positional feedback-training group or a control group. Both groups received physical therapy 5 days per week for the 4 weeks of the study. The positional feedback-training group performed between 20 and 50 contractions per day based on each patient's fatigue level. The pulse duration was set at 220 μs, and the pulse frequency was 30 pps. The contractions were between 8 and 10 seconds in duration with a 2 second ramp-up time, and rest time (off time) set for 20 seconds. The subjects would initiate voluntary knee extension, and using audio and visual feedback, would extend to a position that was about 5 degrees less than their maximum extension. Once that position was reached, the stimulation would begin and complete the knee extension through the available range. Once the subjects achieved 150 degrees of active knee extension or 30 degrees less than the available range, weight was added to the position feedback training in 0.45-kg increments. In addition to the positional feedback stimulation, the experimental subjects underwent cyclical stimulation of the involved quadriceps with the knee in full extension for up to 2 hours per day (while seated in a wheelchair or during standing-weight shifting exercises on the parallel bars). The main outcome measures for this study were maximum isometric torque production and selective and synergistic active range of motion. The subjects who performed the positional feedback stimulation and cyclic stimulation had a significantly greater increase in their knee extension torque production (38 Nm vs. 19.4 Nm) as compared to the control group. The positional feedback subjects also had significantly greater improvements in synergistic knee extension active range of motion (33 vs. 19 degrees). They did not, however, detect a significant difference between groups in the ability to produce selective or isolated knee extension active range of motion. The lack of a difference in selective active range of motion could have been due to the fact that the positional feedback group was not instructed to perform the voluntary knee extension out of the synergy (i.e., in isolation). Unfortunately, this study did not collect functional data or gait characteristics to examine how the changes in strength related to function.

Neuromuscular Electrical Stimulation for Dorsiflexion Assist During Gait

Hemiplegia After Stroke

Only one randomized, controlled trial of electrical stimulation to provide dorsiflexion assist during gait has been conducted in people with hemiplegia after stroke (53). Subjects in this study needed to have hemiplegia at least 6 months, drop-foot on one side as evidenced by foot drag or hip hike/circumduction on the involved side, no mental impairment, and the ability to ambulate 10 m without assistance. Stimulation was applied through surface electrodes placed over the common peroneal nerve at the neck of the fibula, and either the motor point of the tibialis anterior, or a point on the common peroneal nerve proximal to the head of the fibula (Fig. 7.4). A footswitch that was sensitive to force was placed under the heel so that the stimulation was triggered during the swing phase of gait. The footswitch was then used in one of two ways: stimulation was triggered by (i) the heel rise on the affected side, or (ii) by heel strike on the

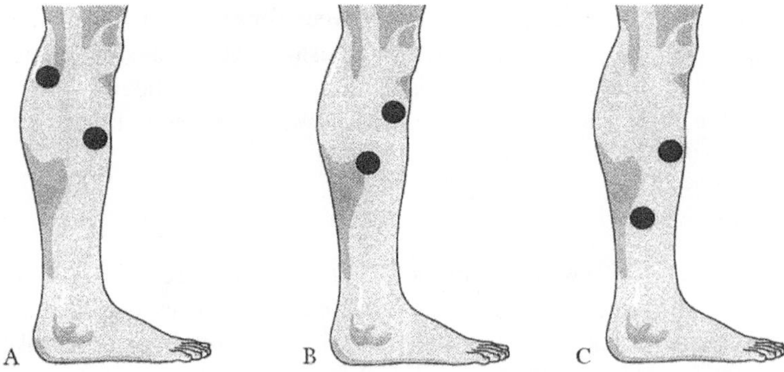

Figure 7.4. Possible electrode configurations that can elicit dorsiflexion of the ankle during swing phase of gait.

unaffected side. The stimulator emitted electrical pulses of 300 μs in duration at a frequency of 40 pps. The subjects were divided into two groups: one group received FES and ten physical therapy sessions (FES group) and the other group received ten physical therapy sessions only (control group). These sessions were provided over the first 4 weeks of the trial. Unfortunately, the authors did not describe the duration and frequency of use of the stimulator by the patients in their home and community environments.

Assessments of 10 m walking velocity and the physiological cost index [(heart rate while walking–resting heart rate)/walking speed] were made at baseline, at 4 to 5 weeks, and at 12 to 13 weeks. For those subjects using the stimulation, walking velocity and the physiological cost index measures were made with and without stimulation. An increase in walking speed was observed in 14 of the 16 FES subjects with the stimulation turned on at the end of the trial as compared with walking without stimulation at the beginning. The physiological cost index demonstrated a similar pattern of change, with 11 of the 16 FES subjects having a lower index at the end of the trial with the stimulation as compared to the start of the trial when not stimulated. The control group that received ten sessions of physical therapy did not experience any significant changes in walking speed or in the physiological cost index (53). Like the Liberson et al. case series (1), only a few of the subjects (3 out of 16) experienced a carryover effect by demonstrating an increased walking speed without the stimulation after the 12-week trial. By not monitoring the subjects' activity with the stimulation (e.g., the amount of continuous walking), we do not know if the improvements seen in the FES group were related to how the device was used by these subjects. It is possible, therefore, that even greater improvements could have been made if the FES subjects had a standardized program of daily use of the stimulation that included walking for least 20 minutes.

Multiple Sclerosis

The use of electrical stimulation to provide dorsiflexion assist during gait in people with multiple sclerosis has not been evaluated in a randomized trial. Taylor et al. (54) reported on the clinical use of stimulating ankle dorsiflexion in 21 people with multiple sclerosis. They used the stimulation in the same manner as described in their study in people after stroke (53). As mentioned above, an important piece of information missing from this report is how much these subjects used the stimulation each day. Using a within-subject design, however, stimulating ankle dorsiflexion significantly improved walking speed by 16% and reduced the physiological cost index by 24% over nonstimulation walking after approximately 18 weeks of training. This report, therefore, demonstrates that further investigation of stimulating ankle dorsiflexion is certainly warranted, and that its clinical use should not be discouraged.

Incomplete Spinal Cord Injury

Electrical stimulation of dorsiflexion has also been studied clinically in people with incomplete spinal cord injury (54–56). In these uncontrolled, pre–post training studies, ankle dorsiflexion was stimulated as described above for stroke and multiple sclerosis, but in some subjects the quadriceps femoris/tibial nerve, hamstrings, or gluteus medius were additionally stimulated to provide knee extension during stance, knee flexion during swing, or pelvic stability during stance. Wieler et al. (55) performed a mulitcenter study and followed 31 subjects for an average of 51 weeks. All subjects could stand, and all but one subject could ambulate some distance without FES. The authors measured the walking speed of subjects throughout the follow-up period with and without the FES system activated. Unfortunately, as in the studies of stroke and multiple sclerosis, the daily use of the electrical stimulation was not described or quantified. The initial walking speed of 0.46 m per second increased significantly by 0.14 m per second over the training period. The slowest walkers, at or below approximately 0.5 m per second, demonstrated the largest percent changes (70%) in walking speed. The faster walkers, at or above approximately 1.0 m per second, demonstrated smaller percentage changes (20%) in walking speed, and by the end of the study, the electrical stimulation no longer increased walking speed due to a possible training effect. The increase in walking speed was explained by an increase in stride length without a change in gait-cycle duration.

Taylor et al. (54) saw similar increases in walking speed in eight subjects, and also demonstrated a decrease in the physiological cost index from 1.06 to 0.84 heartbeats per meter walked. In all, these studies demonstrated that stimulation of the ankle dorsiflexors and other select lower extremity muscles during gait can provide a significant orthotic benefit by increasing walking speed in people with incomplete spinal cord injury, although the effect may be reduced with people who have faster walking speeds (>1.0 m per second).

Cerebral Palsy

Several studies have used electrical stimulation of the lower extremities to improve gait performance in children with cerebral palsy. Carmick (57,58) reported a series of case studies in which she used NMES of the triceps surae combined with motor training in three children with spastic hemiplegic CP to improve walking function. One of the children was 21 months of age and had been receiving physical therapy using a neurodevelopmental treatment approach since he was 7 months old. At the age of 21 months, this child walked with excessive lateral external rotation of the left leg and toe-walked. For the next 5 months the child was treated with NMES to the tibialis anterior during walking activities (triggered during swing phase of gait) using a stimulus frequency of between 30 and 35 pps and a pulse duration of 300 μs. The stimulation amplitude was set to achieve a visible, fused muscle contraction. After 5 months of stimulation of the tibialis anterior, the subject had only achieved an intermittent heel strike and foot-flat during early to mid-stance and demonstrated no carryover to walking without the NMES.

When the child was 26 months of age, Carmick (57) added stimulation of the triceps surae during phase-appropriate portions of gait using a hand-held trigger switch. She observed during the second treatment session that while the triceps surae was stimulated. the child's foot achieved a plantigrade position during stance. This effect, however, was only intermittent, and after several more months of trial and error, it was observed that when only the triceps surae was stimulated, the child attained a plantigrade position during stance and was able to shift his weight onto the left leg. These effects were reported to last for a few days after the weekly training session (15 minutes of stimulation during standing and gait). This case report demonstrates an intriguing concept that stimulation of the triceps surae during the stance phase of gait will produce a more normal foot position during stance as opposed to the traditional approach of stimulating the tibialis anterior during the swing phase.

This concept of stimulating the triceps surae for increasing the frequency of heel strike at initial contact and plantigrade foot position during stance was corroborated by Comeaux et al. (59). In this study, 14 children with CP were monitored through four, 4-week phases of treatment: a pretreatment phase, NMES to the triceps surae, NMES of the tibialis anterior and triceps surae, and a post-treatment phase. At three time points in each treatment phase, the degree of ankle dorsiflexion at initial contact was measured during gait. To minimize the influence of a possible ordering effect between the two stimulation treatment phases, half of the children underwent stimulation of the triceps surae first, and the other half had stimulation of the triceps surae and tibialis anterior first. The stimulation parameters reported included a pulse frequency of 32 pps, a ramp-on time of 0.5 seconds, stimulation amplitude set to elicit a visible muscle contraction, and the delivery of the electrical stimulation controlled by a hand-held trigger switch. Data analysis revealed that both treatments (stimulation of the triceps surae with or without stimulation of the tibialis anterior) improved the amount of dorsiflexion at heel strike equivalently. In addition, a carryover effect was present 4 weeks after treatment withdrawal.

Contrary to the observations by Carmick (57,58) and the data of Comeaux et al. (59) that stimulation of the triceps surae increased dorsiflexion at initial contact during gait, Pierce et al. (60) showed that stimulation of the triceps surae did not improve ankle position at initial contact using three-dimensional motion analysis in a case series on two subjects. Alternatively, they found that stimulation of the tibialis anterior or both tibialis anterior and triceps surae increased dorsiflexion at initial contact. Obviously, further studies are needed to clarify the effects of electrical stimulation on gait in children with CP; however, electrical stimulation does appear to have a role in the treatment of gait dysfunction in CP.

Functional Electrical Stimulation and Locomotor Training

Another new area of research has arisen out of earlier studies of FES for gait correction. The focus of this research is to investigate the effects of combining FES and locomotor training on gait outcomes after stroke and incomplete SCI. Bogataj et al. (61) reported on the use of multichannel FES plus conventional rehabilitation of gait in people with severe hemiplegia (requiring weight-bearing assistance of one or two people for ambulation). Subjects were divided into two groups. One group received FES plus conventional rehabilitation for 3 weeks, followed by conventional rehabilitation alone for 3 weeks. The second group received these same treatments, but in reverse order. FES was administered to up to six muscle groups to promote phase-appropriate ankle dorsiflexion/plantar flexion, knee flexion/extension, hip extension and pelvic stabilization, and elbow extension (to break flexion synergy if present). Stimulation parameters were fixed at a pulse frequency of 30 pps and pulse duration of 200 μs using a rectangular monophasic waveform. Individual foot switches for each channel triggered the onset of stimulation. During the FES sessions, the subjects walked on a 100-m walkway with a therapist's support, and each session ranged from 30 minutes to 1 hour in duration. The results of this study showed that the combined effects of FES and conventional rehabilitation on gait speed, stride length, and Fugl-Meyer score were greater than the effects of conventional rehabilitation alone.

In a slightly different treatment paradigm, Hesse et al. (62) combined multichannel FES with bodyweight-supported treadmill ambulation and compared it to conventional rehabilitation in a group of non-independent ambulatory people with hemiplegia. Seven subjects participated in a single-case research study design (A1-B-A2) during which the A1 phase had 15 treadmill/FES sessions, the B phase had 15 conventional rehabilitation sessions, and the A2 phase had another 15 treadmill/FES sessions. All subjects had strokes more than 3 months previously (range, 13 to 41 weeks). Stimulation was applied by four to six channels and triggered by three different foot switches (heel, lateral metatarsals, medial metatarsals) to activate the ankle dorsiflexors, knee flexors/extensors, hip extensors/abductors, abdominals, or shoulder/elbow extensors. Not all muscle groups were stimulated in each subject. The stimulus pulse duration ranged from 100 to 500 μs and the pulse frequency from 20 to 30 pps. The main outcome measures were the functional ambulation category and 10 m over-ground walking velocity. The functional ambulation category improved during the A1 and A2 phases (treadmill/FES), and remained stable during the B phase (conventional rehabilitation). At the beginning of the study the subjects had functional ambulation categories that ranged from unable to walk to needing continuous or intermittent support from one person for balance and coordination. At the end of the study, the functional ambulation categories ranged from requiring verbal supervision to being completely independent. Additionally, there was an 85% increase in over-ground gait velocity after the A1 phase, a 1% increase after the B phase, and a further 77% increase after the A2 phase. Both of these studies presented exciting possibilities for combining FES with rehabilitation therapies for non-independent ambulatory people with hemiplegia after stroke. However, caution should be exercised with regard to overinterpreting these studies, because neither of them were randomized, controlled trials. Finally, the technology and skill required to use such complex multichannel systems will preclude the widespread use of this technology.

The combined use of bodyweight-supported treadmill locomotion and FES has also been explored in people after incomplete SCI. Field-Fote (63) studied people with chronic (>12 months) incomplete SCI of ASIA C classification (presence of sensory and motor function below level of the lesion). These subjects also demonstrated asymmetric lower-extremity strength and function such that they could advance the stronger limb to take a step. Eighteen subjects completed a 36-session (3 days per week for 12 weeks) program of FES-assisted treadmill locomotion. Each session was a maximum of 1.5 hours in duration, and the subject was allowed to determine the duration of his or her own walk/rest bouts. Electrical stimulation was delivered to the common peroneal nerve during terminal stance to elicit a flexion withdrawal response to assist with stepping using the weaker limb. The stimulation pulse frequency was 50 pps, the pulse duration was 1 ms, and each train of pulses was 500 ms in duration. Before training, over-ground walking velocity was 0.12 m per second, and 6 of the 18 subjects needed manual assistance to advance the weaker limb. After training, over-ground walking velocity increased to 0.21 m per second, and only 2 of the 18 subjects needed manual assistance to advance the weaker limb. Four of the subjects in this study lived locally and were available for long-term follow-up at 2 months and 1 year post-training. Three of these subjects either maintained or improved their over-ground walking velocity. The subject that did not maintain her walking velocity had been not able to ambulate for an extended period secondary to a revision surgery for cervical decompression.

The Field-Fote (63) study shows that FES can be used in combination with bodyweight-supported treadmill locomotion to improve over-ground walking velocity; however, no control group was used, and it is possible that the same results could have been obtained using either treatment alone. Electrical stimulation to elicit a flexion-withdrawal response can provide two advantages to the clinician: a reduction in personnel needed to perform the training because no manual assistance is necessary to advance the weaker limb, and only one channel of stimulation is necessary to elicit the response. Similar results have also been reported for acute, incomplete SCI (64). Researchers have just begun to explore the combination of FES and task-specific training (e.g., locomotor training on the treadmill) to improve function. Look for more studies to appear in the near future that focus on examining the use of combination therapies in people with stroke and SCI.

Functional Electrical Stimulation and Complete Spinal Cord Injury

Electrical stimulation to replace lost lower-extremity function after complete SCI has been limited primarily to use in experimental settings. There are two main types of lower extremity stimulation systems that have been used for standing and ambulation: surface electrode systems and implanted electrode systems (65,66). Restoration of standing and rudimentary locomotion has been achieved in people with complete thoracic-level SCI using between two and eight channels of stimulation, a walker or other assistive device, and ankle–foot orthoses. It has been suggested that for long-term use, implanted electrode systems would provide greater convenience, cosmesis, and reliability over surface electrode systems (65). In fact, children with complete motor SCI, after training and mastery of the system, were able to complete donning the system, stand and reach, high transfer, and inaccessible bathroom transfer faster and with less dependence than with standard knee-ankle-foot orthoses (KAFOs) (67). Although claims of superiority of the implanted systems may ultimately be true, surface and implanted electrode systems have not been directly compared in a controlled trial of lower extremity function and in terms of costs over a long period of time.

Currently only one system, the Parastep I System (Sigmedics, Inc., Fairborn, Ohio), has commercial marketing approval from the Food and Drug Administration. The Parastep I System uses two to six surface electrode channels to stimulate standing and gait when used in combination with assistive devices and ankle-foot orthoses. This system consists of a microprocessor-based NMES device, a belt-clipped battery pack, and a specially adapted walker that contains control switch modules used to regulate the initiation of muscle contractions (Fig. 7.5). The stimulator (Fig. 7.6A) has up to six output channels and produces a pulse with a width of 150 μs, an amplitude up to 300 mA, and a pulse frequency of 24 pps. The switch modules on the walker (Fig. 7.6B, C) allow the user to initiate the timing for standing, sitting, and stepping, and allow for the adjustment of the stimulation amplitude. Standing is typically achieved with simultaneous stimulation of the bilateral quadriceps femoris and gluteus maximus muscles. In some users, the lumbar paraspinals are also stimulated to increase trunk stability (66). Surface electrodes can be placed by the user over these sites and are reported to be reused for approximately 14 days (66). Stepping is achieved by activating the quadriceps of one leg while initiating a flexion withdrawal reflex in the opposite leg. The swing-phase is completed with activation of the quadriceps to extend the knee for heel strike.

In a study by Klose et al. (68) at the Miami Project to Cure Paralysis, training 3 days per week for 11 weeks with the Parastep system allowed an average of 115 m walked at an average pace of 5 m per minute for 15 patients with complete SCI. A similar study performed in Italy trained patients for 85 sessions over 4 months with a mean daily walking time of 90 minutes and achieved an average of 444 m walked at an average pace of 14.5 m per minute (66). This suggests that the frequency of training and possibly its intensity may influence locomotor outcomes of

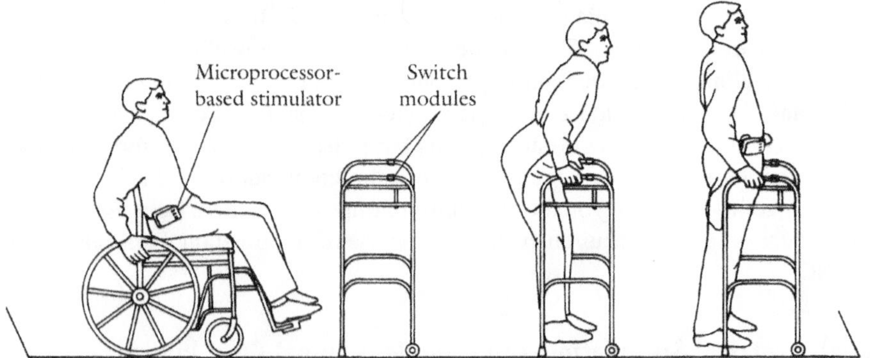

Figure 7.5. The Parastep I System (Sigmedics, Inc., Fairborn, Ohio) for standing and ambulation in people with spinal cord injuries. Microprocessor-based stimulator is belt mounted, and switch modules are located on the handles of the walker.

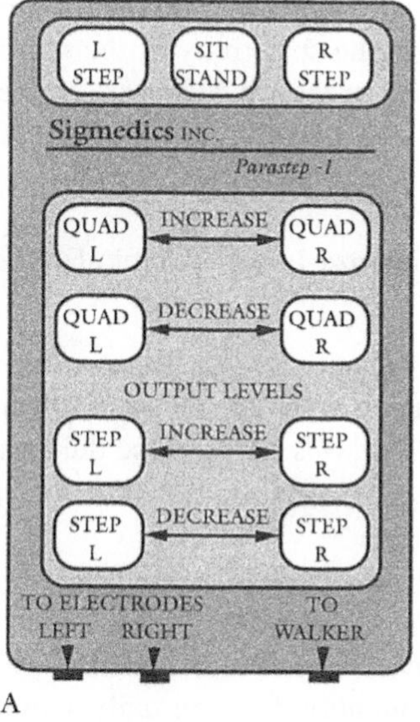

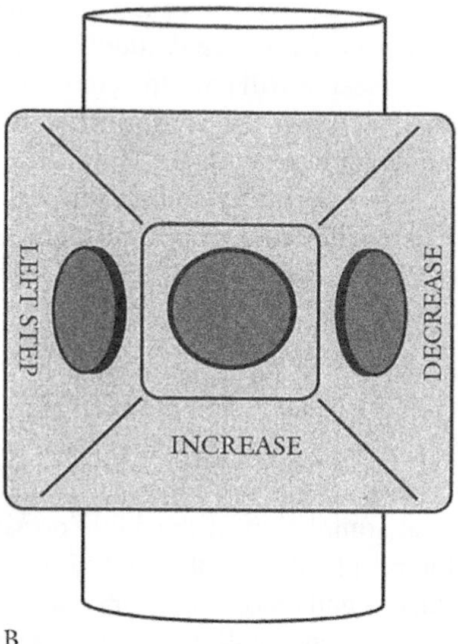

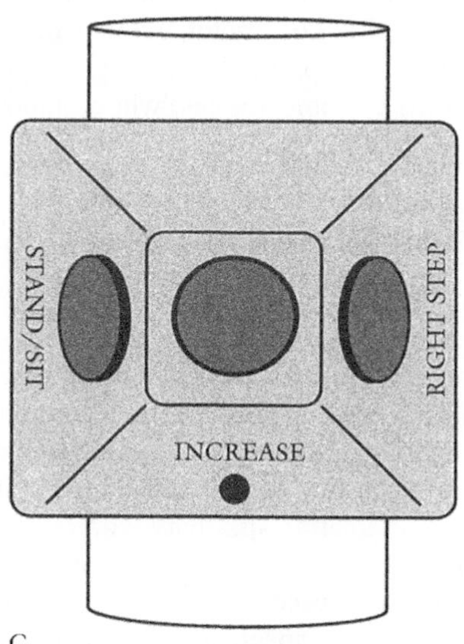

Figure 7.6. Parastep I System. **A:** Control panel of the Parastep I system stimulator. **B:** Parastep I system left switch module mounted on the walker for manual control of the timing of stimulation for stepping on the left. **C:** Parastep I system right switch module mounted on the walker for manual control of the timing of stimulation for stepping on the right and controlling stimulation for sitting and standing.

distance and speed. As of April 2003, the Centers for Medicare and Medicaid Services announced it will pay for approximately 80% of the system acquisition costs and the costs for undergoing the required instruction, therapy, and gait training (about 32 sessions) for qualified patients. Training with the Parastep I System is available at many of the major SCI rehabilitation hospitals in the United States (for a list, see the Sigmedics website (68a)).

Future developments in the area of FES for standing and locomotion will largely depend on the development of components that have long-term reliability and that can use closed-loop feedback to aid in the control of the movement. The use of implantable devices will obviously improve the cosmesis, reduce don/doff times, and improve the selectivity of the muscles to be activated, but research will have to demonstrate that the costs of these systems are outweighed by the functional, physiological, and psychological benefits before they will ever be available commercially to large groups of patients.

Literature-based Guidelines for Using Electrical Stimulation to Improve Lower Extremity Function in People with Stroke, Spinal Cord Injury, and Cerebral Palsy

1. Electrical stimulation can be used to improve force production and active range of motion in people after stroke. Stimulation parameters used were a pulse duration between 200 and 300 μs and a pulse frequency of 30 pps. The ratio of on:off time was 1:2, and the duration of each treatment was approximately 20 minutes. Treatments were performed 5 to 6 days per week for 4 weeks.
2. Electrical stimulation of the ankle dorsiflexors can be used as an orthotic to increase gait speed in people after stroke, SCI, or with MS. Stimulation was triggered to activate the tibialis anterior and peroneals during swing phase by a footswitch. Pulse durations were 300 μs and were delivered at 40 pps. Subjects applied the stimulation for their daily activities.
3. Electrical stimulation of lower extremity muscle can be used in combination with locomotor training to improve over-ground walking velocity without stimulation in people after stroke and in those with incomplete SCI. Locomotor training included over-ground training or training while on the treadmill with partial body weight support. Stimulation of up to six muscle groups was performed in some studies, while others used a brief, high-intensity stimulus to elicit a flexion-withdrawal response to aid limb clearance during swing.

Neuromuscular Electrical Stimulation for Reduction of Spasticity

Muscle spasticity is a clinical phenomenon that is common after CNS disruption. Spasticity has been defined as a velocity-dependent increase in resistance to passive stretch, but many clinicians and scientists also use this term to describe flexion and extension spasms and posturing. The underlying neurophysiologic mechanisms of this phenomenon have not been fully described, but spasticity is thought to be the result of an imbalance of excitatory and inhibitory inputs on the alpha motoneurons such that the net effect results in increased excitability. One problem with most investigations on treating spasticity with electrical stimulation is the lack of use of quantitative methods for measuring the degree of spasticity. This section of the chapter only addresses selected studies that have used quantitative methods to measure spasticity.

Although there are several plausible mechanisms that may explain how NMES reduces spasticity, the exact mechanism has eluded researchers. One possible mechanism is that stimulation of the antagonist muscle to the spastic muscle excites the large-diameter Ia muscle spindle afferents, which in turn excite spinal inhibitory interneurons, which then inhibit the alpha motoneurons (Fig. 7.7). Stimulation of the spastic muscle has also been proposed to reduce spasticity by simply fatiguing the muscle or through the antidromic propagation of stimulated action potentials that may travel up recurrent collateral axons, which are believed to synapse on spinal inhibitory interneurons (Renshaw cells) that will inhibit the alpha motoneuron (see Fig. 7.8).

Neuromuscular Electrical Stimulation of the Antagonist Muscle to Reduce Spasticity of the Agonist

There are only a few studies that have used objective measures of spasticity to test whether NMES of the antagonist muscle will reduce spasticity in the agonist muscle group. Most of the studies have stimulated the tibialis anterior in an attempt to reduce spasticity in the plantarflexors

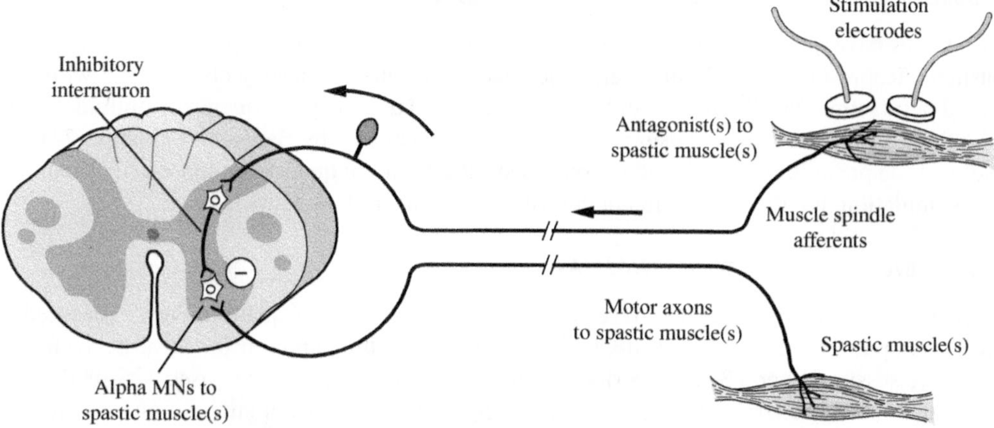

Figure 7.7. Proposed mechanism of action of antagonist stimulation to control spasticity. Stimulation of antagonists Ia afferents reciprocally inhibits motoneurons to spastic muscles.

(69–72). Carnstam and colleagues (69) stimulated the tibialis anterior for 300 ms each second (500-μs pulse duration, 30 pps frequency) for 10 minutes. They measured the force of Achilles tendon reflex immediately before and after the stimulation and found that in some of the subjects the force of the reflex was diminished after stimulation.

Mirbagheri et al. (72) performed a study on the long-term effects of FES for foot-drop on spasticity in people with incomplete SCI. They had developed a methodology to identify the intrinsic (viscoelastic properties of passive tissues and active muscle fibers) and reflex (changes in muscle activation due to sensory responses to stretch) contributions to dynamic stiffness about the ankle. Subjects used FES systems for ambulation for at least 16 months before they were retested. For FES-assisted ambulation, the tibialis or quadriceps muscles were activated during swing or stance, respectively. Mirbagheri et al. observed decreases in both the intrinsic (45%) and reflex (55%) dynamic stiffness in all four subjects that used FES for longer than 16 months.

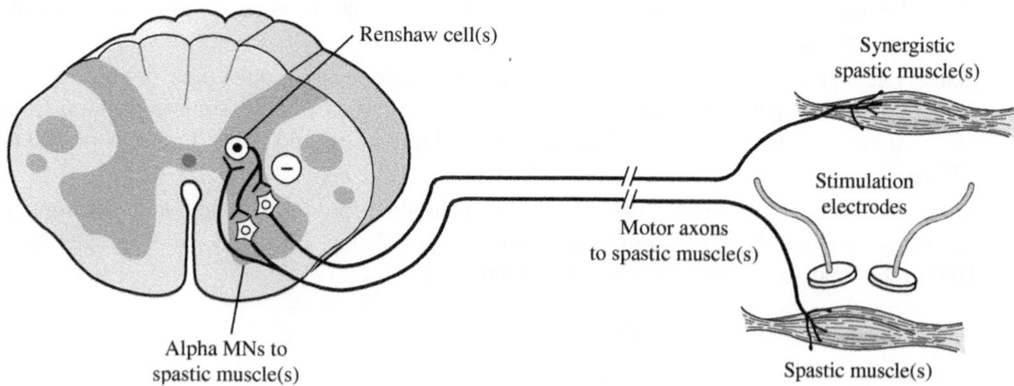

Figure 7.8. Proposed mechanism of action of agonist stimulation to control spasticity. Stimulation over the spastic muscles antidromically activates motoneurons to the spastic muscles. Action potentials propagated toward the spinal cord activate inhibitory interneurons (Renshaw cells), which inhibit alpha motoneurons to the spastic muscles.

Neuromuscular Electrical Stimulation of the Spastic Muscle to Decrease Spasticity

Few studies have quantitatively measured the effects of stimulating the spastic muscle to reduce spasticity. Robinson et al. (73) stimulated the quadriceps muscles in subjects with SCI with a 2.5 second on:off time for 20 minutes (pulse duration of 500 μs, 20 pps frequency, amplitude of 100 mA). Spasticity was quantified using a pendulum test developed by Bajd and Vodovnik (74). The results of the pendulum test showed decreased spasticity of the quadriceps muscles immediately after stimulation, but this effect did not persist when measured 24 hours later.

SENSORY-LEVEL STIMULATION TO DECREASE SPASTICITY

A few studies have used sensory-level electrical stimulation and quantitatively measured its effects on spasticity. Levin and Hui-Chan (75) stimulated the common peroneal nerve for 15, 60-minute sessions over a 3-week period in people with hemiplegia. They used 125-μs duration pulses in a continuous train at a frequency of 99 pps. After 3 weeks of stimulation, inhibition of the soleus H-reflex, increases in dorsiflexion voluntary force, and reductions in the stretch reflex of the triceps surae were observed.

Dewald et al. (76) studied the effects of sensory stimulation over the biceps brachii muscle on the torque responses to passive flexion and extension in nine subjects with poststroke hemiplegia. Sensory stimulation was performed for 10 to 15 minutes at a 20 pps frequency and pulse duration of 100 μs. In seven out of nine subjects, the stimulation of the skin over the spastic muscle reduced the peak torque from passively stretching the flexors and extensors and increased the degree of stretch needed to initiate the reflex response for at least 30 minutes after stimulation.

Literature-based Guidelines for the Use of Electrical Stimulation to Reduce Spasticity

Because few studies have used objective means to quantify spasticity, stimulation parameters have sometimes varied greatly between studies. The guidelines presented below, therefore, mostly include only general stimulation parameters.

1. Stimulation of the antagonist muscle can be used to reduce the spasticity of the agonist muscle. Typical pulse durations (200–600 μs) and frequencies (20–50 pps) for motor-level stimulation have been used. Stimulation can be applied cyclically or can be used in a functional manner (e.g., during gait).
2. Stimulation of the spastic muscle can be used to reduce spasticity in the quadriceps muscles. The pulse duration was 500 μs, pulse frequency was 20 pps, the on:off ratio was 1:1 (2.5 seconds each), and the duration of the session was 20 minutes.
3. Sensory-level stimulation of the afferents over the antagonist or agonist (spastic) muscle can be use to reduce spasticity. Sensory stimulation was applied in a continuous fashion from 10 to 60 minutes, using a pulse frequency from 20 to 99 pps, and pulse durations of 100 to 125 μs.
4. The above stimulation characteristics have been shown to produce immediate reductions in spasticity that may last from minutes to a few hours. Long-term FES users (greater than 16 months) may have longer lasting reductions in spasticity (71).

CLINICAL CASE STUDIES

Case 1

A 54-year-old woman had a hemorrhagic stroke 1 week ago as a result of high blood pressure. She presents with left hemiplegia. In her left upper extremity she has 2+/5 strength in finger, wrist, and elbow flexion/extension, but she has only trace contraction strength (1/5) in the deltoid and scapular muscles. When sitting up, her left shoulder demonstrates a positive sulcus sign, indicating that there is glenohumeral joint subluxation. Plain film radiographs quantify a 10-mm increase in glenohumeral joint subluxation on the left side when compared to the right. From your examination, you conclude that weakness in the deltoid and supraspinatus muscles is putting abnormal strain on the passive ligamentous structures of the glenohumeral joint and is causing subluxation. It is common to have flaccid paralysis followed by partial recovery after stroke. Some of your goals as a clinician are to prevent further strain on the passive ligamentous structures of the glenohumeral joint by ensuring proper positioning and splinting, and to increase the ability to activate the muscular support system around the glenohumeral joint.

Interventions

1. Therapeutic exercise to address upper extremity range of motion and muscle strength.
2. Retraining for ADL.
3. Task-oriented motor training for the upper extremity.
4. Implement and teach caregivers proper positioning and splinting use to prevent further subluxation.
5. Neuromuscular facilitation techniques to enhance volitional activation of the musculature around the glenohumeral joint
6. NMES of the middle deltoid, posterior deltoid, and supraspinatus to reduce glenohumeral joint subluxation.

Detailed Electrotherapeutic Intervention

Mode of stimulation: Tetanic muscular contraction; pulse frequency approximately 30 to 40 pps; pulse duration 200 to 600 μs; current amplitude enough to produce a palpable reduction of the glenohumeral subluxation

Duration of stimulation: The duration of the stimulation sessions and the on:off times will be progressively increased based on whether full reduction of the subluxation can be attained at the end of each session. The duration of the sessions will start at 1.5 hours and will progress to 6 hours, and the on:off times will be initiated at 10:12 seconds and gradually progress to 30:2 seconds. NMES should be performed 5 to 7 days per week for approximately 6 weeks.

Type of stimulator: Portable NMES so client can attend other therapies and activities while NMES is reducing the subluxation.

Electrode placement: Channel 1—two small electrodes placed along the length of the middle deltoid; channel 2—two small electrodes placed over the motor points of the posterior deltoid and supraspinatus muscles.

Rationale

This NMES program was devised based on the study by Faghri et al. (28) with one modification: the addition of NMES to the middle deltoid (31). NMES to the affected muscle may enhance volitional activation and therefore reduce the amount of glenohumeral joint subluxation. In addition, the NMES will provide an orthotic benefit and reduce any strain on the passive supportive structures and thus prevent further increases in subluxation.

Outcomes

1. Plain film radiographs to quantify the side-to-side difference in glenohumeral joint subluxation
2. Fugl-Meyer test for upper extremity function
3. Wolf Motor Function Test
4. Amount of external shoulder rotation before onset of shoulder pain
5. Manual muscle testing
6. Ability to complete selected activities of daily life tasks for the upper extremity

Case 2

In the case presented above, this client also has left lower extremity impairments. In her left lower extremity, manual muscle testing reveals the following: hip flexion 3/5, hip extension 3+/5, knee flexion 2+/5, knee extension 4/5, ankle plantarflexion 2/5, ankle dorsiflexion 2−/5. She can ambulate with contact guard assistance with a wide-base quad cane; however, she demonstrates left sided leg circumduction during swing to compensate for impaired foot clearance, and she has a greatly reduced walking speed. From your clinical examination you conclude that the weakness and the impaired ability to control some of the lower extremity musculature is contributing to her impaired gait. Some of your goals as a clinician are to improve the patient's strength and ability to voluntarily activate the impaired musculature during tasks such as walking.

Interventions

1. Therapeutic exercise to address range of motion and muscle strength
2. Retraining of activities of daily life tasks that involve the lower extremities
3. Task-oriented motor training of the lower extremity
4. Neuromuscular facilitation techniques to enhance volitional activation of selected musculature
5. NMES for strengthening selected lower extremity muscles
6. NMES during gait to the muscles that control ankle dorsiflexion to improve foot clearance during swing phase

Detailed Electrotherapeutic Intervention of NMES for Dorsiflexion Assist

Mode of stimulation: tetanic muscular contraction; pulse frequency approximately 30 to 50 pps; pulse duration 200 to 600 μs; current amplitude high enough to produce dorsiflexion with a balanced amount of inversion and eversion

Duration of stimulation: total of at least 20 minutes of stimulation during locomotion on a treadmill, and an additional 20 minutes of stimulation during over-ground locomotion performed 5 to 7 days per week while in inpatient rehabilitation; the patient or a caregiver, if capable, may be trained to don and doff the system to allow stimulation during all ambulatory activity throughout the day after discharge

Type of stimulator: portable NMES with an external trigger system (either handheld or footswitch)

Electrode placement: a single channel with two small electrodes placed over the motor points of the tibialis anterior and the peroneus longus

Rationale

The main rationale is to use NMES for dorsiflexion assist during gait. Massed practice of locomotion on the treadmill and over ground may increase the representation of the impaired limb within the primary motor cortex and thus increase its movement capabilities. The basis for the use of NMES for dorsiflexion assist comes partially from Burridge (53), and the main goal is to achieve a carryover effect so that gait is improved when the stimulation is not present. In the study by Burridge (53), no information was reported on the actual use of the electrical stimulation, and the lack of controlled training conditions may have influenced the result that only 3 out of 16 subjects demonstrated a carryover effect.

Outcomes

1. Walking velocity
2. Physiological cost index
3. Fugl–Meyer test for lower extremity function

Case 3

A 29-year-old man sustained a cervical spinal cord injury as a result of a traumatic blow to the posterior cervical spine. Initially the patient had quadriparesis, but as the inflammatory response subsided, nearly all upper extremity function and left lower extremity function returned (ASIA C). Twelve weeks have passed since the initial injury, and the patient is able to initiate a step with the left lower extremity, but has minimal ability to do so on the right due to poor hip, knee, and ankle flexion. He can ambulate 10 m in 83 seconds (~0.12 m per second) using a walker and wearing an ankle-foot orthosis on the right. Your patient's main goal is to be able to ambulate independently for short distances in the home environment in functionally reasonable timeframes.

Interventions

1. Therapeutic exercise to address range of motion and muscle strength of the right lower extremity
2. Task-oriented motor training/locomotor training on the treadmill and over ground using body weight support
3. NMES for strengthening selected lower extremity muscles
4. Electrical stimulation to the sural or common peroneal nerves to cause a lower extremity flexion withdrawal response during terminal stance phase of gait while performing locomotor training on the treadmill or over ground

Detailed Electrotherapeutic Intervention of NMES for Dorsiflexion Assist

Mode of stimulation: brief sensory stimulation; pulse frequency 50 to 100 pps; pulse duration 200 to 1000 μs; current amplitude high enough to elicit a flexion withdrawal response

Duration of stimulation: on time is brief (<1 second) and is determined by how long the external trigger is held in the on position.

Type of stimulator: portable NMES with a handheld external trigger system

Electrode placement: a single channel with two small electrodes placed over the sural nerve distribution on the lateral aspect of the heel and foot; a single channel with two small electrodes placed over the common peroneal nerve

Rationale

The use of a single channel of stimulation to elicit a flexion withdrawal response to assist the advancement of the limb during swing phase is useful because it reduces the complexity of stimulation with multiple channels, and it allows for activation of the hip flexors, which are otherwise inaccessible to surface NMES. This treatment uses a task-oriented motor training approach and has been shown by Field-Fote (63) to improve over-ground walking velocity in this specific population.

Outcomes

1. Walking velocity
2. Lower extremity manual muscle test scores
3. Six-minute walk test
4. Berg balance scale

SUMMARY

This chapter reviewed the theoretical concepts, general application principles, and the evidence for using NMES to control movement and posture in people with CNS dysfunction. There is a wealth of literature on the use of NMES to control movement and posture, and it is continually growing. In the time from publication of the last edition of the book, more evidence has mounted that NMES for the control of movement and posture can improve functional outcomes in certain patient populations. This evidence base is constantly growing, and clinicians are encouraged to keep up with changes as the evidence evolves. The almost universal access to the Internet makes this task easier than it has ever been in the past. Through continued efforts by clinicians and researchers, our knowledge of how to treat CNS dysfunction with NMES should continue to grow in order to better restore the functional capabilities of our clients.

LABORATORY EXERCISES

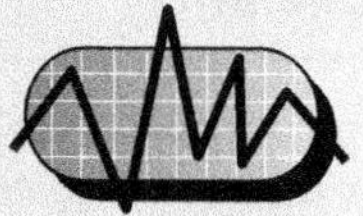

Exercise 1

Electrical stimulation of dorsiflexion with balanced inversion and eversion

Objective

Find the proper electrode placement to get ankle dorsiflexion without either excessive inversion or eversion using a single stimulation channel

Equipment

Electrical stimulator that allows control of pulse frequency and pulse duration; two to four small, self-adhesive electrodes (2.5 × 2.5 cm or 5 × 5 cm)

Description

1. Palpate for the common peroneal nerve as it courses around the fibular neck. Place one electrode over the common peroneal nerve at this location.
2. Place the second electrode over the motor point for the tibialis anterior. Use a motor point chart or electrical stimulation to locate the motor point.
3. Connect the electrodes to the stimulator, set the pulse duration to 300 μs, pulse frequency to 30 pps, on time to 5 seconds with a 2-second ramp on, and off time of 20 seconds.
4. Turn up the current amplitude to evoke a motor response.
5. Did you get dorsiflexion with a balanced inversion and eversion?
6. If you had too much inversion, locate the motor point of the peroneous longus muscle and move the electrode that is over the common peroneal nerve to the peroneous longus motor point. Test the stimulation again to see if you get a balanced dorsiflexion.
7. You may need to move the electrodes several times to find the optimal placement that produces a balanced dorsiflexion.

Exercise 2

Electrical stimulation of the supraspinatus and posterior deltoid muscles for subluxation

Objective

Find the proper electrode placement to get activation of the supraspinatus and posterior deltoid muscles without activation of the upper trapezius using a single channel of stimulation

Equipment

Electrical stimulator that allows control of pulse frequency and pulse duration; two to four small, self-adhesive electrodes (5 × 5 cm); scissors

Description

1. Locate by palpation where the acromion process intersects with the spine of the scapula.

2. Find the point on the spine of the scapula that is approximately 5 to 10 cm from the acromion process. This is the approximate location of the supraspinatus motor point. Confirm position by stimulation of this motor point and place an electrode over this point.
3. Use a motor point chart or electrical stimulation to locate the posterior deltoid motor point, and place an electrode over this point.
4. Connect the electrodes to the stimulator, set the pulse duration to 300 μs, pulse frequency to 25 pps, on time to 10 seconds with a 2-second ramp on, and off time to 20 seconds.
5. Turn up the current amplitude to evoke a motor response.
6. Did you get activation of the upper trapezius? In a person with glenohumeral joint subluxation, you do not want to activate the upper trapezius because the upward/lateral rotation of the scapula may cause further subluxation of the glenohumeral joint.
7. To reduce the activation of the upper trapezius, cut the 5 × 5 cm electrode that is over the supraspinatus motor point into a 2.5 × 5 cm electrode (be sure not to cut the lead wire within the electrode).
8. Replace the electrode so that the longer portion of the electrode is over the spine of the scapula. This smaller electrode should avoid stimulating the upper trapezius while still activating the supraspinatus.
9. Turn up the current amplitude to evoke a motor response to see if your adjustment was correct.

SELF-STUDY QUESTIONS

For answers, see Appendix B.

1. What is the general definition of functional electrical stimulation?
2. Which two motor control theories may be used as a foundation for treatment effects related to FES?
3. What are some important patient considerations that need to be examined before incorporating NMES for the control of movement into a treatment program?
4. Which five medical conditions are most commonly treated with FES?
5. Which impairments may need to be addressed before using NMES for the control of movement?
6. Which stimulator control features are ideal for FES applications?
7. Which intervention is more effective than NMES at halting idiopathic scoliosis curves that are between 20 degrees and 45 degrees?
8. The glenohumeral joint relies most on which two muscles to prevent inferior humeral head subluxation?
9. What are the two major drawbacks to using slings to prevent or control glenohumeral joint subluxation?
10. Which alternative muscle group can be stimulated to decrease glenohumeral joint subluxation?
11. How long should NMES for glenohumeral joint subluxation be applied each day?
12. Which two treatments produced a synergistic effect in the recovery of hand function in people with poststroke hemiplegia?
13. Does the evidence show that EMG-triggered NMES of wrist and finger extension could be performed in a clinically feasible timeframe to improve hand function?
14. Which two grasps can be produced with the implantable neuroprothesis studied by Peckham et al. (47)?
15. What motor level of spinal cord injury is appropriate for using the implantable neuroprothesis for restoration of grasp?
16. What are some of the problems associated with the Bionic Glove surface stimulation system for grasping function?
17. What were the two main effects reported by Burridge et al. (53) in the only randomized clinical trial of FES for the correction of dropped-foot in people with poststroke hemiplegia?
18. What was a major weakness of the Burridge et al. (53) study?
19. What are the two major limitations to using multichannel FES in nonfunctionally ambulatory people with poststroke hemiplegia?
20. List two factors that could make it possible to use FES as a training technique in patients with incomplete SCI or poststroke hemiplegia.

21. Describe how the ParaStep I System functions to produce standing and stepping.

22. Describe two types of electrode placements that can be used to reduce spasticity.

REFERENCES

1. Liberson W, Holmquest H, Scott M. Functional electrotherapy: stimulation of the common peroneal nerve synchronized with the swing phase of gait in hemiplegic subjects. *Arch Phys Med Rehabil.* 1961;42:202–205.
2. Nudo RJ, Milliken GW, Jenkins WM, et al. Use-dependent alterations of movement representations in primary motor cortex of adult squirrel monkeys. *J Neurosci.* 1996;16:785–807.
3. Biernaskie J, Chernenko G, Corbett D. Efficacy of rehabilitative experience declines with time after focal ischemic brain injury. *J Neurosci.* 2004;24:1245–1254.
4. Wolf SL, Blanton S, Baer H, et al. Repetitive task practice: s critical review of constraint-induced therapy in stroke. *Neurologist.* 2002:8:325–338.
5. Winstein CJ, Rose DK, Tan SM, et al. A randomized controlled comparison of upper-extremity rehabilitation strategies in acute stroke: a pilot study of immediate and long-term outcomes. *Arch Phys Med Rehabil.* 2004:85:620–628.
6. Lovely RG, Gregor R, Roy RR, et al. Effects of training on the recovery of full-weight bearing stepping in the adult spinal cat. *Exp Neurol.* 1986;92:421–435.
7. Wernig A, Müller S, Nanassy A, et al. Laufband locomotion with body weight support improved walking in persons with severe spinal cord injuries. *Paraplegia.* 1992;30:229–238.

7a. Sullivan KJ, Knowlton BJ, Dobkin BH. Step training with body weight support: effect of treadmill speed and practice paradigms on poststroke locomotor recovery. *Arch Phys Med Rehabil.* 2002;83:683–691.

8. Cauraugh J, Light K, Sangbum K, et al. Chronic motor dysfunction after stroke recovering wrist and finger extension by electromyography-triggered neuromuscular stimulation. *Stroke.* 2000: 31:1360–1364.
9. Brown JC, Axelgaard J, Howson DC. Multicenter trial of a noninvasive stimulation method for idiopathic scoliosis. *Spine.* 1984;9:382–387.
10. McCullough NC. Nonoperative treatment of idiopathic scoliosis using surface electrical stimulation. *Spine.* 1986;11:802–804.
11. Nachemson AL, Peterson LE. Effectiveness of treatment with a brace in girls who have adolescent idiopathic scoliosis: a prospective, controlled study based on data from the brace study of the scoliosis research society. *J Bone Joint Surg Am.* 1995;77-A:815–822.
12. Allington NJ, Bowen JR. Adolescent idiopathic scoliosis: treatment with the Wilmington Brace: a comparison of full-time and part-time use. *J Bone Joint Surg Am.* 1996;78-A:1056–1062.
13. Bradford DS, Tanguy A, Vanselow J. Surface electrical stimulation in the treatment of idiopathic scoliosis: preliminary results in 30 patients. *Spine.* 1983;8:757–764.
14. Swank SM, Brown JC, Jennings MV, et al. Lateral electrical surface stimulation in idiopathic scoliosis—experience in two private practices. *Spine.* 1989;14:1293–1295.
15. Fisher DA, Rapp GF, Emkes M. Idiopathic scoliosis: transcutaneous muscle stimulation versus the Milwaukee brace. *Spine.* 1987;12:987–991.
16. Goldberg C, Dowling FE, Fogarty EE, et al. Electro-spinal stimulation in children with adolescent and juvenile scoliosis. *Spine.* 1988;13:482–484.
17. O'Donnell CS, Bunnell WP, Betz RR, et al. Electrical stimulation in the treatment of idiopathic scoliosis. *Clin Orthop Relat Res.* 1988;229:107–113.
18. Durham JW, Moskowitz A, Whitney J. Surface electrical stimulation versus brace in treatment of idiopathic scoliosis. *Spine.* 1990;15:888–891.

19. Poulin de Courval L, Barsauskas A, Berenbaum B, et al. Painful shoulder in the hemiplegic and unilateral neglect. *Arch Phys Med Rehabil.* 1990;71:673–676.
20. Fitzgerald-Finch OP, Gibson IIJM. Subluxation of the shoulder in hemiplegia. *Age Aging.* 1975;4:16–18.
21. Najenson T, Pikielny SS. Malalignment of the glenohumeral joint following hemiplegia: a review of 500 cases. *Ann Phys Med.* 1965;8:96–99.
22. Taktoni Y. Observation of the subluxation shoulder in hemiplegia. *Phys Ther.* 1975;55:39–40.
23. Smith RG, Cruikshank JG, Shelagh D, et al. Malalignment of the shoulder after stroke. *Br Med J.* 1982;284:1224–1226.
24. Basmajian JV, Bazant FJ. Factors preventing downward dislocation of the adducted shoulder joint: an electromyographic and morphological study. *J Bone Joint Surg Am.* 1959;41:1182–1186.
25. Basmajian JV, Deluca CJ. *Muscles Alive: Their Function Revealed by Electromyography.* 5th ed. Baltimore, Md: William & Wilkins; 1985:239–276.
26. Brooke MM, de Lateur BJ, Diana-Rigby GC, et al. Shoulder subluxation in hemiplegia: effects of three different supports. *Arch Phys Med Rehabil.* 1991;72:583–586.
27. Baker LL, Parker K. Neuromuscular electrical stimulation of the muscles surrounding the shoulder. *Phys Ther.* 1986;66:78–85.
28. Faghri PD, Rodgers MM, Glaser RM, et al. The effects of functional electrical stimulation on shoulder subluxation, arm function recovery, and shoulder pain in hemiplegic stroke patients. *Arch Phys Med Rehabil.* 1994:75:73–79.
29. Chantraine A, Baribeault A, Uebelhart D. Gremion G. Shoulder pain and dysfunction in hemiplegia: effects of functional electrical stimulation. *Arch Phys Med Rehabil.* 1999:80:328–331.
30. Linn SL, Granat MH, Lees KR. Prevention of shoulder subluxation after stroke with electrical stimulation. *Stroke.* 1999:30:963–968.
31. Kobayashi H, Onishi H, Ihashi K, et al. Reduction in subluxation and improved muscle function of the hemiplegic shoulder joint after therapeutic electrical stimulation. *J Electromyogr Kinesiol.* 1999:9:327–336.
32. Wang RY, Chan RC, Tsai MW. Functional electrical simulation on chronic and acute hemiplegic shoulder subluxation. *Am J Phys Med Rehabil.* 2000:79:385–390.
33. Long C, Masciarelli V. An electrophysiological splint for the hand. *Arch Phys Med Rehabil.* 1963;44:499–503.
34. Rebersek S, Vodovnik L. Proportionally controlled functional electrical stimulation of the hand. *Arch Phys Med Rehabil.* 1973;54:378–382.
35. Merletti R, Acimovic R, Grobelnik S, et al. Electrophysiological orthosis for upper extremity in hemiplegia: feasibility study. *Arch Phys Med Rehabil.* 1975;56:507–513.
36. Baker LL, Yeh C, Wilson D, et al. Electrical stimulation of wrist and fingers for hemiplegic patients. *Phys Ther.* 1979:59:1495–1499.
37. Bowman BR, Baker LL, Waters RL. Positional feedback and electrical stimulation: an automated treatment for the hemiplegic wrist. *Arch Phys Med Rehabil.* 1979:60:497–502.
38. Chae J, Bethoux F, Bohine T, et al. Neuromuscular stimulation for upper extremity motor and functional recovery in acute hemiplegia. *Stroke.* 1998:29:975–979.
39. Powell J, Pandyan D, Granat M, et al. Electrical stimulation of wrist extensors in post stroke hemiplegia. *Stroke.* 1999:30:1384–1389.
40. Roby-Brami A, Fuchs S, Mokhtari M, et al. Reaching and grasping strategies in hemiparetic patients. *Motor Control.* 1997;1:72–91.
41. Francisco G, Chae J, Chawla H, et al. Electrogram-triggered neuromuscular stimulation for improving the arm function of acute stroke survivors: a randomized pilot study. *Arch Phys Med Rehabil.* 1998:79:570–575.
42. Cauraugh JH, Kim S. Two coupled motor recovery protocols are better than one: electromyogram-triggered neuromuscular stimulation and bilateral movements. *Stroke.* 2002;33:1589–1594.

43. Han BS, Jang SH, Chang Y, et al. Functional magnetic resonance image finding of cortical activation by neuromuscular electrical stimulation on wrist extensor muscles. *Am J Phys Med Rehabil.* 2003:82:17–20.

44. Scheker LR, Chesher SP, Ramirez S. Neuromuscular electrical stimulation and dynamic bracing as a treatment for upper-extremity spasticity in children with cerebral palsy. *J Hand Surg.* 1999:24B:226–232.

45. Wright PA, Granat MH. Therapeutic effects of functional electrical stimulation of the upper limb of eight children with cerebral palsy. *Dev Med Child Neurol.* 2000:42:724–727.

46. Hanson RW, Franklin MR. Sexual loss in relation to other functional losses for spinal cord injured males. *Arch Phys Med Rehabil.* 1976;57:291–293.

47. Peckham PH, Keight MW, Kilgore K, et al. Efficacy of an implanted neuroprosthesis for restoring hand grasp in tetraplegia: a mulitcenter study. *Arch Phys Med Rehabil.* 2001:82:1380–1388.

48. Creasey GH, Kilgore KL, Brown-Triolo DL, et al. Reduction of costs of disability using neuroprostheses. *Assist Technol.* 2000:12:67–75.

49. Popovic D, Stojanovic A, Pjanovic A, et al. Clinical evaluation of the bionic glove. *Arch Phys Med Rehabil.* 1999;80:299–304.

50. Alon G, McBride K. Persons with C5 or C6 tetraplegia achieve selected functional gains using a neuroprosthesis. *Arch Phys Med Rehabil.* 2003;84:119–124.

51. Merletti R, Zelaschi F, Latella D, et al. A control study of muscle force recovery in hemiparetic patients during treatment with functional electrical stimulation. *Scand J Rehab Med.* 1978; 10:147–154.

52. Winchester P, Montgomery J, Bowman, Hislop H. Effects of feedback stimulation training and cyclical electrical stimulation on knee extension in hemiparetic patients. *Phys Ther.* 1983;63:1096–1103.

53. Burridge JH, Taylor PN, Hagan SA, et al. The effects of common peroneal stimulation on the effort and speed of walking: a randomized controlled trial with chronic hemiplegic patients. *Clin Rehabil.* 1997;11:201–210.

54. Taylor PN, Burridge JH, Dunkerley AL, et al. Clinical use of the Odstock dropped foot stimulator: its effect on the speed and effort off walking. *Arch Phys Med Rehabil.* 1999;80:1577–1583.

55. Wieler M, Stein RB, Ladouceur M, et al. Multicenter evaluation of electrical stimulation systems for walking. *Arch Phys Med Rehabil.* 1999;80:495–500.

56. Ladouceur M, Barbeau H. Functional electrical stimulation-assisted walking for persons with incomplete spinal injuries: longitudinal changes in maximal over ground walking speed. *Scand J Rehabil Med.* 2000;32:28–36.

57. Carmick J. Clinical use of neuromuscular electrical stimulation for children with cerebral palsy, part 1: lower extremity. *Phys Ther.* 1993;73:505–513.

58. Carmick J. Managing equinus in children with cerebral palsy: electrical stimulation to strengthen the triceps surae muscle. *Dev Med Child Neurol.* 1995;37:965–975.

59. Comeaux P, Patterson N, Rubin M, et al. Effect of neuromuscular electrical stimulation during gait in children with cerebral palsy. *Pediatr Phys Ther.* 1997;9:103–109.

60. Pierce SR, Laughton CA, Smith BT, et al. Direct effect of percutaneous electric stimulation during gait in children with hemiplegic cerebral palsy: a report of 2 cases. *Arch Phys Med Rehabil.* 2004;85:339–343.

61. Bogataj U, Gros N, Kljajic M, et al. The rehabilitation of gait in patients with hemiplegia: a comparison between conventional therapy and multichannel functional electrical stimulation therapy. *Phys Ther.* 1995;75:490–502.

62. Hesse S, Malezic M, Schaffrin A, et al. Restoration of gait my combined treadmill training and multichannel electrical stimulation in non-ambulatory hemiparetic patients. *Scand J Rehabil. Med.* 1995;27:199–204.

63. Field-Fote EC. Combined use of body weight support, functional electric stimulation, and treadmill training to improve walking ability in individuals with chronic incomplete spinal cord injury. *Arch Phys Med Rehabil.* 2001;82:818–824.

64. Postans NJ, Hasler JP, Granat MH, et al. Functional electric stimulation to augment partial weight-bearing supported treadmill training for patients with acute incomplete spinal cord injury: a pilot study. *Arch Phys Med Rehabil.* 2004;85:604–610.

65. Creasey GH, Ho CH, Triolo RJ, et al. Clinical applications of electrical stimulation after spinal cord injury. *J Spinal Cord Med.* 2004;27:365–375.

66. Graupe D. An overview of the state of the art of noninvasive FES for independent ambulation by thoracic level paraplegics. *Neurol Res.* 2002;24:431–442.

67. Johnston TE, Betz RR, Smith BT, et al. Implanted functional electrical stimulation: an alternative for standing and walking in pediatric spinal cord injury. *Spinal Cord.* 2003;41:144–152.

68. Klose KJ, Jacobs PL, Bronton JG, et al. Evaluation of a training program for persons with SCI paraplegia using the Parastep-I ambulation system, Part 1: ambulation performance and anthropometric measures. *Arch Phys Med Rehabil.* 1997;78:789–793.

68a. Sigmedics. Parastep I Clinical Programs http://www.sigmedics.com/Clinics/clinics.html. Accessed May 13, 2007.

69. Carnstam B, Larsson LE, Prevec TS. Improvement of gait following functional electrical stimulation. 1. Investigations on changes in voluntary strength and proprioceptive reflexes. *Scand J Rehabil Med.* 1977;9:7–13.

70. Peterson T, Klemar KB. Electrical stimulation as a treatment of lower limb spasticity. *J Neuro Rehabil.* 1988;2:103–108.

71. Apkarian JA, Naumann S. Stretch reflex inhibition using electrical stimulation in normal subjects and subjects with spasticity. *J Biomed Eng.* 1991;13:67–73.

72. Mirbagheri MM, Ladouceur M, Barbeau H, et al. The effects of long-term FES-assisted walking on intrinsic and reflex dynamic stiffness in spastic spinal-cord-injured subjects. *IEEE Trans Neural Syst Rehabil Eng.* 2002;10:280–289.

73. Robinson CJ, Kett NA, Bolam JM. Spasticity in spinal cord injured patients. 1. Short-term effects of electrical stimulation. *Arch Phys Med Rehabil.* 1988;69:598–604.

74. Bajd T, Vodovnik L. Pendulum testing of spasticity. *J Biomed Eng.* 1984;6:9–16.

75. Levin MF, Hui-Chan CWY. Relief of hemiparetic spasticity by TENS is associated with improvement in reflex and voluntary motor functions. *Electroencephalogr Clin Neurophysiol.* 1992;85:131–142.

76. Dewald JP, Given JD, Rymer WZ. Long-lasting reductions of spasticity induced by skin electrical stimulation. *IEEE Trans Rehabil Eng.* 1996;4:231–242.

CHAPTER 8

Electrical Stimulation to Augment Healing of Chronic Wounds

Andrew J. Robinson

Chronic nonhealing wounds are a common complication of disease, injury, and aging. Chronic vascular leg ulcers are found in about 1% of the general population, and in approximately 10% of persons in health care facilities (1,2). There are numerous factors that contribute to the occurrence of chronic wounds, including circulatory disease, metabolic disease, nutritional deficits, tissue trauma, poor tissue perfusion, excessive inflammation, and failure or delay of the healing components. Elderly individuals and individuals with neurological injury (e.g., spinal cord injury) are more prone to developing a nonhealing wound because immobility and impaired sensation are two of the most important factors that contribute the development of chronic wounds. Nonhealing wounds in many cases prolong hospitalizations, retard rehabilitation efforts, risk limb loss, interrupt the ability for independent living, and, in some cases, may threaten life.

Nonhealing wounds are routinely referred to as *chronic wounds*. A chronic wound is a wound that fails to heal within an expected time given the underlying etiology (3). Others have defined a chronic wound as a wound that does not heal in the expected sequence of repair in terms of time, appearance, and response to aggressive and appropriate treatment (4). Preventing and treating chronic wounds can be frustrating, costly, and labor intensive. However, treatment of chronic wounds with electrical stimulation (ES) has been shown to be a safe, effective, and efficient solution for many individuals. The clinical use of electrical stimulation of tissue to directly or indirectly enhance the rate of tissue healing has been referred to as *ESTHR* (electrical stimulation for tissue healing and repair). The use of electrical stimulation to treat wounds is not new. Reports on the use of electricity date back to the 17th century (5). The use of ES for wound management, however, was not commonly used in the medical community even through the first 80 years of the 20th century. With the resurgence in interest in electrotherapy and a better understanding of the physiology of tissue healing and the effects of electrical currents on tissues, interest in studying and applying ES for wound healing was renewed in the 1970s. The demonstrated efficacy of ESTHR in published reports from clinical trials during this time has led to a much more widespread use of this intervention in the management of chronic wounds. After a lengthy review process, these positive findings led to the approval of the use of ESTHR for treatment of lower-extremity pressure ulcers, vascular insufficiency ulcers, and diabetic ulcers in the United States in 2002 (6).

Given the apparent value of ESTHR. the objectives of this chapter are to (i) define and describe the types of chronic wounds; (ii) provide an overview of the wound healing process and factors that may impede wound healing; (iii) describe the basics of clinical wound assessment; (iv) discuss the physiological effects of ES relevant to wound healing; (v) outline the commonly-used stimulation procedures and parameters of stimulation for chronic wound healing; (vi) review the literature on the effectiveness of ESTHR in chronic wounds; (vii) outline the precautions and contraindications for ESTHR; and (viii) present case studies that illustrate the use of ESTHR in contemporary practice.

OVERVIEW OF WOUND HEALING PROCESS

Phases of Normal Wound Healing

The normal process of wound healing is generally viewed as occurring in three ongoing and overlapping phases (Fig. 8.1): inflammatory, proliferative, and remodeling (or maturation). A detailed description of each of these phases of healing is beyond the scope of this chapter. The following subsections provide an overview of some of the key elements in each of these healing phases that are particularly relevant to the effects of electrical stimulation in the management of chronic nonhealing wounds. More in-depth discussion of the processes taking place during the phases of wound healing can be found in Kloth and McCulloch's comprehensive text on wound healing [see Kirsner and Bogensberger (7)].

Inflammatory Phase

The *inflammatory phase* of normal wound healing is characterized by the body's initial responses to a wound. The processes occurring first in response to a wound include *hemostasis* (stopping bleeding), *autolysis* (removal of damaged cellular debris), and *phagocytosis* (engulfment of bacteria). These responses are initiated at the time of injury and normally occur over a period of 2 to 7 days from the onset of the wound, depending in part on the wound severity. Hemostasis is mediated by the activation of blood platelets. These platelets bind or adhere to collagen in the wound to occlude small blood vessels in order to reduce or stop bleeding. Another key role of platelets in the inflammatory phase relates to their ability to attract cells (chemotactic influence) to the wound. Activated platelets release a number of different chemotactic substances broadly referred to as growth factors (e.g., transforming growth factor-beta, platelet-derived growth factor) that attract numerous cells including macrophages, monocytes, and neutrophils. These cells are responsible for the processes of autolysis and phagocytosis during which they enclose and break down cellular debris and pathogens in the wound to combat infection. By releasing chemotaxic agents and growth factors, platelets and macrophages stimulate the formation of connective tissue (collagen, granulation tissue) by fibroblasts and stimulate the formation of new blood vessels (*angiogenesis*) by endothelial cells to the healing wound.

Proliferative Phase

The *proliferative phase* of wound healing generally spans from 2 or 3 days to 3 weeks after the onset of the wound. The proliferative phase of wound healing is characterized by cellular activity that leads to formation of a granulation tissue (*fibroplasia*), a new epithelial layer (*re-epithelialization*), the development of a new vascular supply (*neovascularization* or angiogenesis), and wound contraction. Granulation tissue is normally pink or beefy red in appearance and

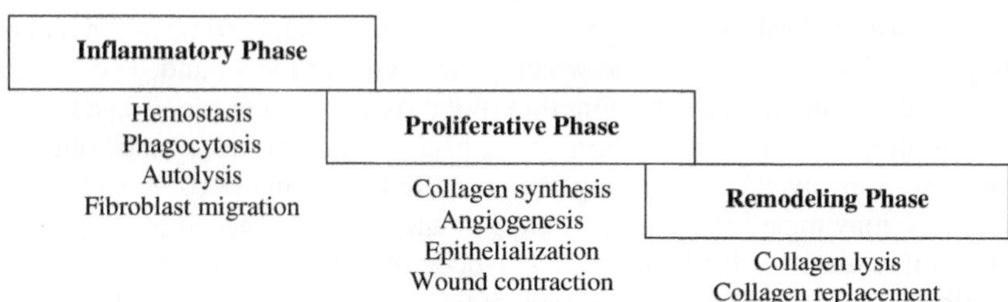

Figure 8.1. Phases of wound healing and the processes that occur in each phase that produce wound repair.

is formed by the migration of dermal fibroblasts into the wound. *Fibroblasts* produce collagen fibers, elastin, proteoglycans, and ground substance. The *collagen* for the matrix provides tensile strength to the wound, whereas the *elastin* has elastic qualities that help maintain the shape of the wound and resist stretch of the wound. The *proteoglycans* serve several roles, including stimulation of fibroblast proliferation and migration and retention of water in the wound. The *ground substance* is gel-like and reduces friction between collagen fibers when the wound sustains mechanical stress. Fibroblasts also differentiate into myofibroblasts with contractile properties like those of muscle. The *myofibroblasts* are primarily responsible for wound contraction.

The regrowth of the blood vessels into the wound results from the migration of endothelial cells from the margins of the wound. The new vasculature supplies the necessary oxygen and nutrients to the proliferating cells within the wound.

Epithelialization of wounds results from the migration of epidermal cells from the margins of the wound. A single layer of epithelial cells may completely cover a wound in as little as a few days if the wound is protected from stress and strain. Once this thin epithelial layer is closed, the epithelial cells begin to proliferate to increase the skin thickness. The purpose of re-epithelialization is to re-establish a functional barrier of skin over the wound to protect it from external pathogens and substances that would compromise wound healing.

Remodeling Phase

The *remodeling phase* of wound healing can extend from 3 weeks up to 2 years. This phase of healing is characterized by the degradation of the collagen formed in the initial two phases of healing with replacement and proliferation of new collagen. In the early phases of wound healing, collagen similar to that in fetal tissues (type III) is formed. In the remodeling phase, type III collagen is broken down by the action of an enzyme called collagenase in a process called *collagen lysis*. This process is coincident with the formation of adult collagen (type I) that replaces the fetal form of collagen formed early in healing. Adult collagen has greater tensile strength than fetal collagen and hence forms a stronger healed wound than would exist if the type III collagen were not replaced. The scar formed by the proliferation of adult collagen, however, is generally not as strong as the collagen in the tissue before injury. Over time the new adult collagen can remodel in a manner to provide the most appropriate resistance to compressive and tensile forces that are applied to the wound in everyday activities. The vascular supply to newly formed collagen gradually decreases with time, giving rise to the typical lighter appearance of a mature scar as compared to the surrounding intact skin.

Factors That Impede Wound Healing

Wound healing does not always proceed in the normal manner described above. In such cases, wound healing may be either markedly delayed or may not occur, leading to a chronic wound. A large number of factors can contribute to impairment of wound healing. Table 8.1 lists a variety of conditions that may impair wound healing. For the clinician responsible for the treatment of wounds, of particular importance are those conditions that may be altered, minimized, or eliminated to facilitate wound healing. Among the most important factors to be addressed are wound infection, impaired blood perfusion of the wound, and drying of the wound. The development of wound infection results in bacterial consumption of the oxygen and nutrients needed by the cells producing the healing response. In addition, some bacteria may produce metabolic by-products that are toxic to cells involved in the healing response. Reduction in the volume of blood circulating to wounds also may impair the supply of oxygen and nutrients needed to support the cellular activity in the inflammatory, proliferative, and remodeling phases of healing. In addition, poor perfusion of blood through healing wounds may impair the removal of carbon dioxide and the by-products of cellular metabolism, and hence slow the activity of cells responsible for tissue healing.

Table 8.1. Selected Conditions or Factors That Impede Wound Healing (9)

Condition/Factor	*Example/Effect*
Some systemic medications	Examples: corticosteroids , aspirin , and indomethacin Suppress inflammatory phase response
Some topical medications	Example: iodine Can kill cells that produce healing
Malnutrition	Reduces supply of nutrients to healing wound
Prolonged pressure or stretch	Reduces capillary blood supply to tissues
Infection	Counteracts healing processes
Immunodeficiency	Impairs inflammatory response to infection
Smoking	Impairs supply of nutrients and oxygen and removal of carbon dioxide and wastes by reducing capillary circulation to wound
Dryness or necrotic tissue	Impedes migration of cells in inflammatory and proliferative phases of healing

Drying of open wounds has several consequences that impede healing. Moisture in the wound is essential for the migration of cells into the wound through each of the phases of healing. Moisture in the wound creates the interface between the cells producing the healing response and the capillary blood, allowing the exchange of oxygen and nutrients and the by-products of cellular metabolism. Fluid in the wound contains the growth factors and enzymes that promote cellular migration and cellular function in healing. The moisture in the wound is important for efficient cellular migration. Some the basic principles that guide treatment of chronic wounds follow from the above discussion: control infection, stimulate or restore circulation, and keep the wound environment moist.

Categorization of Chronic Wounds

A variety of classification systems are used in clinical practice to differentiate between the various types of chronic wounds. The Centers for Medicare and Medicaid Services (CMMS) characterize a chronic wound as one that has not healed within 30 days of occurrence. Examples of wounds categorized by etiology include ulceration associated with arterial insufficiency, venous insufficiency, diabetic neuropathy, and chronic tissue pressure. These are the types of chronic wounds included for coverage by CMMS.

ASSESSMENT OF CHRONIC WOUNDS

The results of wound evaluation provide valuable information that guides decisions regarding the treatment approaches used to address chronic wounds. The scope of wound evaluation can include a wide array of techniques that may be administered by providers from many disciplines. For more detailed discussions of the various dimensions of contemporary wound evaluation, the reader is referred to more comprehensive resources (8,9). Of particular importance to the topic of this chapter on ES for wound healing are the quantitative and qualitative measures that reflect the relative efficacy of the intervention. These measures include wound size, a description of the wound base and boundaries, characterization of wound drainage, and a description of the surrounding tissues.

Wound size is quantified in several ways. The surface area of the wound defect is most commonly measured. At the simplest level, clinicians use a tape measure to record the greatest length and width of the wound. Alternatively, the wound surface area may be traced or photographed and the surface area determined by manual planimetry or computer-assisted methods. In addition to the measurement of surface area, wound depth is routinely measured. This generally involves placing a sterile cotton swab to the base of the wound and measuring the length of the swab to point where the swab reaches the surface opening. Swabs may also be used to document the depth of tunnels, undermining of tissues or fistulas in wounds. Knowledge of the surface area and depth of a wound can provide a sense of the volume of a wound.

More accurate measures of wound volume have been developed. Volumetric measurement of wounds may be performed by determining the amount of either sterile saline or hydrogel required to fill the wound. Wound volume may also be determined by making a positive mold of the wound using an alginate hydrocolloid in saline that is poured into the wound and sets up as a firm gel. This mold is removed from the wound and its volume is determined by water displacement.

Documentation of the changes in appearance of the wound base and surrounding tissues can reveal whether a wound is responding positively to treatment. Observation of the wound can reveal the presence of active infection, necrotic tissue, and eschar that may impede wound healing. Alternatively, observation may reveal the proliferation of granulation tissue (red or pink moist tissue) or epithelial tissue (translucent or white thin sheets over granulation tissue) that reflects progress in healing.

Assessment of the periwound tissues includes a determination of the skin hydration (dryness or excessive moisture), regularity and configuration of the edges of the wound, color and texture of skin, and presence or absence of swelling. The appearance, consistency, volume, and odor of wound drainage should be assessed. Clear or pink watery drainage without significant odor is indicative of the inflammatory or proliferative stages of healing. In contrast, yellow-green cloudy drainage is frequently associated with significant wound infection that may impede healing.

A number of instruments have been developed to guide the health care provider in the process of wound healing. These instruments include the Pressure Sore Status Tool (10), the

Table 8.2. Common Types of Chronic Wounds (8)

Type of Chronic Wounds	*Definition*	*Common Locations of Wounds*	*Etiology*
Pressure sores	Areas of local tissue loss subsequent to prolonged tissue compression between bony prominences and an external surface	Sacrum, heels, over ischial tuberosities, over the greater trochanter, over malleoli	Compression of tissues reduces tissue blood perfusion and produces tissue necrosis
Arterial insufficiency ulcers	Area of local tissue loss subsequent to arterial blood supply deficiency	On the foot, over malleoli, over toe joints, over lateral foot border	Arteriosclerosis, arterial occlusion (e.g., thrombosis), arterial disruption
Venous insufficiency ulcers	Area of local tissue loss subsequent to venous drainage deficiency	Above the ankle, on the medial lower leg	Sustained venous hypertension, venous valvular dysfunction
Diabetic ulcers	Area of local tissue loss subsequent to sensory neuropathy and arterial blood supply deficiency	Plantar surface of foot, over the heel, lateral foot border, over the metatarsal heads on plantar surface	Tissue trauma in insensate area, peripheral vascular disease

Table 8.3. Pressure Ulcer Stages (14)

Pressure Ulcer Stage	*Definition*
Stage I	Nonblanchable erythema of intact skin, the heralding lesion of skin ulceration. In individuals with darker skin, discoloration of the skin, warmth, edema, induration, or hardness may also be indicators
Stage II	Partial-thickness skin loss involving the epidermis or dermis, or both. The ulcer is superficial and presents clinically as an abrasion, blister, or shallow crater.
Stage III	Full-thickness skin loss involving damage or necrosis of subcutaneous tissue, which may extend down to but not through the underlying fascia. The ulcer presents clinically as a deep crater with or without undermining of adjacent tissue.
Stage IV	Full-thickness skin loss with extensive destruction, tissue necrosis, or damage to muscle, bone, or supporting structures (such as tendon, joint capsule) and may be associated with undermining or sinus tracts.

Sussman Wound Healing Tool (11), the Pressure Ulcer Scale for Healing (12), and the Wound Healing Scale (13). The validity, reliability, and sensitivity of these and other tools have yet to be definitively established with respect to healing in the various types of chronic wounds.

The comprehensive assessment of chronic wounds involves much more than observation and measurements of the wounds alone. Comprehensive assessment includes the past and current medical history, current medications, nutritional status, identification of risk factors, evaluation of circulatory status (both arterial and venous), and even the psychological status of the individual with a chronic wound.

Types of Chronic Wounds

Upon completion of a thorough evaluation of a chronic wound, the evaluator may categorize the wound with respect to suspected etiology and severity. Among the most prevalent types of chronic wound are pressure sores, arterial insufficiency ulcers, venous insufficiency ulcers, and diabetic ulcers. *Ulcers* are wounds that involve the tissues deep to the epidermis of the skin. Definitions of each of these types of chronic wounds are presented in Table 8.2. *Pressure sores* are typically staged with respect to severity based upon the depth of the ulcer and its appearance using a system developed in 1989 by the National Pressure Ulcer Advisory Panel (14). Establishment of the stage of pressure ulcers (Table 8.3) is particularly important in the consideration of the use of ES for management because, in the United States, the CMMS has approved the use of ES only in the management of stage III and stage IV ulcers. Staging systems have not yet been developed for arterial insufficiency, venous insufficiency, or diabetic chronic wounds.

PHYSIOLOGICAL EFFECTS OF ELECTRICAL STIMULATION RELEVANT TO WOUND HEALING

Galvanotaxis

Electrical stimulation using DC or monophasic pulsed current appears to be capable of attracting cells to wounds to augment healing. This process is called *galvanotaxis* and is defined as the attraction of electrically charged (positively or negatively charged) cells toward an electrical

Table 8.4. Galvanotaxis of Cells During the Three Phases of Wound Healing

Phase of Healing	Cell: Cell Polarity	Roles in Healing
Inflammatory	Macrophages: negative	Phagocytosis
	Neutrophils: negative	Autolysis
Proliferative	Fibroblasts: positive	Collagen formation
Remodeling	Myofibroblasts: positive	Wound contraction
(maturation)	Keratinocytes: positive	Epithelialization
	Epidermal: negative	

Adapted with permission from Kloth LC. Electrical stimulation for wound healing: a review of evidence from in vitro studies, animal experiments and clinical trials. *Lower Extremity Wounds* 2005;4:23–44

conductor of opposite polarity. Galvanotaxic effects of DC or monophasic pulsed current may be important during each main phase of healing (see Table 8.4). Although a number of researchers have demonstrated that cells associated with wound healing may be made to migrate toward electrodes of opposite polarity (15,16), evidence for augmentation of galvanotaxis in human chronic wounds in response to ES is limited. In a study evaluating the effects of ES on cell migration in human skin exudate, Eberhardt et al. (17) produced small (0.5 cm^2) partial thickness wounds on the forearms of 10 young males. Each subject received three wounds made once every 10 days. Wound exudate was examined at 2, 4, 6, 9, and 12 hours after making the wounds. The second wound in the series was exposed to ES using rectangular pulsed current (frequency, 100 pps; pulse duration, 1 ms; treatment duration, 30 minutes) at an amplitude adjusted to produce minimal perceptible paresthesia before collecting the exudates. The third wound was stimulated with the same form of current at an amplitude just below pain threshold. In the subjects exposed to the higher level of stimulation, researchers found an increase in the number (34% greater) of granulocytes (neutrophils) in stimulated wound exudate as compared to control wound exudates and minimally stimulated wound exudates. This relative increase in the neutrophils in the maximally stimulated wound 12 hours after treatment was attributed to an improvement in circulation to the wound, which may contribute to the activation of chemotactic processes. Clearly, the limitation of this study with respect to the significance of the outcome as it pertains to the treatment of chronic wounds is that it was conducted on acute wounds of partial thickness.

Augmentation of Collagen Synthesis and Proliferation of Fibroblasts

Fibroblasts normally migrate into the healing wound, especially during the proliferative phase. Research has demonstrated that fibroblast activity can be influenced by exposure to electrostatic fields. Fibroblast cultures exposed to electrostatic fields respond with increases in both DNA synthesis and collagen synthesis.

Bourguignon and Bourguignon (18) stimulated a human fibroblast cell culture using 20 minutes of high-voltage pulsed current (HVPC) applied at various voltages and pulse frequencies, placing the cathode over the fibroblasts. After 2 hours of stimulation, the rate of protein synthesis was increased in the fibroblasts by 160% over the control specimens. Maximum synthesis occurred at 50 to 75 V and 150 pulses per second (pps). When the fibroblasts were positioned below the anode, the maximum rate of protein synthesis was 120% of the unstimulated control specimens, using a stimulus of 150 V. There was a significant increase in DNA production between 2 and 24 hours after stimulation; maximum synthesis occurred closer to the cathode at

75 V and 100 pps. These findings indicate that as a result of increasing protein and DNA synthesis by HVPC stimulation, collagen synthesis and fibroblast proliferation also increase.

Subsequent experiments have revealed that the increase in activity of fibroblasts in response to monophasic pulsed-current stimulation may arise from an increase in calcium ion uptake and an associated increase in the insulin receptors on fibroblasts (19). Increased ability to bind insulin may have the effect of enhancing protein and DNA synthesis by enhancing glucose and amino acid uptake in fibroblasts. In addition, other researchers have demonstrated that ES as described above increases the number of receptors for transforming growth factor-beta (TGF-β) (20). TGF-β bound in greater amounts would facilitate connective tissue growth factor, enhancing collagen synthesis in fibroblasts, leading ultimately to the formation of scar tissue. In addition, TGF-β also appears to enhance cell proliferation, cell differentiation, and matrix production (21).

Stimulation of Angiogenesis and Wound Microperfusion

For wounds to successfully heal, the cells involved in the healing process must be supplied with the oxygen and nutrients required for the support of their roles in combating infection, removal of necrotic tissue, proliferation of connective tissue, and covering the wound with new epithelium. As cells involved in the healing process migrate into the wound, the vasculature (blood vessels) that supplies nutrients and oxygen to these cells also regrows into the wound. This is the process of angiogenesis. To date, one study provides evidence of enhanced microcirculation in chronic wounds in response to ES (22) This study treated chronic venous ulcers (mean duration, 79 months) in 15 individuals using a form of monophasic pulsed current (pulse duration, 140 μs; frequency, 128 or 64 pps; treatment time, 30 minutes daily for 38 days). Initial treatments employed the cathode over the wound (7–14 treatments), followed by treatments with the anode over the wound (3–10 days), and in the final treatments the cathode was again placed over the wound. Junger et al. (22) reported an increase in capillary density (44%) that was accompanied by an increase (82%) in the transcutaneous oxygen partial pressure in the tissue around the edges of the wound. These measured changes were thought to be the result of stimulation of capillary regrowth into the wound.

Killing or Impeding the Growth of Bacteria in the Wound

Chronic wounds may become infected by a wide array of bacteria that can either impede wound healing or actually cause further tissue damage. For these reasons, control of bacterial infection becomes a primary focus in chronic wound care whenever any signs or symptoms of infection become apparent. Many studies have been performed to examine the effects of electrical currents on bacteria grown in cultures in the laboratory. In a summary of the literature by Kloth (23), the majority of these studies have demonstrated that ES using either low intensity (voltage) direct current (LIDC) or high voltage (intensity) pulsed current (HVPC, a monophasic pulsed current) inhibit the growth of bacteria but do not necessarily kill colonies of bacteria. Both LIDC and HVPC have been shown to have bacteriostatic effects on *Escherichia coli*, *Pseudomonas aeruginosa*, and *Staphylococcus aureus*. In addition, LIDC has been shown to have a bacteriostatic effect on gram-positive bacteria when placed below the anode and a bactericidal effect on gram-negative bacteria when placed beneath the cathode. Studies designed to examine the effects of biphasic pulsed currents or alternating currents on bacteria in vitro have generally failed to detect either bacteriostatic or bactericidal effects on *E coli* (24). Studies to assess the effect of electrical currents on bacterial growth in living animals or humans (25) are limited.

For many years it has been maintained that the cathode of a DC circuit or the cathode of a monophasic pulsed current circuit produce inhibition of bacterial growth, while the anode of these two circuits had no influence on bacteria. A recent study on the effects of DC, pulsed current, and AC on *S. aureus* growth in vitro calls that belief into question. Merriman et al. (26)

demonstrated inhibition of bacterial growth at both the cathode and anode of electrical circuits passing both LIDC (500 μA) and HVPC (250 V, 100 pps) delivered for 1 hour daily for 3 days.

Enhancing the Rate of Epithelialization

In a study examining the effects of ES on the rate of epithelialization, Mertz et al. (27) applied monophasic pulsed current (current density, 0.513 mA per cm^2; peak amplitude, 30 mA; pulse duration, 140 μs; 128 pps for 30 minutes twice a day for 7 days) to partial thickness wounds produced with a modified electrokeratome in pigs. In wounds treated with the anode (positive polarity) for the subsequent 7 days, or wounds treated with the cathode on the first day and the anode for the remaining 6 days, the re-epithelialization was complete in 6 days. Pig wounds treated with only the cathode over the wounds or alternating the polarity daily resulted in only 62% and 29% of wounds being completely re-epithelialized in 6 days. In fact, wounds treated with only the cathode or with alternating polarity daily healed more poorly than wounds in control animals that were not treated with electrical stimulation. Studies of the effect of electrical stimulation on the rate of re-epithelialization in chronic wounds have yet to be conducted.

Enhancing Blood Flow to Wounds

Recently a report published by Petrofsky et al. (28) addressed the issue of enhancing blood flow to wounds by the use of ES applied near the wound. Seven patients with wounds of mixed etiology, location, and duration participated. In this study, a rectangular, balanced, biphasic pulsed current with a 250-μs pulse duration and frequency of 30 pps was used for just 5 minutes. Amplitude of stimulation was adjusted to approximately the sensory threshold for subjects with intact sensation, or to 15 mA if skin sensation was impaired. Electrodes were placed such that stimulation was applied across the wounds. Blood flow before and after stimulation was measured with a laser Doppler flow imager both within the wound and just outside the wound. The results revealed an average increased blood flow approximately 50% greater than before stimulation, and the increases in blood flow were sustained for a short period after stimulation was stopped. Whether this short-term increase in blood flow to the wound is an important effect of ES that contributes to an enhanced rate of healing has yet to be determined.

In summary, substantial evidence exists that ES using low amplitude direct current or monophasic pulsed current may enhance cellular activity in each of the phases of wound healing (29). In the inflammatory phase, this cellular activity results in antibacterial effects and the attraction of cells to begin wound healing. In the proliferative phase, ES increases the migration and activation of fibroblasts, endothelial cells, and epithelial cells to heal and cover the wound. In the maturation phase, ES appears to facilitate the conversion of new wound connective tissue into the mature adult form of collagen that is characteristic of normal tissue. The net result of the effects of ES on wound healing processes is faster deposition of collagen tissue, improved revascularization of wound tissues, faster close rates, and improved wound tensile strength.

PRINCIPLES AND PROCEDURES OF ELECTRICAL STIMULATION FOR WOUND HEALING

Preparation of the Wound

Before the initiation of the use of electrical stimulation to promote wound healing, chronic wounds should be properly managed using standard wound management procedures (30). Conditions in and around wounds that should be routinely addressed before beginning ES for chronic wounds include management of necrotic tissue, infection, and edema. Necrotic tissue impedes wound healing because it serves as a medium for bacterial growth and may be a physical barrier to the formation of granulation tissue and re-epithelialization. Dry necrotic tissue may also prevent the passage of electrical currents within the wound, and hence mitigate the wound responses to electrical currents that promote wound healing. Removal of necrotic tissue is important if the maximum benefits of ES in wound healing are to be achieved. At the simplest level, removal of necrotic tissue may be achieved by the facilitation of autolysis (break down of necrotic tissue by cellular enzymes and white blood cells) through the use of moisture-retaining dressings in the wound. Management of necrotic tissue often also includes some form of mechanical debridement (e.g., wound irrigation), enzymatic debridement, or even sharp debridement.

Although ES may have antibacterial effects in chronic wounds, other infection management approaches should be undertaken either before or simultaneously with the use of ES for augmentation of healing. Among the procedures used to manage wound infection are wound cleansing (e.g., normal saline irrigation), use of topical agents to either inhibit or kill bacteria (antiseptics) and or fungi (antifungals), and use of systemic antibacterial drugs.

Types of Current Used in Electrical Stimulation for Wound Healing

At the time of writing, ES to promote wound healing is provided using either monophasic pulsed currents, relatively low amplitude direct currents, or biphasic pulsed currents. The optimal parameters of stimulation for wound healing have not yet been definitively identified for these forms of stimulation for each type of chronic wound. The published research on ESTHR in human wounds does allow one to identify the range of stimulation parameters that have been used with success in wound management.

Low-Intensity Direct Current for Wound Healing

Direct current is the continuous unidirectional flow of charged particles for >1 second (31). Direct current stimulation was one of the first forms of current studied for the treatment of chronic wounds. The rationale for using direct current for wound healing is in part associated with the finding that wounds have a negative polarity as compared to intact surrounding skin. This change in polarity has been proposed as a stimulus to initiate the physiological responses that produce wound healing. Wounds that fail to heal are thought to have reduced polarity as compared to wounds that heal at a normal rate. Healing processes that may be facilitated in chronic wounds by direct currents include phagocytosis and autolysis in the inflammatory phase, followed by fibroplasias, epithelialization, and wound contraction in the subsequent phases of healing (23). The passage of direct current through the wound is thought to facilitate the attraction of electrically charged cells such as leukocytes and neutrophils, and stimulate the proliferation and activity of fibroblasts to increase collagen synthesis in the wound. In contemporary clinical practice, the polarity that should be selected for the electrode initially placed over the opening of the wound has not been definitively established. Some authors outline protocols whereby the cathode of the DC circuit is placed directly over the wound during initial treatments (1 to 5 days) (32). This recommendation appears to be associated with the protocols used in clinical trials that have resulted in significant improvements in the rate of wound healing. Other authors recommend setting the initial polarity of the electrodes over the wound based on the specific findings from wound evaluation (23). For example, the negative electrode should be selected initially if the wound is infected with organisms sensitive to cathodal stimulation, such as *E. coli* and *P. aeruginosa*. Alternatively, if the wound is infected with bacteria such as *S. aureus*, the positive pole may be a more appropriate choice.

Kloth (23) suggested that the polarity of the electrode placed over the wound should be selected based on the types of healing processes the clinician wants to facilitate. For example, the anode should be selected if one wants to attract macrophages and neutrophils to stimulate phagocytosis and autolysis. In contrast, if one wants to enhance the formation of granulation tissue mediated by fibroblasts, enhance wound contraction by myofibroblasts, or increase the rate of re-epithelialization by keratinocytes, the cathode should be used over the wound.

At times the choice of electrode polarity may be based on the electrochemical responses of tissues to the exposure to direct currents. For example, the cathode of DC circuits may solubilize, liquefy, or soften necrotic tissue, which may secondarily facilitate the migration of cells that characterize the inflammatory or proliferative phases of wound healing. At this time, the clinical trials and laboratory research have not clearly defined whether it is most appropriate to begin treatment with either the anode or the cathode placed over the wound. As discussed later in this chapter, a number of clinical trails using DC or monophasic pulsed current for wound healing have applied the cathode for a few sessions and then switched the polarity to the anode. Several trials periodically reverse the polarity of the electrode over the wound when the rate of healing of the wound appears to be diminishing or when it plateaus.

After 1 to 3 days of stimulation with the cathode over the wound, the anode of the DC circuit is placed over the wound. Anodal stimulation following cathodal stimulation may stimulate epithelialization. These and other potential effects on cellular migration and/or cellular activity may account for the wound healing effect of direct current. It is important to note, however, that these theories are primarily based on experimental results derived from laboratory experimentation on bacterial and tissue cultures or in experimentally induced wounds in animals.

Polarity of the active treatment electrode over the chronic wound is commonly reversed every 3 days during the treatment period. As already mentioned, this change in polarity of the treatment electrode is at times prompted by what appears as a slowing or plateau in the rate of healing of the chronic wound.

The general parameters of DC stimulation used for chronic wound healing are shown in Table 8.5. The amplitude of stimulation using DC in chronic wound treatment has been consistently maintained at <1 mA (<1000 μA). In the clinical trials that have been published, the amplitude of stimulation has ranged from 200 to 800 μA. Only in one of the three clinical trials was the amplitude of stimulation expressed in terms of current density (amperage per square centimeter of active treatment electrode area). In that study (33), the current density was 30 to 110 μA per cm^2. In some but not all patients, this level of stimulation may produce a very mild tingling sensation. Amplitudes of DC stimulation are adjusted downward during the course of treatment if the stimulation induces bleeding in the wound.

The duration of ES treatments of chronic wounds using DC is generally on the order of 2 hours for each treatment session with two treatment sessions per day. Some recommended protocols stipulate 30 to 45 minutes of stimulation in each session with only one treatment session per day. Treatments are applied 5 to 7 days per week.

Electrodes applied over open wounds (referred to as "active electrodes") have included stainless steel or aluminum foil and carbon rubber electrodes. Electrodes used with DC treatment

Table 8.5. Stimulation Parameters for Use of Direct Current for Chronic Wounds

Type of Current	*Continuous Direct Current*
Amplitude of current	200–800 mA; <1000 mA
Treatment duration	1–2 hours
Treatments per day	1–3 per day
No. of treatment days/week	5–7 per week

of chronic wounds are generally fabricated from heavy-duty aluminum foil folded into three to four layers and cut in a shape slightly smaller (0.5-cm margin) than the opening of the wound. Conduction of currents from the electrode over the wound is achieved by loosely placing sterile gauze pads into the wound and saturating them with sterile saline. Alternatively, some clinicians may use gauze saturated with an electrically conductive hydrogel. The electrode of the DC circuit required to complete the stimulation circuit (at times called "dispersive") that is not placed over the wound may be fabricated in a manner like the electrode over the wound, or may be commercially available self-adhesive electrodes. In general, this second electrode is approximately the same size as the active electrode and is placed at 15 to 30 cm away from the wound opening.

The practical limitation to the application of DC to treat chronic wounds is that DC stimulators with the capability of delivering accurate microamperage DC are not readily commercially available. This limitation in availability of stimulators capable of producing microcurrent-level DC, along with the successful outcome of trials using monophasic pulsed current (see below), may explain why no randomized clinical trials on the use of DC for chronic wound healing have been reported since 1985. In addition, this limitation in DC stimulator availability may in part explain why this particular approach to ES care of chronic wounds never became commonplace in clinical practice.

Monophasic Pulsed Currents for Wound Healing

Monophasic pulsed current is defined as the brief, unidirectional flow of charged particles that is interrupted for longer periods of time. The brief periods of current flow are called pulses, and each pulse has a duration that is typically on the order of 20 to 100 μs. These pulses of current are delivered in a series of pulses that are each separated by a much longer period of no flow of charged particles (called the interpulse interval). Intervals between pulses are determined by the frequency of pulses delivered.

Two forms of monophasic pulsed current have been regularly used in chronic wound healing applications (Table 8.6). These two forms of monophasic pulsed current are usually differentiated based on the shape of the current waveform, either spikelike or rectangular in appearance. The most readily available monophasic pulsed current is referred to as HVPC. In standardized terms, this form of current should be described as twin-spike or paired-spike, monophasic pulsed current. The duration of these twin spikes is very short (typically 10 to 50 μs for each spike and $>$100 μs from the beginning of the first spike to the end of the second spike). The peak voltages applied to produce this form of pulsed current may be up to 500 V but have not exceeded 250 in clinical studies, and typically are in the 100 to 150 V range. This relatively large driving force (electromotive force) produced by the stimulators has led to this current being commonly

Table 8.6. Stimulation Parameters for High Voltage Monophasic Pulsed Current (HVPC) and Rectangular Monophasic Pulsed Current (PC) in Wound Healing

Type of Current	*HVPC*	*Rectangular Monophasic PC*
Pulse amplitude	100–200 V peak	30–35 mA peak
Pulse duration	100 μs	150 μs
Pulse frequency	30–130 pps	64–128 pps
Mode	Continuous	Continuous
Treatment duration	30–60 min	30 min
No. of treatments/day	1–2	2
Treatment frequency	5–7 days/wk	7 days/wk

Table 8.7. Stimulation Parameters for Biphasic Pulsed Current in Wound Healing

Type of Current	Rectangular Asymmetric Biphasic Pulsed Current
Pulse amplitude	Strong sensory; just less than motor level
Pulse duration	100 μs
Pulse frequency	50 pps
Mode	Continuous
Treatment duration	30 min
No. of treatments/day	3
Treatment frequency	5–7 days/wk

referred to as "high volt" units in clinical settings. The peak amplitude of stimulation is commonly adjusted to sensory level, which may produce a mild tingling (*paresthesia*) beneath the electrodes. In wound healing applications, the frequency of delivery of the twin-spike waveforms generally ranges from 30 to 130 twin-spike pulses per second. Treatment times have ranged from 20 to 60 minutes per session with one to two treatment sessions per day.

Rectangular monophasic pulsed currents employed for wound healing typically use amplitudes that are lower than those used with HVPC. The pulse duration of rectangular monophasic waveforms (100 to 150 μs), in contrast, is longer than those of the twin-spike waveforms (10 to 30 μs per spike) of HVPC. Other parameters of stimulation are similar to those used with HVPC (Table 8.6).

The electrode placement with ES for wound healing using HVPC and rectangular monophasic PC is generally one electrode over the wound and a second electrode 15 to 20 cm proximal over normal tissue. The type of electrodes used has varied, but generally clinicians are using electrodes fabricated from heavy-duty aluminum foil and cut to a size just larger than the wound opening. Alternatively, some clinicians use commercially manufactured carbon rubber electrodes that may be trimmed to approximate the wound size. Saline-soaked gauze is loosely placed within the wound to allow for conduction of current between the electrode over the wound and the wound tissue.

The polarity of the electrode placed over the wound has varied in clinical studies. Frequently, the treatments are initiated with the cathode as the active electrode. After several days of treatment the electrode polarity is reversed to the positive charge. Thereafter, the polarity has often been reversed again until the wound is completely healed whenever the rate of healing appears to have significantly slowed throughout the remainder of treatments.

Biphasic Pulsed Currents for Wound Healing

Only a few studies have been performed using biphasic pulsed currents. The waveform shape in two of the more successful clinical trials was rectangular, asymmetric, balanced biphasic pulsed current. Parameters of stimulation for use of this form of current in chronic wound healing are shown in Table 8.7. This form of current is applied with electrodes placed just proximal and distal to the edges of the opening of the wound. Electrodes used are commercially available carbon rubber electrodes. The dimensions of these electrodes have not been specified.

EVIDENCE ON THE EFFECTIVENESS OF ELECTRICAL STIMULATION FOR HEALING OF CHRONIC WOUNDS

A substantial body of literature has developed over the past three decades regarding the efficacy of electrical stimulation as an adjunctive therapy in the treatment of wounds. Many of these studies have examined the effects of ES on experimentally induced wounds in both animals and humans. In such cases, the wounds are acute, and the relevance of the results of these studies to the effects of ES on chronic wounds is questionable. Summaries of the studies on the effects of ES on acute wounds can be found in several reviews (23,29,34–36). The review of the literature in this chapter is confined to the clinical trials on the effects of ES on chronic wounds in humans.

Low-Intensity Direct Current for Wound Healing

The modern era of investigation of electrical stimulation for wound healing arose in the late 1960s and early 1970s. Some of the earliest studies examined the effects of continuous, low-amplitude direct current on chronic wounds. In 1969, Wolcott and et al. (37) reported on the effects of LIDC on healing of chronic wounds of various etiologies in a descriptive clinical trial. Wound volumes were estimated by either the manual measurement of the largest wound dimensions (length × width × depth) or, if possible, by the instillation of measured amounts of normal saline into the wound. Wolcott et al. used amplitudes of stimulation in the range of 200 to 800 μA DC applied daily for periods of 2 hours, 3 times per day for a total of 6 hours of stimulation per day. Subjects had 4 hours of rest between stimulation sessions. The amplitude of stimulation was adjusted in the treatment of each wound to avoid excessive harmful levels as revealed by bleeding in the wound during or after treatment. Electrodes (2 inches × 2 inches) were fabricated from copper mesh and placed over several layers of gauze saturated in Ringer solution (an isotonic solution of sodium chloride, potassium chloride, and calcium chloride in water). The cathode of the DC circuit was placed directly over the chronic wound in initial treatments. The anode was placed over Ringer-saturated gauze pads 15 cm proximal to the wounds. When the wound appeared to be uninfected, the polarity was reversed such that the anode was placed over the wound. If healing reached a growth plateau, the cathodal stimulation was reinstituted over the wound. Late in the course of treatment the polarity of the electrodes over the wound was switched each day. Using this protocol on 75 ulcers produced an average healing rate of 13.4% per week, with complete healing occurring in more than 40% of the ulcers treated. The healing rate of those ulcers that healed completely was 18.4% per week. Eight of the patients in this study had bilateral ischemic ulcers. In this group, one of the ulcers was treated with the LIDC protocol and the other ulcer served as a control. The mean healing rate was 27% per week for the treated ulcers, and the mean healing rate for the control untreated ulcers was less than 5% per week. It is interesting to note that the electrodes in this study were fabricated from copper mesh, and some people believe that copper, when exposed to electrical currents, may produce toxic effects on healing wounds. This study did not indicate which estimates of wound volume (dimension measurement or saline instillation volume) were used with each patient to determine the percentage of wound healing. In spite of this shortcoming, the study served as a model for at least two subsequent studies by other groups.

In a descriptive clinical trial published in 1976, Gault and Gatens (38) applied LIDC to 100 ischemic skin ulcers in 76 patients with multiple primary diagnoses. Using the same stimulation protocol outlined above in the Wolcott et al. study (37), 100 ulcers were treated. Six individuals had bilateral ulcers, and one of the ulcers in each of these people served as control, untreated ulcers. Gault and Gatens reported a mean healing rate of 28% in treated ulcers, with an approximate 15% healing rate in the untreated control ulcers ($n = 6$). Complete healing was achieved in about half of the treated ulcers over the 4- to 5-week treatment period.

In the mid-1980s, Carley and Wainapel (33) applied LIDC to chronic ulcers in a randomized clinical trial. Thirty individuals with chronic dermal ulcers were pair matched according to age, diagnosis, wound location, and wound size. One of the members of each pair was then randomly assigned to receive LIDC and standard wound care, and the second pair member received only standard wound care. LIDC was applied in the treatment group for 2 hours, twice each day for 5 days each week. Amplitude of stimulation was in the range of 300 to 700 μA, with the cathode initially over the wound, switching to anodal stimulation over the wound after several days of treatment. Average rate of healing per week was about 18%, and only about half that rate (9%) in control-group wounds (39).

Monophasic Pulsed Current for Wound Healing

As described previously, two forms of monophasic pulsed current have been used in ES for treatment of chronic wounds: twin-spike monophasic pulsed current (also known as HVPC) and rectangular monophasic pulsed current.

In 1988, Kloth and Feedar (40) reported the results of a small-scale trial using twin-spike monophasic pulsed current for the treatment of long-term recalcitrant, stage IV ulcers. Patients were assigned to a stimulation group ($n = 9$) or to a sham-stimulated, control group ($n = 7$) by the results of a coin toss. Amplitude of stimulation was adjusted to a level just below that required to produce muscular contraction in the area of the wound. A frequency of stimulation of 105 pps was used in single, daily treatment sessions lasting 45 minutes. Stimulation was provided using the anode over the wound, with the cathode placed 15 cm proximally over intact skin. Treatment was continued until wounds in the ES group healed completely. The polarity of the electrode over the wound was reversed if the wound healing appeared to plateau. Wound size was determined by tracing the opening of the wound and transferring the tracing to metric graph paper. The number of square millimeters of the wound tracing was counted manually. The authors reported a mean healing rate of 45% in the treated group, although the exact method by which they calculated this healing rate was not described. Possibly the most significant finding arising from this study is that all of the long-term chronic wounds in the treated group healed completely, whereas the wounds in the sham-treated group on average actually increased in size. This study provided a catalyst to the research into the effectiveness of monophasic pulsed current treatment of chronic wounds.

In 1991 Feedar et al. (41) published the results of a multicenter, double-blind, randomized controlled clinical trial of rectangular monophasic pulsed current for chronic wound treatment. Forty-seven patients with stage II, III, or IV chronic dermal ulcers who met their selection criteria were randomly assigned to either an ES treatment group ($n = 26$) or a sham-treated control group ($n = 24$). Wounds in individuals in the ES group were treated with rectangular monophasic pulsed current with the cathode initially placed over the wound. Amplitude of stimulation was 29.2 mA with a pulse duration of 132 μs and a frequency of either 64 pps or 128 pps for a treatment time of 30 minutes. These treatments were delivered twice per day, every day, for 4 weeks. Before treatment was started and weekly during the course of the study, wound appearance was monitored and recorded, along with the wound opening size [wound longest dimension (length) times the width of the wound perpendicular to the length measurement]. The wound size measured weekly was expressed as a percentage of the wound size before treatment. The study revealed that after 4 weeks of daily treatment, the average rate of healing was 14% for the treated group and about 8% for the unstimulated control group. On average, the wounds in the stimulated group were 56% smaller, while in the control group wounds on average were only 33% smaller. After completion of this first phase of the study, 14 of the 24 wounds in the original control group were treated with ES for 4 weeks. These wounds at the end of this 4-week treatment period healed by approximately 50% and at a rate (12.8% per week) similar to that in the original treatment group.

In 1991, Griffin et al. (42) reported on the results of using HVPC on the healing of stage II, III, or IV pressure ulcers (over either the sacrum or greater trochanter) in a clinical trial on 17 individuals with spinal cord injury. The subjects were randomly assigned to either a stimulation group ($n = 8$) or a sham-stimulated control group ($n = 9$). The stimulation program consisted of placement of the cathode of the stimulator over the wound with a large anode over the thigh of one leg. The cathode was fabricated from aluminum foil and cut to a size slightly larger than the opening of the ulcer. Ulcers were packed with saline or gauze soaked with Ringer solution. The frequency of twin-spike monophasic pulsed current was set to 100 pps, and the amplitude of stimulation was gradually increased to 200 V. This level of stimulation did not evoke muscular contraction in any of the treated subjects and did not produce discomfort. Continuous stimulation was applied daily for 1 hour for a period of 20 days. Wounds were photographed every 5 days, and the size of each wound opening was determined using digitization of projected wound tracings and computer software. The study found that those ulcers treated with HVPC were reduced in size by 80% (median percent change), while ulcers in the sham-stimulated, control group were reduced by approximately 50%. The rate of healing per week was not reported and cannot be calculated from the data provided in the report.

In 2001, Peters et al. (43) reported the results of a double-blind, randomized, placebo-controlled clinical trial of the effect of twin-spike monophasic pulsed current on the healing of foot ulcers in individuals with diabetes. Forty patients with uninfected foot ulcers ranging in severity from superficial wounds to wounds penetrating to tendon or joint capsule were randomly assigned to either receive ES treatment or sham ES treatment. In this study, stimulation using HVPC was applied at 50 V (subsensory level), a pulse duration of 100 μs, and a frequency of 80 twin-spikes per second for 10 minutes, followed by 10 minutes of treatment at a frequency of 8 pps. This treatment was followed by 40 minutes of no stimulation. This pattern of stimulation (20 minutes on/40 minutes off) was repeated for an 8-hour period each night for 12 weeks. Wound size was measured using digital techniques from video pictures of the wound. An analysis of the changes in wound size revealed no significant difference in the rate of wound healing between treated and sham-treated ulcers. One might speculate that this negative outcome may be related to the relatively low amplitude of stimulation (subsensory level, 50 V peak amplitude applied to a garment electrode that was markedly larger in surface area than those used in other studies evaluating the efficacy of HVPC in the management of chronic wounds).

A unique feature of the Peters et al. (43) study was the method of delivery of the current. The active treatment electrode was a Dacron-mesh silver nylon stocking with a surface area of about 176 square inches. The stocking electrode is apparently designed to allow the passage of current over the entire surface area in contact with the skin of the foot and ankle. Before application of this stocking electrode, a slowly evaporating electrolytic fluid was applied to the foot to facilitate conduction of current. The use of such a large electrode with such a low amplitude of stimulation would have resulted in current density beneath the electrode that was much lower than that achieved in previous studies with successful outcomes.

In 2003, Houghton et al. (2) published the results of a study using HVPC for the treatment of 42 chronic leg ulcers in 27 individuals. The chronic wounds in these patients were categorized as either diabetic ulcers, venous insufficiency ulcers, or arterial ulcers. Participants were divided into subgroups based on the type of chronic wound and were then randomly assigned to a stimulation group ($n = 14$) or a sham-stimulation group ($n = 13$). All subjects in the ES group received HVPC with the cathode placed directly over the wound three times per week for 4 weeks. Electrode polarity was not changed during the 4-week course of treatment. Stimulation parameters included an amplitude of stimulation of 150 V, twin-spike pulse duration of 100 μs, and pulse frequency of 100 pps. Wound surface area was measured by tracing the wound opening and determining the area of the tracing with planimetry. The wound surface area was determined during the initial screening evaluation, after 1 to 2 weeks of conventional wound care before initiation of ES or sham ES, after the 4-week ES treatment program, and 1 month after ES had been discontinued. The percentage decrease in wound surface areas was calculated at each of these times. The percentage decrease in wound area in the ES group was approximately 47% (12% per week), whereas the percentage decrease in wound area for the sham-stimulated group was about 22% (5% per week).

Biphasic Pulsed Current for Wound Healing

In 1992 Lundeberg et al. (44) published the result of a study on the treatment of diabetic ulcers due to venous stasis using a rectangular biphasic pulsed current (amplitude sufficient to produce paresthesia; pulse duration, 1 ms; frequency, 80 pps). It is unclear from this study whether the waveform used was symmetric or asymmetric. Sixty-four patients were randomly divided into two groups. Patients in the stimulated group received standard care plus stimulation for 20 minutes two times per day for 12 weeks. Patients in the control group received standard care plus placebo stimulation for the same period. Before initiation of treatment, ulcer surface openings were traced, and wounds were categorized as superficial or deep. Surface area of each wound was determined using computer graphics programs. Electrodes in this study were placed outside the ulcer surface area as opposed to placing one electrode directly over the wound and the second on the surrounding intact tissue. The healing rate per week for treated ulcers was 5% per week, whereas the healing rate for ulcers in the sham-treated group was 3.4% (39). These rates of healing appear to be markedly lower than those found with the use of LIDC or monophasic pulsed current when applied directly over the wound, and in many studies patients were treated for a longer period of time than was used in this study.

In 1997, Baker et al. (45) reported on the use of both rectangular, balanced, asymmetric, biphasic, pulse current and rectangular, balanced, symmetric biphasic pulsed current on the healing of 114 diabetic ulcers in 80 patients. Patients were randomly assigned to receive the asymmetric biphasic pulsed current (amplitude less than motor level, 65 mA on average; pulse duration, 100 μs; frequency, 50 pps; on:off time, 7 seconds:7 seconds); symmetric biphasic pulsed current (amplitude less than motor level, 63 mA on average; pulse duration, 300 μs; frequency, 50 pps; on:off time: 7 seconds:7 seconds); symmetric biphasic pulsed current (amplitude less than motor level, 4 mA on average; pulse duration, 10 μs, frequency, 1 pps, on:off time, 7 seconds:7 seconds) or were assigned to a nonstimulated control group. Electrodes in patients in the stimulated groups were placed just proximal to and just distal to the open wound. For subjects receiving one of the three forms of stimulation, three 30-minute treatment sessions were provided each day with a brief break between each treatment session. The primary outcome measure was the area of the opening of the wound that was measured from tracings of the wounds on a weekly basis. The findings revealed that the rate of healing was greatest in the group of patients receiving the asymmetric biphasic pulsed current (27%), and this was significantly greater than that of the merged control group (17%) (initial control subjects plus the minimal stimulation subjects). Subjects in the group stimulated with the symmetric biphasic pulsed current did not heal at a rate that was significantly different from individuals in the merged control group. It may be that the superior response found in this study by comparison to that of Lundberg resulted from either the longer duration of treatment (90 minutes vs. 40 minutes) or to some as yet unknown difference between the different waveforms used in each study.

Baker et al. (46) used nearly the same treatment protocol described above in the treatment of chronic wounds in individuals with spinal cord injury. The major difference in the stimulation program was that the treatment duration was 45 minutes each day. In contrast to the approximately 30% per week rate of healing seen in the treatment of chronic diabetic ulcers, this study found a 64% per week rate of healing.

In both studies, Baker et al. (45,46) proposed that the increase in the rates of healing of ulcers was likely due to an increase in the blood flow to the wound, a proposed mechanism that is given some support by the previously discussed work of Petrofsky et al. (28)

Meta-Analysis of Studies on Electrical Stimulation for Tissue Healing and Repair

In 1999, Gardner et al. (39) reported the results of a meta-analysis of 15 studies on the effects of electrical stimulation of chronic wounds on the rate of wound healing. Each of these studies were conducted with human subjects and provided stimulation directly over the wounds or to tissues immediately around the wounds and included wounds classified as pressure ulcers, venous ulcers, arterial ulcers, or neuropathic ulcers. In addition, each of the studies reported data on wound size before and after treatment, as well as the rate of wound healing expressed as the percentage of healing per week. The studies reviewed included placebo-controlled, randomized clinical trials ($n = 8$); nonrandomized, placebo-controlled clinical trials ($n = 1$); nonrandomized clinical trials ($n = 5$); and one study with a descriptive design. The forms of electrical stimulation varied and included LDIC, continuous monophasic pulsed current (e.g., HVPC), and continuous biphasic pulsed current (either symmetric or asymmetric waveforms). Stimulation parameters such as polarity of electrodes placed over the wounds (for LIDC or monophasic pulsed current), frequency of stimulation (for PC), duration of each treatment, and frequency of treatments varied among the studies examined. In addition, in some of the studies some of the information that characterizes the dosage of treatment was not reported. For each of the included studies, the mean percentage healing per week (PHW) was determined for both treated and control wounds.

The analysis revealed that the mean PHW was 22.5% for wounds treated with ES and 9% for untreated wounds. The net effect of ES to chronic wounds was reported to be a mean PHW of 13.5%, which represented a 144% increase over the control wound rate of healing. These findings were similar for both placebo-controlled studies or for all the studies reviewed including nonplacebo-controlled studies. The meta-analysis did not provide insight into the relative effectiveness of the different forms of stimulation used (which form or dosage of ES was best for wound healing), or which types of wounds responded best to the electrical stimulation treatment.

CONTRAINDICATIONS AND PRECAUTIONS TO THE USE OF ELECTRICAL STIMULATION TO AUGMENT HEALING OF CHRONIC WOUNDS

As in much of electrotherapy, the delineation of conditions that represent contraindications from those that represent precautions is difficult. Among those conditions that would preclude the use of ES for wound healing are osteomyelitis or malignancy in or around the wound. Some authors have not used ES for wounds in patients with cardiac conductivity disorders or in the presence of any implanted stimulation device. Others have suggested that stimulation may be used if the current produced by the stimulation will not pass in the vicinity of the implanted electrodes or the stimulator producing the current.

Reduction of cutaneous sensation is at times identified as a contraindication to the use of ES. Many of the patients who develop chronic wounds, however, have diminished ability to perceive the stimulation applied to wounds. Diminished or absolute loss of the sensation in the area of the wound does not appear to be an absolute contraindication, because none of the clinical trials reviewed in this chapter reported any adverse clinical response. It may be that the relatively low levels of stimulation, sensory level or subsensory level, have a low probability of producing adverse tissue responses.

Close observation of the patient responses both during and after treatment is advisable. In some patients it may be wise to monitor blood pressure during the first few treatments to determine if the stimulation produces any significant changes (increases or decreases). The response of the wound or periwound tissues should be monitored routinely during the course of treatment. The initiation of bleeding within the wound, as has been seen with LIDC applications, is an example of an adverse response that calls for reduction in the amplitude of stimulation in subsequent treatments, not cessation of treatment.

Some topical medications that may be used in the standard treatment of chronic wounds should be removed from the wound before the initiation of stimulation because of the potential electrophoretic effect of treatment currents on ions in the medication. These medications may include those containing ions such as zinc, mercury, or silver.

CLINICAL CASE STUDIES

Case Study 1

History

The patient is a 35-year-old man who sustained a spinal cord injury in a motor vehicle accident 8 years ago. He has been confined to a wheelchair since his accident. He is currently employed as a computer programmer, which is associated with long periods of time spent sitting in his wheelchair. Several months ago he developed a small ulceration over his left buttocks. He has seen a number of clinicians for standard wound care since he developed the wound. In spite of this care, the wound has now progressed to become a stage III pressure sore.

Examination

An open wound approximately 3 cm in diameter is present over the patient's left ischial tuberocity. The wound does not appear to be infected at this time. No undermining of tissues is present.

Assessment

Left ischial stage III pressure ulcer

Plan

Instruction in periodic unweighting activities to be performed every hour while seated in his wheelchair, new wheelchair seat cushion, and ESTHR for wound healing.

Detailed Electrotherapeutic Plan

Mode of stimulation: sensory-level HVPC with cathode initially over the wound

Type of stimulator: portable (battery-operated)

Electrodes and electrode placements: heavy-duty aluminum foil cut to the size and shape of the wound opening; saline-soaked gauze loosely packed into the open wound

Duration and frequency of treatment: 30 to 45 minutes, 2 to 3 times each day at home and at work

Rationale

Patient has both the physical ability and intelligence to perform ESTHR independently. He did not want to receive treatment either on an inpatient or outpatient basis. Battery-operated HVPV stimulators are commercially available and easy to operate. This choice was based on the outcomes of clinical trials by Kloth and Feedar (40) and Griffin et al. (42).

Case Study 2

A 65-year-old woman with a 45 year history of type I diabetes presents with a persistent (2 years) ulcer over the right calcaneous.

Examination

Observation reveals a moderately obese woman with a wide-based gait. She does not recall any specific incident that led to the onset of the wound. Sensory testing with monofilaments reveals a stocking-type sensory deficit to the mid-lower leg bilaterally. Ankle brachial index is >1.00.

The patient has a well-circumscribed, erythematous, draining, and foul-smelling chronic ulcer, measuring 3 cm × 2 cm over her heel Wound culture is positive for *Staphylococcus aureus.*

Assessment

Infected stage IV diabetic ulcer on right heel, polyneuropathy, and decreased circulation with possible arterial calcification.

Plan

1. Cleaning with surgical Water Pik
2. Debridement as needed
3. HVPC for wound healing
4. Occlusive dressing
5. Referral to nutritionist for weight management program and blood glucose control

Detailed Electrotherapeutic Plan

Mode of stimulation: sensory-level HVPC

Type of stimulator: clinical HVPC stimulator

Electrodes and placement: heavy-duty aluminum foil cut to the size and shape of the wound opening; saline-soaked gauze loosely packed into the open wound. Initial placement is cathode in the wound, anode (regular electrode) placed proximal to the wound. After wound is uninfected, switch polarity of electrodes.

Duration of treatment: 1 hour, once per day

Rationale

HVPC current has been chosen to promote wound healing. The negative electrode is placed over the wound initially for purported antibacterial effects. When the wound looks uninfected, the positive electrode is used to facilitate the proliferative phase of healing. This patient is not capable of performing the treatment at home, and her family is unwilling to assist in the provision of the treatment. She lives only a short distance from the clinic and can be seen daily on an outpatient basis. This treatment was selected based on the outcomes of the study by Houghton et al. (2).

SUMMARY

The purpose of this chapter was to review the use of electrical stimulation to augment healing of chronic wounds. The review of the literature revealed that three types of currents (direct current, monophasic pulsed currents, and asymmetric biphasic pulsed currents) have been successfully used in the management of chronic wounds of various etiologies. The clinical benefit of electrical stimulation to treat chronic wounds becomes particularly apparent from the results of studies in which wounds that were unresponsive to conventional or standard wound-care techniques were healed when ES was added to the treatment program.

Although clinical trials have demonstrated that the healing rate of chronic wounds may be increased with electrical stimulation, many important questions regarding ESTHR in the treatment of chronic wounds remain unanswered. Research is needed to identify and define the optimal form and dosage of electrical stimulation treatment. Many of the studies reviewed in this chapter have expressed important parameters of stimulation such as amplitude in terms of the peak voltage of the monophasic pulsed current waveforms, or the amount of the absolute magnitude of the current (microamperes or milliamperes). In some reports using monophasic pulsed currents, the magnitude of stimulation has been expressed in terms of the electrical charge within each pulse. Seldom have the publications on ES for wound healing expressed the dosage of current in terms of the density of current (μA per cm^2), a measure that takes into account the size of the electrodes that are often placed directly over the open wounds. It may also be important in future studies to consider expressing the dosage of the treatment in terms of the rate of application of charge (Coulombs per second) with respect to the size of the treatment (active) electrodes.

Large-scale studies are needed on the use of ES for wound healing of specific types of chronic wounds. Many of the clinical trials reviewed in this chapter examined the effects of ES on wounds of mixed etiologies, an approach that may limit the ability to identify and define the optimal parameters of stimulation (charge density, current density, frequency of stimulation, duration and frequency of treatments) to produce the optimal rate of wound healing.

More research is required regarding the physiological effects of ES on chronic wounds. Understanding the wound-healing processes that may be enhanced with electrical stimulation may provide better guidance to clinicians and researchers in selecting treatment parameters and forms of treatment (e.g., the most appropriate type of current for a specific class of wounds, the most appropriate polarity of electrodes to stimulate galvanotaxis).

Given the accumulated evidence to date and the quality of that evidence, clinicians should consider electrical stimulation as an important tool to be integrated into the comprehensive plan of care for chronic nonhealing wounds.

SELF-STUDY QUESTIONS

For answers, see Appendix B.

1. Define a chronic wound.
2. List the typical phases of normal wound healing and provide a brief description of the processes that characterize each phase.
3. Identify several factors that may impede wound healing and describe how each may affect healing.
4. Identify and define the four types of chronic wounds and describe the etiology of each type of chronic wound.

5. Identify and define the four stages of pressure ulcers.

6. Identify six purported physiological effects of electrical stimulation that may enhance the rate of healing in chronic wounds.

7. Describe the activities that may be undertaken to prepare the wound before the application of electrical stimulation to augment healing.

8. a. Define direct current and characterize the stimulation parameters that have been used in the application of low-intensity direct current for wound healing. b. Compare and contrast the stimulation parameters of high voltage pulsed current and rectangular, monophasic, pulsed current that have been used in clinical trials on electrical stimulation for wound healing.

9. Where are electrodes typically placed in the treatment of chronic wounds with either LIDC or monophasic pulsed currents?

10. Identify the stimulation parameters of the rectangular symmetric biphasic pulsed current and rectangular asymmetric biphasic pulsed current used for the treatment of chronic wounds in patients with diabetes and in patients with spinal cord injury.

11. Where are treatment electrodes placed when using biphasic pulsed currents for healing of chronic wounds?

12. Why is LIDC seldom used in contemporary clinical treatment of chronic wounds?

13. What are the contraindications and precautions to the use of electrical stimulation in the treatment of chronic wounds?

14. Provide some suggestions for ongoing research in the area of electrical stimulation for wound healing.

REFERENCES

1. Callum MJ, Ruckley CV, Harper DR, et al. Chronic ulceration of the leg: extent of the problem and provision of care. *BMJ.* 1985;290:1855–1856.
2. Houghton PE, Kincaid CB, Lovell M, et al. Effect of electrical stimulation on chronic ulcer size and appearance. *Phys Ther.* 2003;83:17–28.
3. Lazarus GS, Cooper DM, Knighton DR, et al. Definitions and guidelines for assessment of wounds and evaluation of healing. *Arch Dermatol.* 1994;130(4):489–493.
4. Mulder GD, Jeter KF, Fairchild PA, eds. *Clinicians Guide to Chronic Wound Repair.* Spartanburg, SC: Wound Healing Publications; 1991.
5. Robertson W. Digby's receipts. *Ann Med Hist.* 1925;7:216.
6. Centers for Medicare and Medicaid Services. *National Coverage Determination for Electrical Stimulation (es) and Electromagnetic Therapy for the Treatment of Wounds.* NCD 270.1. Washington, DC: Centers for Medicare and Medicaid Services; 2004.
7. Kirsner RS, Bogensberger G. The normal process of healing. In: Kloth LC, McCulloch JM, eds. *Wound Healing Alternatives in Management.* Philadelphia: F. A. Davis; 2002:3–29.
8. Lampe KE. Methods of wound evaluation. In: Kloth LC, McCulloch JM, eds. *Wound Healing Alternatives in Management.* Philadelphia: F. A. Davis; 2002:151–200.
9. Sussman C. Assessment of skin and wound. In: Sussman C Bates-Jensen BM, eds. *Wound Care: A Collaborative Practice Manual for Physical Therapists and Nurses.* Gaithersburg, Md: Aspen Publishers; 1998:49–82.

10. Bates-Jensen BM. Indices to include in wound healing assessment. *Adv. Wound Care.* 1995; 8:25–33.
11. Sussman C, Swanson G. The utility of the Sussman wound healing tool in predicting wound healing outcomes in physical therapy. *Adv. Wound Care.* 1997;10:74–77.
12. Thomas DR, Rodeheaver GT, Bartolucci AA, et al. Pressure ulcer scale for healing: derivation and validation of the PUSH tool. *Adv. Wound Care.* 1997;10(5):96–101.
13. Krasner D. WHS. Wound healing scale. Version 1.0: A proposal. *Adv. Wound Care.* 1997;10:82.
14. National Pressure Ulcer Advisory Panel. Pressure ulcer prevalence, cost and risk assessment: consensus development conference statement. *Decubitus.* 1989;2:24.
15. Fukushima K, Senda N, Inui et al. Studies of galvanotaxis of leukocytes. *Med J Osaka Univ.* 1953;4:195–208.
16. Orida N, Feldman J. Directional protrusive pseudopodial activity and motility in macrophages induced by extra-cellular electric fields. *Cell Motil.* 1982;2:243–255.
17. Eberhardt, Szczypiorski P, Korytowski G. Effect of transcutaneous electrostimulation on cell composition of skin exudates. *Acta Physiol Pol.* 1986;37:41–46.
18. Bourguignon G, Bourguignon L, Khorshed A, et al. Effect of high voltage pulsed galvanic stimulation on human fibroblasts in cell culture [abstract]. *J Cell Biol.* 1986;103:344a.
19. Bourguignon G, Wenche J, Bourguignon L. Electrical stimulation of human fibroblasts casues an increase in Ca2+ influx and the exposure of additional insulin receptors. *J Cell Phsyiol.* 1989;140(2):379–385.
20. Falanga V, Bourguignon G, Bourguignon L. Electrical stimulation increases the expression of fibroblast receptors for transforming growth factor-beta. *J Invest Dermatol.* 1987;88:488–492.
21. Braddock M, Capbell CJ, Zuder D. Current therapies for wound healing: electrical stimulation, biological therapeutics and the potential for gene therapy. *Int J Dermatol.* 1999;38:806–817.
22. Junger M, Zuder D, Steins A, et al. Treatment of venous ulcers with low frequency pulsed current (Dermapulse): effects on cutaneous microcirculation. *Der Hautarzt.* 1997;48:897–903.
23. Kloth L. Electrical stimulation for wound healing: a review of evidence from in vitro studies, animal experiments and clinical trials. *Lower Extremity Wounds.* 2005;4:23–44.
24. Rowley B. Electrical current effects on *E. coli* growth rates. *Proc Soc Exp Biol.* 1972;139:929–934.
25. Rowley B, McKenna J, Chase G, et al. The influence of electrical current on an infecting microorganism in wounds. *Ann N Y Acad Sci.* 1974;238:543–551.
26. Merriman HL, Hegyi CA, Albright-Overton CR, et al. A comparison of four electrical stimulation types on *Staphylococcus aureus* growth in vitro. *J Rehabil. Res. Dev.* 2004;41(2):139–146.
27. Mertz P, Davis S, Cazzaniga A, et al. Electrical stimulation: acceleration of soft tissue repair by varying the polarity. *Wounds.* 1993;5:153–159.
28. Petrofsky J, Schwab E, Taiken L, et al. Effects of electrical stimulation on skin blood flow in controls and in and around stage III and IV wounds in hairy and non-hairy skin. *Med Sci Monitor.* 2005;11:CR309–316.
29. Houghton PE, Campbell KE. Choosing adjunctive therapy for the treatment of chronic wound. *Ostomy Wound Manage.* 1999;45:43–53.
30. Loehne HB. Wound debridement and irrigation. In: Kloth LC, McCulloch JM, eds. *Wound Healing Alternatives in Management.*) Philadelphia: F.A. Davis; 2002:201–231.
31. American Physical Therapy Association. *Electrotherapeutic Terminology in Physical Therapy.* Alexandria, Va: Section on Clinical Electrophysiology, American Physical Therapy Association; 2000.
32. Unger PG. Update on high-voltage pulsed current research and application. *Top Geriatr Rehabil.* 2000;16:35–46.
33. Carley PJ, Wainapel SF. Electrotherapy for acceleration of wound healing: low intensity direct current. *Arch Phys Med.* 1985;66:443–446.
34. Houghton PE. Effects of therapeutic modalities on wound healing: a conservative approach to the management of chronic wounds. *Phys Ther Rev.* 1999;4:167–182.

35. Markiov MS. Electric current and electromagnetic field effects on soft tissue: implications for wound healing. *Wounds.* 1995;7:94–110.
36. Bogie KM, Reger SI, Levine SP, et al. Electrical stimulation for pressure sore prevention and wound healing. *Assist Technol.* 2000;12:50–66.
37. Wolcott LE, Wheeler PC, Hardwicke HM, et al. Accelerated healing of skin ulcers by electrotherapy. *South Med J.* 1969;62:795–801.
38. Gault WR, Gatens PF. Use of low intensity direct current in management of ischemic skin ulcers. *Phys Ther.* 1976;56:265–269.
39. Gardner SE, Frantz, RA, Schmidt FL. Effect of electrical stimulation on chronic wound healing: a meta-analysis. *Wound Rep. Regul.* 1999;7:495–503.
40. Kloth LC, Feedar JA. Acceleration of wound healing with high voltage pulsed current. *Phys Ther.*1988;68:503–508.
41. Feedar JA, Kloth LC, Gentskow GD. Chronic dermal ulcer healing enhanced with monophasic pulsed electrical stimulation. *Phys Ther.* 1991;71:639–649.
42. Griffin JW, Tooms RE, Mendius RA, et al. Efficacy of high voltage pulsed current for healing of pressure ulcers in patients with spinal cord injury. *Phys Ther.* 1991;71:433–444.
43. Peters EJ, Lavery LA, Armstron DG, et al. Electric stimulation as an adjunct to heal diabetic foot ulcer: a ramdomized clinical trial. *Arch Phys Med Rehabil.* 2001;82:721–725.
44. Lundeberg TCM, Eriksson SV, Malm M. Electrical nerve stimulation improves healing of diabetic ulcers. *Ann Plast Surg.* 1992;29:328–330.
45. Baker LL, Chambers R, DeMuth SK, et al. Effects of electrical stimulation on wound healing in patients with diabetic ulcers. *Diabetes Care.* 1997;20:405–412.
46. Baker LL, Rubayi S, Villar F, et al. Effect of electrical stimulation waveform on healing of ulcers in human beings with spinal cord injury. *Wound Rep Regul.* 1996;4:21–28.

CHAPTER 9

Electrical Stimulation and Biofeedback for Genitourinary Dysfunction

Rebecca G. Stephenson and Elizabeth R. Shelly

The objective of this chapter is to make the reader aware that electrical stimulation and biofeedback treatments are being used clinically as a component of a comprehensive conservative management program for specific pelvic floor disorders. The chapter presents a brief overview of the neuromuscular anatomy of the pelvic floor, a summary of the normal process of micturition (storage and release of urine), identification of pelvic floor disorders and associated impairments, an overview of the types of anatomical or physiological disorders that may produce the urogenital impairments, and an introduction to the electrical stimulation and biofeedback interventions that have been used in the management of some common impairments of pelvic floor function. Case studies and clinical laboratory exercises are provided to help the reader to appreciate how the theory underlying selected interventions is applied to clinical practice in the care of genitourinary disorders. Bowel and rectal dysfunctions may also be treated with electrical stimulation; however, it is not within the scope of this chapter to review treatment of bowel dysfunction.

Based on Nagi's (1) model on the origin of disability, common problems in genitourinary disorders result in functional limitations that restrict a person's ability to perform physical tasks or activities in an efficient, expected. or competent manner (2). These functional limitations occur in disorders of sphincteric and supportive function. Disorders of sphincteric function such as incontinence (fecal or urinary), difficulty initiating urination, sexual dysfunction, and disorders of supportive function such as organ prolapse may result from pathological processes or from lesions in anatomical structures or in physiological or psychological functions. A comprehensive discussion of the full scope of diseases and disorders that may lead to genitourinary dysfunction is beyond the scope of this chapter. However, examples of impairments that can lead to common urogenital problems include weakness in pelvic musculature, incoordination of pelvic muscle contraction, spasm in pelvic floor or urinary tract musculature, and pelvic pain will be given. Muscle weakness, muscle spasm, muscle incoordination, and pain in musculoskeletal disorders are often managed with conservative, nonsurgical interventions, including electrical stimulation and biofeedback. When found in pelvic structures, these same impairments may also be managed with these conservative interventions.

The prevalence of pelvic floor dysfunctions is best understood by breaking down the statistics by general diagnosis. More than 13 million adults in the United States are affected by incontinence (see Table 9.1 for definition). Incontinence is twice as common in women as in men, and 1 in 10 Americans over the age of 65 are affected (3). A U.S. telephone survey of 5,263 women aged 18 to 50 revealed a prevalence of chronic pelvic pain of 15% (4). Comparatively, the incidence of chronic pelvic pain measured with clinical criteria was 14%. The prevalence of vaginismus [spasm of the pelvic floor muscles (PFM)] in sexual dysfunction clinics is 5% to 17%. Community-based studies of occurrence rate of dyspareunia (painful penetration) ranged from 8% to 23% (4).

Table 9.1. Types of Urinary Incontinence

Type	Result
Stress	Involuntary leakage occurs on effort, or exertion, or on sneezing, or coughing
Urge	Involuntary leakage accompanied by or immediately preceded by an urge to urinate
Mixed	Involuntary leakage associated with urgency and also with exertion, effort, sneezing, or coughing
Overflow	Unexpected leakage of small amounts of urine due to a full bladder
Functional	Untimely urination because of physical disability, external obstacles, or problems in thinking or communicating that prevent a person from reaching a toilet quickly
Transient	Leakage that occurs temporarily because of a condition that will pass (infection, medication)

Adapted from the International Continence Society. Available: International Continence Society (ICS) http://www.continet.org/, with permission.

ANATOMY AND PHYSIOLOGY OF MICTURITION

Anatomy of the Pelvic Floor Musculature

The genitourinary (GU) system in the female includes the uterus, vagina, bladder, urethra, PFM, and external structures of the perineum. Many ambiguous terms have been used in the medical literature to identify pelvic floor structures. This section outlines the most current terminology used by most clinicians. Female anatomy is discussed in detail in this chapter, as 14% of patients with urinary in continence are women and 5% are men (5). However, the pelvic diaphragm layers and intrapelvic hip rotators are fundamentally the same in both sexes.

In this chapter, PFM refers to the entire group of perineal muscles as shown in Fig. 9.1 (6). The PFM, skeletal in composition, can be divided into four layers, from superficial to deep (see Table 9.2 for the muscle attachments and nerve innervations arranged by layer) (6):

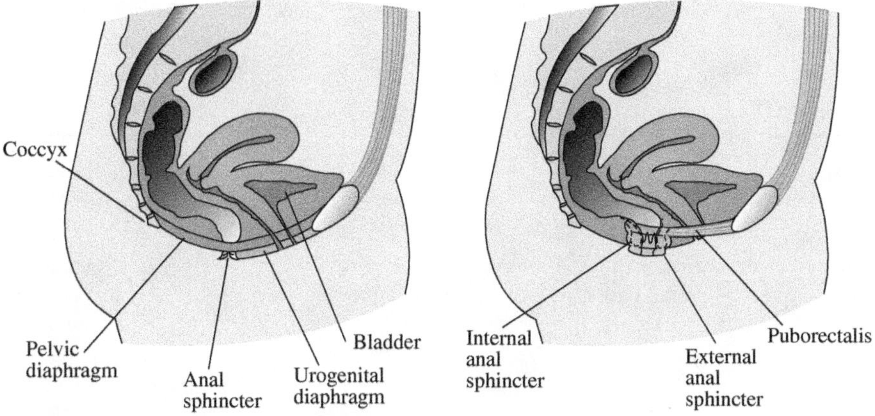

Figure 9.1. The skeletal muscles of the pelvic floor in four layers: anal sphincter, superficial perineal muscles, urogenital diaphragm, and pelvic diaphragm. (Adapted with permission from Shelley, E. The pelvic floor. In: Hall CM, Brody LT, eds. *Therapeutic Exercise: Moving Toward Function.* 2nd ed. Philadelphia: Lippincott Williams & Wilkins; 2005:402–435.)

Table 9.2. Muscle Attachments and Nerve Innervation by Layer

Muscle	Origin	Insertion	Innervation	Function
Layer 1: Anal Sphincter				
Internal anal sphincter (smooth muscle)	Circular muscle at the anorectal junction	Surrounds upper 3/4 of anal canal	S4 and inferior branch of the pudendal nerve	Fecal continence
External anal sphincter (skeletal muscle)	Surrounds whole length of anal canal	Both sphincters fuse superiorly with puborectalis sling of pelvic diaphragm muscle	S4 and inferior branch of the pudendal nerve	Fecal continence
Layer 2: Superficial Perineal Muscles also known as Superficial Senital Muscles				
Bulbocavernosus	Corpus cavernosum of the clitoris	Perineal body	Perineal branch of pudendal S2–S4	Clitoral erection
Ischiocavernosus	Ischial tuberosity and pubic rami	Crus of the clitoris	Perineal branch of pudendal S2–S4	Clitoral erection
Superficial transverse perineal	Ischial tuberosity	Central perineal tendon	Perineal branch of pudendal S2–S4	Stabilizes perineal body
Layer 3: Urogenital Diaphragm also known as Perineal Membrane				
Urethrovaginal sphincter	Vaginal wall	Urethra	Perineal branch of pudendal S2–S4	Compression of the urethra
Sphincter urethrea	Upper 2/3 of urethra	Trigone ring	Perineal branch of pudendal S2–S4	Compression of the urethra
Compressor urethrea	Ischiopubic rami	Urethra	Perineal branch of pudendal S2–S4	Compression of the urethra
Layer 4: Pelvic Diaphragm				
Coccygeus muscle	Spine of the ischium	Anterior portion of the coccyx and S4	Sacral nerve roots S3–S5	Flexes the coccyx
Levator ani muscle	Posterior os pubis, medial surface of the ischial spine, arcus tendinous	Perineal body, vaginal walls, anterior coccyx and lateral rectum	Sacral nerve roots S3–S5	Supports the pelvic viscera, continence mechanism by constricting the rectum and vagina

Adapted from Shelly B. The pelvic floor. In Hall CM, Brody LT. *Therapeutic Exercise, Moving Toward Function*. 2nd ed. Philadelphia: Lippincott Williams & Wilkins; 1999.

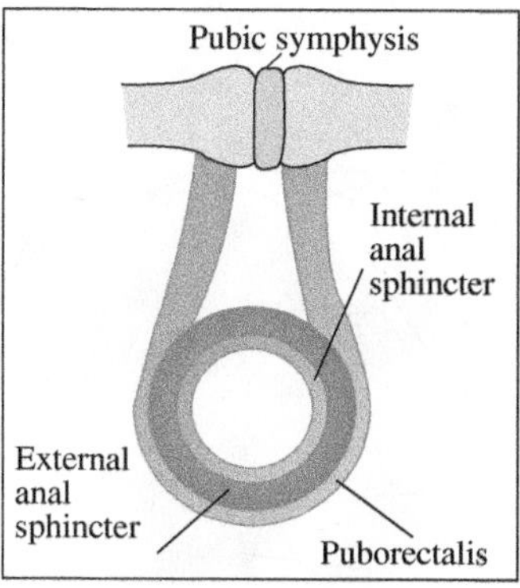

Figure 9.2. The anal sphincter, consisting of the internal anal sphincter and external anal sphincter (From Shelley, E. The pelvic floor. In: Hall CM, Brody LT. *Therapeutic Exercise: Moving Toward Function.* 2nd ed. Philadelphia: Lippincott Williams & Wilkins; 2005:402–435.)

Layer 1: The *anal sphincter* (Fig. 9.2) is the most superficial muscle, composed of the internal anal sphincter (smooth muscle) and the external anal sphincter (skeletal muscle). These sphincters function together to provide fecal continence by maintaining closure of the distal rectum.

Layer 2: The *superficial perineal muscles or superficial genital muscles* (Fig. 9.3) (6), include the bulbocavernosus and ischiocavernosus, which have a role in the final phase of micturition and maintain clitoral erection. The third muscle in this layer, the superficial transverse perineal muscle, supports the perineal body, thereby giving support to the entire pelvic floor.

Layer 3: The *urogenital diaphragm or the perineal membrane* incorporates the urethrovaginal sphincter, the compressor urethrae muscle, and the sphincter urethrae muscle (7–9) (Fig. 9.4). These are important skeletal muscles in maintaining urinary continence. These muscles are mostly composed of slow-twitch muscle fibers. The urethral sphincters in this

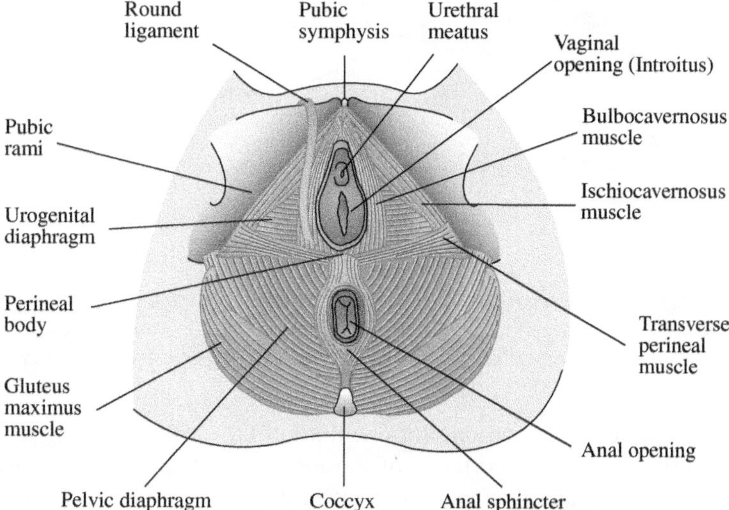

Figure 9.3. The superficial perineal muscles: bulbocavernosus, ischiocavernosus, and the superficial transverse muscles (From Shelley, E. The pelvic floor. In: Hall CM, Brody LT. *Therapeutic Exercise: Moving Toward Function.* 2nd ed. Philadelphia: Lippincott Williams & Wilkins; 2005:402–435.)

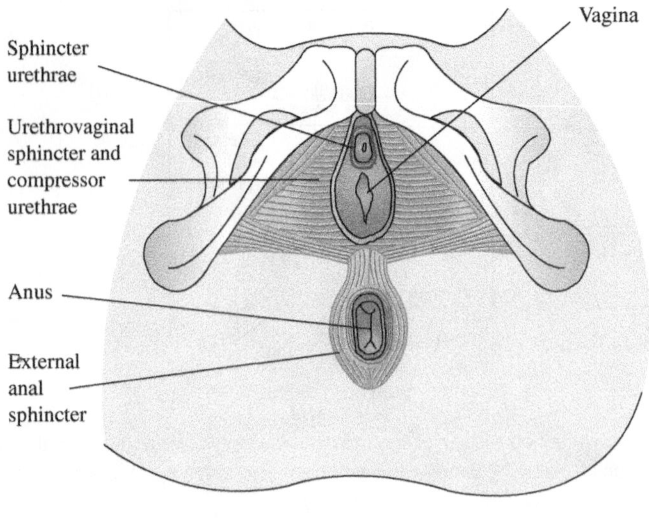

Figure 9.4. The urogenital diaphragm, showing the urethrovaginal sphincter, compressor urethrae muscle (formerly known together as the deep transverse perineal), and sphincter urethrae muscle. (Used with permission from Schussler B, Laycock J, Norton P, Stanton S, eds. *Pelvic Floor Re-education Priciples and Practice*. New York: Springer-Verlag; 1994.)

layer are thought to be responsible for one-third of the urethra's resting tone (5). Current research is showing the importance of the urogenital diaphragm than was previously thought because age and dysfunction result in decreasing fiber count, which decreases strength and continence (10).

Layer 4: The *pelvic diaphragm* is the largest muscle group in the pelvic floor and is responsible for assisting in control of continence and support of pelvic floor organs. This large

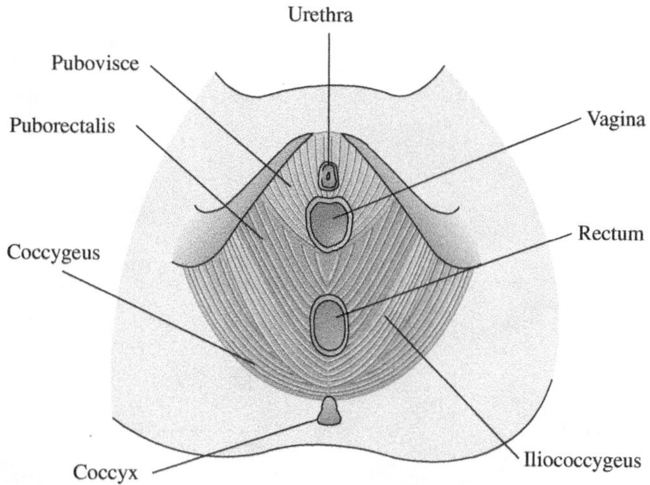

Figure 9.5. The pelvic diaphragm, showing the coccygeus muscle and the levator ani muscles. (From Shelley, E. The pelvic floor. In: Hall CM, Brody LT. *Therapeutic Exercise: Moving Toward Function.* 2nd ed. Philadelphia: Lippincott Williams & Wilkins; 2005:402–435.)

layer is best understood in its two divisions of muscle: the coccygeus muscle and the levator ani muscles (Fig. 9.5). There is some controversy regarding the innervation of the levator ani muscles. It has long been thought that the innervation of the levator ani muscles was the inferior rectal branch of the pudendal nerve. However, in 2002, Barber et al. (11) found, through gross dissections, that the levator ani nerve originates from sacral nerve roots S3-5 and innervates the pelvic diaphragm superiorly. Gross dissection was unable to locate innervation of the pelvic diagram by the pudendal nerve in all 12 cadavers (11).

The pelvic diaphragm muscles are made up of approximately 70% slow-twitch muscle fibers (type 1) and 30% fast-twitch muscle fibers (type 2) (7). Muscle type is important in determining the type of biofeedback needed for pelvic floor dysfunction, addressed later in the chapter. Fiber types have specificity of function in the pelvic floor, and a comprehensive exercise program should train both types of muscle fibers. The physiology of these muscles is similar to that of other skeletal muscles. The PFM respond to quick stretch and have extensive fascia throughout the muscle layers (see Fig. 9.1). The PFM contract as a unit to achieve pelvic support and urethral and anal closure. Impairments can occur in a single layer or throughout the entire skeletal muscle layers unilaterally or bilaterally.

Physiology of Micturition

Micturition is the process of storage and release of urine. Storage and intermittent release of urine is accomplished by the lower urinary tract and is controlled by voluntary, autonomic, and spinal reflex mechanisms. The lower urinary tract consists of the urinary bladder, the urethra, and the muscles in or around these structures (sees Fig. 9.6) (12).

The urinary bladder serves as a reservoir for urine, which is continuously produced by the kidneys at a rate of 15 drops a minute. The urethra is a tubular structure that forms the outflow pathway for the release of urine from bladder storage. Three primary muscles associated with control of micturition are

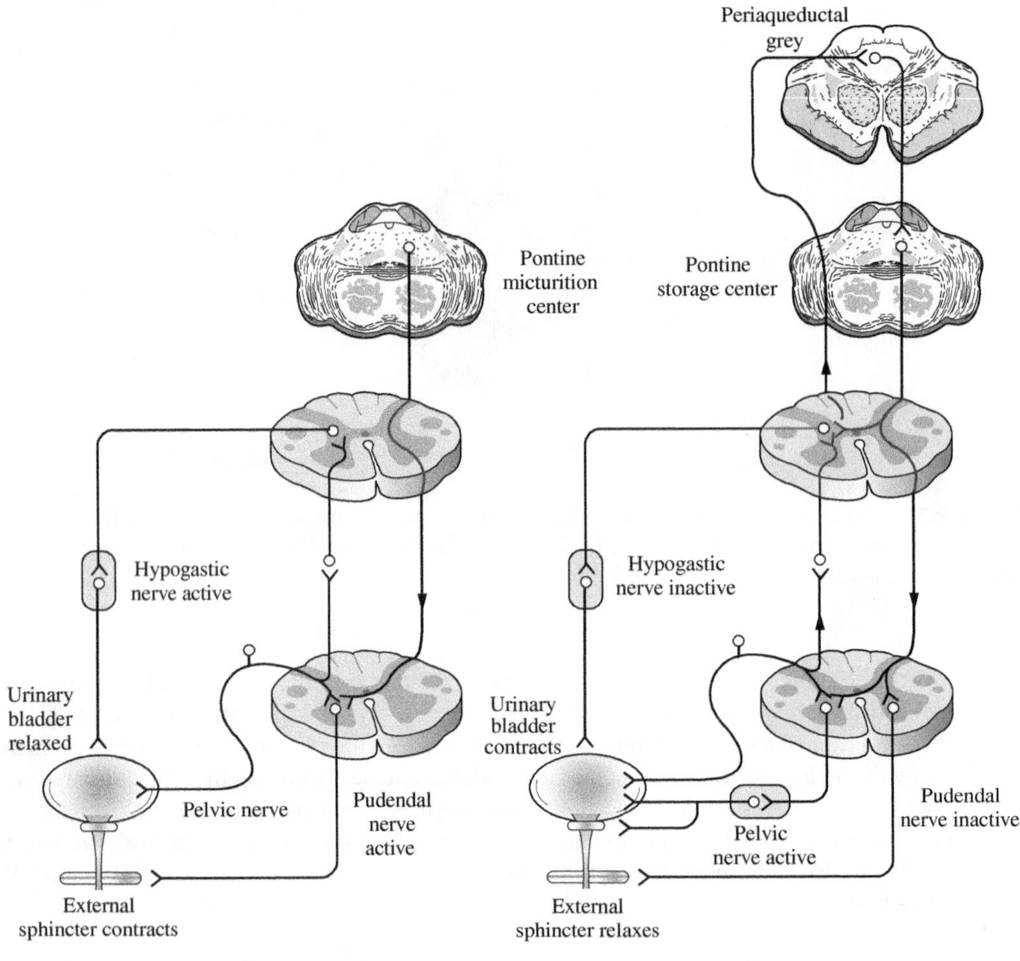

Figure 9.6. A: During urine storage, activity in the hypogastic nerve inhibits the detrusor muscle, allowing the bladder to fill, and contracts the bladder outlet (internal sphincter) to prevent urine release. Activity in the pudendal nerve contracts the external urethral sphincter and pelvic floor musculature to also prevent urine release. **B:** Release of urine from the bladder (voiding) occurs when activity in the pelvic nerve contracts the detrusor while simultaneously relaxing the bladder outlet. In addition, the activity in the pudendal nerve to the external urethral sphincter and pelvic floor muscles is reduced.

1. The *detrusor muscle* (smooth muscle) layer of the bladder
2. The *internal urethral sphincter* (smooth muscle) at the base of the bladder where the urethra begins
3. The *sphincter urethrea* (striated muscle) located around the urethra as it passes through the pelvic floor.

Three nerves innervate these muscles of the urinary tract and control the level of contraction in these muscles to allow for either bladder filling or bladder emptying. The *hypogastric nerve* innervates both the detrusor muscle of the bladder and the internal urethral sphincter. This nerve represents the sympathetic innervation to the urinary tract, and its activity is primarily controlled by inputs to its neurons at the T12 to L2 levels of the spinal cord arising from the *pontine micturition center*. Activation of the hypogastric neurons produces detrusor muscle relaxation and internal urethral sphincter contraction. The *pelvic nerve* innervates the detrusor muscle and represents the parasympathetic innervation of the urinary tract. Finally, the *pudendal nerve* and the levator ani nerve, both somatic nerves with motor and sensory input, innervate the PFM (12).

The activity of the parasympathetic neurons contributing to the pelvic nerve is also under the control of the pontine micturition center. Activity in the pelvic nerve axons produces detrusor contraction. The pudendal nerve innervates the urogenital diaphragm. This is a somatic nerve (as opposed to autonomic nerve), and hence its activity is under voluntary control from the cerebrum. Activity in the pudendal axons produces contraction in the urogenital diaphragm.

The last important neurons associated with the control of micturition are sensory axons, which arise from stretch receptors that lie in the wall of bladder. These neurons are activated as the wall of the bladder is stretched when urine volume in the bladder rises. These sensory axons that travel through the pelvic and hypogastric nerves make synaptic connections at the lumbar and sacral levels of the spinal cord and are associated with reflex control of the sympathetic and parasympathetic outputs to the urinary tract (12). In addition these neurons transmit information regarding bladder filling to the pontine micturition center and the cerebral cortex, which results in control of voiding and conscious perception of bladder fullness.

Storage of Urine

A layer of smooth muscle in the bladder wall, the detrusor muscle, is a layer of the bladder. During the storage phase of micturition, the detrusor is normally relaxed, allowing for the expansion of the bladder as urine volume gradually increases. Two circular muscles are present at the proximal and distal ends of the urethra. These are known as the internal urethral sphincter and sphincter urethrea, respectively. In addition, the sphincter urethrea encircles the entire length of the urethra. While urine is being stored, these two muscles are normally in a state of tonic low-level contraction, closing the urethra and preventing the release of urine from the bladder. The relaxation of the detrusor muscle to allow filling of the bladder and the contraction of the internal urethral sphincter result from sympathetic axon activity in the hypogastric nerve. The contraction of the sphincter urethrea during urine storage is produced by somatic axon activity in the pudendal nerve. Under normal conditions, while the bladder fills, the activity in the parasympathetic pelvic nerve axons to the detrusor is very low if not absent. As the bladder expands to 150 mL of urine, stretch receptors stimulate the brain with a signal to void. The bladder will hold up to 300 mL, at which point a strong sensation of urgency is experienced. At 400 to 550 mL, a severe urge to void is felt (9).

Release of Urine: Voiding

Voiding results from a reversal of the activity of autonomic and somatic neurons to the bladder and urethra (see Table 9.3) (13). As urine accumulates in the bladder and the bladder expands, sensory stretch receptors located in the bladder wall are activated. Action potentials initiated in the axons of these stretch receptors are carried to and terminate at two primary locations, the spinal cord and the brainstem pons. At the spinal cord level, bladder-stretch afferent axons form reflex connections that excite the bladder's parasympathetic innervation of the detrusor, while simultaneously inhibiting both the sympathetic and somatic neurons to the bladder and the urethral sphincters. If this reflex effect is great enough, the net effect will be relaxation of the urethral sphincters accompanied by bladder contraction, leading to voiding. This reflex is counteracted by activation from the cerebral cortex, which acts to decrease the detrusor contraction and increase the skeletal muscle activity, which in turn decreases the effect of the reflex and maintains continence.

Table 9.3. Autonomic Activity of Bladder Storage and Emptying

Bladder	*Detrusor Muscle*	*Parasympathetic*	*Sympathetic*	*Pelvic Floor Muscle*
Storing	Relaxed	Inactive	Active	Contracted
Emptying	Contracted	Active	Inactive	Relaxed

Adapated from Shelly B. *Beginner Gynecological Therapy*. Coursework presented for Women's Hospital of Baton Rouge, La; 1998.

Bladder stretch receptors also give input to the level of the pons and activate the pontine micturition center. This center in turn projects to the lumbosacral spinal cord, where the spinal reflexes are augmented. As can be seen from the description above, control of voiding is mediated at two separate levels of the central nervous system. The spinal-level reflex control is called the micturition or detrusor reflex, and it operates mainly in infants and in individuals with spinal cord injury that impairs ascending activation of the pontine micturition center. The pontine micturition center is a site that is closely associated with one's ability to voluntarily control the timing of voiding from childhood through adulthood.

Micturition is controlled by many complex reflexes. Storage reflexes involve the sympathetic output of the hypogastric nerve and the somatic output of the pudendal nerve (pudendal to hypogastric). During normal urine storage, a small activation of the detrusor stretch receptors signals the hypogastric nerve to fire, resulting in continued relaxation of the detrusor muscle and continued contraction of the internal urethral sphincter. The pudendal nerve will also signal continued tension in the pelvic floor muscle, thus resulting in storage of urine. The pudendal to pudendal reflex is a simple somatic reflex in which stimulation of the tissue innervated by the pudendal afferent nerve results in contraction of the muscles innervated by the pudendal efferent. For example, compression of the clitoris results in contraction of the PFM. This maintains continence by closing the urethra as well as increasing the pudendal to hypogastric reflex.

In contrast, voiding reflexes are the result of parasympathetic output from the pelvic nerve with inhibition of the pudendal nerve (pudendal to pelvic). During normal micturition, a significant activation of the detrusor stretch receptors will signal the need to void. When an appropriate location is reached, the cortical pathways inhibit the pudendal nerve, resulting in a relaxation of the PFM. This is quickly followed by activation of the pelvic nerve, which results in contraction of the detrusor muscle. It is postulated that artificial stimulation of the pelvic nerve using vaginal or rectal electrical stimulation will result in the opposite action, that of inhibition of the parasympathetic nerve (see "Proposed Mechanism of Action of Electrical Stimulation for Bladder Inhibition" for more details).

Functionally, as one voids, either in a standing or sitting position, the pelvic floor muscles relax, the detrusor muscle contracts, and urine is released without voluntary pushing (8). At the termination of urination, the PFM again returns to resting tone. Postvoid residual studies show that there is usually 5 to 50 mL of urine remaining in the bladder. Normal voiding frequencies are seven to nine times within 24 hours, occurring every 2 to 5 hours (6)

Role of Pelvic Floor Muscles in Normal Micturition

Besides the sphincter urethrea, other muscles of the pelvic floor contribute to the control of micturition. The bulbocavernosus in males aids in the expulsion of urine from the urethra after the bladder is emptied by detrusor contraction. The levator ani muscle acts to support the bladder and urethra. An elevated and well-supported urethra will resist increased intra-abdominal pressure and thereby result in less incontinence. A strong levator ani contraction can also assist in inhibiting the micturition reflex.

DYSFUNCTION OF NORMAL MICTURITION

Symptoms of urinary dysfunction include but are not limited to incontinence, postmicturition dribbling, frequency, slow voiding, difficulty in initiating voiding, sense of urgency, and pain at rest or during voiding. These problems can arise from many different causes, including side effects of medications, urinary tract obstruction (e.g., tumors, polyps, prostatic hypertrophy, abscesses), fistulas, and neuromuscular disorders. A comprehensive discussion of the full range of disorders that may compromise urogenital function is beyond the scope of this chapter.

The focus of electrotherapeutic interventions for genitourinary disorders is management of the effects arising from neuromuscular dysfunction. Before electrical stimulation interventions are applied to manage the problems arising from neuromuscular dysfunction, a thorough medical evaluation should be conducted to rule out causes that are not amenable to electrotherapeutic interventions.

Dysfunction of the neural pathways and the muscular components that control urination may lead to urinary disorders. Compromise of neural function in either the afferent pathway leading from bladder or the urethral stretch receptors may disrupt voluntary and/or autonomic control of urine storage and release. Neurological disorders may arise from either peripheral nerve or spinal cord damage or diseases (Table 9.4). Injury to the peripheral nerve (pudendal, hypogastric, or pelvic) may occur with lower abdominal surgery, such as hysterectomy in women or prostatectomy in men.

Lesions of the spinal cord proximal to the sacral levels may disrupt or disturb pontine micturition center control of storage and voiding. Because both autonomic (hypogastric and pelvic nerves) and somatic (pudendal nerve) activity is partially controlled by the pontine micturition center, disruption of these inputs will alter the normal level and timing of impulses that regulate bladder muscle and urethral sphincter contraction. Typically, this will result in incomplete bladder emptying and urinary incontinence.

Trauma to urinary tract musculature or muscles of the pelvic floor can interfere with normal contraction of these muscles and lead to incontinence. Table 9.1 summarizes the types of incontinence. Stress incontinence is the most common type of incontinence, accounting for 50% of cases. Childbirth has been proven to result in injury to the PFM, resulting in stress urinary incontinence (5). Muscle injuries result from tears, incisions (via an episiotomy), stretching of the PFM, and/or stretching of the perineal nerves. Obesity, chronic constipation, and chronic cough result in increased intra-abdominal pressure, which weakens the PFM and connective tissue supports. If a person contracts the abdominal and respiratory diaphragm muscle, as in a Valsalva

Table 9.4. Neurological Disorders Effecting Micturition

Neurologic Condition	*Effect on Micturition*
Lumbar disc prolapse	Acute urinary retention
Cauda equine compression	Increased detrusor contractility, increased bladder capacity, and urinary incontinence
Sacral lesions	Bladder areflexia, low compliance bladder, high detrusor leak point pressures
Suprasacral lesions	Bladder overactivity, detrusor sphincter dysynergy, low bladder compliance, high detrusor leak point pressure
Spinal cord injury above T7	Overactive bladder
Lumbar spinal stenosis	Elevated post void residual, reduced flow rates
Multiple sclerosis	Urgency, frequency, urge incontinence due to overactive bladder
Alzheimer disease	Overactive bladder

maneuver, this causes increased intra-abdominal pressure and pressure on the exterior of the bladder (see "Coordination Impairment," below).

Hysterectomy is associated with both stress and urge incontinence due to possible pelvic nerve damage, estrogen deficiency, damage to bladder ligaments, and postoperative catheter use. Prostatectomy is the most common cause of stress urinary incontinence in men. In this procedure, many of the support structures of the bladder and urethra are removed, including the prostate, the bladder neck, and sometimes part of the urogenital diaphragm. External anal sphincter weakness contributes to the occurrence of fecal incontinence. Weakness of the anal sphincters and the urinary sphincters in men is treated in the same way that female urinary incontinence is treated.

Pathophysiology of an overactive bladder is more difficult to determine, and it seems to have a large neural component. It is the second most common type of incontinence (20% to 40%), and is most common in the elderly. Damage to autonomic pelvic nerves and the central nervous system is a possible etiology for increased bladder activity. The term *detrusor hyperreflexia* is used when overactive bladder activity occurs in a patient with documented neurological events such as stroke, Parkinson disease, or multiple sclerosis. Urinary tract infections also stimulate and irritate bladder symptoms. Habit has also been indicated as a cause (i.e., poor fluid intake and voiding too frequently or not voiding often enough).

PELVIC FLOOR MUSCLE IMPAIRMENT

All skeletal muscles, including the PFM, are classified using the impairment model. These impairments are briefly reviewed here to give the reader a more complete understanding of the application of electrical stimulation to these conditions. Many of these impairments fit into musculoskeletal practice pattern C: impaired muscle performance, from the *Guide to Physical Therapy Practice* (2). PFM impairments are treated using similar methods to those used to treat the muscle impairments in other areas of the body. These impairments include weakness, poor endurance, pain, and disruptions in coordination.

Weakness Impairment

The performance of the PFM can become compromised for many reasons. These include injury during vaginal delivery, pelvic pain, central nervous system or peripheral nervous system neurologic dysfunction, surgical procedures, decreased consciousness of PFM, disuse, prolonged increased intra-abdominal pressure, pelvic congestion or swelling, and back or pelvic pain (6). Weakness is usually the primary impairment in the *supportive dysfunction* diagnostic classification. When weakened muscles do not support the pelvic organs, a supportive dysfunction of the PFM results. Pain and pressure in the perineum may also result as the lengthened muscles disrupt the ligamentous supports, which results in stretch on the nerves. Treatment for weakness includes active pelvic floor exercises (14–16), EMG or pressure biofeedback, electrical stimulation, and facilitation and overflow techniques for extremely weak PFM.

Endurance Impairment

Endurance impairment is the second most common PFM impairment that practitioners see clinically. The PFM are composed of 70% slow-twitch muscle fibers. They provide a baseline tone for long periods of time and support pelvic organs against gravity in upright positions. Consequently, the PFM function as postural muscles. Poor endurance of the PFM is a common finding in many women before they display symptoms of PFM dysfunction. Prophylactically teaching pelvic floor exercises (PFE) to all adults may help prevent PFM dysfunctions in the future. This is especially true in prenatal (10) and postpartum women and women before gynecologic surgery or at the onset of menopause. Endurance impairments are treated with PFE and electrical stimulation (7).

Pain and Hypertonic Impairment

Pain and hypertonia impairments are usually the primary impairments of hypertonia dysfunctions, also referred to as overactive pelvic floor muscles, and commonly are seen together. These impairments may be caused by lumbopelvic joint mobility impairment, tonic holding patterns of the PFM, hip muscle imbalance, spasm, abdominal adhesions, and adhered scars in the trunk and perineum, fissures, and fistulas. PFM dysfunction may directly or indirectly cause PFM spasm (6). Consequently, PFM spasm with or without muscle shortening occurs in response to many situations. Coccyx pain can be a result of sacrococcygeal joint mobility impairment and or referred pain from spasm and/or trigger points from the PFM, obturator internus, and piriformis muscles (17).

Treatment of PFM spasm includes manual soft-tissue manipulation of PFM vaginally, rectally, or externally around the ischial tuberosities and coccyx. Surface EMG biofeedback and PFE may also help restore the normal tone of the PFM. In some cases, the PFM become contracted with a high resting tone, confirmed by EMG testing, and these muscles cannot relax fully or contract effectively. Physical interventions such as electrical stimulation, ultrasound, heat, and cold are used on the perineum to treat spasm. Due to the proximity of the bacteria in the vagina in applying physical interventions, the practitioner should learn the logistics of applying the modality to the perineum (6).

Coordination Impairment

Coordination impairment of the PFM is the inability of the collective PFM to contract and relax at the appropriate times. Evaluation of the PFM strength through manual and biofeedback training can reveal the client's inability to produce and maintain a muscle contraction. This problem is usually related to decreased awareness of the PFM contraction (6). In conditions that are not neurologically based, the client can be taught how to properly contract and hold the PFM through biofeedback (e.g., surface EMG, pressure, or internal stimulation).

Coordination impairment is related to inappropriate timing and recruitment of the PFM (6). This impairment includes incoordination of the PFM contraction, incoordination of the abdominal contraction, incoordination of the PFM during activities of daily life, and incoordination of the PFM with the abdominals (18).

During daily activities, the patient may notice urine leaking when lifting objects, coughing, and sneezing. Weakness of the PFM and/or improper contraction of the PFM at the time of activity can cause this leaking. Training patients to contract the PFM before and during increased intra-abdominal pressure when coughing, lifting, and sneezing can decrease or prevent leakage up to 70% (19,20).

Subjectively, most people feel a stronger PFM contraction when the abdominals are correctly pulled inward toward the spine, especially when there is PFM weakness. Fine-wire EMG research done in women with no symptoms of PFM dysfunction show that the abdominal muscles participate in contraction with the PFM (21,22). The PFM cannot contract effectively with a Valsalva maneuver when the abdominals are distended or lengthened, or during bearing down. In PFM training, it is especially important not to bear down and bulge the abdominals outward with the PFM contraction. A goal of therapy is to ensure that patients learn to coordinate the PFM and the abdominal muscles through the use of biofeedback.

Although a complete discussion on bowel function and dysfunction is beyond the scope of this chapter, there are some general considerations in understanding the coordination of the PFM

Table 9.5. Clinical Classifications of Pelvic Floor Muscle Dysfunctions

Dysfunction	*Etiology*	*Common Impairments*	*Functional limitations*
Supportive dysfunction (also known as underactive PFM)	Birth trauma-stretch to muscle/nerve, nerve compression, muscle tear, CNS or PNS trauma Pelvic surgery: nerve injury, stretched connective tissue Prolonged increased intra-abdominal pressure: organ prolapse Obesity	Impaired muscle performance: PFM weakness, muscle atrophy, connective tissue length Endurance impairment Abdominal muscle performance: increased weakness and muscle length	Stress incontinence Mixed incontinence Organ prolapse Limited social and work activates due to fear of leakage Urinary frequency may decrease capacity to sleep or participate in activities Pain with pelvic organ prolapse may limit choices of recreational, social, and work activities
Hypertonia dysfunction (also known as overactive PFM)	Lumbopelvic joint dysfunction: coccyx injury, pubic symphysis strain Tonic holding pattern of the PFM in response to pain or stress Connective tissue dysfunction in disease (i.e., fibromyalgia) Painful conditions: fistula, fissure, vulvadynia, interstitial cystitis, endometriosis, episiotomy adhesions	Altered tone of the PFM with muscle spasm, trigger points Altered tone and spasm of the associated hip and trunk muscles Mobility impairment of scars and connective tissue Mobility impairment of pelvic and lumbar joints Faulty posture leading to joint and muscle strain Pain in the perineum and trunk	Decreased sitting, standing and lifting ability Decreased ability to perform work and household duties Decreased ability to wear jeans or ride a bike Decreased ability to tolerate penetration in intercourse, gynecological examinations, tampons
Incoordination dysfunction	Neurological disease, spinal cord lesion Non-neurological: muscle atrophy, disuse, decreased awareness of PFM, pain inhibited	Coordination impairment of the PFM with ADLs, PFM with abdominal control	Stress incontinence Obstructed voiding or defecation Fear of leakage limits social and work activities Decreased ability to sleep or participate in activities Pain with pelvic organ prolapse limits choices of recreational, social, and work activities

CNS, central nervous system; PNS, peripheral nervous system; PFM, pelvic floor muscles; ADLs, activities of daily living.
Adapted from Shelly B. The pelvic floor. In Hall CM, Brody LT. *Therapeutic Exercise, Moving Toward Function.* 2nd ed. Philadelphia: Lippincott Williams & Wilkins; 1999.

during defecation. During bowel evacuation, the PFM relax to allow complete elimination. Coordination impairment results if there is a PFM contraction during defecation. Accordingly, difficulty can occur in passing feces, which can cause constipation and pain, resulting in obstructed defecation. The challenge is to instruct the patient to relax the PFM with the proper timing associated with abdominal contraction necessary for defecation.

Table 9.5 (6) summarizes the above clinical classifications of PFM dysfunction by etiology, common impairments, and functional limitations. As the practitioner gains skill in examination and prescription for treatment, the type of dysfunction will become evident.

ELECTRICAL STIMULATION FOR GENITOURINARY DYSFUNCTION

General Considerations for Electrical Stimulation of Pelvic Floor Musculature

Early in the history taking, screening questions can assist the practitioner in identifying dysfunctions of micturition that need further medical intervention and referral. These questions can easily be incorporated into all initial evaluations. Screening questions to ask all patients include (6):

Do you ever leak urine or feces?

Do you ever wear a pad because of leaking urine?

Do you have vaginal pain during and/or after penetration?

Several dedicated electrical stimulation units for pelvic floor strengthening are available in the United States for treatment of stress and urge incontinence. Most are preprogrammed, battery operated, and fairly easy to use. Many companies have developed and tested their own protocols, and many patients have benefited from preprogrammed, generic protocol treatments.

Electrical Stimulation for Urinary Incontinence and Supportive Dysfunction in Pelvic Floor Muscle Weakness

The primary objectives of electrical stimulation for urinary incontinence and supportive dysfunction, also referred to as underactive pelvic floor muscles, with PFM weakness are to increase sensory feedback and increase muscle strength to restore urinary continence.

Patient Selection and Indications

Patients with severe PFM weakness (0/5 to 1/5 on a 0 to 5-muscle grading system) and decreased pelvic floor proprioception may benefit from electrical stimulation. Significant weakness often results in the patient's poor sensation of contraction. Electrical stimulation can assist in increasing sensory input to the muscle. Patients with very weak PFM may have symptoms of urinary stress incontinence, fecal incontinence, or pelvic organ prolapse. Patients with incoordination may also benefit from electrical stimulation to create rhythmical contraction and relaxation and a neuromodulation effect. Some studies have shown increased urethral closure pressure with vaginal electrical stimulation (23,24).

Electrical stimulation may be of limited benefit in cases of severe internal sphincter deficiency, urethral hypermobility, and severe organ prolapse (25). Damage to sensory or motor nerves in this region will also result in a less than ideal outcome. Several studies have attempted to identify factors that predict the effectiveness of pelvic floor stimulation (26–28). However, all these studies found it was not possible to accurately predict outcome. A trial of electrical stimulation is suggested if the patient satisfies the following criteria:

At least partial innervation of the PFM
Intact reflexes (intact sensation and motor innervation of the PFM implies intact reflexes)
Ability of the patient to feel the electrical stimulation
Cognitive ability to understand the procedure.

Treatment position for patients using electrical stimulation may be supine, reclined, or sitting, depending on the electrode. Patients with uterine prolapse may get better results if they are positioned supine with the buttocks elevated on several pillows, so that the effect of gravity moves the uterus away from the electrode.

Contraindications to electrical stimulation include use of internal sensors in patients with acute perineal infections (vaginal, urethral, bladder, or rectal) or with patients that have pessaries (an internal device to support a displaced uterus, bladder, or rectum), as many have metal parts. Most patients can tolerate an appropriate level of stimulation. However, those with atrophic vaginitis may complain of constipation and/or vaginal irritation. Electrical stimulation should not be used if the patient is under the influence of any substance such as alcohol or medications that alter perception of sensation. If the patient's sensation is decreased, then perception of electrical intensity may be inaccurate, and sensitive tissues may burn. In women, electrical stimulation should not be performed during heavy menstrual flow, as hot spots in the vagina may occur, causing pain. Additionally, menstrual flow may increase as a result of electrical stimulation.

Electrical Stimulation Parameters for Pelvic Floor Muscle Weakness

Optimal stimulation parameters for electrical stimulation of weak PFM have not yet been established. Generally accepted parameters of intravaginal or intra-anal electrical stimulation for PFM weakness, stress incontinence, and overactive bladder are summarized in Table 9.6.

Lower amplitude (<35 mA) should be used for afferent (sensory) stimulation and higher amplitude (>65 mA) for efferent (motor) stimulation. Clinically, the amplitude is increased to patient tolerance or when an anal wink is observed, indicating external sphincter contraction. The levator ani is believed to also contract when the anal wink is visualized. The sensation is usually described as tingling, tickling, or throbbing. If the patient experiences pulsing, burning, or stinging, the intensity is too high. To use this parameter, instruct the patient to slowly turn up the stimulation amplitude (intensity) while you observe the anal opening. When a contraction is visualized, tell the patient to stop. The patient is then instructed in subsequent sessions to turn the

Table 9.6. Parameters of Intravaginal or Intra-anal Electrical Stimulation Parameters for Pelvic Floor Muscle Weakness, Stress Incontinence, and Overactive Bladder (33)

Client Position	*Reclined*
Frequency	5–50 Hz weakness, 5–20 Hz detrusor instability
Pulse duration	100–250 μs
Amplitude	To anal wink
On:off time	Equal rest or double rest
Waveform	Symmetrical or asymmetrical biphasic, pulsed current
Electrode	Internal vaginal or rectal
Duration of treatment	15–30 min
Frequency of treatment	Twice a day, 7 days a week
Duration of treatment	6–8 mo

intensity of the stimulation to the initially perceived level. The anal wink method is especially helpful with patients who have decreased sensory awareness or a high tolerance for pain. Clinical experience has shown that electrical stimulation at very high intensities may result in worsening of symptoms for both urge and stress incontinence.

The frequency should be 5 to 20 Hz for bladder inhibition and 5 to 50 Hz for strengthening. Urinary retention has been treated using 200 Hz (29). Regarding pulse duration, Plevnik et al. (30) found 200 μs to be the most effective pulse duration for pelvic floor stimulation. Research by Ohlsson et al. (31) favored longer pulse durations (5000 μs). Most current commercial electrical stimulation units for PFM dysfunction are set at 350 μs. Shorter pulse duration activates motor nerve fibers, whereas long pulse duration activates pain nerve fibers (31). Practitioners have had good results with a variety of pulse durations. The waveform is symmetrical or asymmetrical biphasic pulsed. The on:off time should be adjustable. For moderate weakness, the stimulation is 5 seconds on:5 seconds off. For very weak muscles, the stimulation is 5 seconds on:10 seconds off.

Treatment time varies widely. Long-term stimulation (8 to 10 hours a day) is not currently being used to treat the pelvic floor. Treatment sessions usually last from 10 to 40 minutes depending on patient tolerance. Shorter stimulation times are used for very weak muscles. Some patients may need only one or two electrical stimulation treatments to re-educate the muscles and gain sensory awareness. Detrusor instability and pelvic floor weakness often require extended periods of twice-daily treatments (2 to 4 months and 4 to 6 months, respectively), although some practitioners are having success with office treatments one to three times per week for 4 to 6 weeks. Patients may be asked to contract the pelvic floor with the stimulation. If the patient is very weak, adding a voluntary contraction with every other stimulated contraction can increase their sensory awareness. Appropriate active pelvic floor exercise programs are given to do at home in addition to electrical stimulation treatments.

SENSORY-LEVEL ELECTRICAL STIMULATION FOR PELVIC FLOOR MUSCLE WEAKNESS

Varying intensity and/or frequency dictates the type of nerve activated and thus the structures affected. Low amplitude (<35 mA) pulsed current introduced vaginally or rectally stimulates the afferent (sensory) branch of the pudendal nerve (29). The impulse travels back to the spinal cord (S2 to S4) and synapses with the pudendal efferent neurons. It then travels along the efferent pudendal nerve axons to the muscle fibers of the urogenital diaphragm, causing muscle contraction in innervated muscles. Contraction of the urogenital diaphragm muscles improves urethral closure pressure, which decreases the incidence of incontinence.

PROPOSED MECHANISM OF ACTION OF SENSORY-LEVEL STIMULATION

Activating muscle contractions through sensory stimulation, as described above, results in reflex recruitment of motor units. This decreases fatigue and allows the pelvic floor muscles to tolerate longer stimulation times with less recuperation. Additionally, through reflex stimulation, all components of the pelvic floor muscle can be stimulated from a single site, and electrode placement is less critical, in contrast to direct motor nerve stimulation (32).

Pudendal-to-pudendal reflex stimulation results in a simultaneous contraction of all the pelvic floor muscles (32). Physiological pelvic floor muscle contraction by electrical stimulation enhances sensory awareness of pubococcygeus muscles, resulting in more effective voluntary muscle contractions. The ideal goal is for patients to be able to contract the pelvic floor muscles adequately without stimulation. As discussed at the end of the chapter, biofeedback-triggered electrical stimulation may be the most desirable combination of active and passive strengthening. This treatment modality allows the practitioner to set a threshold of active muscle contraction, which the patient must achieve before the stimulation occurs. At present, internal vaginal and rectal electrodes are not approved by the Food and Drug Administration for this type of unit.

MOTOR-LEVEL ELECTRICAL STIMULATION FOR PELVIC FLOOR MUSCLE WEAKNESS

Higher current amplitudes (>65 mA) directly depolarize the efferent pudendal nerve, which in turn causes contraction of the pelvic floor muscles (29). Intensities high enough to depolarize efferent nerves may be too painful for some patients to tolerate without anesthesia. In the past, physicians performed high-intensity electrical stimulation on anesthetized patients with mixed results. Today, patients with decreased or absent sensory innervation may benefit from high-intensity efferent nerve stimulation. The frequency used for strengthening varies widely (5 to 50 Hz). Some practitioners feel that 50 Hz is most effective, while others have good results with 20 Hz (4). The above peripheral neural pathways must be intact for neuromuscular electrical stimulation to be effective. Upper motor neuron input to lower motor neuron outputs such as the bladder and urethral sphincters is not necessary (32). Clinical studies are mixed, and research in this area is limited.

Evidence on Electrical Stimulation for Pelvic Floor Muscle Strengthening for Incontinence and Supportive Dysfunction

Caldwell (34) introduced genitourinary electrical stimulation in 1963 to correct urinary incontinence. He proposed the use of an implantable radio-linked electrical stimulator with electrodes fixed to the periurethral musculature for direct stimulation. This method proved to be too technically complicated and had poor results (34). In 1966, Hopkinson and Lightwood (35) experimented with electrical stimulation using an anal plug similar to the electrodes used today. In 1968, Alexander and Rowan (36) created an electronic pessary [a flat device used internally to support a displaced uterus (37)], but the success rates were low. Bladder inhibition was attempted with stimulation at very high intensities while the patient was under general anesthesia (38). Numerous studies that followed focused on long-term stimulation (8 to 12 hours per day) and on choosing an appropriate electrode (39–41). Fall et al. (42) published several studies that showed the effectiveness of electrical stimulation on bladder inhibition. They differentiated between the frequencies necessary for bladder inhibition and those for strengthening (42).

Three papers have been published evaluating the effectiveness of electrical stimulation in producing a PFM contraction. All studies measured urethral pressure, a measure of the urogenital diaphragm contraction. If the pudendal nerve only innervates the urogenital diaphragm, then electrical stimulation would specifically target it, and contraction of the levator ani muscles is not as crucial. Bernier et al. (23) and Yamanishi et al. (24) found maximal urethral pressure increased more with electrical stimulation than with voluntary PFM contraction. Bo and Talseth (43) found maximal urethral pressure was further enhanced with voluntary PFM contraction. Many electrical stimulation protocols require assurance that the external sphincter or levator ani muscle are contracting. Electrical stimulation of the pudendal nerve should result in a contraction of the rectal sphincter.

From the research to date, it does not appear necessary to achieve a PFM contraction for electrical stimulation to effectively decrease symptoms of urinary incontinence. Current research on electrical stimulation theories focuses on the stimulation of sensory afferents S2, S3 in the modulation of unwanted detrusor contractions. These studies are helpful in clarifying the role of electrical stimulation in detrusor instability, but do not address the issue of PFM weakness. Practitioners should remember that PFM strength is not the only mechanism of continence. Many patients achieve significant decreases in incontinence without any change in PFM strength. This may result through increased sensory stimulation. The role of PFM strengthening in continence training is not fully understood.

Currently, most neuromuscular electrical stimulation of the pelvic floor is done vaginally or rectally. Externally strengthening the PFM has been attempted using a biphasic or interferential wave (44,45). Often, skin resistance is too great, and the patient experiences extreme pain before a PFM contraction occurs. External strengthening stimulation provides a possible alternative to internal electrodes. Interferential current devices are not commonly used in current practice because of poor outcomes. External stimulation for overactive bladder may be effective and is covered later in this chapter.

Research on electrical stimulation for PFM weakness is difficult to compare, as parameters vary and are not always reported. Sample sizes are often small, and parameters used may not be based on current research knowledge. Placebo-controlled studies appear to be the most valuable because the placebo effect can be quite high. Bo (46) and Yasuda and Yamanishi (47) have published summary papers on the use of electrical stimulation in incontinence. Bo (46) reports nine randomized placebo-controlled studies on stress incontinence and one on urge incontinence. Several are summarized below. Randomized, controlled trials of electrical stimulation with stress incontinence are summarized in Table 9.7.

Electrode Issues in Stimulation for Urogenital Disorders

Considerations for Internal Electrodes

Electrodes are chosen based on the electrical stimulation machine used, patient comfort, and cost. Electrode use should result in little or no adverse tissue reaction to minimize the potential for burns and irritation. It is important for electrodes to be placed in proximity to the pudendal afferent nerve at the level of the pubococcygeus muscle for maximum effect. Patients must remove their pessary or diaphragm before inserting the electrode.

Table 9.7. Summary of Randomized, Controlled Trials of Electrical Stimulation with Stress Incontinence

Researchers	***Year***	***Treatment Parameters/ Stimulation Site***	***Frequency/ Duration***	***Outcomes***
Sand et al. (48)	1996	Multicenter, 7 visits over 15-week trial comparing the use of an active pelvic floor stimulator with a sham device	50 Hz and 12.5 Hz settings used; first two weeks 5 s on: 10 s off for 15 min; varying schedules up to 5 s on: 5 s off for 30 min	62% improved among stimulation subjects; 19% improved in sham group
Luber and Wolde-Jsadih (49)	1997	Vaginal stimulation BID 15 min for 12 weeks	Pulse width 2000 μs, work 2 s, rest 4 s, frequency 50 Hz, intensity to olerance	25% improvement in object measures with stimulation; 29% improvement with sham
Yamanishi et al. (24)	1997	Anal electrode in men, vaginal electrode in women. BID or TID treatments, 15 min for 4 weeks	50 Hz, 1000 μs pulse duration, maximum tolerable intensity,	60% subjective improvement with stimulation; 8% subjective improvement with sham
Brubaker et al. (50)	1997	Vaginal electrode BID 20 min for 8 weeks	20 Hz, 2 s on, 4 s off, 100 μs, intensity to tolerance	No statistical difference between sham and stimulation groups

Irritation may result if the probe is poorly positioned. Most often, it is not inserted far enough. The patient or practitioner may have to hold the probe in place for the duration of the treatment. Vaginal infection is possible but rarely documented in the literature. Sand et al. (48) report 11% to 12% vaginal infection rates and 3% to 12% urinary tract infection rates. Electrical stimulation may not be the treatment of choice for patients prone to infections.

Vaginal versus Rectal Stimulation

Kiesswetter and Flamm (28) tested mucosal electrosensitivity threshold (MST) rectally and vaginally. They found that 65.8% had rectal sensation and 34.1% had vaginal sensation at 7.5 volts (one 9-V battery). These practitioners believe that patients with a positive MST have better results with electrical stimulation. Therefore, if the patient cannot feel the stimulation vaginally, you may have better success with rectal stimulation. However, the rectal mucosa may inhibit current flow (48,49,50), thus decreasing the effectiveness of stimulation Ohlsson (51) also found rectal sensitivity to be higher than vaginal. However, his study clearly states that most female patients find vaginal stimulation more acceptable and more comfortable. Better compliance may occur with a more comfortable electrode. Intra-anal stimulation has resulted in rectal and lower extremity pain in some patients. Referred pain has not been reported in intravaginal stimulation (51). A literature search found no clinical outcome studies comparing vaginal and rectal stimulation.

Conductive Material of Vaginal or Rectal Electrodes

The two types of conductive material are metal or carbon-filled silicone. Metal is durable and corrosion resistant, but it is also hard and sometimes uncomfortable. Carbon-filled silicone is soft and pliable and may be more comfortable, but it may break down with long-term use. Sand et al. (48) reported a 12% to 14% incidence of skin irritation with their carbon-filled silicone electrode. The type of conductive material does not seem to make a significant difference in the outcome of treatment.

Electrode Design Considerations

Electrodes can be arranged in a horizontal or circumferential design (Fig. 9.7). Horizontal strips must be positioned in proximity to the nerve. Slight rotation of the electrode often results in a significant difference in contraction strength. Some practitioners believe that horizontal strip electrodes are more likely to be positioned in proximity to the PFM, resulting in a more effective contraction.

Concentric rings also must be positioned in proximity to the nerve. This is important in relationship to the depth at which the electrode is placed in the vagina or rectum. However, it seems easier for patients to place these accurately. Perry (44) reported that concentric rings are more appropriate for stimulation and horizontal strips are better for EMG monitoring. This is not substantiated in any other studies. There are no clinical studies comparing horizontal strips to circumferential band configurations on the electrode.

Ohlsson (51) found that doubling the electrode area significantly decreased the voltage needed to reach sensory threshold, therefore increasing the patient's comfort. Theoretically, larger electrode surfaces would require lower intensities to activate the pudendal afferent nerve, with less edging effect.

Electrode Shape Considerations

There are two shapes of electrodes: dumbbell and cylindrical. The vaginal vault is usually shaped like an hourglass, and the PFM is located at the thin, intersecting area. The dumbbell-shaped electrode fits into the hourglass with some consistency in placement from treatment to treatment.

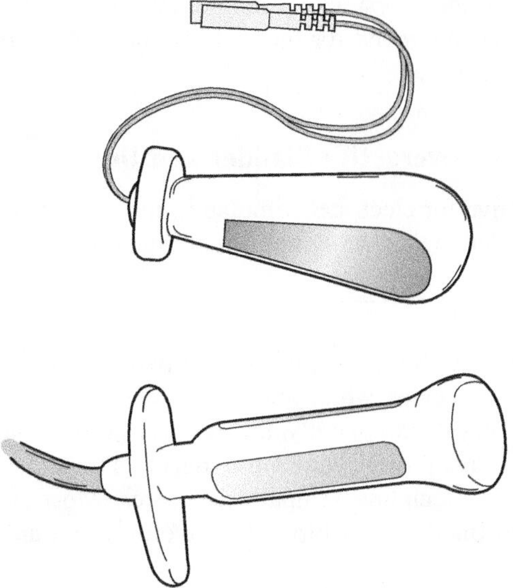

Figure 9.7. Electrodes used for electrical stimulation for urogenital dysfunction.

When the PFMs are very weak, the vagina is more cylindrical in shape, and the dumbbell shape may not necessarily provide consistent stimulation.

Cylindrical electrodes are uniform in circumference. This electrode may be more difficult for patients to place consistently in proximity to the pudendal nerve. In the clinic, the electrode is moved slightly in and out of the vagina until the patient feels a maximal contraction. This provides more precise placement. In patients who have a large vaginal vault, this electrode may provide better contact with the vaginal walls.

Electrode Size Considerations

For a very small vagina, a rectal electrode can be used either vaginally or rectally. The clinician should also consider a rectal electrode if the vagina is not able to accommodate an electrode due to pain, prolapse, atrophic vaginitis, or other factors. For a large or lax vagina, the practitioner or patient can hold the electrode in place during treatment or choose an electrode with a larger circumference.

Some electrodes extend outside the canal, while some are completely internal. Longer electrodes can be angled toward the weaker pelvic floor muscle. Some practitioners believe this increases the benefit of stimulation to an asymmetrical muscle; however, there is no physiological basis for this statement.

Other Considerations

All internal electrodes are single user and cannot be transferred from patient to patient.

Electrodes should be easy to use by patients and easily cleaned. Follow manufacturer's recommendations for cleaning.

High-volt pulsed current is delivered through the Sohn's electrode used rectally or vaginally.

This electrode is intended for multiple use and is autoclaved between patients.

Patients should be instructed to inspect the electrode for cracks before using.

Lead wires should be durable, resist cracking, and be long enough to facilitate ease of electrode insertion.

Lubrication on the electrode is best with water-soluble gel, warm water, or other commercial electroconductive gels approved for internal use, but not petroleum jelly. Follow manufacturer's recommendations.

Electrical Stimulation for Overactive Bladder and Urge Incontinence

The overall primary objective for electrical stimulation for overactive bladder and urge incontinence is to inhibit the bladder so that the symptoms of urgency are relieved.

Internal Sensory-level Stimulation

Simulation of sensory afferent S2, S3 neurons modulate unstable bladder contractions and inhibit the pontine micturition center, which abolishes excessive inputs to the detrusor and hence decreases the sense of urgency. Consequently, this restores normal micturition reflex and effects a reflex-mediated inhibition of the hypogastric nerve. The sensory accommodation then decreases the excitability of ascending sympathetic nerves. Most electrical stimulation for an overactive bladder is performed with a biphasic waveform and an internal vaginal or rectal electrode.

External Sensory-level Stimulation

Several focused studies have been published on the use of external stimulation using a standard biphasic pulsed current with overactive bladder (52–58). This modality is gaining popularity, and additional studies are expected. External stimulation can be used to modulate the bladder through the stimulation of the S2, S3 nerves. The most common frequency is 10 Hz, although 150 Hz has also been used. Electrode placement varies and includes suprapubic, over the S3 nerve root, and the S3 dermatome. Stimulation is worn for 1 to 4 hours twice a day. No specific intensity is reported, but moderate to high sensory level is usually adequate. Unfortunately, stimulation may need to be continued for several days before the patient is able to determine its benefit. Studies show decreased urgency and increased bladder filling (54). Walsh et al. (57) showed increased bladder capacity with decreased detrusor pressures during stimulation. This type of stimulation is not widely used in physical therapy clinics but warrants further investigation to determine its benefit.

Internal Motor-level Stimulation

To date there is no evidence for the use of motor-level vaginal or rectal electrical stimulation for the treatment of overactive bladder.

Proposed Mechanism of Action of Electrical Stimulation for Bladder Inhibition

As mentioned previously, stimulation of the sensory afferents of sacral nerves S2 and S3 is the goal for modulation of bladder overactivity. Table 9.8 outlines the proposed actions of stimulation of these nerves. Exactly how these actions occur is still under investigation. Electrical stimulation for overactive bladder may produce central inhibition of the parasympathetic nerves. Studies have also shown that active contraction of the PFM results in decreased detrusor contractions. Micturition reflex number three (Bradley loop) is sometimes referred to as the *detrusor inhibition reflex*. Contraction of the PFM results in relaxation of the bladder. This may be one mechanism for bladder inhibition by electrical stimulation.

Low-frequency stimulation (5 to 20 Hz) inhibits bladder contractions through the *pudendal to hypogastric reflex* (29,32). The hypogastric plexus carries sympathetic autonomic nerve fibers. Some researchers also believe that stimulation at 20 Hz inhibits bladder contractions

Table 9.8. Effects of Stimulation of Sensory Afferent S2, S3

- Modulates unstable bladder contractions
- Inhibits the pontine micturition center which abolishes excessive inputs to the detrusor
- Restores normal micturition reflex
- Reflex mediated inhibition of the hypogastric nerve
- Sensory accommodation which decreases excitability of ascending sympathetic nerves

Adapted from Wilder E. *The Gynecological Manual.* 2nd ed. Alexandria, Va: Section on Women's Health, American Physical Therapy Association; 2002.

using the pudendal to pelvic reflex (59). The pelvic nerve carries parasympathetic nerve fibers. Lindstrong et al. (60) reported optimal frequency for bladder inhibition as 10 Hz. Soomro et al. (61) theorized that stimulation-activated endorphin pathways in the spinal cord lead to a decrease in detrusor activity.

High intensities may also directly depolarize the efferent hypogastric nerve, causing contraction of the smooth muscle of the internal urinary sphincter and inhibition of the bladder (32). Researchers have documented several permanent changes in neurotransmitters and other biological substances after electrical stimulation (32). These changes are thought to be the reason for the long-term benefit of electrical stimulation for detrusor instability (52,62,63,64).

Evidence on Efficacy of Electrical Stimulation Interventions for Overactive Bladder

Research on electrical stimulation for overactive bladder (Table 9.9) most often shows a positive benefit in decreasing symptoms. Brubaker et al. (50) showed 50% improvement in the stimulation group and no significant change in the sham group. Yamanishi (24) showed 81% improvement with stimulation as opposed to 35% with sham treatment.

Electrical Stimulation for Pelvic Pain and Hypertonus

Hypertonus is a dysfunction of the urogenital system that results from increased tension in PFM, causing musculoskeletal pain and or dysfunction (18). Because pelvic pain and PFM hypertonus accompany each other, they are considered here as one dysfunction.

Table 9.9. Research on Electrical Stimulation for Overactive Bladder

Researchers	*Type of Incontinence*	*Outcomes*
Brubaker et al. (50)	All	Detrusor instability: 50% decrease in activity, no change in sham; no change in stress incontinence; subjective improvement in stimulation, 35%, sham, 17%
Luber and Wolde-Jsadih (49)	Stress	Objective improvement: 15% stimulation, 12.5% sham; subjective improvement: 25% stimulation, 29% sham
Yamanishi et al. (24)	Stress	Subjective improvement: 60% stimulation, 8% sham; cure: 45% stimulation, 7.7% sham
Geirsson and Fall (64)	Urgency	Subjective improvement: 54% improved, 5% cured (no control)
Seigal et al. (65)	Urge and mixed	41% improved, 29% cured (no control)

The pathophysiology of pelvic pain and hypertonus dysfunction is a topic of much debate and discussion among health professionals. Few research studies have investigated the origin of pelvic pain syndromes. Possible etiology for pelvic pain include joint dysfunction (5), trigger points (5,16,65), chronic muscle holding patterns, psychogenic factors, visceral or systemic factors, nerve entrapment during pelvic surgery, and other neurological events locally and centrally. The primary objectives for electrical stimulation in pelvic pain and hypertonus is to decrease pain, decrease the increased muscle tone in the PFM, and eliminate symptoms.

Increased tone of the PFM may result in vaginal, rectal, or coccyx pain present in diagnoses such as levator ani syndrome, tension myalgia, vaginismus, and proctalgia fugax. Urinary retention and constipation may result from PFM hypertonus. Identification of increased tone is best achieved with EMG testing. Palpation of the muscle inside the vaginal or rectal canal can assist in identifying trigger points and tight muscles. Electrical stimulation inside the vaginal and rectal canals can be beneficial in treatment of these patients. Hypertonus of the PFM may or may not be part of other pelvic pain syndromes. These syndromes include endometriosis, dysmenorrhea, pelvic inflammatory disease, coccygodynia, vulvodynia, interstitial cystitis, and many more. Electrical stimulation may be directed at decreasing PFM tension or at overall pain management. Some patients with increased uterine cramping may find vaginal stimulation aggravating.

Internal and External Sensory-level Stimulation for Pelvic Pain and Pelvic Floor Muscle Hypertonus

Electrical stimulation for pelvic pain and hypertonus may be administered externally or internally through the vagina or rectum. Dysfunctions localized to the perineum and bladder should be considered for internal treatment. As described previously, the treatment frequency is usually 100 Hz; all other parameters remain the same. If the patient cannot tolerate an internal electrode, or if one is not available, external stimulation should be used. A "crisscross pattern" for electrode placement over the sacrum or over the S3 dermatome has been shown in clinical practice to decrease pain in the perineum. Stimulation around the rectum does not appear to have satisfactory results in decreasing pain or dysfunction.

Pain found elsewhere in the pelvis is treated using conventional treatments for pain management. The clinician who is familiar with the various modes of transcutaneous electrical stimulation (TENS) will determine the best parameters of treatment depending on the patient's condition, age, and severity of pain. Parameters are usually set at a conventional TENS setting of submotor sensory amplitude and frequency, from 60 to 100 pps. Pulse duration of 100 to 150 μs, for 20 to 30 minutes, one to five times per day, is standard treatment. Some patients find relief using TENS almost continuously during the first 2 or 3 days of their menstrual flow. Setting of continuous, burst, or modulated modes may be used according to patient preference. Low-rate (2 to 4 pps) motor-level TENS may also be beneficial. Related acupuncture points are useful, such as spleen 6 (Sp 6), which is one hand width above the medial malleolus, just behind the edge of the tibia. Spleen 10 (Sp 10) is 2 inches above the medial aspect of the patellar base, and large intestine 4 (LI 4), which is located in the web space of the thumb (Fig. 9.8).

Levator ani syndrome is a collection of symptoms including pain, pressure, or discomfort in the rectum and is more frequent in women. Discomfort is usually aggravated by sitting and often radiates to the coccyx, left gluteal area, vagina, and thighs (66,67). This syndrome may accompany other conditions such as anal infection. The proximity of the lymphatic drainage to the pelvic musculature may be responsible for myositis or reflex spasm of the levator ani muscles (68). Thiele (69) also noted associated spasm of the piriformis muscle in 43.7% of 324 patients he examined with levator ani syndrome. Some practitioners use this syndrome as a catch-all term. To benefit from high-voltage stimulation (a monophasic waveform), the patient must have true symptoms of levator ani syndrome. Clinically, tenderness and spasm are found on palpation of one or both levator muscles. The left levator muscle is often the site of involvement (67).

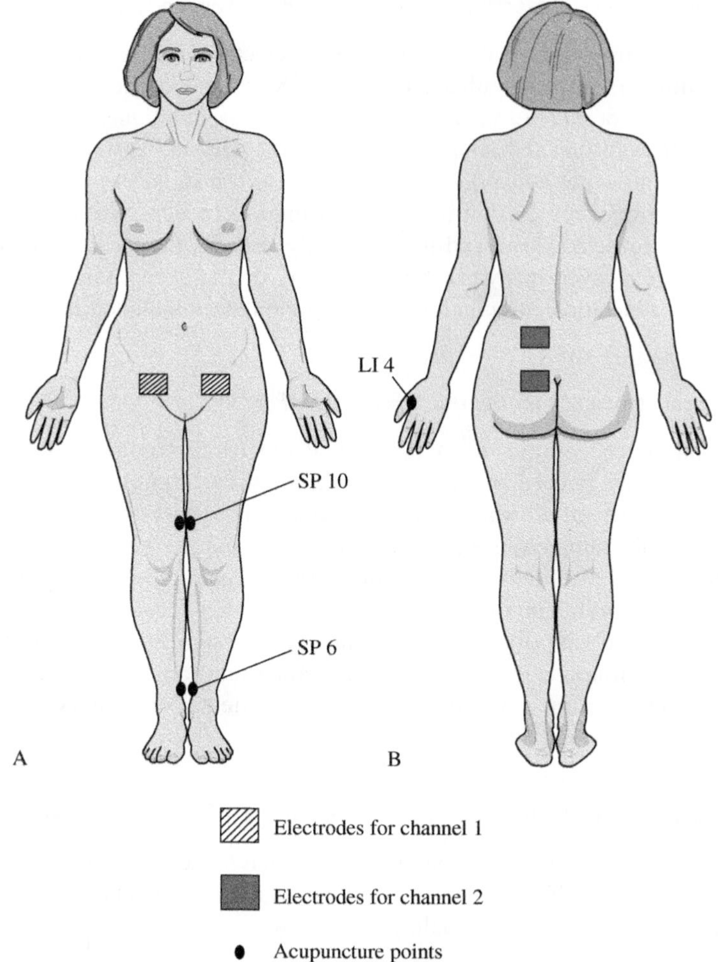

Figure 9.8. Placement of electrodes for pain modulation in bilateral pain A and unilateral abdominal pain B (54).

Levator ani syndrome often occurs in individuals who sit for long periods on the toilet, straining or reading. Usually the pain is unrelated to bowel function; however, defecation may exacerbate the pain.

Several studies have documented the use of high-voltage pulsed current in patients with levator ani syndrome. There are three models of probes: vaginal, rectal, or the Shon multi-user electrode. Patient comfort and preference determine which one to use. Treatments vary from 15 to 60 minutes every other day for five treatments, and then patients should be reassessed (66,67,70). Sohn reported that the negative pole was used but gave no rationale. Pulse frequency is usually 80 Hz, with the amplitude increased gradually until the patient experiences mild discomfort. Amplitude is then reduced to a level that the patient finds comfortable (71a). Usually, amplitude can be progressively increased to 250 to 400 V depending on patient tolerance (66,70). The amplitude is increased for severe muscle spasm and reduced in subsequent treatments as the patient improves and spasm decreases. Morris found better results with a 60-minute treatment time and increased the frequency to 120 Hz, as this gave more relief of chronic pain (67). Follow-up treatments may need to be made based on the clinician's assessment and severity of symptoms.

Proposed Mechanism of Action of Electrical Stimulation for Pelvic Pain and Hypertonus

To date, no study has investigated the mechanism of electrical stimulation for pelvic pain or hypertonus. Practitioners have postulated that the success of electrical stimulation could be attributed to at least one or more of the following factors: muscle fatigue, motor neuron suppression and/or accommodation, and adaptation of central nervous system pathways (such as interneural or motor neuronal networks or neurochemical transmission) (70). Scott and Hsuek (67) wrote that low-frequency current applied to a muscle induces fasciculation and fatigue, thereby breaking the muscle spasm, and it additionally benefits the local tissue circulation and reduces edema (70). However, many practitioners today do not accept this theory. Mechanisms underlying the use of electrical stimulation for pain modulation included in Chapter 4 apply to this area as well.

Evidence on Electrical Stimulation for Control of Pelvic Floor Pain

Little research has been conducted on the use of electrical stimulation and pelvic pain. Dysmenorrhea (menstrual pain) alone accounts for more than 140 million lost working hours a year and affects about 50% of all women in their childbearing years.

Dysmenorrhea and endometriosis can be effectively managed with TENS. In a 1990 study, Daywood and Ramos (71) found that TENS alone provided pain relief in approximately 40% of subjects. TENS with ibuprofen produced pain relief in 75% of subjects. The literature notes 25% to 90% of cases improved with dramatic results and without significant side effects in the treatment of levator ani syndrome with high-voltage pulsed current (66,67,70). Suprapubic pain was resolved and bladder function normalized in 53% of patients with interstitial cystitis using intravaginal electrical stimulation (72).

Recent Developments in Conservative Management of Genitourinary Disorders

Since the 1990s there has been a large resurgence in research and development in all types electrical stimulation treatments. These forms of stimulation are included here with a brief description of each. New types of stimulation include:

Pericutanous peripheral afferent nerve stimulation (manufacturer, SANS)
Sacral nerve stimulation (manufacturer, Interstim)
Magnetic stimulation (manufacturer, Neotonus)
Clitoral nerve stimulation

Percutaneous Peripheral Afferent Nerve Stimulation

In percutaneous peripheral afferent nerve stimulation, a needle electrode inserted posterior to the lateral malleolus in the posterior tibialis nerve delivers stimulation (73–75). This results in direct stimulation of the S3 nerve root, thus modulating unwanted bladder contractions. Treatments are provided in the physician's office once per week for 12 weeks. The SANS (73) device is the only device currently approved in the United States. It delivers a low-voltage, low-amplitude current. Using urodynamic data, Vandoninck et al. (75) showed a 63% subjective success rate.

Sacral Nerve Stimulation

Sacral nerve stimulation has successfully reduced fecal and refractory urinary urge incontinence (76–80). The Interstim implantable stimulator provides stimulation directly to the S3 nerve root at 10 to 21 Hz, 210 μs, with amplitude variations of 0.1 to 7.9 V. The stimulation is tested with external placement of needle electrodes into the S3 foramen. If test stimulation of 3 to 7 days provides at least 50% decrease in symptoms, then the patient is appropriate for surgical implantation. The surgery involves open insertion of a needle electrode into the S3 foramen. The stimulation unit is placed in a subcutaneous flank pocket. An external device (similar to those used for cardiac pacemakers) is used to activate and modify the parameters. The patient has a small controller to modify the stimulation intensity and a control switch. This treatment is only used in severe urgency, frequency, or retention when conservative management has failed. Equipment malfunctions are possible, and stimulator battery life varies up to 10 years before a revision is needed. Studies show properly chosen patients have very good results (78).

Magnetic Stimulation

The Neotonus chair offers a nonsurgical therapy for the treatment of stress, urge, and mixed incontinence in women (81–84). It has a drum emitting a magnetic field that is imbedded in the chair seat. The magnetic field produces an ion flow with nerve activation in the adjacent tissue. Patients remain fully clothed during treatment; direct skin contact is not necessary. The pulse width is set at between 275 μs to 720 μs, and the frequency varies from 5 to 50 Hz. Treatments are given one to three times per week for 16 sessions. Clinical studies have shown that 66% of patients have significant improvement (84). This percentage can be increased if patients are taught pelvic floor muscle exercises in addition to receiving stimulation. Most patients note a contraction in the gluteal and hamstring muscles. Some can confirm a pelvic floor muscle contraction as well. It is unclear whether a pelvic floor muscle contraction is necessary for the success of this treatment. Insurance reimbursement of this treatment varies, and the device is costly (81–84).

Dorsal or clitoral nerve stimulation is another form of external stimulation for overactive bladder. Two silver/sliver chloride electrodes placed 1 cm apart at the base of the penis or clitoris give stimulation. Oliver et al. (85) showed that 57% of patients had an increase in overall bladder capacity on cystometry. This represents another method of activating the S2, S3 nerve, resulting in neuromodulation of the bladder (86).

BIOFEEDBACK FOR UROGENITAL DISORDERS

General Consideration for Use of Biofeedback Interventions

Types of Biofeedback

Evaluation and treatment of PFM function is challenging because the muscle is deep inside the pelvis. Biofeedback can take many forms and is helpful in providing information about the muscle in order to enhance the training process. Simple biofeedback includes using a mirror to visualize the inward or lifting movement of the perineal body during PFM contraction. Also, palpation of the perineal body from outside gives feedback as to the correct contraction or relaxation. Palpation inside the vagina or rectum by the patient or clinician provides additional information and refinement of PFM contraction quality. Instrumented biofeedback of the PFM includes *vaginal weights* (87), *pressure biofeedback* or manometry (88), and *EMG biofeedback.*

Kegel (88) was the first to describe the inward lift of the perineum during PFM contraction. External observation of this lift during PFM contraction is a form of evaluation and is best used in combination with other evaluation tools (89). Patients frequently have poor perineal excursion during PFM contraction. Mirror observation and palpation can identify bearing down, an incorrect method of contraction. Although mirror observation and external palpation are simple forms of biofeedback, they have not been proven to be reliable.

Palpation inside the vagina or the rectum is helpful in determining if the patient is performing the PFM contraction correctly (89). Van Kampen et al. (90) found 25 different methods of vaginal

PFM evaluation. Many practitioners use vaginal palpation to quantify the strength and endurance of the contraction. Patients can use internal palpation as a form of self-feedback for PFM contraction.

When properly positioned in the upright position, vaginal weights sit just above the PFM. Low-level contraction of the muscle is needed to keep the weight in place. Relaxation of the PFM will result in slipping of the weight, thus signaling the need to increase PFM contraction. Anecdotally, clinicians find that vaginal weights can be helpful in women with relatively small vaginas and fairly good strength. Research has not shown vaginal weights to be any more effective than PFM exercise alone (87).

Kegel (91) reported subjective improvements of 89% with a perineometer pressure biofeedback device. This simple pressure device registers a pressure reading of a PFM contraction that is interpreted as a force measurement (89). Pressure biofeedback devices are widely available. All pressure biofeedback devices have a pressure sensor, which is placed inside the vagina or the rectum. The sensor is connected to a manometric device by tubing and measures changes in pressure. The pressure reading is displayed by dial, bar graph, colored lights, or LCD images. These devices have some limitations and are not recommended for use in patients with hypertonus dysfunction, as they do not measure resting tone accurately (92). Patients must also be carefully instructed to perform the contractions correctly, as bearing down will also result in an increased pressure reading and may be mistaken for a correct PFM contraction.

EMG muscle training has application in supportive dysfunction, hypertonus dysfunction, and incoordination dysfunction of the PFM. It is used by many clinicians for the treatment of a wide variety of diagnoses and will be the focus of the remainder of this section.

Sensors in EMG Biofeedback for Urogenital Dysfunction

Clinical EMG measurements of PFM activity are best obtained with surface electrodes. Kieswetter (93) and Siroky (94) both reported that vaginal electrodes produce EMG patterns comparable to those obtained with needle EMG of the PFM. Surface EMG of the PFM can be obtained using a vaginal sensor, a rectal sensor, or skin-patch electrodes adhered to the skin over the external rectal sphincter. Barrett (95) found that surface electrocardiogram electrodes were as reliable as wire or pressure sensors in 400 clinical evaluations.

Internal vaginal sensors are placed in proximity to the levator ani muscle group. Rectal sensors are usually placed more superficially to measure both the external sphincter and the rectal portion of the levator ani muscle (puborectalis). Skin-patch electrodes are a better choice in patients with contraindications for internal sensor use (see "Electrical Stimulation for Genitourinary Dysfunction"), severe vaginal or rectal pain on penetration, significant prolapse in which the organ occupies the vault, or in cases were vaginal dilators may be used for training. Infant EKG electrodes are typically used for skin-patch electrodes of the PFM. They are placed on the skin over the external sphincter (96). These electrodes are reported to provide accurate information for clinical EMG training in many patients (95).

Most commercially available electrodes are made of silver–silver chloride. Frequently these sensors are specific to one machine and are not interchangeable. They are oriented in small longitudinal bands or larger circumferential sensors. Binnie (97) compared longitudinal bands with circular bands and found better clinical data and better correlation with fine-wire electrodes using the longitudinal bands. In general, specificity of muscle measurements is best with smaller EMG electrodes (longitudinal bands are usually smaller that circular bands). In contrast, electrical stimulation is better provided with a larger surface area electrode. Many vaginal and rectal sensors can be used for both electrical stimulation and EMG treatments. Despite the data provided by Binnie (97), many clinicians do not believe that electrode orientation significantly affects clinical EMG or electrical stimulation treatment. The type of sensor may play a small role in the choice of EMG machine.

EMG Evaluation of Pelvic Floor Muscle Dysfunction

A basic EMG evaluation consists of a 1- or 2-minute resting baseline and a 5- or 10-second holding set, repeated for 10 contractions. In many cases, a single-channel measurement is sufficient. However, dual-channel measurements are often used to monitor the activity of the abdominal muscles simultaneously with a PFM contraction. An increase in adipose layer precludes accurate EMG measurements of the abdominals. Palpation of the abdominal and gluteal muscles can provide valuable information about the occurrence of overflow contraction in these muscles.

Additional measurements may be made during quick contraction, Valsalva test, and long-endurance contraction testing. Clinicians often choose the tests based on the patient presentation. Quick contractions are performed by asking the patient to quickly and maximally recruit the PFM and then quickly relax the muscle without holding. The mastery of this skill is particularly important to decrease the occurrence of stress incontinence (particularly, urine leaks occurring with sneezing).

Valsava testing is helpful in patients with constipation. During bearing down, the PFM should relax below resting tone. Obstructive defecation is documented when PFM activity increases during bearing down. Long endurance testing can be done in 30-second intervals or at 50% of maximal contraction for up to 2 minutes (98). The value of these tests has not been examined in research studies.

The range of audio and video feedback displays is varied. Elderly patients may need bold lines and colors, while children may be more motivated with fun graphics and games. A display with high sensitivity is necessary to display small microvolt levels in very weak patients. Audio feedback is also helpful in some cases, especially with visually impaired patients. Goals can be used to enhance learning and motivation.

The beneficial calculations for EMG evaluation are average work and average rest, measured in microvolts. No research was found on the expected or average peak and holding microvolt levels for continence. Cram and Kasman (99) document a benchmark of 17.5 μV for a "strong contraction" without reference to source. They also point out that EMG amplitude closely correlates with muscle force (99). It is important to remember that microvolt levels recorded during PFM contractions depend on many variables such as skin impedance, amount of adipose tissue, electrode placement, muscle fatigue, length–tension relationship, and contraction velocity. Resting tone of the PFM is rarely flat (94), and many practitioners strive for a level <2 μV. However, there is no research basis for this. Average work and rest values can be tracked as treatment proceeds, and they often increase. More important, patients should improve the holding capacity of the muscle (number of seconds of holding), its coordination (with the abdominals and during daily activities), and the quality of the EMG tracing (see Table 9.10).

Some devices display other calculations, such as each individual work and rest and peak and minimum values. Individual work and rest values can be helpful in documenting the consistency

Table 9.10. Qualities Evaluated in a Pelvic Floor Muscle Contraction

- Quick recruitment
- Steady holding capacity
- Smooth and quick relaxation
- Return to normal baseline between each contraction
- Repeatability of contractions
- Minimal use of overflow muscles (abdominals, gluteals, and legs)
- Normal breathing during contraction

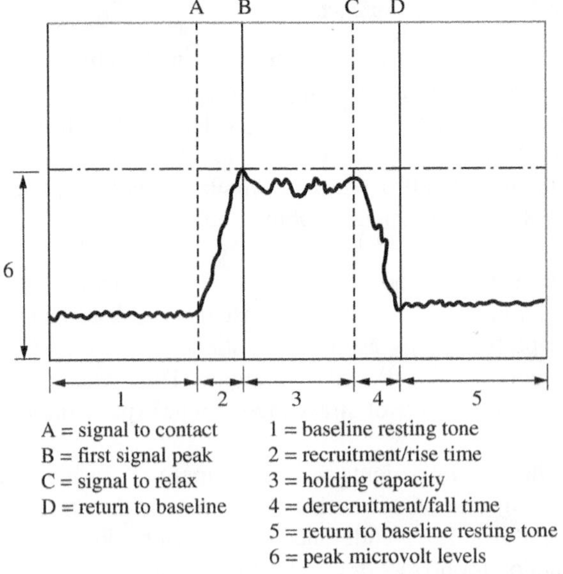

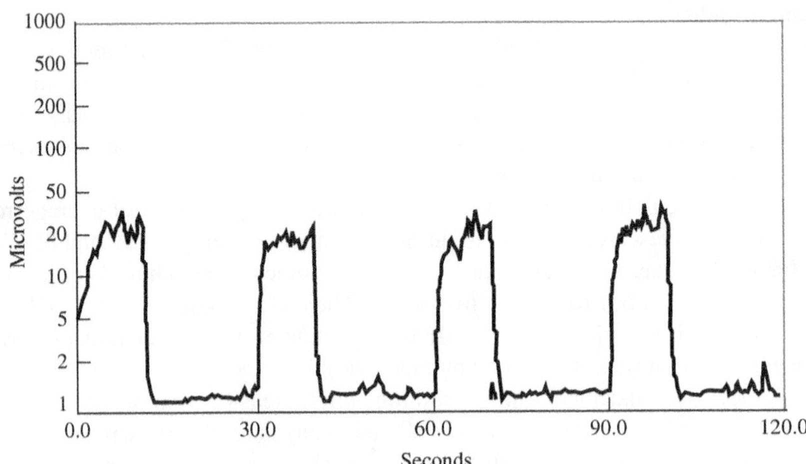

Figure 9.9. Normal EMG biofeedback tracing.

of the patient's contraction. Standard deviation is a measure of the variation of the signal and can be significant in the rest phase in hypertonic patients. Glazer (100) uses standard deviation in monitoring improvements in vulvodynia patients. He has shown that with a decrease in pain, there is improvement in muscle stability during rest. Rise time (time from contraction signal to peak recruitment) and fall time (time from relaxation signal and lowest relaxation) can also give objective measures that can be traced during treatment (Fig 9.9).

Incorrect technique can be mistaken for proper PFM EMG tracings if not closely monitored. A combination of evaluation and training techniques is best (89,94). Overflow from abdominal, gluteal, and adductor muscles should be carefully monitored for activity. In patients with severe weakness, it may be acceptable to include overflow muscles, and, hence, EMG tracings will be artificially elevated. Progression should move toward elimination of overflow muscle activity (101). Bearing down can be registered in some cases as an increase in microvolt output during an attempted contraction. Knight and Laycock (101) theorize that this may be due to electrode movement or minor PFM recruitment against the intra-abdominal pressure. In either case, bearing down is not acceptable and should be avoided. It is not recommended that practitioners rely solely on EMG measurements to determine muscle function (89), and initial training should confirm proper contraction by palpating vaginally or rectally. Periodic checks are recommended to confirm continued correct contraction. This can be accomplished by feeling for the inward movement of the sensor by palpating the external portion of the sensor during a contraction.

PFM EMG evaluation inter-rater reliability between examiners is significant ($r = 0.86$) (102). This form of evaluation has also been shown to have a statistically significant predictive validity ($p < 0.05$) for lower EMG values in patients with all forms of urinary incontinence, parity (refers to one or more live births), and peri- or postmenstrual status (without hormone replacement therapy) (102). An additional study shows shorter EMG holding ability and lower maximum voluntary contraction in all patient groups (stress, urge, mixed) with urinary infections as compared to controls, with good reproducibility and repeatability (103).

EMG Biofeedback for Urinary Incontinence and Supportive Dysfunction in Pelvic Floor Muscle Weakness and Incoordination

Primary Objective

EMG biofeedback provides increased information about the electrical output of the PFM during voluntary contraction and relaxation. The PFM sensory innervation can become impaired through childbirth, surgery, and neurological disease. Decreased visualization of the muscle contraction and impaired sensation make learning the correct contraction challenging. EMG measurements are used as an examination tool and can provide information necessary for proper treatment planning. For example, increased resting tone is present in some people with urinary incontinence. This increased tone can sometimes be identified on palpation, but it is better quantified and qualified with EMG measurements. Patients with increased resting tone must learn both contraction and relaxation. Clinically, patients find EMG information very helpful in increasing recruitment and maintaining the contraction.

Treatment Procedures During EMG Biofeedback for Urinary Incontinence and Supportive Dysfunction

A brief review of training principles of the PFM is provided here, as they are the same with or without biofeedback. All treatment protocols begin with a comprehensive instruction in correct

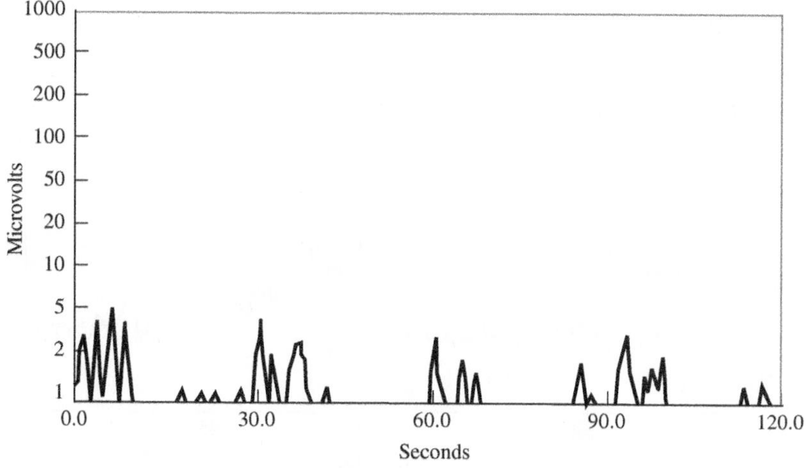

Figure 9.10. EMG biofeedback tracing of supportive and incoordination dysfunction.

Table 9.11. Common Findings in Supportive/Incoordination Dysfunction

- Slow recruitment
- Low peak microvolt readings
- Poor holding capacity
- Increased accessory muscle activity (especially abdominals, gluteals, and adductors)
- Normal resting tone (although a small percentage of patients have dysfunctional resting tone, which must be treated for good clinical outcome)
- Normal derecruitment
- Inconsistent contraction ability

PFM contraction technique. Bump (104) has shown that as many as 30% of patients verbally instructed in PFM contraction are performing them incorrectly. Many training protocols have been suggested (105–119).

Bo (120) evaluated training from an exercise science perspective and suggests three sets of 8 to 12 contractions, at least three to four times per week for 15 to 20 weeks, with continued independent exercises up to 6 months. Holding time varies from 2 to 3 seconds to 30 to 40 seconds. In all situations, exercise prescriptions are individualized for each patient.

Patient position usually begins as supine, as this is a gravity-minimized position for the PFM. As strength increases, it is important to progress the patient to sitting and standing positions. Initial training is completed without distractions and with displays that maximize information. As training progresses, distractions are provided and less clear feedback is given. This may take the form of conversations with the patient as the session is proceeding, or using distracting displays on the biofeedback monitor.

PFM holding time is increased as endurance improves. Typically, resting time is double work time or equal work time (i.e., 5 seconds work and 10 seconds rest, 10 seconds work and 10 seconds rest). A longer rest is chosen for weaker patients and for patients who have hypertonus. Patients should be taught to contract the PFM before and during sneezing, coughing, and laughing. This can be practiced with the EMG by having the patient make a sound ("ffff," "ssss," "ch,ch,ch") or by having her pretend to cough or sneeze during the contraction.

The number of repetitions in one session is increased as function improves. Often, sets of 10 are used to provide block training for increased motor learning. Hold time may be varied in

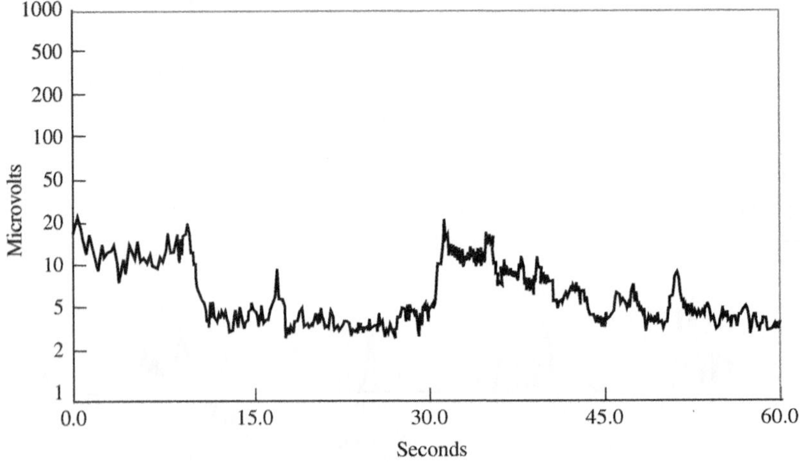

Figure 9.11. EMG biofeedback tracing of hypertonus dysfunction.

Table 9.12. EMG Characteristics of Hypertonus Dysfunction

- Elevated resting tone as reflected by increased electrical activity in PFM at rest
- Irregular resting tone
- Slow derecruitment
- Slow peak microvolt readings
- Inconsistent contraction ability
- Increase in accessory muscle activity
- Poor holding capacity

PFM, pelvic floor muscles.

different sets within one session (i.e., 10-second hold 10 times, 7-second hold 10 times, 5-second hold 10 times). Home sessions are completed two to four times per day depending on how many repetitions can be performed in one session. Clinically, practitioners often use a target of 60 to 80 contractions per day (121).

Over the years, much discussion has been given to the role of the abdominals in EMG training of the PFM. Research has shown that increasing intra-abdominal pressure contributes to increased stress urinary incontinence and prolapse (122). In the past, it was thought that any abdominal muscle contraction would result in undesirable increases in intra-abdominal pressure. Several good current studies document the importance of the transversus muscle contraction during PFM contraction (21,123–125). Careful instruction is needed to ensure proper use of the abdominals. Bo et al. (124) showed that direct PFM contraction is better in the management of urogenital dysfunction than abdominally-activated PFM contraction.

Most clinicians provide treatments in the clinic at 1- to 2-week intervals until the patient has shown some improvement in PFM function and experienced a decrease in her symptoms. Treatment frequency then decreases to eventual discharge as the patient becomes independent with home exercises. EMG home trainers are available and are used for those people who are unable to perform the exercise accurately without feedback, or in cases were the person cannot attend therapy on a regular basis. No quality studies comparing PFM exercise with and without an EMG home trainer have been done to date. Studies comparing PFM exercise with and without a pressure biofeedback device have failed to show significant benefit (126), although many still advocate their use (127,128).

Table 9.13. Factors to Consider for Developing PFM Training Program

- PFM contraction quality
- Hold time
- Rest time
- Number of repetitions
- Number of sets per session
- Number of sessions per day
- Patient position
- Accessory muscle activity: facilitation or isolation of primary muscle
- Integration of PFM and abdominal muscles
- Focused versus distracted training
- Quick contractions

PFM, pelvic floor muscles.

Evidence on Biofeedback for Control of Urinary Incontinence, Supportive Dysfunction, and Incoordination Dysfunction

Several randomized, controlled trials have shown that PFM training is more effective than no treatment or placebo in the treatment of stress urinary incontinence (15,121,129–131). Many studies support the claim that PFM exercises with biofeedback are effective in treating all types of urinary incontinence (105–113), fecal incontinence (114–116), postprostatectomy urinary incontinence (117), and pediatric voiding dysfunctions (118,119). The Urinary Incontinence in Adults: Clinical Practice Guidelines (121) rate PFM rehabilitation with biofeedback as an "A," supported by scientific evidence. However, multiple randomized, controlled trials comparing the results of exercises with and without EMG biofeedback (105,107,111–113) have failed to show a statistically significant difference, leaving clinicians to decide for themselves if biofeedback is really necessary in this patient population. The research does not give much insight.

Morkved et al. (105) performed a randomized, controlled trial comparing two groups: EMG versus PFM exercises alone. They found that both groups improved (58% and 46% objective cure rate, respectively), with no statistically significant difference between the groups. Burgio et al. (106) performed a nonrandomized and non-blinded study, which showed EMG training to be significantly more effective than verbal PFM instruction in decreasing urinary incontinence and in increasing PFM strength. Burns (109) found a negative correlation with EMG scores to urine loss. An increase in EMG score resulted in a decrease in reported urine loss. However, these findings did not reach statistical significance in comparison to the control group.

Pages et al. (110) performed a randomized, nonblinded clinical trial comparing the outcome of patients undergoing intensive group physical therapy treatment with or without biofeedback training. They reported patients' subjective cure rates after 3 months to be 28% in the physical therapy group and 62% in the individual biofeedback group. This result may reflect the fact that participants in the biofeedback group received individual treatment, and the other group did not. Burns et al. (111) found significant improvement in quick and sustained PFM contraction in the EMG-trained group compared with the group trained without biofeedback, but there was no significant difference in urinary incontinence reported between the groups. Berghmans et al. (112) showed improvements in PFM strength that were statistically significant at 3 and 6 months, but there was no difference in cure rates. The study by Glavind et al. (113) is the only randomized, controlled trial to show significant long-term results in the EMG group. However, the training schedules for the two groups were different.

EMG biofeedback treatment is an approach used in combination with other modalities. Some practitioners have combined EMG and electrical stimulation for treatments. Sung (132) compared these two groups. The first group received electrical stimulation and EMG biofeedback in an alternating pattern. The other group performed video-led PFM group exercises at home and came into the clinic periodically to have manual confirmation of correct PFM contraction technique. Sung found that the group receiving EMG and electrical stimulation had statistically less urinary incontinence. In another study using EMG biofeedback and electrical stimulation, patients reported overall satisfaction rating of 70%, with 96% of patients noting improvement 4 months after treatment was completed, though no comparison group was studied (133).

Studies of postprostatectomy EMG training yield similarly confusing results. Hunter et al. (117) looked at five trials and found biofeedback better than no treatment or sham treatment for short-term recovery. Nevertheless, comparison at 12 months did not show a statistically significant difference between the groups. Jackson et al. (134) also studied EMG treatment after radical prostatectomy, without a control group, and found 48% had complete success and 26% significantly improved. "Complete success" was defined as the ability to discard all incontinence devices in all situations and "significantly improved" was defined as >50% decrease in the number of incontinence pad changes (134). Enck (115) reported on 13 studies using EMG and pressure biofeedback to treat fecal incontinence. The overall success rate was 79.8%.

EMG Biofeedback for Pain and Hypertonus Dysfunction

The primary objective of EMG training for patients with hypertonus dysfunction is to normalize the PFM resting tone and improve the contractility of the muscle. In addition, hypertonus patients have generalized tension syndromes and can benefit from generalized relaxation biofeedback training (see Chapter 11 for more details). As noted earlier, many practitioners use a normal rest level of 2 μV as a goal with EMG. The ultimate goal of treatment is to facilitate complete bladder and bowel emptying, pain-free penetration, increase sitting tolerance, and decrease pain in the pelvis.

EMG Biofeedback Treatment Procedures and Evidence for Treatment of Hypertonus Dysfunction

Specific PFM relaxation techniques for pelvic pain and hypertonus dysfunctions are listed in Table 9.14. Characteristics of the PFM in patients with vulvodynia are elevated resting tone; low overall rise; increased EMG standard deviation during rest, poor relaxation after contraction; and low frequency on spectral analysis (135). Many other groups of patients with PFM hypertonus also have these same findings. Many practitioners document the use of EMG treatment with PFM hypertonus (4,136,137), but few have conducted research studies.

Glazer et al. (138) used EMG biofeedback to treat vestibulitis and vulvodynia. These researchers theorized that instability of the PFM at rest irritates the sympathetic nerves and results in skin changes and perpetuation of pain. This mechanism is not well understood, but, Glazer et al. (138) have documented a decrease in pain with improvement in the stability of the PFM using EMG biofeedback training. Their protocol is individualized to each patient's needs and is based on a hold–relax sequence. These maximal contractions often encompass overflow muscles, long holds, and multiple repetitions.

Paradoxical PFM contractions occurring at the time of attempted defecation effectively limit evacuation of feces for many patients, resulting in pain and constipation. This is readily seen on defecography, a test that allows visualization of the pelvis with x-ray during defecation of a radio-opaque material. Many studies have documented the success of EMG training in the treatment of constipation (115,139, 140). Rao (139) analyzed the results of 14 studies and reported 44% to 100% symptomatic improvement in constipation. This treatment involves training the patient to relax the PFM during bearing down. Wexner et al. (141) studied painful paradoxical PFM contractions and found a 89% success rate with EMG biofeedback training.

Table 9.14. Specific PFM Relaxation Techniques
Diaphragmatic breathing: purposeful descent of the respiratory diaphragm is said to encourage relaxation of the PFM diaphragm (21)
Visualization: visualize a relaxing place; imagine that you are heavy and warm, that the ischial tuberosities are separating (especially helpful in sitting), that a hole is getting larger, that the PFM are sagging
Perineal bulging: have patient place a hand over the anal cleft with the middle finger in the cleft and gently push out as if expelling gas. The patient should feel the tissues bulge, at their finger. This bulging is evidence of PFM relaxation.
Quiet environment, music, low lights, comfortable, warm
Education with pictures of the muscle may help visually-oriented patient
Contract relax, or hold relax
Total body relaxation: head to toes, toes to head
Body scanning touch the area and breath in the relaxation frequently throughout the day.

Dyspareunia (painful intercourse) and vaginismus (spasm of the muscles around the vaginal opening) are often the result of increased PFM tension during attempted penetration. Husted (142) published a protocol for the sexual desensitization of patients with dyspareunia. This protocol involves learning relaxation of the PFM and then visualizing intercourse. Clinicians have taken this treatment a step further by having the patient "practice" penetration using progressively larger vaginal dilators (136). Skin-patch electrodes can be used in combination with EMG biofeedback and dilators. The patient or the practitioner inserts the vaginal dilator. The patient remains as relaxed as possible checking her progress with the EMG feedback. In this way, the patient has control of the insertion and is able to decrease some of the possible apprehension of intercourse until she is comfortable. She can stop at any time and allow her vaginal opening to accommodate. This greatly decreases anxiety and improves confidence.

EMG biofeedback training is used extensively, although not exclusively, to treat PFM dysfunction. Clinically, EMG training is a very valuable clinical tool. To date, few standard protocols have been developed, and research is conflicting as to the benefit of EMG training over well-taught PFM exercise. Relaxation of the PFM is harder for patients to learn, and they often benefit from EMG training.

CLINICAL CASE STUDIES

Case Study 1

Examination

History

The patient is a 42-year-old woman referred to physical therapy for PFM strengthening. Approximately 3 years ago she had symptoms of organ prolapse. Four months ago she underwent a vaginal hysterectomy with a repair of anterior and posterior vaginal wall laxity. She continues to have a feeling of perineal sagging. Her medical history includes three vaginal deliveries; otherwise there is no other significant history.

Demographics

The patient is a nurse manager who has no lifting duties at work. Before surgery she was active in volleyball, Pilates, and weight training. She has not gone back to these activities but would like to and is looking for guidance.

Tests and Measures

Integumentary: at the introitus there is significant posterior scarring with pain and adhered tissue on palpation. External genitalia skin is within normal limits and demonstrates no pain to palpation.

Muscle performance: external perineal descent is minimal and the introitus (entrance to the vagina) is slightly open at rest. Muscle strength on her right PFM internally is 2/5 and 2+/5 on her left. Muscle endurance is 3 seconds. Muscle bulk is significantly decreased no the right.

Motor function: quality of PFM contraction is poor and coordination is poor.

Pain*:* on palpation at the introitus 6/10 on a verbal analog scale of 0 to 10.

EMG biofeedback training: with a vaginal electrode she is able to hold 3 seconds, rest 10 seconds, and able to complete 10 repetitions. Work averages 9.5 μV and rest averages 4.4 μV.

Quality of recruitment is slow, and holding is poor. Her ability to derecruit is average.

Consistency of contraction is poor, and her baseline contraction is irregular. Patient uses leg adductors as accessory muscles when contracting PFM.

Evaluation

Significant weakness of the PFM

Perineal scar adherence

Decreased PFM strength 2/5

Decreased PFM endurance to 3 seconds per contraction

Poor knowledge of proper PFM contraction and proper posture and body mechanics

Slow PFM recruitment and poor PFM support

Poor coordination of PFM with daily activities

Pendulous, weak abdominal muscles −2/5

Poor trunk stability

Pain on palpation of PFM at intervals

Diagnosis

Impaired muscle performance with connective tissue dysfunction

Prognosis

Patient has good potential to improve with conservative management. Over 2 months she will achieve the anticipated goals and expected outcomes of the interventions:

PFM strength 3/5 and PFM endurance 10 seconds per contraction

Normal PFM recruitment

Good coordination of PFM during daily activities

Minimal to no tenderness on palpation of PFM

Good scar mobility

Demonstrate good knowledge of proper posture and body mechanics

Intervention

Frequency of treatment: 1 time per week for 6 to 8 weeks

Neuromuscular re-education: EMG biofeedback for 15- to 20-minute sessions to increase endurance and coordination

PFM strengthening program during static supine exercise sessions and later during dynamic exercise

Manual scar therapy

Education on body mechanics, posture, and PFM contractions

Assessment of outcome: higher quality of PFM contraction and increased endurance (to 10 seconds) with EMG biofeedback training, resulting in elimination of perineal sagging sensation

Patient achieved with small improvement of BIM strength, 2+/5. She will likely realize additional increase in strength if she can continue with aggressive home exercise program for PFM and abdominal strengthening for another 3 to 4 months.

Case Study 2

Examination

History

The patient is a 78-year-old male who underwent a quadruple bypass heart surgery 1 year ago. After the surgery the patient noted urinary leakage. He has been evaluated and tried on medication (Ditropan XL). Patient is referred to physical therapy for conservative management. Past medical history is positive for prostate cancer, with a prostatectomy 8 years ago. He reports no difficulty with urinary incontinence after his prostate surgery. No bowel dysfunction noted. Patient had back pain in the past that resolved with an L5 fusion 2 years ago. He complains of urinary leakage with coughing, sneezing, laughing, lifting, and jumping with a strong urge to urinate. The patient also has urgency of two to three times per night.

Demographics

The patient is retired and fairly active.

Tests and Measures

EMG biofeedback*:* with rectal electrode, work average 11.9 μV and rest average 9.2 μV. Abdominal electrode used to detect contraction of the abdominal muscles 5-second hold and 10-second rest for 10 repetitions. The patient has an average work of 8.9 contraction seconds and an average rest of 3.2 contraction seconds. Quality of recruitment was fair, quality of hold was fair, derecruitment was average, and consistency was fair. His baseline was slightly elevated, and he used some gluteal muscles as accessory muscles.

Muscle performance*:* strength of external rectal sphincter demonstrates minimal tone and resting position slightly open. Muscle strength of external sphincter and rectal pelvic floor muscles is 1/5.

Motor function*:* muscle endurance of external sphincter and rectal pelvic floor muscles is poor (able to hold 1 second), and quality of the contraction is poor. Significant overflow to gluteal muscles when performing a PFM contraction.

Pain*:* no complaints on contraction or palpation.

Evaluation

Severe PFM weakness probably related to prostate surgery. Symptoms started after heart surgery.

Prognosis

Patient has fair potential to improve with conservative management. Goals:

PFM strength 3/5

PFM endurance 10 second per contraction

Good knowledge of proper PFM contraction without overflow to gluteal muscles

Normal PFM recruitment

Two- to 4-hour voiding pattern

Six to eight nonirritating fluids per day

Good coordination of PFM during daily activities

Intervention

Neuromuscular re-education training of PFM with abdominal muscle contraction and no overflow to the gluteal muscles

Electrical stimulation rectally with anal electrode at 50 Hz with a treatment phase of 5-second hold and 10-second rest for 10 minutes

Assessment of outcome: The patient has improved the accuracy of the PFM contractions and has decreased irritating fluids to 1/day. When he incorporates the abdominal muscles, the quality of the contraction of the PFM improves. Continue with therapy for neuromuscular rehabilitation, including electrical stimulation and therapeutic exercise.

SUMMARY

Treatment of urogenital dysfunctions is within the scope of practice of physical therapy for therapists with specialized training. Electrical stimulation and biofeedback treatments are being used clinically as a component of a comprehensive conservative management program for specific pelvic floor disorders. The man or woman with a pathophysiological dysfunction of the pelvic floor can be impaired due to compromised force or strength of the PFM, and disabled because of leakage and or pain. The reader is encouraged to read the article by Bø and Sherburn (143) published in the journal *Physical Therapy*. This article gives an overview of methods used to assess PFM function and strength responsiveness, their reliability and validity obtained with the methods that are available for clinical practice and research today. It is the intent of this chapter to encourage the reader to consider treatment of urogenital dysfunctions once the therapist has received specialized training.

ACKNOWLEDGMENT

The authors are grateful to the Section on Women's Health of the American Physical Therapy Association, who gave permission for parts of this chapter that originally appeared in their text *The Gynecological Manual* (18).

LABORATORY EXERCISES

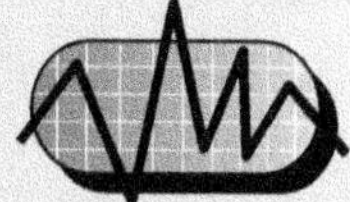

Exercise 1

Changes Occurring with Incontinence

Objective

To understand the social and physical changes that can occur with urinary incontinence

Equipment

A journal to keep track of answers to questions

Description

A 32-year-old woman presents with the primary complaints of a strong urge to urinate every 1 to 2 hours and occasionally urine leakage before reaching the toilet. One year ago she delivered her first baby vaginally after a 24-hour labor. Forceps and a large episiotomy were needed to deliver the 10-lb 1-oz baby. This patient is an emergency room nurse and reports that she frequently leaks a small amount of urine when lifting patients in and out of bed. Other significant medical history includes right low-back pain since pregnancy and increased back pain with intercourse. The patient reports voiding 10 to 14 times each day and gets up two to three times each night. She wears maxi pads (two per shift) to work because she is unsure whether she will be able to leave a patient to urinate. The urologist has tried medication without success and feels the patient may have a permanent dysfunction.

Imagine you are this patient. Examine how you would feel about your situation. Describe the impact on your life in the areas of work, family, social interactions, and emotional life. List four things you would be forced to change because of your condition.

Exercise 2

Patient Experiences while filling out a Bladder Diary

Objective

To understand what a patient experiences as they catalogue their urinary frequency and to begin to interpret bladder diary findings

Equipment

Seven blank bladder diaries.

Description

Record the number of times you urinate in a 24-hour period, your fluid intake, and incontinence episodes. Keep track for 4 to 7 days. Compare your finding to the norms listed. Determine if you have frequency or are not urinating often enough. Do you drink six to eight 8-oz glasses of nonirritating fluids per day?

Exercise 3

The Relevance of Urinary Dysfunction to Clinical Physical Therapy Practice

Objective

To understand and explain in understandable terms why urinary dysfunction is relevant to clinical physical therapy practice.

Equipment

A journal to keep track of answers to questions and willing friends or relatives to practice your explanation.

Description

Practice asking a patient if they have urinary dysfunction and explain why it is important for you to know the function of their bladder when treating various orthopedic conditions.

Exercise 4

Transcutaneous Electrical Stimulation for Patients with Pain

Objective

To set up TENS for pain relief during menstruation for patients referred for dysmenorrhea and to practice alternative settings.

Equipment

A TENS unit with two leads and four electrodes.

Description

For menstrual cramping, try TENS in a criss-crossed pattern over the abdomen. The most frequently used setting is 100 Hz, continuous. Experiment with alternative settings and record Visual Analog Scores every hour from the day cramping starts to the end of menstrual flow for three cycles and compare results.

SELF-STUDY QUESTIONS

For answers, see Appendix B.

1. What is the prevalence of incontinence in the United States?
2. What are the four major pelvic floor muscle groups?
3. What are the three nerves that innervate the primary muscles of the urinary system, and what happens when these nerves are activated?
4. What are the symptoms of urinary dysfunction?
5. Identify and define the six types of urinary incontinence.
6. What are the three clinical classifications of pelvic floor muscle dysfunctions?
7. Identify the four types of pelvic floor muscle impairments.
8. What are the criteria associated with determining whether a trial of electrical stimulation for urinary incontinence and supportive dysfunction is appropriate?
9. Identify the contraindications to electrical stimulation in pelvic floor dysfunction.
10. Describe the proposed mechanism of action of sensory-level electrical stimulation for pelvic floor muscle weakness.
11. Identify the various kinds of issues the clinician must consider in the application of electrical stimulation via internal electrodes for urogenital dysfunction.
12. What is the primary objective of the use of electrical stimulation for the management of overactive bladder and urge incontinence?
13. Why does hypertonus dysfunction occur?
14. Define levator ani syndrome.
15. Identify four relatively recent alternative stimulation approaches that have been developed for the management of genitourinary disorders.
16. What are the types of biofeedback approaches that have been used to manage pelvic floor muscle dysfunction?
17. EMG biofeedback training may be used for which types of pelvic floor muscle dysfunctions?
18. What is the primary objective of EMG biofeedback in the management of urinary incontinence in supportive dysfunction?
19. What is the primary objective of EMG biofeedback training in individuals with pain and hypertonic dysfunction?
20. Identify and describe the EMG characteristics of hypertonus dysfunction.

REFERENCES

1. Nagi S. Some conceptual issues in disability and rehabilitation. In: Sussman M, ed. *Sociology and Rehabilitation*. Washington, DC: American Sociological Association; 1965:100–113.
2. Guide to physical therapist practice, 2nd ed. *Phys Ther*. 2001;81(1):9–744.

3. International Continence Society. Home page. Available at: http://www.continet.org/. Accessed April, 2006.

4. Shelly B, Knight S, King P, et al. Treatment of pelvic pain. In: Laycock J, Haslam J, eds. *Therapeutic Management of Incontinence and Pelvic Pain*. London: Springer; 2002:157–192.

5. Laycock J, Haslam J. *Therapeutic Management of Incontinence and Pelvic Pain*. London: Springer; 2002.

6. Shelly B. The pelvic floor. In Hall CM, Brody LT. *Therapeutic Exercise, Moving Toward Function*. Philadelphia, Pa: Lippincott Williams & Wilkins; 1999:353–386.

7. Schussler B, Laycock J, Norton P, et al. *Pelvic Floor Re-Education Principles and Practice*. New York: Springer-Verlag; 1994.

8. DeLancey J, Richardson A. Anatomy of genital support. In Benson T, ed. *Female Pelvic Floor Disorders*. New York: Norton Medical Books; 1992.

9. Sapsford RR. The pelvic floor and its related organs. In Sapsford R, Bullock-Saxton J, Markwell S, eds. *Women's Health*. Philadelphia, Pa: WB Saunders; 1998:56–86.

10. Perucchini D, DeLancey JO, Ashton-Miller JA, et al. Age effects on urethral striated muscle. II. Anatomic location of muscle loss. *Am J Obstet Gynecol*. 2002;186:356–360.

11. Barber MD, Bremer, RE, Thor KB, et al. Innervation of the female levator ani muscles. *Am J Obstet Gynecol*. 2002;187:64–71.

12. Abrams P, Cardozo L, Khoury S, et al. *Incontinence*. Vol 1. *Basics and Evaluation* [Proceeding of the 3rd International Consultation on Continence]. Monaco: Health Publications Ltd.; 2005.

13. Shelly B. *Beginner Gynecological Therapy*. Coursework presented for Women's Hospital of Baton Rouge, La; 1998.

14. Pages I, Jahr S, Schaufele MK, et al. Comparative analysis of biofeedback and physical therapy for treatment of urinary incontinence in women. *Am J Phys Med Rehabil*. 2001;80:494–502.

15. Bo K, Talseth T, Hulme I. Single blind, randomized controlled trial of pelvic floor exercise, electrical stimulation, vaginal cones and no treatment in management of genuine stress incontinence in women. *BMJ*. 1999;318:487–493.

16. Arvonen T, Fiano-Johnson A, Tyni-Lenne R. Effectiveness of two conservative modes of physical therapy in women with urinary stress incontinence. *Neurourol Urodynam*. 2001;20:591–599.

17. Travell JG, Simons DG. *Myofascial Pain and Dysfunction, the Trigger Point Manual*. Vol 2. Baltimore, Md: Williams &Wilkins; 1992:110–186.

18. Wilder E. *The Gynecological Manual*. 2nd ed. Alexandria, Va: Section on Women's Health, American Physical Therapy Association; 2002.

19. Miller JM, Ashton-Miller J, Delancey J. A pelvic muscle pre-contraction can reduce cough-related urine loss in selected women with mild stress urinary incontinence. *J Am Geriatr Soc*. 1998;46:870–874.

20. Miller JM, Perucchini D, Carchidi LT, DeLancey JO, et al. Pelvic floor muscle contraction during a cough and decreased vesical neck mobility. *Obstet Gynecol*. 2001;97:255–260.

21. Sapsford RR, Hodges PW, Richardson CA, et al. Co-activation of the abdominal and pelvic floor muscles during voluntary exercises. *Neurourol Urodynam*. 2001;20:31–42.

22. Neuman P, Gill V. Pelvic floor and abdominal muscle interaction: EMG activity and intra-abdominal pressure. *Int Urogynecol J*. 2002;13:125–132.

23. Bernier F, Jenkins P, Davila G. Does functional electrical stimulation elicit a pelvic floor muscle contraction? Conference notes Society of Working Nurses and Associates. New Orleans, LA. April 14, 1999.

24. Yamanishi T, Yasuda K, Sakakibara R, Hattori T, Ito H, Murakami S. Pelvic floor electrical stimulation in the treatment of stress incontinence: an investigational study and a placebo controlled double-blind trial. *J Urol*. 1997;158:2127–2131.

25. Plevnik S, Janez J. Maximal electrical stimulation for urinary incontinence. *Urology* 1979; 14:638–645.

26. Merrill D. The treatment of detrusor incontinence by electrical stimulation. *Urology* 1979; 122:515–517.

27. Edwards L, Malvern J. Electronic control of incontinence: a critical review of the present situation. *Br J Urol.* 1972;44:467–462.

28. Kiesswetter H, Flamm J. The muscosal electrosensitivity threshold (MST): a test for the use in conjunction with electronic stimulation in urinary incontinence in women. *Br J Urol.*1978;50:262–263.

29. Kralj, B. The treatment of female urinary incontinence by functional electrical stimulation. In: Ostergard BA, Bent DR, eds. *Urogynecology and Urodynamics.* 3rd ed. Baltimore, Md: Williams & Wilkins; 1991:508–517.

30. Plevnik S, Vodusek B, Vrtacnik P, et al. Optimization of pulse duration for electrical stimulation in treatment of urinary incontinence. *World J Urol.* 1986;4:22–23.

31. Ohlsson B, Lindstrom S, Erlandson BE, et al. Effects of some different pulse parameters on bladder inhibition and urethral closure during intravaginal electrical stimulation: an experimental study in the cat. *Med Biol Eng Comput.* 1986;24:27–33.

32. Eriksen B. Nonsurgical therapies, electrical stimulation. In: Benson T, ed. *Female Pelvic Floor Disorders.* New York: W.W. Norton; 1992:219–231, chapter 11.

33. Shelly ER, Stephenson RG. Electrical stimulation. In: Wilder E, ed. *The Gynecological Manual.* 2nd ed. Alexandria, Va: Section on Women's Health, American Physical Therapy Association; 2002:165–200.

34. Caldwell K. The electrical control of sphincter incompetence. *Lancet.* 1963;2:174.

35. Hopkinson BR, Lightwood R. Electrical treatment of anal incontinence. *Lancet.* 1966;1:297–298.

36. Alexander S, Rowan D. An electronic pessary for stress incontinence. *Lancet.* 1968;1: 7–28.

37. Dox I, Melloni BJ, Eisner GM. *Melloni's Illustrated Medical Dictionary.* Baltimore, Md: Williams & Wilkins; 1979.

38. Mover T, Skofied P. Treatment of stress incontinence by maximal perineal, electrical stimulation. *BMJ.* 1967;3:150–151.

39. Godec C, Cass A, Ayala G. Electrical stimulation for incontinence: technique, selection, results. *Urology.* 1976;7:388–397.

40. Merrill D, Conway C, Dewolf. Urinary incontinence: treatment with electrical stimulation of the pelvic floor. *Urology.* 1975;4:67–72.

41. Fall M, Carlsson C, Erlandson B. Electrical stimulation in interstitial cystitis. *J Urol.* 1980;192–195.

42. Fall M, Erlandson B, Carlson C, et al. Effects of electrical intravaginal stimulation on bladder volume, an experimental and clinical study. *Urol Int.* 1978;33;440–442.

43. Bo K, Talseth T. Change in urethral pressure during voluntary pelvic floor muscle contraction and vaginal electrical stimulation. *Int Urogynecol J.* 1997;8:3–7.

44. Perry JD. *Therapist Instructions for the Orion/Perry Pelvic Muscle Software Cartridge.* Ft. Lauderdale, Fla: Self Regulation System; 1993.

45. Laycock J, Green RJ. Interferential therapy in the treatment of incontinence. *Physiotherapy.* 1988;74:161–168.

46. Bo, K. Effects of electrical stimulation on stress and urge urinary incontinence. *Acta Obstet Gynecol Scand.* 1998;168:3–11.

47. Yasuda, K. Yamanishi T. Critical evaluation of electro-stimulation for management of female urinary incontinence. *Curr Opin Obstet Gynecol.* 1999;11:503–507.

48. Sand PK, Richardson DA, Staskin DR, et al. Pelvic floor stimulation in the treatment of genuine stress incontinence: a multicenter, placebo-controlled trial. *Am J Obstet Gynecol.* 1995;173:72–79.

49. Luber K, Wolde-Jsadih G. Efficiency of functional electrical stimulation in treating genuine stress incontinence: a randomized clinical trial. *Neurourol Urodynam.* 1997;16:543–551.

50. Brubaker L, Benson T, Bent A, et al. Transvaginal electrical stimulation for female urinary incontinence. *Am J Obstet Gynecol.* 1997;177:536–540.

51. Ohlsson BL. Effects of some different pulse parameters on the perception of intravaginal and intra-anal electrical stimulation. *Med Biol Eng Comput.* 1986;26:508–508.

52. Plevnik S, Janez J. Short-term electrical stimulation: home treatment for urinary incontinence. *World J Urol.* 1986;4:24–26.

53. Empi Inc. *Instruction Manual for TENS*. Empi Inc.;1994.
54. Bower W, Moore K, Adams R, et al. A urodynamic study of surface neuromodulation versus sham in detrusor instability and sensory urgency. *J Urol.* 1998;160:2133–2136.
55. Oliver, S. What does neuromodulation do for the sensations of urinary urge and urgency? *Neurourol Urodynam.* 1999;18:403–404.
56. Hoebeke P. Transcutaneous neuromodulation in non-neuropathic bladder sphincter dysfunction in children: preliminary results. *Neurourol Urodynam.* 1999;18: 263–264.
57. Walsh IK, Thompson T, Loughridge WG, et al. Non-invasive antidromic neurostimulation: a simple effective method for improving bladder storage. *Neurourol Urodynam.* 2001;20:73–84.
58. Bower W, Moore K. A pilot study of transcutaneous neuromodulation in children with urgency of urge incontinence. ICCS Abstr.1999;60.
59. Empi Inc. *The Fundamentals of Pelvic Floor Stimulation Manual.* Empi Inc.; 1994.
60. Lindrom S, Fall M, Carlsson CA, et al. The neurophysiological basis of bladder inhibition in response to intravaginal electrical stimulation. *J Urol.* 1983;129:405–410.
61. Soomro NA, Khadra DL, Robson W, et al. A crossover randomized trial of transcutanous electrical nerve stimulation and oxybutynin in clients with detrusor instability. *J Urol.* 2001;166:146–149.
62. McGuire EJ, Shi-Chun Z, Horwinski ER. Treatment of motor and sensory detrusor instability by electrical stimulation. *Urology.* 1983;129:78–79.
63. Godec C. Cass AS, Ayala GF. Bladder inhibition with functional electrical stimulation. *Urology.* 1975;6:663–666.
64. Geirsson, G. Fall M. Maximal functional electrical stimulation in routine practice. *Neurourol Urodynam.* 1997;16:559–565.
65. Siegel S, Richardson DA, Miller KL, et al. Pelvic floor electrical stimulation for the treatment of urge and mixed urinary incontinence in women. *Urology.*1997;50:934–940.
66. Nicosia JF, Abcarian J. Levator syndrome, a treatment that works. *Dis Colon Rectum.* 1985;28:406–408.
67. Scott R, Hsuek G. A clinical study of the effects of galvanic vaginal muscle stimulation in urinary stress incontinence and sexual dysfunction. *Am J Obstet Gynecol.* 1979;135:663–665.
68. Oliver G, Rubin RJ, Salvatia EP, Eisentat JE. Electrogalvanic stimulation in the treatment of levator syndrome. *Dis Colon Rectum.* 1985;28:662–662.
69. Thiel G. Coccygodynia. *Dis Colon Rectum.*1963;6;6:422.
70. Morris L, Newton R. Use of high voltage pulsed galvanic stimulation for clients with levator ani syndrome. *Phys Ther.* 1987;67:1522–1525.
71. Daywood MY, Raymos J. Transcutaneous electrical nerve stimulation (TENS) for the treatment of primary dysmenorrhea: a randomized crossover comparison with placebo TENS and ibuprofen. *Obstet Gynecol.* 1990;75:656–660.

71a. Sohn N, Weinstein MA, Robbins R. The levator syndrome on its treatment with high-voltage electrical electrogalvanic stimulation. *Amer J Surg* 1982;144(11):580–582.

72. Eriksen BC. Painful bladder disease in women—effect of maximal electrical pelvic floor stimulation. *Neurourol Urodynam.* 1989;8:362–363.
73. Hubert J, Rüedi C, Kötting S, et al. A new high frequency electrostimulation device to treat chronic prostatitis. *J Urol.* 2003;170:1257–1277.
74. Littwiller S, Govier F, Kreder K, et al. Pericutaneous peripheral nerve stimulation for urgency/ frequency syndrome. *Neurourol Urodynam.* 1999;18:380.
75. Vandoninck V, van Balken MR, Agro EF, et al. Percutaneous tibial nerve stimulation in the treatment of overactive bladder: urodynamic data. *Neurourol Urodynam.* 2003;22:227–237.
76. Weil E, Ruiz-Cerda J, Eerdmans P, et al. Clinical results of sacral neuromodulation for chronic voiding dysfunction using unilateral sacral foramen electrodes. *World J Urol.* 1998;16: 13–321.
77. Schmidt R, Jonas U, Oleson KA, et al. Sacral nerve stimulation for treatment of refractory urinary urge incontinence. *J Urol.*1999;162:352–357.

78. Janknengt R, Schmidt R., Jonas U, et al. Sacral nerve stimulation (SNS) as treatment for refractory urge incontinence: long term results after proper client selection in a prospective, randomized study. *J Urol.* 1999;162:352–357.

79. Thon W, Baskin L, Jonas U, et al. Neuromodulation of voiding dysfunction and pelvic pain. *World J Urol.* 1991;9:138–141.

80. Shaker H, Loung D, Balbaa L, et al. Sacral root neuromodulation induces inhibition of the hyperactive c-afferent fibers in a hyperactive animal model. *Neurourol Urodynam.* 1999;18:278.

81. Yamanishi T, Yasudak K., Suda S, et al. Effects of functional continuous magnetic stimulation on urethral closure in healthy volunteers. *Urology.* 1999;54:652–655.

82. Ishikawa N, Suda S, Sasaki T, et al. Development of a non-invasive treatment system for urinary incontinence using a functional continuous magnetic stimulator. *Med Biol Eng Comput.* 1998;36:704–710.

83. McFarlane J, Folys S, Winter P, et al. Acute suppression of idiopathic detrusor instability with magnetic stimulation of the sacral nerve roots. *Br J Urol.* 1997;80:734–741.

84. Galloway N, El-gallery R, Sand P, et al. Extracorporeal magnetic innervation therapy for stress urinary incontinence. *Urology.* 1999;53:1108–1111.

85. Oliver S, Fowler C, Mundy A, Craggs M. Measuring the sensation of urge and bladder filling during cystometry in urge incontinence and the effects of neuromodulation. *Neururol Urodynam.* 2003;22:7–16.

86. Nakamura M, Sakurai. Bladder inhibition by penile electrical stimulation. *Br J Urol.* 1984; 56:413–415.

87. Herbison P, Mantle J. Weighted vaginal cones for urinary incontinence. *Cochrane Database Syst Rev.* 2000;2(CD 002114).

88. Kegel A. Progressive resistance exercise in functional restoration of perineal muscle. *Am J Obstet Gynecol.* 1948;56:238–248.

89. Bo, K, Sherburn M. Evaluation of female pelvic floor muscle function and strength. *Phys Ther.* 2005;85:269–282.

90. Van Kampen M, De Weerdt W, Feys H, et al. Reliability and validity of a digital test for pelvic muscle strength in women. *Neurourol Urodynam.* 1996;15:338–339.

91. Kegel AH. Physiologic therapy for urinary stress incontinence. *JAMA.* 1951;146:915–917.

92. Assad L. Biofeedback Air Pressure. In: Wilder E, ed. *The Gynecological Manual.* Alexandria, Va: Section on Women's Health, American Physical Therapy Association; 2002.

93. Kiesswetter H. EMG-patterns of the pelvic floor muscles with surface electrodes. *Urol Int.* 1976;31:60–69.

94. Siroky MB. Electromyography of perineal floor. *Urol Clin N Am.* 1996;23:299–307.

95. Barrett DM. Disposable (infant) surface electrocardiogram electrodes in urodynamics: a simultaneous comparative study of electrodes. *J Urol.* 1980;124:663–665.

96. O'Donnell P, Doyle R. Biofeedback therapy techniques for treatment of urinary incontinence. *Urology.* 1991;37:432–436.

97. Binnie N. The importance of the orientation of the electrode plates in recording the external anal sphincter EMG by non-invasive anal plug electrodes. *Int J Colorectal Dis.* 1991;8:8–11.

98. Corcos J, Drew S, West L. Urinary and fecal incontinence: the use of electromyographic biofeedback for training pelvic floor musculature. *Phys Ther Prod.* 1993:26–29.

99. Cram JR, Kasman GS. *Introduction to Surface Electromyography.* Gaithersburg, Md: Aspen Publication; 1998:378.

100. Glazer H, Rodke G, Swencionis C, et al. Treatment of vulvar vestibulitis syndrome with electromyography biofeedback of pelvic floor muscular. *J Reprod Med.* 1995;40: 283.

101. Knight S, Laycock J. The role of biofeedback in pelvic floor re-education. *Physiotherapy.* 1994;80:145–148.

102. Glazer H. Pelvic floor muscle surface electromyography reliability and clinical predictive validity. *J Reprod Med.* 1999;44:779–782.

103. Gunnarsson M. Circumvaginal surface electromyography in women with urinary incontinence and in healthy volunteers. *Scand J Urol Nephrol.* 157:89–95.

104. Bump R, Hurt G, Fantly J, et al. Assessment of Kegel pelvic muscle exercise performance after brief verbal instructions. *Am J Obstet Gynecol.* 1991;165:322–329.

105. Morkved S, Bo K, Fjortoft T. Effect of adding biofeedback to pelvic floor muscle training to treat urodynamic stress incontinence. *Obstet Gynecol.* 2002;100:730–739.

106. Burgio K, Robinson J, Engel B. The role of biofeedback in Kegel exercise training for stress urinary incontinence. *Am J Obstet Gynecol.* 1986;154:58–64.

107. Taylor K, Henderson J. Effects of biofeedback and urinary stress incontinence in older women. *J Gerontol Nurs.* 1986;12:25–30.

108. Susset J, Balla G, Read L. Biofeedback therapy for female incontinence due to low urethral resistance. *J Urol.* 1990;143:1205–1208.

109. Burns PA, Pranikoff K, Nochajski TH, et al. Treatment of stress incontinence with pelvic floor exercise and biofeedback. *J Am Geriatr Soc.*1990;38:241–244.

110. Pages I, Jahr S, Schaufele MK, et al. Comparative analysis of biofeedback and physical therapy for treatment of urinary incontinence in women. *Am J Phys Med Rehabil.* 2001;80:494–502.

111. Burns PA, Pranikoff K, Nochajski TH, et al. A comparison of effectiveness of biofeedback and pelvic muscle exercise treatment of stress incontinence in older community dwelling women. *J Gerontol.* 1993;48:167–74.

112. Berghmans LCM, Frederiks CMA, deBie RA, et al. Efficacy of biofeedback, when included with pelvic floor muscle exercise treatment, for genuine stress incontinence. *Neurourol Urodyn.* 1996;15:37–52.

113. Glavind K, Nohr S, Walter S. Biofeedback and physiology vs. physiology alone in the treatment of genuine stress incontinence. *Int Urogynecol Jl.* 1996;7:339–343.

114. Weiss Coffey S, Wilder E, Majsak M, et al. The effects of a progressive exercise program with surface electromyographic biofeedback on an adult with fecal incontinence. *Phys Ther.* 2002;82:798–811.

115. Enck P. Biofeedback training in disordered defecation. A critical review. *Dig Dis Sci.* 1993;38:1953–1960.

116. Rieger NA, Wattchow DA, Sarre RG, et al. Prospective trial of pelvic floor retraining in patients with fecal incontinence. *Dis Colon Rectum.* 1997;40:821–826.

117. Hunter K, Moore K, DJC, Glazener C. *Conservative Management for Prostprostatectomy Urinary Incontinence* (Cochrane Review). Chichester, UK: John Wiley and Sons; 2004.

118. Wennergren H, Oberg B. Pelvic floor exercises for children: a method of treating dysfunctional voiding. *Br J Urol.* 1995;76:9–15.

119. McKenna PH, Herndon CD, Connery S, et al. Pelvic floor muscle retraining for pediatric voiding dysfunction using interactive computer games. *J Urol.* 1999;162:1056–1062.

120. Bo K. Pelvic floor muscle exercises for treatment of stress urinary incontinence: an exercise physiologist perspective. *Int Urogynecol J.* 1995;6:282–291.

121. Urinary Incontinence Guideline Panel. *Urinary Incontinence in Adults: Clinical Practice Guidelines.* AHCPR Pub. No. 92-0038. Rockford, MD: Agency for Health Care Policy and Research, Public Health Services, U.S. Department of Health and Human Services; 1992.

122. DeLancey JOL. Anatomy and biomechanics of genital prolapse. *Clin Obstet Gynecol.* 1993;36:897–909.

123. Sapsford R. Rehabilitation of the pelvic floor muscles utilizing trunk stabilization. *Manual Ther.* 2004;9:3–12.

124. Bo K, Sherburn M, Allen T. Transabdominal ultrasound measurement of pelvic floor muscle activity when activated directly or via a transversus abdominis muscle contraction. *Neurourol Urodynam.* 2003;22:582–588.

125. Neumann P, Gill V. Pelvic floor and abdominal muscle interaction: EMG activity and intra-abdominal pressure. *Int Urogynecol J.* 2002;13:125–132.

126. Laycock J, Brown J, Cusack C, et al. A multicenter, prospective, randomized, controlled group, comparative study of efficiency of vaginal cones and PFX. *Neurourol Urodynam.* 1999;18:301–302.

127. Perry J, Hullet L. The role of home trainers in Kegel's exercise program for treatment of incontinence. *Ostomy Wound Manage.* 1990;30:1–8.

128. Smith B, Boileau MA, Buan LD. A self-directed home biofeedback system for women with symptoms of stress, urge, and mixed incontinence. *J Wound Ostomy Continence Nurs.* 2000;27:240–246.

129. Henalla SM, Hutchins CJ, Robinson P, et al. Non-operative methods in the treatment of female genuine stress incontinence of urine. *J Obstet Gynecol Neonatal Nurs.* 1989;222–225.

130. Berghmans LCM, Hendricks HJM, Bo K, et al. Conservative treatment of stress urinary incontinence in women: a systematic review of randomized clinical trails. *Br J Urol.* 1998;82:181–191.

131. Lagro-Janssen A, Debruyne F, Smiths A, et al. The effects of treatment of urinary incontinence in general practice. *Fam Pract.* 1992;9:284–289.

132. Sung MS, Hong JY, Choi YH, et al. FES biofeedback versus intensive pelvic floor muscle exercise for the prevention and treatment of genuine stress incontinence. *J Korean Med Sci.* 2000;15:303–308.

133. Abdelghany S. Biofeedback and electrical stimulation therapy for treating urinary incontinence and voiding dysfunction: one center's experience. *Urol Nurs.* 2001;21:401–410.

134. Jackson J, Emerson L, Johnston B, et al. Biofeedback: a noninvasive treatment for incontinence after radical prostatectomy. *Urol Nurs.* 1996;16:50–54.

135. White G, Jantos M, Glazer H. Establishing the diagnosis of vulvar vestibulitis. *J Reprod Med.*1997;42:157–160.

136. Herman H. Conservative management of female patients with pelvic pain. *Urol Nurs.* 2000;20:393–417

137. Costello K. Myofascial syndromes. In: Stegge J, Metzger D, Levy B, eds. *Chronic Pelvic Pain: An Integrated Approach.* Philadelphia: WB Saunders; 1998:251–265.

138. Glazer HI, Rodke G, Swencionis C, et al. Treatment of vulvar vestibulitis syndrome with electromyographic biofeedback of pelvic floor musculature. *J Reprod Med.* 1995;40:283–290.

139. Rao SSC. Technical aspects of biofeedback therapy for defecation disorders. *Gastroenterologist.* 1998;6:96–103.

140. Nogueras J, Wexner S. Biofeedback for non-relaxing puborectalis syndrome. *Dis Colon Rectum.* 1992;3:120–123.

141. Wexner S, Cheape JD, Jorge JMN, et al. Prospective assessment of biofeedback for the treatment of paradoxical puborectalis contraction. *Dis Colon Rectum.* 1992;35:145–149.

142. Husted J. Desensitization procedures in dealings with female sexual dysfunction. *Counsel Psychol.* 1975;5:30–37.

143. Bo K, Sherburn M. Evaluation of female pelvic-floor muscle function and strength. *Phys Ther.* 2005; 85:269–282.

CHAPTER 10

Electrical Stimulation for the Delivery of Medications: Iontophoresis

Charles D. Ciccone

Iontophoresis is the use of electric current to enhance the transcutaneous administration of pharmacologically active substances. These substances typically consist of medications such as anti-inflammatory steroids and local anesthetics, as well as a variety of other prescription and nonprescription agents. In theory, iontophoresis uses electric current to facilitate movement of the medication through the skin and into the underlying tissues. This procedure may provide a relatively safe and painless way to deliver clinically significant amounts of medication to cutaneous and subcutaneous tissues.

The basic principles underlying iontophoresis techniques were first described more than a century ago (1,2), and iontophoresis has been used as a clinical intervention for the past 60 years. Regarding physical therapy practice, iontophoresis is typically used as a therapeutic intervention to administer a medication to a specific site or tissue. Unfortunately, relatively few experimental studies exist that document the clinical effects of iontophoresis when this technique is used to deliver drugs locally to such tissues. The rehabilitation literature consists largely of case reports and a small number of clinical trials that describe the potential uses and effects of various iontophoresis techniques. Although it is regrettable that more studies have not been conducted, preliminary evidence does suggest that iontophoresis can be considered an intervention in the treatment of certain conditions that occur in patients seen commonly by physical therapists.

More recently, iontophoresis techniques have been advocated as a way to deliver medications into the systemic circulation. That is, electric current can be used to facilitate transdermal drug delivery so that the drug permeates the skin and is ultimately delivered throughout the body. This technique could serve as a noninvasive method for administering drugs that are typically given by injection. By adjusting the amount of electric current during administration, iontophoresis could likewise provide a method for controlling systemic drug delivery of certain medications. The use of iontophoresis for systemic drug delivery is not typically as relevant for physical therapists as the iontophoretic delivery of medications to local tissues such as tendons, muscle, and so forth. Nonetheless, the fact that electricity might be used to facilitate systemic drug delivery has renewed interest in determining the mechanisms and biophysical properties that affect iontophoresis. Hence, there has been a recent upsurge in the research literature of reports on how to effectively use electricity to facilitate transdermal drug delivery.

The purpose of this chapter is to provide an overview of how iontophoresis can be used to help achieve specific therapeutic goals, especially with regard to how physical therapists can use this intervention. The chapter will first present some of the basic principles that govern the use of direct current to enhance drug administration. A discussion of some of the practical issues involved in iontophoresis, including the selection of appropriate instrumentation and the clinical methods typically used during iontophoresis application, follows. Finally, medications that have been applied iontophoretically to achieve specific outcomes are discussed.

BASIC PRINCIPLES OF IONTOPHORESIS APPLICATION

How Does Iontophoresis Enhance Transdermal Drug Delivery?

Iontophoresis can potentially enhance the movement of drugs across the skin via three mechanisms: *electromigration*, *electroporation*, and *electro-osmosis* (3). These mechanisms are addressed briefly below.

Electromigration

Electromigration occurs when the ionized (charged) form of the drug is repulsed and driven into the skin by a similarly charged electric field. This process (also called electrophoresis; see Chapter 1) is based on the fact that many drug compounds are composed of positively and negatively charged structural units called *ions*. When these compounds are placed in an appropriate solution, they dissociate into these polar (electrically charged) components and assume a positive charge or a negative charge depending on whether the atom loses or gains an electron. While in a charged state, each ion can be influenced by an electrical field created within the solution. Positively charged ions (cations) will be attracted to the negative pole (cathode) and repelled from the positive pole (anode). Negatively charged ions (anions) will be attracted to the anode and repelled from the cathode. The electrostatic repulsion of like charges is the primary driving force for iontophoresis (Fig. 10.1).

Many drugs placed in an aqueous solution are ionic compounds that dissociate into positive and negative components. When drugs ionize in solution, the drug portion of the molecule will assume either a negative charge or a positive charge, while some ionic side group will assume the opposite charge. For instance, the anti-inflammatory preparation dexamethasone sodium

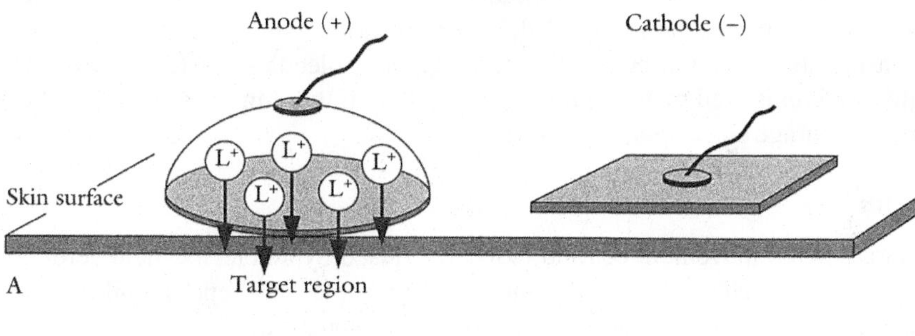

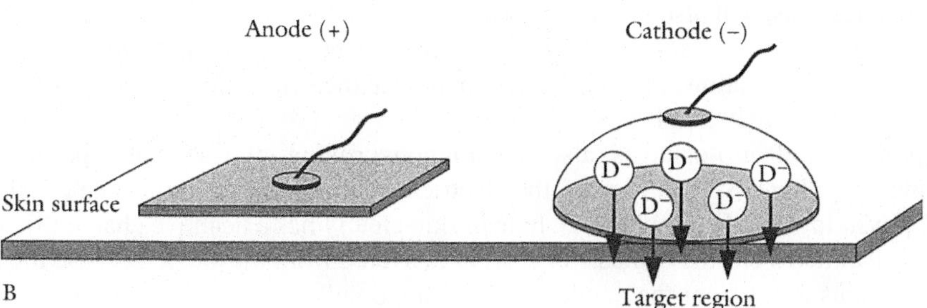

Figure 10.1. Schematic diagram of ion transfer during iontophoresis. Positive ions such as lidocaine (L+) are driven away from the anode, and negative ions such as dexamethasone (D−) are driven away from the cathode.

phosphate will ionize in an aqueous solution to form the negatively charged dexamethasone phosphate ion and the positively charged sodium ion (see Fig. 10.1). Other drugs, such as lidocaine hydrochloride, typically assume a positive ionic charge in aqueous solution. Identification of the drug's polarity dictates the polarity of the electrode used to drive the ion toward underlying tissues. Positive drugs are placed under the positive electrode (anode), and negative drugs are placed under the negative electrode (cathode). The electrode containing or overlying the drug is typically referred to as the "active" or "delivery" electrode, with the opposite electrode often called the "return" or "dispersive" electrode.

Table 10.1 lists some of the drugs commonly used during iontophoresis, the polarity of the ionized form of each drug, and indications for the use of each drug. These drug indications are addressed in more detail later in this chapter.

Electroporation

Electroporation is the formation of temporary channels or pores within the outer layer of the skin (stratum corneum) (4–6). Normally the stratum corneum is impervious to water and to water-soluble (hydrophilic) medications. It appears, however, that certain types of electrical current can create transient structural changes in the stratum corneum, resulting in the formation of pores that facilitate movement of substances through the skin (7–9). Although the exact structure and size of these pores remains to be determined, it is generally believed that these pores represent aqueous channels (i.e., water-filled pathways) through the lipid bilayer between the cells (keratinocytes) that make up the stratum corneum (5).

Much of the evidence for electroporation has been obtained from in vitro studies using excised portions of human or animal skin that are suspended between experimental chambers. Likewise, it has also become apparent that these pores can be optimally induced using electrical stimulation parameters that are different from the parameters typically used in clinical iontophoresis (4) (see "Electricity as a Drug Administration Vehicle," below). Nonetheless, it is clear that iontophoresis can produce temporary changes in skin structure that further enhance cutaneous permeability and transdermal delivery of various substances (4,10). This idea has received considerable attention because large nonpolar molecules (proteins, hormones, and so forth) might be administered by iontophoresis, especially if the skin is first treated with electrical currents that encourage electroporation (4,11,12).

Electro-osmosis

Electro-osmosis is the movement of fluid (solvent) caused by an electric field acting on ions in the solvent. Current discharged from the anode, for example, will repel mobile cations such as sodium, and the movement of sodium away from the anode will create an osmotic force that draws fluid away from the anode. Presumably, any other substances dissolved in that fluid, including medications, will also be carried away from the anode via the overall (bulk) flow of the solvent. The bulk flow of the solvent therefore has the potential to contribute to transdermal drug delivery, presumably by allowing the solvent to permeate the skin via pre-existing pathways such as hair follicles and sweat glands (13).

The process of electro-osmosis (also called ionohydrokinesis) has some important implications during iontophoresis. In particular, the electrical charge of the skin must be considered. At neutral or physiological pH (around 7.0), human skin clearly has a negative charge (3). This negative charge facilitates electro-osmosis of solvent delivered from the anode because the skin will help draw cations away from the anode and encourage bulk fluid movement into the skin (3). Conversely, delivery from the cathode will be inhibited because the negatively charged skin will repel anions in the solvent (3). This situation becomes reversed if skin pH decreases. As skin pH approaches 5.0 or lower, the skin potential reverses so that the skin assumes a positive charge.

Table 10.1. Medications Commonly Administered by Iontophoresis

Drug	Principal Indication(s)	Treatment Rationale	Iontophoresis
Acetic acid	Calcific tendonitis; myositis ossificans	Acetate is believed to increase solubility of calcium deposits in tendons and other soft tissues	2%–5% aqueous solution from negative pole
Calcium chloride	Skeletal muscle spasms	Calcium stabilizes excitable membranes; appears to decrease excitability threshold in peripheral nerves and skeletal muscle	2% aqueous solution from positive pole
Dexamethasone	Inflammation	Synthetic steroidal anti-inflammatory agent	4 mg/mL in aqueous solution from negative pole
Iodine	Adhesive capsulitis and other soft-tissue adhesions; microbial infections	Iodine is a broad-spectrum antibiotic; the sclerolytic actions of iodine are not fully understood	5%–10% solution or ointment from negative pole
Lidocaine	Soft-tissue pain and inflammation (e.g, bursitis, tenosynovitis)	Local anesthetic effects produce transient analgesia	4%–5% solution or ointment from positive pole
Magnesium sulfate	Skeletal muscle spasms; myositis	Muscle relaxant effect may be caused by decreased excitability of the skeletal muscle membrane and decreased transmission at the neuromuscular junction	2% aqueous solution or ointment from positive pole
Hyaluronidase	Local edema (subacute and chronic stage)	Appears to increase permeability in connective tissue by hydrolyzing hyaluronic acid, thus decreasing encapsulation and allowing dispersement of local edema	Reconstitute with 0.9% sodium chloride to provide a 150 μg/mL solution from positive pole
Salicylates	Muscle and joint pain in acute and chronic conditions (e.g, overuse injuries, rheumatoid arthritis)	Aspirin-like drugs with analgesic and anti-inflammatory effects	10% trolamine salicylate ointment or 2%–3% sodium salicylate solution from negative pole
Zinc oxide	Skin ulcers, other dermatologic disorders	Zinc acts as a general antiseptic; may increase tissue healing	20% ointment from positive pole

Adapted from Ciccone CD. *Pharmacology in Rehabilitation* 3rd ed. Philadelphia: F.A. Davis; 2002.

In this situation, electro-osmosis facilitates the movement of solvent delivered from the cathode because the skin will attract anions in the solvent (3).

Hence, the contribution of electro-osmosis during iontophoresis must be considered according to specific conditions. Electro-osmosis will assist the delivery of drugs from the anode when skin pH is >5.0, but it might retard drugs delivered from the anode when skin pH is <5.0 (14). The opposite is true for cathodal delivery: electro-osmosis facilitates delivery at conditions of lower skin pH, but it will impair drug delivery from the cathode if skin pH is >5.0 (14). Under the correct conditions, electro-osmosis might be used to facilitate the movement of certain drugs, including delivery of relatively large molecules that are carried by the solvent medium (3).

Relative Contributions of Electromigration, Electroporation, and Electro-osmosis During Iontophoresis

Although all three mechanisms can influence drug movement, it is generally accepted that electromigration is the primary force that influences iontophoresis (15,16). At the stimulation parameters used during clinical iontophoresis, electroporation and electro-osmosis probably play a secondary and complementary role (3); that is, these latter mechanisms have the potential to enhance the transdermal delivery of drugs caused by electromigration.

One could consider these relative contributions somewhat analogous to the forces acting on a billiard ball. The primary force (electromigration) occurs when one billiard ball strikes and repels a second ball, much like the appropriate electrical field used during iontophoresis will repel a similarly charged drug molecule. Electroporation would be analogous to a process that temporarily enlarged the size of the pockets/holes on the billiard table, thereby making it easier for the repelled ball to enter the pocket. Under the appropriate conditions, electro-osmosis would be analogous to providing a slight "downhill" tilt to the billiard table, so that the repelled ball will roll more easily to the other end of the table. As discussed earlier, electro-osmosis can also retard bulk solvent flow under certain conditions, similar to the billiard table being tilted in the opposite or "uphill" direction in our analogy.

The exact contribution of each mechanism during iontophoresis must, of course, be considered for each medication and the stimulation parameters used to deliver that medication. Nonetheless, clinicians must be aware that all three mechanisms can affect drug delivery, and that electricity can influence drug movement by not only repulsion of like charges (electromigration), but also by inducing temporary changes in skin structure (electroporation), and by affecting bulk fluid movement (electro-osmosis).

Electricity as a Drug Administration Vehicle

The primary role of electric current during iontophoresis is to help transmit medication to a target site. In this sense, electricity can be viewed as a vehicle for transdermal drug administration much in the same way that a hypodermic syringe serves as the vehicle to administer a drug via subcutaneous or intravenous injection. Specific parameters of electricity should be selected to optimize iontophoretic effects much in the same way that a certain size and caliber syringe are chosen for different types of injections. These optimal electric parameters for iontophoresis are summarized in Table 10.2 and are presented in more detail here.

Table 10.2. Summary of Typical Current Parameters During Clinical Iontophoresis

Type	Direct current
Amplitude	1.0–4.0 mA
Duration	20–40 min
Total current-dosage	40–80 mA•min

Table 10.3. Summary of Reactions at the Anode and Cathode

Cathode	Anode
Attraction of positive ions	Attraction of negative ions
Alkaline reaction by formation of NaOH	Acidic reaction by formation of HCl
Decreased density of proteins (sclerolytic)	Increased density of proteins (sclerotic)
Increased nerve excitability via depolarization	Decreased nerve excitability via hyperpolarization (anode block)
Vasodilation	Coagulation of microcirculation (capillary coagulation)

Type of Current

Traditionally, direct (galvanic) current has been used for clinical iontophoresis. Direct current creates a constant, unidirectional electrostatic field between the electrodes to allow continuous transmission of the medication. General aspects of DC were discussed in Chapter 1, and types of DC generators that can supply the appropriate current for iontophoresis are discussed in Chapter 2 and later in this chapter. One aspect of DC that is particularly important during iontophoresis is the tendency for specific clinical and electrophysiological effects to occur beneath each electrode (Table 10.3). Even in the absence of any medication, an alkaline reaction occurs at the cathode due to the formation of sodium hydroxide, whereas an acidic reaction occurs at the anode due to the formation of hydrochloric acid. These reactions are especially important when the cathode is used as the delivery electrode because alkaline reactions are usually more caustic to human skin during application of DC. Likewise, other effects on protein density and nerve excitability can influence the patient's ability to tolerate repeated applications of iontophoresis. Finally, changes in pH at the site of the delivery electrode may affect drug stability and ionization, thus having the potential to dramatically affect the amount of drug delivered. This issue of pH and drug stability is discussed in more detail later in this chapter.

Current Amplitude

Most clinical studies using iontophoresis have reported using current amplitudes ranging from 1.0 to 5.0 mA (17–23). Contemporary iontophoresis devices typically provide a maximum current of 4.0 mA, with the minimum amplitude ranging from 0.01 to 1.0 mA. Manufacturers of these devices advocate amplitudes in the range of 1.0 to 4.0 mA. The exact current amplitude used during an iontophoresis treatment, however, is dictated by several factors, including patient tolerance, polarity of the active electrode, size of the active electrode, and duration of treatment.

Duration of Current Application

The length of time (duration) that the current is applied during iontophoresis varies greatly from study to study. Durations as short as 5 minutes or as long as several hours have been reported (24–26). Generally, the length of time the current is applied is inversely proportional to the magnitude of the current. Larger amplitude currents (approaching or exceeding 4.0 mA) are typically applied for shorter periods of time, whereas smaller currents are applied for longer durations.

Alternative Methods of Current Application

ALTERNATING CURRENT

It has been suggested recently that alternating current might also be useful in iontophoresis. The basic characteristics of AC were described in Chapter 1. Whereas DC applies a constant current in one direction (from the anode to the cathode or vice versa), AC provide a sinusoidal pulse that alternates between positive and negative according to a set frequency (e.g., 1 kHz). Preliminary evidence suggests that AC might facilitate transdermal drug delivery by temporarily altering the conductance of the skin, thereby allowing medications to penetrate the skin more easily (10). It has also been suggested that AC might create an electric field that causes vibration of the drug molecule with subsequent breakdown of bonds between the drug molecule and surrounding water molecules (27). This effect would enhance the ability of drug molecules to diffuse across membranes by reducing the effective size (radius) of the drug molecule when it is stripped of surrounding water molecules (27).

Use of AC during iontophoresis remains experimental at this time. One in vitro study suggested that AC applied at 20 V over a range of frequencies increased the transport of a local anesthetic (lidocaine) through excised rat skin (28). Another study found that AC-assisted application of local anesthetics to the plantar surface of the foot of human volunteers resulted in decreased sensation, suggesting that transdermal administration of this drug might be enhanced by this technique (29).

If AC can facilitate transdermal delivery, this type of current offers certain advantages over traditional DC methods. In particular, AC might provide a more predictable and less variable method for administering drugs into the systemic circulation (10). Prolonged application of DC at a given current amplitude often results in variable and unpredictable changes in skin conductance and pH (10). Use of AC could potentially maintain relatively constant skin conductance for prolonged periods and thereby provide a more constant drug flux than DC (10,30). Low intensities of AC are also less damaging to the skin than equivalent application of DC (see Chapter 2).

For these reasons, AC could potentially be used for the systemic administration of various compounds, including those containing larger molecules that are either charged or neutral. This idea continues to be investigated as a method for systemic administration of substances such as hormones, cardiovascular drugs, and other medications. Further research will indicate if this technique can be used commercially for the safe and predictable administration of various substances.

HIGH-VOLTAGE, SHORT-DURATION DC

As indicated earlier, certain electrical currents may cause electroporation—that is, creation of temporary pores within the stratum corneum that enhance drug permeation through the skin. Although traditional iontophoresis DC currents may cause some degree of electroporation (31), it has been suggested that higher voltages (≥100 V) applied for very short time periods (a few microseconds or milliseconds) might be much more successful in creating such pores (4,8). Again, the evidence for this effect has been obtained primarily from in vitro experiments or studies on excised or in situ animal skin. At present, there is little evidence that these currents can be used effectively in clinical situations.

Nonetheless, there is considerable interest in determining if these electroporation currents can be used to facilitate drug delivery in humans (4,5). Clearly, there is a need for additional studies to determine if these higher voltage currents can be used safely and effectively to help deliver medications locally or systemically to treat various pathologies and impairments. Likewise, devices used to administer clinical iontophoresis must be developed to safely and conveniently apply the voltages and durations of DC currents that are advocated in electroporation (4). It will be interesting to see if various stimulation protocols might someday be used to provide optimal drug delivery. One could envision a protocol where high-voltage, short-duration current is applied initially to promote pore formation, followed by more traditional application of DC current to provide the actual vehicle for drug delivery through the newly created pores (7,11).

Concept of Current-Dosage During Iontophoresis

Both the current amplitude and duration are factors that influence how much electricity will be provided to facilitate drug administration during traditional iontophoresis. Rather than referring to these two parameters independently, it is much more practical to consider the product of these factors as the total electrical "dosage" used to facilitate drug application. That is, the current amplitude (mA) is multiplied by the duration (minutes) to provide the *current-dosage* in units of mA•min. For instance, a current applied at an amplitude of 2 mA for a duration of 20 minutes would yield a dosage of 40 mA•min.

Many contemporary iontophoresis protocols describe treatment parameters in terms of a mA•minutes dosage. Dosages ranging from 40 mA•min to 80 mA•min have often been suggested for treating conditions such as pain and inflammation (17,18,32–34). Many clinical studies, however, reported using a current–duration combination that resulted in dosages that approach the upper end of this dosage range (17,18,35–37). That is, it may be worthwhile to use dosages of 70 or 80 mA•min whenever possible to achieve optimal effects. Clearly, an ideal current-dosage for iontophoresis treatments remains to be determined, and clinicians should adjust current-dosage as needed for each individual patient.

It should also be noted that any given current-dosage can be achieved by an infinite number of amplitude–duration combinations. For instance, a dosage of 40 mA•min could be achieved by applying 1 mA for 40 minutes, 2 mA for 20 minutes, 3 mA for 13.3 minutes, or 4 mA for 10 minutes. This illustrates how the concept of current-dosage can be very helpful in standardizing the amount of electrical current that is used as a drug vehicle during iontophoresis. Patients who are not able to tolerate higher current amplitudes can still be given a designated current-dosage by prolonging treatment duration accordingly.

Clinicians should be aware, however, that different combinations of amplitude and duration might not provide equivalent amounts of ion transfer, even if the current-dosages are mathematically identical. It is unclear, for example, if 1 mA applied for 40 minutes will actually deliver the same amount of medication as 4 mA applied for 10 minutes. This issue was examined in a series of experiments conducted by Anderson et al. (24). These investigators compared administration of an anti-inflammatory steroid (dexamethasone) under two current-dosage protocols: a high-current, short-duration (HCSD) protocol of 4.0 mA for 10 minutes, and a low-current, long-duration (LCLD) protocol of 0.1 mA for 400 minutes. Theoretically, these two protocols should deliver equivalent amounts of drug because they both use a current dosage of 40 mA•min. This study, however, suggested that the total amount of drug delivered to an in vitro measurement device (agarose gel columns) might be greater (although more variable) using LCLD compared to HCSD (24). Likewise, the physiological effect of the drug on human cutaneous circulation in vivo appeared to be greater and more prolonged when applied by the LCLD protocol (24).

The study described above suggests that different combinations of current amplitude and duration can affect the amount of drug delivered and the subsequent physiological effects, even if the overall current-dosage is the same. Clearly, additional laboratory and clinical studies are needed to definitively address issues regarding the amplitude and duration combinations that will ultimately provide optimal drug delivery in clinical situations.

INSTRUMENTATION FOR IONTOPHORESIS

DC Generators

Any DC generator capable of delivering direct current with fine control in the 0 to 5 mA range could be used to administer iontophoresis. Several commercial devices are available, however, that are designed to be used exclusively for iontophoresis. These iontophoresis-dedicated devices are typically small, battery-powered units that provide one or two channels for current application. Manufacturers of these devices have included additional control features to assist in providing iontophoresis treatments. For instance, many devices provide an automatic current ramp-up at the beginning of the treatment and current ramp-down at the end of the treatment. Some devices also allow the therapist to preset the parameters of current amplitude and total desired dosage (in mA•minutes), and the treatment duration is then adjusted automatically within the device. Other features such as a built-in timer, automatic shut-off at the end of the treatment, and an audible warning signal that indicates an interruption in current delivery are also available on some devices. Individuals interested in using these devices should compare these units based on cost, ease of use, and various other features.

Electrodes

Types of Electrodes for Iontophoresis

Electrodes used for iontophoresis can either be constructed by the clinician or they can be obtained commercially (Fig. 10.2). Noncommercial electrodes are typically made from some type of malleable metal such as tin, aluminum, or copper. Sheets of tin or copper foil can be purchased and cut to fit over the treatment site. Alternatively, several folds of heavy-duty aluminum foil can be cut and pressed into a treatment electrode. The metal delivery electrode is placed over gauze pads or paper towels that have been soaked in the drug that is being applied. Towels or gauze soaked in tap water are placed beneath the return electrode. The electrodes are then held in place by weights, rubber straps, or elastic bandages, and alligator clips are used to connect the electrodes to wires coming from the DC generator.

Several types of commercial electrodes have been introduced for use during iontophoresis (Fig. 10.2). These self-adhesive electrodes usually come in a package containing a delivery and a return pad. The delivery electrode typically consists of a fiber pad or gel matrix that can be impregnated with the desired medication. The return electrode may be either a fiber pad that must be filled with tap water or a gumlike polymer that does not need filling. These electrodes have some specific connector to allow attachment of wires leading to the DC generator (usually a commercial iontophoresis device). Some commercial electrodes are designed for a single application, while others may be used for two to three applications of the same drug.

A popular commercial electrode used in the past consisted of a reservoir that could be filled with the drug solution. These reservoir or "bubble" electrodes were difficult to apply properly and tended to cause skin irritation in some patients. These electrodes have essentially been replaced by the gel or fiber electrodes described above.

There are advantages and disadvantages to using noncommercial and commercial electrodes. Commercial electrodes come in fixed sizes, and the maximum area of drug delivery will be limited by the size and shape of the delivery electrode. Self-constructed electrodes of tin or aluminum are very inexpensive and can be custom made for each patient. This may be beneficial for treating rather large areas (i.e., areas that cannot be covered adequately by the commercial electrodes). Disadvantages of self-constructed electrodes include the fact that it might be difficult to conform the electrode to irregularly shaped areas of the body, and burning can occur because uniform contact of the electrode to the skin may be difficult to maintain.

Commercial electrodes offer advantages of convenience and ease of application, but these electrodes are often quite expensive (one set of electrodes may cost upwards of $10.00 U.S.). Commercial electrodes may, however, have other features that could make these more attractive for use in some patients. For instance, certain commercial electrodes contain a chemical feature such as a buffering agent or silver chloride that helps regulate pH at the electrode site during the treatment. This buffering effect helps moderate the acidic and alkaline reactions that typically occur at the anode and cathode, respectively, thus helping decrease the chance of skin irritation

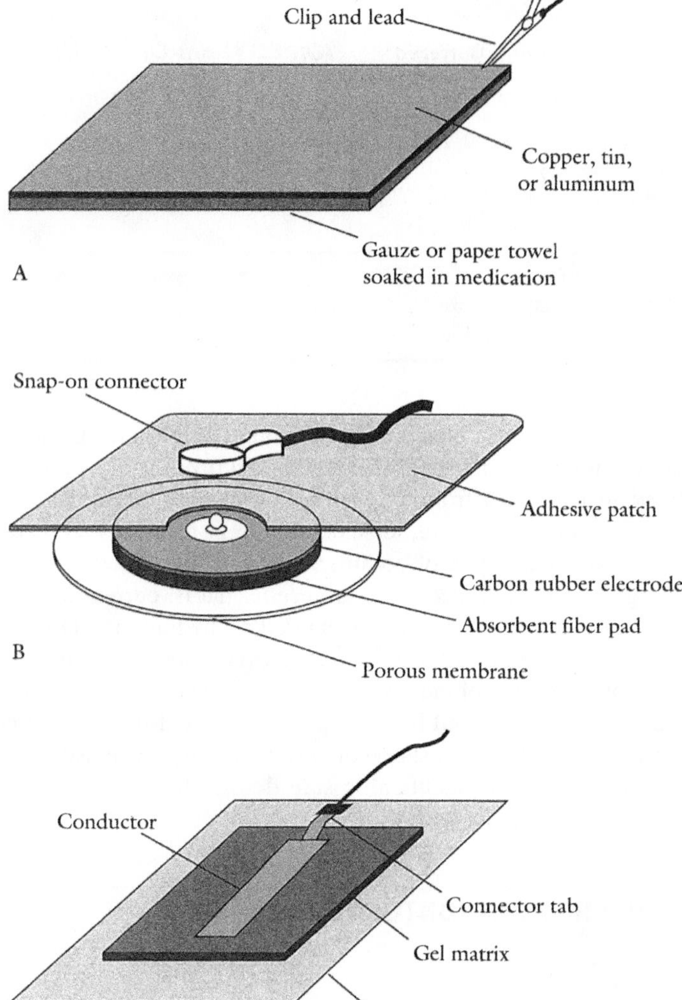

Figure 10.2. Electrodes used for drug delivery during iontophoresis. Types of electrodes shown here are self-constructed electrodes **(A),** and commercially available fiber pads **(B)** and gel pads **(C).**

and burns. No real evidence exists, however, that these features help prevent burns in a clinical setting. Hence, clinicians must continue to make a decision between commercial electrodes or some type of self-constructed electrode based on their own experience and practical issues such as time and cost.

Electrode Size and Current Density

Current density is the magnitude of the applied current (in milliamperes) divided by the conductive surface area of the electrode (in square centimeters). It has been suggested that current density should not exceed 0.5 mA/cm^2 if the cathode is used as the delivery electrode, and current density should not exceed 1.0 mA/cm^2 if the anode is used to apply the drug (38). These parameters must be considered during iontophoresis to minimize skin irritations and burns.

Table 10.4. Examples of Current Density Using Small Commercial Electrodes

	Empi Buffered[a]	*IOMED (Trans-O)*[b]	*Life-Tech Meditrode*[c]
Active area (cm^2)	11.0	7.2	6.5
Density at 4.0 mA/cm^2	0.36	0.56	0.62
Current (mA) that will generate current density of 0.5 mA/cm^2	5.5	3.6	3.25

[a]Empi, Inc., 599 Cardigan Rd, St. Paul, Minn 55126-4099.
[b]IOMED, Inc., 3385 West 1820 South, Salt Lake City, Utah 84104.
[c]Life-Tech, Inc., 4235 Greenbriar Dr, Stafford, Tex 77477-3995.

Self-constructed electrodes can be made large enough to provide an adequate current density even when larger current amplitudes are used (3.0–4.0 mA). The commercially available electrodes have fixed areas ranging from 6.5 cm^2 for the smaller electrodes to >30 cm^2 for the largest electrodes. It is critical, therefore, to select a current that does not exceed the maximal current density when using each type of commercial electrode. This is usually not a problem when medium or large commercial electrodes are used. That is, current density will fall below 0.5 mA/cm^2 even when a current of 4.0 mA is applied at medium and large commercial electrodes. Current densities exceeding 0.5 mA/cm^2 may occur, however, when higher amplitudes (4.0 mA) are applied through some of the smaller commercial electrodes (see Table 10.4). Again, this could precipitate skin irritation and burns, especially if the drug is delivered from the cathode. Thus, clinicians should consider the issue of current density when using iontophoresis techniques and be especially aware of maintaining safe density levels when applying drugs with cathodal current through smaller electrodes.

APPLICATION PRINCIPLES IN IONTOPHORESIS

Drug Concentrations

As indicated in Table 10.1, specific doses and concentrations have been reported for the various medications administered via iontophoresis. These doses tend to be fairly low or contain relatively low concentrations of the drug. Increasing the concentration of drugs administered by iontophoresis does not appear to increase in the amount of the drug delivered (38). This is probably due to the fact that increasing the ionic strength of the drug at the delivery site will increase the interionic attraction of the ions in solution; that is, the drug ions will tend to be attracted more strongly to one another at higher concentrations and retard the ability of the active electrode to drive the drug into the underlying tissues. Likewise, iontophoresis is often described as being "current limited," meaning that the amplitude and duration of the applied current is the primary factor that influences how much drug will be applied through the skin (38). Hence, the doses and concentrations listed in Table 10.1 should probably remain as the standard convention for clinical practice.

Simultaneous Use of Two Drugs

Several studies have reported using two drugs simultaneously at the same delivery electrode (17,18,35,36,39). Typically this is done by combining lidocaine (a local anesthetic) with dexamethasone (an anti-inflammatory steroid). It was originally believed that both of these drugs were positively charged and that both could be delivered from the anode to achieve a concomitant reduction in pain and inflammation. It has since been realized that dexamethasone is negatively charged, and this drug should be administered from the cathode for optimal penetration (40). Studies that applied these two medications from the anode may have produced some movement of dexamethasone away from the delivery electrode by the process of ionohydrokinesis (electro-osmosis) (38). This is a phenomenon where the bulk flow of the solution containing the iontophoresed ion (lidocaine) carries other substances, including the opposite ion (dexamethasone), into the underlying tissue. It has been estimated, however, that this process of ionohydrokinesis is only about one-tenth as effective as delivering the ion from the proper electrode (38).

Using two drugs of opposite polarity has therefore prompted some clinicians to reverse the polarity of the delivery electrode at some point during the iontophoresis treatment. For instance, Gangarosa et al. (39) advocate beginning the treatment with 2 mA for 10 minutes from the anode (to facilitate lidocaine delivery), and then switching to the cathode for 20 minutes at 2 mA (to facilitate dexamethasone delivery). There is some discussion, however, that providing two drugs at the same time may not be beneficial, even if both drugs are similarly charged. This idea relates to the issue discussed above about drug concentration. Including two drugs in the delivery solution increases the concentration of the ions at the delivery site. In addition, the fact that iontophoresis is current limited means that the two drugs must compete for the available current when both drugs are delivered simultaneously from the same electrode (38). This competition could potentially limit the amount of each medication that is phoresed. It may therefore be advisable for clinicians to select only one medication during iontophoresis to achieve optimal transfer of that particular drug.

Use of Other Physical Agents to Accentuate Iontophoretic Effects

Some studies and clinical reports have proposed that other physical agents may be useful as an adjunct to iontophoresis. For instance, ultrasound has been used directly over the site after iontophoresis to facilitate further drug entry by phonophoresis (19). Heating agents (continuous ultrasound, diathermy) have also been applied after iontophoretic drug delivery to increase the dispersal and penetration of the drug. It must be realized, however, that one of the benefits of using iontophoresis is that the drug is administered to a fairly localized and specific site. Use of heating agents or other interventions (exercise, massage) that might hasten drug dispersal by increasing blood flow may be counterproductive if the intention is to keep the drug localized at the target site.

Effects of pH at the Delivery Electrode

The degree of alkalinity or acidity (pH) at the delivery electrode can directly influence the amount of ion transfer during iontophoresis. Many drugs are weak acids or weak bases, and the ionization potential of these drugs is directly influenced by the pH of the drug solution. As the pH of the solution decreases, acidic compounds will begin to lose their ability to ionize. Basic compounds will lose their ionization potential as pH increases. Because DC produces an acidic reaction at the anode and an alkaline reaction at the cathode (38) (see Table 10.3), these changes in pH at the delivery electrode may facilitate or impair the amount of drug available for ion transfer. For instance, applying an acidic drug from the anode (acidic reaction) could reduce the amount of drug available for ion transfer because the drug molecule begins to become less ionized and more neutral. Conversely, a basic drug applied from the cathode could result in decreased ionization and less drug available for transfer.

The potential effect of iontophoresis and buffering systems on skin pH was illustrated in a study by Guffey et al. (41). These investigators measured skin pH when administering normal saline from the cathode using several current-dosages and buffer systems. They found that skin surface pH only changed significantly when no buffer was used at the higher current-dosage (80 mA•min). Addition of either a simple phosphate buffer to the saline, or use of an immobile resin buffer similar to the buffering systems found in some commercial electrodes resulted in no significant pH changes even at the higher current-dosage. Skin surface pH remained relatively stable at lower current-dosages (20 and 40 mA•min), even when no buffer was used.

The study by Guffey et al. (41) suggests that iontophoresis can cause changes in skin-surface pH and that these changes might be blunted by using some type of buffer system. Controlling pH at the delivery electrode could prevent unexpected changes in the ionization potential of the drug, thereby maintaining drug stability and the amount of the drug available in a charged/ionized state. As indicated earlier, maintaining skin pH at a relatively neutral state (around 7.0) should also help maintain the normal negative charge of the skin, thereby helping account for any drug movement that might occur via electro-osmosis.

More information is needed to determine how buffer systems might influence the actual amount of drug delivered. Although it might be advantageous to control pH at the delivery electrode, adding immobile resins or buffer solutions to the delivery electrode could potentially impair drug delivery by altering the osmotic gradient at the delivery site. That is, high concentrations of buffer at the delivery electrode could create a local osmotic environment that retains the drug and impairs movement away from the electrode. Future laboratory and clinical studies should shed some light on the optimal way to control pH during iontophoresis treatments.

CLINICAL PROCEDURES OF IONTOPHORESIS APPLICATION

Patient Screening, Indications, and Contraindications

A thorough examination should verify that iontophoresis of a specific medication has the potential to help alleviate the patient's condition without producing any untoward effects. Patients should be queried about drug allergies or adverse drug reactions. The patient's physician should be contacted before proceeding with iontophoresis if the patient has experienced a problem with the type of drug selected for iontophoresis. Conditions amenable to iontophoresis should be fairly localized so that the active electrode can adequately cover the affected area. For example, conditions involving a single tendon (bicipital, supraspinatus) have been reported to respond more favorably to iontophoresis of dexamethasone than those involving larger areas such as adhesive capsulitis of the shoulder (35).

The target tissues of iontophoresis generally include the skin and relatively superficial tissues, including muscle, tendon, and bursae. Maximum depth of penetration of iontophoresed drugs has not been established, because studies of drug penetration in humans are difficult to perform. Likewise, depth of penetration in individual patients will be influenced by a number of factors, including the type of drug used, current-dosage, and current density. Various anatomical factors such as skin thickness, subcutaneous adipose tissue, and the size of other structures such as skeletal muscle will also influence the depth of penetration from patient to patient. It may, for example, be much more difficult to reach the supraspinatus tendon in an athletic patient who has a hypertrophied deltoid muscle than it is in a patient whose supraspinatus tendon is relatively more accessible. Hence, each patient must be evaluated carefully to determine if iontophoresis might be a viable intervention.

Iontophoresis is contraindicated if the skin at the treatment site is damaged or broken (42,43). A decrease in skin sensation at the treatment site may also be a contraindication to iontophoresis, although several studies have reported using iontophoresis with caution to help resolve scar tissue and other conditions where sensation may be impaired (44–46). Sensitivity to the drug being administered or sensitivity to direct current (excessive skin irritation) may also contraindicate iontophoresis treatments. Iontophoresis should not be applied if the direct current will affect cardiac pacemakers or some other implanted electrical device (43).

Skin Preparation and Electrode Placement

Most sources advocate preparing the skin by vigorous rubbing with isopropyl alcohol (42,47). This action is believed to lessen the chance of skin irritation by removing any oils and impurities. The skin should be shaved if excessive hair is present. The solution or preparation containing the drug is usually impregnated into gauze or paper towels, or it is placed directly onto the delivery electrode if an absorbable commercial electrode is used. Medications contained in thicker creams (zinc oxide, salicylate ointments) may be placed directly on the skin and then covered by a few thicknesses of gauze or paper towels soaked in warm tap water. The amount of drug applied varies according to each preparation and according to the size of the delivery electrode and area being treated.

The delivery electrode is placed over the desired site of application with care taken to maintain uniform contact between the skin and electrode throughout the treatment. The return electrode is placed at a nearby site on the same limb or on an adjacent body segment. Some sources advocate a minimum distance of 18 inches between the delivery and return electrodes (42), but there does not appear to be any evidence that this will enhance drug application. Commercial electrodes typically have a fixed distance between the delivery and return electrodes, and this distance usually dictates how far the return electrode can be placed away from the delivery electrode. Efforts should be made, however, to separate the delivery and return electrodes as much as possible to minimize the chance of irritation and burns. Placing these electrodes too close to one another increases the risk of irritation and burns because the direct current may tend to bridge across the skin's surface rather than penetrate into the underlying tissues.

Connection to the DC Generator and Application of Current

After verifying that the current source is turned off, wire leads should be attached to the treatment electrodes. The leads are then connected to the DC generator, with care taken to match the polarity of the delivery electrode to the polarity of the drug being administered. Current is then slowly increased (ramped up) to the initial desired amplitude. Most protocols advocate fairly low amplitudes (1–2 mA) for the initial part of the treatment (5–10 minutes). If tolerated well, current can then be increased to higher levels (3–4 mA) for the remainder of the treatment. As discussed earlier, total treatment duration depends on the desired current-dosage. Increasing the current will shorten the overall treatment time, whereas longer treatment duration is needed if current is maintained at lower levels.

Completing the Treatment

Current should be slowly decreased (ramped down) at the end of the treatment. Electrodes are then removed, and the skin at each electrode site should be carefully inspected. Some redness may be present at the skin of the treatment site, especially if the drug is delivered from the cathode. Likewise, small blisterlike vesicles may be present on the skin where the drug is delivered. These signs of redness and irritation typically disappear within several minutes to several hours. Failure of these signs to resolve may indicate a more serious reaction, and subsequent treatments may be contraindicated because the patient is not able to tolerate the direct current, the drug, or a combination of current and drug.

Many clinicians conclude iontophoresis treatments by applying a skin lotion containing lanolin, aloe vera, or a similar ingredient. This may help alleviate any redness and accelerate recovery of the skin.

CLINICAL INDICATIONS FOR IONTOPHORESIS

Treatment of Inflammation

Evidence of Clinical Efficacy Using Anti-inflammatory Agents

Iontophoresis has often been reported to be helpful in treating inflammation of the skin and subcutaneous tissues. Anti-inflammatory steroids, known also as *glucocorticoids*, are often used in this situation. Glucocorticoids consist of a group of chemically related compounds that includes hydrocortisone, methylprednisolone, dexamethasone, and several similar medications. The most common glucocorticoid currently used for iontophoresis is dexamethasone sodium phosphate (Decadron). It was originally believed that this drug formed a positive ion and should be administered from the anode. Contemporary thought is that this drug forms a negative ion when administered as dexamethasone sodium phosphate, and this preparation should be delivered from the negative pole (43,48).

Several studies have noted that glucocorticoid iontophoresis may be beneficial in treating musculoskeletal inflammation. Bertolucci (35) used dexamethasone combined with a local anesthetic (lidocaine) to treat patients who had various inflammatory conditions, including lateral epicondylitis, sacroiliitis, and tendinitis in the shoulder area (35). Results suggested that patients who actually received the drug responded more favorably than those receiving a placebo (sodium chloride), and that patients were more apt to respond favorably if they were younger (<45 years old) and if they did not also have degenerative conditions involving the shoulder or neck. Similar results were noted by Harris (36), who used dexamethasone and lidocaine to treat conditions of tendinitis and bursitis at various anatomical sites. Delacerda (18) reported that iontophoresis of dexamethasone with lidocaine was superior to systemic medications (analgesics, antispasmodics) or physical agents (hydrocollator packs, ultrasound) in resolving soft-tissue inflammation around the shoulder girdle.

Several investigators have reported that various glucocorticoids can be introduced iontophoretically into the temporomandibular joint (TMJ), and that this intervention combined with other drugs (lidocaine) and exercise may be especially helpful in alleviating TMJ pain and inflammation (17,19,39,43). Glucocorticoid iontophoresis has also been advocated for the treatment of carpal tunnel syndrome (CTS). In one prospective, nonrandomized clinical trial, a regimen of dexamethasone iontophoresis and wrist splinting was associated with positive responses in 11 of 19 hands (58 %) (49). The lack of a control group in this study, however, prevented any definitive conclusion about the effectiveness of dexamethasone iontophoresis in these patients. Nonetheless, the subjects in this study had already failed to respond to a treatment using splints and orally administered nonsteroidal anti-inflammatory medications, suggesting that dexamethasone iontophoresis might be a reasonable course of action for people with CTS that fails to respond to oral medications.

Some preliminary evidence has indicated that chronic inflammatory conditions such as rheumatoid arthritis (RA) may also respond favorably to iontophoresis. Case reports document the application of dexamethasone iontophoresis, used either alone or in conjunction with exercise, to help manage inflammation in the knees of patients with RA (37,50). The effects of dexamethasone iontophoresis on people with RA was likewise examined in a small randomized, controlled trial (51). Five patients with RA received three treatments of dexamethasone iontophoresis to the knee joint, while another five patients received placebo treatments of saline iontophoresis. This study found that pain at rest and during movement was significantly improved in the treated group, suggesting that dexamethasone iontophoresis is more effective than placebo in relieving symptoms associated with RA (51).

Iontophoresis of glucocorticoids has also been used to decrease inflammation in tenosynovitis. In a case report, a 61-year-old woman with de Quervain tenosynovitis was treated with a regimen that included superficial heat, ice, transverse friction massage, joint mobilization, and dexamethasone iontophoresis (40 mA•min) (32). This regimen was evidently successful in resolving this patient's pain and impairment. We cannot, of course, attribute these benefits solely to the dexamethasone intervention, but this case report is a good example of how glucocorticoid iontophoresis can be incorporated into a comprehensive treatment regimen for conditions such as tenosynovitis.

Glucocorticoid iontophoresis has been studied as a method for treating lateral epicondylitis/epicondylalgia, or elbow pain that is commonly referred to as tennis elbow. Runeson and Haker (52) treated 64 people with lateral epicondylalgia, with half the group receiving dexamethasone iontophoresis and the other half receiving a placebo treatment of saline iontophoresis. Four treatments were provided over an 8-day period, using a protocol of 0.4 % dexamethasone at 4 mA for 10 minutes (40 mA•min) during each treatment. Treatments were provided by assistant nurses, and a physical therapist who was blinded to the treatment groups evaluated the results of the treatment regimen. These researchers found no significant difference in pain between the two groups immediately after the final treatment. Outcomes in the two groups were likewise similar at 3 and 6-month follow-up examinations. These results therefore failed to support the use of four treatments of dexamethasone iontophoresis at 40 mA•min in treating lateral epicondylalgia.

Nirschl et al. (34) studied 199 patients with lateral epicondylitis. Half the group received active treatment of dexamethasone iontophoresis (2.5 mL of 0.4% solution), using a current-dosage of 40 mA•min. Six treatments were applied over a 15-day period. The other half of the patients (control group) received a placebo treatment using saline solution. Pain and tenderness improved significantly in the treatment group compared to the control group 2 days after concluding the iontophoresis treatments. Global improvement was likewise generally better in the treated versus control group 2 days after concluding treatment. Differences seen between the two groups at the short-term (2-day) follow-up were generally lost when patients were studied 1 month after the treatments. These researchers concluded that dexamethasone iontophoresis was effective in the short-term reduction of symptoms associated with lateral epicondylitis.

It is not clear why Nirschl et al. (34) were able to document short-term beneficial effects of dexamethasone iontophoresis, while Runeson and Haker (52) failed to see a definitive effect of this treatment. Apparently, the primary difference between these studies is that Nirschl et al. applied six treatments over approximately a 2-week period, whereas Runeson and Haker applied only four treatments over approximately 1 week. Perhaps applying an additional two treatments (i.e., six total treatments) over a slightly longer period of time (2 weeks) provided enough drug and enough time for that drug to exert its anti-inflammatory effects. Hence, the discrepancy between these two studies might be explained by the fact that patients in the Runeson and Haker study simply did not receive enough treatments, and that the short-term benefit of these treatments was not observed because the drug had not been given enough time to exert meaningful effects.

Glucocorticoid iontophoresis seems to be effective in treating inflammation associated with plantar fasciitis. In a study by Gudeman et al. (33), 36 patients with plantar fasciitis that affected 40 feet (some patients had bilateral fasciitis) were divided randomly into a treatment group that received dexamethasone iontophoresis ($n = 20$ feet), and a placebo group that received iontophoresis of buffered saline ($n = 20$ feet). Patients in both groups also received ice pack and stretching treatments. Six treatment sessions were applied over a 2- to 3-week period, using 0.4% dexamethasone sodium phosphate applied at current amplitude up to 4.0 mA depending on each subject's sensitivity. A total current-dosage of 40 mA was applied over 20 minutes to each subject. Immediately after the treatments, subjects in the dexamethasone group had significantly better improvement compared to the placebo group as measured by the Maryland Foot Score. There was no difference, however, between the groups 1 month after concluding treatment. These researchers suggested that dexamethasone iontophoresis should be considered as an intervention for plantar fasciitis when a more rapid reduction in symptoms is needed, as might be the case for athletes and active patients (33).

In summary, there is considerable evidence that glucocorticoid iontophoresis, using agents such as dexamethasone, is associated with beneficial effects in various inflammatory conditions. Nonetheless, questions still arise concerning the ability of this technique to provide meaningful amounts of the active form of the drug to subcutaneous tissues. A study by Smutok et al. (53), for example, applied dexamethasone iontophoresis to the volar surface of the wrist of six healthy subjects, and then measured the amount of dexamethasone and dexamethasone phosphate in the venous blood of the ipsilateral antecubital vein (i.e., the venous blood draining the wrist area). Presumably, successful transdermal administration of dexamethasone would result in the appearance of measurable amounts of this drug in the venous blood immediately proximal to the administration site. These researchers, however, did not detect any form of dexamethasone in the venous blood during or after iontophoresis. Although many factors need to be considered in this study, this finding raises questions about the ability of typical treatment parameters used during clinical iontophoresis to deliver meaningful amounts of dexamethasone through the skin.

Mechanism of Glucocorticoid Effects

Glucocorticoids such as dexamethasone exert a number of effects that decrease inflammation (Fig. 10-3). In particular, these drugs act directly on macrophages and lymphocytes that promote inflammation. Within these cells, glucocorticoids bind directly to a cytoplasmic glucocorticoid

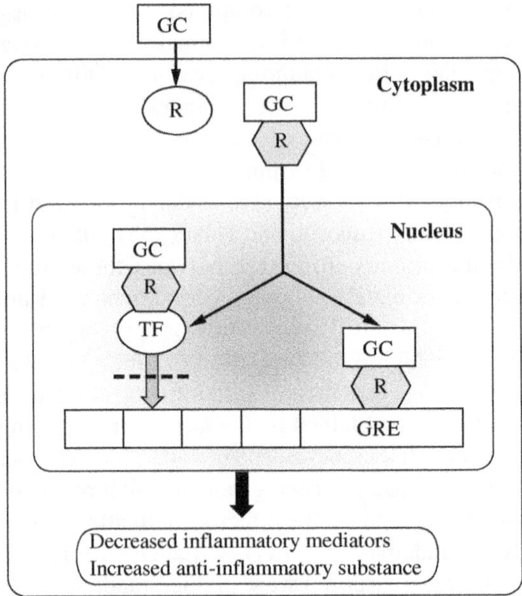

Figure 10.3. Mechanism of glucocorticoid effect. Glucocorticoids (GC) enter cell and bind to cytoplasmic receptor (R) to form a complex. This complex travels to the nucleus, where it inhibits the action of proinflammatory transcription factors (TF). The complex also binds directly to glucocorticoisd response elements (GRE) on specific genes and directly inhibits the production of inflammatory components and increases the production of anti-inflammatory substances in the cell.

receptor, and the drug-receptor complex then travels to the cell's nucleus, where it exerts several actions. The activated drug–receptor complex inhibits certain proteins, such as nuclear factor-κB and activator protein 1 (54–56). These proteins, known also as transcription factors, normally activate genes that promote the expression of inflammatory mediators. By inhibiting these transcription factors, glucocorticoids prevent the activation of genes that would otherwise produce cytokines and enzymes that promote the inflammatory response (55). In addition, the drug–receptor complex can act as a gene transcription factor because it binds directly to specific gene segments and either inhibits the expression of proinflammatory substances, or increases the expression of anti-inflammatory proteins (55,56). Thus, glucocorticoids exert their rather powerful anti-inflammatory effects by directly affecting gene transcription, or by inhibiting other transcription factors so that the production of proinflammatory mediators is inhibited and the production of anti-inflammatory substances is increased.

Potential Side Effects

Although glucocorticoids are very effective in decreasing the symptoms of inflammation, these drugs are associated with a number of side effects. Primary among these is the potential for causing breakdown (catabolism) of muscle, tendon, bone, and other collagenous tissues in the body (57,58). Likewise, prolonged administration of glucocorticoids can inhibit the body's endogenous production of these hormones, thus producing a potentially serious problem known as adrenocortical suppression (58,59). These side effects are very common when high doses of glucocorticoids are given systemically for prolonged periods of time. The use of iontophoresis to administer these drugs to specific local tissues at relatively lower doses should diminish the risk of these serious side effects. Still, indiscriminate and repeated use of glucocorticoid iontophoresis could expose the patient to some potentially serious side effects.

To avoid these potential adverse effects, it has been suggested that treatments should not be given every day and that at least one recovery day should be provided between each iontophoresis session (36,37). Lark and Gangarosa (43) recommend a 3- to 7-day interval between each treatment. They believe that this allows the drug to exert anti-inflammatory effects without producing a sustained inhibition of collagen synthesis, thus minimizing the catabolic effects. In addition, the total number of glucocorticoid treatments should probably be limited during any given treatment sequence. Several sources suggest that beneficial effects should begin to occur within three or four treatments (17,36,43). The lack of any positive effects after three or four treatments may indicate that glucocorticoid iontophoresis is not going to be effective in that patient, and an alternative intervention should be considered.

Treatment of Pain

As discussed above, iontophoresis can be used to reduce inflammation and thus reduce pain typically associated with the inflammatory process. It may also be desirable, however, to iontophorese drugs that have direct analgesic effects. Iontophoresis has been used to administer analgesic agents such as local anesthetics, salicylates, opioids, and other drugs. Examples are provided here describing how iontophoresis of these agents can be used to decrease pain.

Iontophoresis of Local Anesthetics

Local anesthetics such as lidocaine have been used frequently during iontophoresis. These drugs produce an anesthetic effect by blocking transmission of impulses along peripheral nerve axons. Lidocaine and similar drugs bind to sodium channels in the nerve membrane and prevent sodium from entering the axon (60,61). The affected portion of the axon is not able to initiate an action potential, and anesthesia occurs in the tissues innervated by that neuron because afferent impulses cannot reach the central nervous system.

As indicated earlier, several studies reported simultaneously administering a local anesthetic (lidocaine) and an anti-inflammatory steroid (dexamethasone) to decrease pain and inflammation in various musculoskeletal disorders (17,18,35,36). Although this protocol has been used by clinicians in the past, there seem to be some obvious problems with this technique. For instance, these drugs are now regarded as having opposite polarity, with lidocaine being positively charged and dexamethasone being negatively charged. Some clinicians believe that both drugs can be administered from the positive pole because lidocaine will pull the negatively charged dexamethasone by the process of electro-osmosis (i.e., bulk flow of the solvent containing both drugs). Other clinicians report that these drugs can be given simultaneously, but the polarity of the delivery electrode should be reversed at some point during the treatment to allow optimal delivery of both drugs (39). This has practical implications because it prolongs the treatment time and may increase the chance for skin irritation.

Another important issue regarding lidocaine iontophoresis is the fact that local anesthetics may cause a decrease in sensation by anesthetizing the skin at the delivery site. An interesting paradox is created by this approach to pain control because decreased skin sensation is usually considered a contraindication to iontophoresis treatment. Lidocaine iontophoresis could put the patient at a greater risk for an electrical burn if sensation is decreased at the delivery site. To diminish the chances of electrical burns, clinicians who elect to administer local anesthetics either alone or in combination with other drugs should probably avoid using higher current amplitudes.

Finally, clinicians should consider what constitutes appropriate clinical use of iontophoresis using local anesthetics. Ample evidence exists that lidocaine iontophoresis can be used to produce local anesthesia to allow some relatively minor surgical or diagnostic procedure. For instance, iontophoresis has been used to administer lidocaine or a similar drug to the eardrum before myringotomy, to the teeth before tooth extraction, or to other cutaneous tissues to allow some other minor surgical procedures to be performed (40,62–65). In particular, lidocaine iontophoresis has been advocated as a simple and noninvasive method for producing local skin anesthesia to reduce the pain and apprehension before hypodermic injections and venous or arterial blood sampling, especially in children (66–68). Lidocaine iontophoresis was also used to treat acute, localized soft-tissue injuries in patients admitted to an emergency room, and this intervention was reported to be more effective in short-term (within 30 minutes) pain reduction compared with patients receiving more traditional treatment using orally administered nonsteroidal anti-inflammatory drugs (69).

The benefits of iontophoresis of local anesthetics in the management of subacute and chronic musculoskeletal disorders, however, seem questionable. These drugs create an anesthetic effect by inhibiting the excitation of sensory nerve membranes, but they do not really influence the actual source of pain. This could have beneficial effects if this transient decrease in pain allows some intervention to be performed (e.g., a vigorous manual technique like transverse friction massage), or if the intent is to try to interrupt some type of cycle such a pain–spasm syndrome. Therapists should realize, however, that local anesthetics are typically used only to produce a temporary decrease in sensation so that some other procedure can be performed; use of these agents may not have any long-term effects.

Rather than using lidocaine iontophoresis as a primary intervention, it has been suggested that this technique could be used as a tool to determine the efficacy of subsequent iontophoresis treatments. Clinicians considering iontophoretic administration of other drugs to treat pain and inflammation (e.g., dexamethasone) could administer an initial treatment of lidocaine to see if iontophoresis is successful in delivering the drug to the appropriate tissues. If pain is temporarily diminished after lidocaine iontophoresis, this is a fairly good indication that iontophoresis is successful in driving the drug to the affected tissues (43). Subsequent treatments with drugs that may have a more lasting effect should then be attempted. This assumes, of course, that these other drugs will penetrate to the same depth as lidocaine, a fact that may or may not be true. Still, failure of lidocaine iontophoresis to decrease pain suggests that iontophoresis may not be successful in reaching the target tissue and that alternative treatments may be more appropriate.

Salicylate Iontophoresis

Non-narcotic analgesics such as the salicylates are weak acids that produce several therapeutic benefits including analgesic and anti-inflammatory effects because of their ability to inhibit the biosynthesis of prostaglandins (70,71). Prostaglandins are hormonelike substances produced locally in injured tissues, and excessive production of these substances potentiates pain and inflammation in the affected tissues (72). Salicylates and similar nonopioid analgesics are potent inhibitors of the enzyme that produces prostaglandins, and these drugs are effective in controlling pain and inflammation in a variety of conditions. Likewise, these drugs may be ideally suited for iontophoretic administration in conditions such as bursitis, tendinitis, and similar musculoskeletal problems. Regrettably, there is little information about the clinical efficacy of salicylate iontophoresis. One case study documented the successful use of salicylate iontophoresis in treating residual thigh pain after hip arthroplasty (73). Additional research is needed to determine if iontophoresis of these drugs is effective in treating a variety of patients who have other types of problems.

Salicylate iontophoresis might also be useful in treating conditions other than pain. Plantar verrucae (plantar warts), for example, are sometimes treated with local application of sodium salicylate. In a case report, five patients with plantar verrucae were treated once each week with 10% sodium salicylate, applied from the cathode at a dosage of 10 mA•min (74). The verrucae disappeared after two treatments in four of these patients, and the fifth patient was treated three times before the verrucae disappeared (74). Use of salicylate iontophoresis to treat plantar verrucae was also investigated in a prospective, nonrandomized trial (75). Nineteen subjects with plantar verrucae were given three treatments of 2% sodium salicylate at a current dosage of 22.5 mA•min over a 6- to 9-day period. The size (area) of verrucae decreased in 15/19 subjects, increased in 2/19 subjects, remained unchanged in one subject, and the verrucae disappeared in one subject. These results suggested that salicylate iontophoresis might be a more convenient and less invasive alternative to other treatments for plantar verrucae, such as electrocautery, cryotherapy (freezing), or medicated patches (75).

Other Nonsteroidal Anti-inflammatory Drugs

Nonsteroidal anti-inflammatory drugs (NSAIDs) are a diverse group of medications that includes sodium salicylate (aspirin) and other agents (naproxen, ibuprofen, ketoprofen, and so forth) (70). Like the salicylates, NSAIDs decrease pain and inflammation by inhibiting the production of prostaglandins. Because electric current might be useful in facilitating transdermal salicylate administration, several studies have also investigated the possibility of administering other NSAIDs via iontophoresis.

One clinical trial included local transdermal naproxen administration as part of a comprehensive regimen for the treatment of lateral epicondylitis (76). One group of patients in the trial ($n = 32$) received naproxen iontophoresis, and the other group ($n = 29$) received naproxen administered with ultrasound (naproxen phonophoresis). Both groups also received other interventions such as cryotherapy, stretching, and strengthening exercises. Pain score, grip strength, and epicondylitis grading system scores improved significantly in both groups, but the improvements were similar between the groups. The authors concluded that naproxen iontophoresis and phonophoresis were equally effective in treating lateral epicondylitis (76). The lack of a control group in this study, however, prevents making any definitive judgment about the ability of naproxen iontophoresis to resolve lateral epicondylitis when included in a comprehensive regimen for treating this condition.

Iontophoresis of other NSAIDs continues to be examined using animal models and other experimental techniques. Ketoprofen iontophoresis, for example, resulted in increased concentration of drug (compared with passive delivery) into the outer layers of the medial thigh musculature of a pig (77). Indomethacin has likewise been administered via iontophoresis into rat abdominal skin, and the ability of electrical current to enhance transdermal delivery was estimated using this model (78). In a study using human volunteers, iontophoresis was reported to increase the amount of piroxicam administered to the stratum corneum compared with passive delivery (79). Future research should lend more definitive insight into the ability of iontophoresis to facilitate NSAID administration and perhaps identify specific protocols that could be used in specific clinical situations.

Opioid Iontophoresis

Pain after extensive surgery or severe trauma is often treated with opioid analgesics such as meperidine or morphine. These drugs are powerful analgesics that have traditionally been used to act on neurons in the central nervous system (brain and spinal cord) to impair the transmission and perception of painful stimuli. Recent evidence also suggests that peripheral opioid receptors exist and that administration of these drugs directly into peripheral tissues (e.g., an inflamed joint) may be helpful in decreasing pain (80). Opioids are usually administered orally or by some type of injection (intravenous, intramuscular). Certain opioids such as morphine and fentanyl can also be administered by medicated transdermal patches that provide steady passive delivery of the analgesic into the systemic circulation (81).

It has been suggested that opioids may also be administered iontophoretically to provide adequate postoperative analgesia (25,82). In one study, patients who had undergone hip or knee arthroplasty were able to decrease their need for other analgesic drugs if they received morphine iontophoresis (25). Morphine was delivered postoperatively for an extended period of time (6 hours) by an electrode placed on the patient's anterior forearm. Morphine iontophoresis was used in this situation to provide a slow, continuous supply of the drug into the patient's bloodstream rather than applying the drug to a specific site or tissue. Electric current might also facilitate the transdermal delivery of other opioids such as fentanyl, especially when traditional iontophoresis techniques are combined with electric currents that promote electroporation (82).

Although the use of opioid iontophoresis is still experimental at this time, perhaps this technique will gain acceptance and be used in more clinical situations in the future. Therapists may want to consult with physicians about the possibility of including opioid iontophoresis as a means of providing postoperative pain relief in certain patients.

Vinca Alkaloid Iontophoresis

Postherpetic neuralgia (PHN) is the severe pain that typically occurs in specific dermatomes following herpes zoster infection. Several studies have documented that PHN may be resolved in many patients by iontophoretic administration of drugs known as vinca alkaloids (83–85). Vinca alkaloids are a group of nitrogen-based compounds including vincristine and vinblastine. These drugs are usually classified as cancer chemotherapy agents, and they are administered systemically to inhibit cell replication in certain forms of cancer (86). These drugs may also be administered by iontophoresis over the affected dermatomes in patients with PHN. Vinca alkaloids work by inhibiting cellular microtubule function. Hence, their ability to resolve pain in PHN seems to be due to inhibition of retrograde axoplasmic transport in sensory neurons of the affected dermatome (83). This inhibition supposedly causes degenerative changes in afferent pain pathways so that painful stimuli are not able to reach central areas of pain perception (87).

Most of the reports documenting the benefits of vinca alkaloid iontophoresis originated more than two decades ago, and this technique has not gained overwhelming acceptance in contemporary practice. More recently, a randomized, controlled trial suggested that iontophoresis using vincristine was no more effective in reducing pain than a placebo treatment using saline iontophoresis (88). As a result, the effectiveness of this technique seems questionable when treating patients with PHN. Unless more definitive evidence is forthcoming, clinicians should consider alternative treatments for patients with PHN.

Resolution of Soft-tissue Mineralization

It has been suggested that iontophoresis may be helpful in dissolving and dispersing painful mineral deposits such as calcium deposits and urate crystal deposits (89,90). Acetic acid appears to be the drug of choice for treating calcium deposits. Iontophoresis of acetic acid from the cathode induces the negatively charged acetate ion to combine with the relatively insoluble calcium carbonate to form a more soluble compound, calcium acetate. The use of acetic acid to resolve calcium deposits is summarized by the following chemical reaction:

$$\underset{\text{calcium carbonate (insoluble)}}{CaCO_3} + \underset{\text{acetic acid}}{2H(C_2H_3O_2)} \rightarrow \underset{\text{calcium acetate (soluble)}}{Ca(C_2H_3O_2) + H_2O + CO_2}$$

Because it is more soluble, calcium acetate can then be more easily dispersed from the affected tissues by local blood flow.

As with many iontophoresis techniques, there is little documentation of the clinical effectiveness of acetic acid iontophoresis. One rather convincing case report describes how this technique can be used to successfully resolve the soft-tissue mineralization that occurs in myositis ossificans (47). In this study, a series of nine iontophoresis treatments using 2% acetic acid was applied over a 3-week period. This treatment was helpful in resolving a large ossified mass in the patient's thigh, suggesting that acetic acid iontophoresis may be useful in treating some types of soft-tissue calcification. Clinicians should consider using this technique in patients with myositis ossificans.

The effectiveness of acetic acid iontophoresis was questioned, however, in a small randomized, controlled trial involving patients with calcific tendonitis of the shoulder (91). Patients with calcified lesions in the shoulder were divided randomly into treatment ($n = 11$) and control groups ($n = 10$). The treatment group received nine sessions of a regimen that included acetic acid iontophoresis and continuous-wave ultrasound; the control group was not treated. The size and density of the calcium deposits decreased significantly in both groups, but there was no difference between the groups in terms of resorption of these deposits or other outcomes such as pain and range of motion. The fact that the control group improved to the same extent as the treatment group suggested that calcium deposit resorption occurred by a natural process rather than the regimen that included acetic acid iontophoresis (91).

With regard to other types of soft-tissue mineralization, lithium iontophoresis has been documented in a case report as being useful in treating urate deposits that typically occur in gouty arthritis (89). Gouty arthritis is characterized by the precipitation of sodium urate crystals in specific areas such as the first metatarsalphalangeal joint. Administration of lithium from the anode supposedly replaces sodium in these deposits, thus forming lithium urate, which is more soluble in the blood (89). Once again, there is no experimental evidence documenting the effectiveness of this procedure. Still, therapists should be aware that this may be a plausible course of action in patients with localized, painful urate crystal deposits.

Treatment of Wounds and Infection

Iontophoresis has been reported to be useful in administering several types of drugs to treat infections and to facilitate wound healing. Zinc oxide administered from the positive pole has been reported to have several beneficial properties, including bactericidal effects and an ability to accelerate tissue growth and repair. Like many heavy metals, zinc may exert an antibacterial effect by interfering with critical metabolic activities in microbial cells, and tissue healing may be facilitated by zinc's ability to precipitate proteins. The use of zinc oxide iontophoresis in treating recalcitrant skin ulcers has been documented in several case reports appearing in the literature (44,92).

Other antibacterial drugs (penicillin, gentamicin) have been administered by iontophoresis to treat certain types of infection. In particular, these agents have been described as being beneficial in treating chondritis after burns of the ear (21,93). Iontophoresis appears to offer the advantage of administering fairly high doses of antibacterial drug through eschar into the underlying avascular tissue (26,93). Clinicians who treat patients with burns may want to pursue the possibility of using antibacterial iontophoresis in managing conditions such as ear chondritis.

Finally, it has been suggested that iontophoresis of certain antiviral drugs could be a possible means of controlling cutaneous herpes virus infections. Iontophoresis has been used to administer vidarabine from the negative pole to treat herpes simplex virus in experimental animals (94). More recently, cathodal application of idoxuridine has been shown to be beneficial in treating herpetic infection of the finger in two patients (95). Perhaps future reports will continue to document iontophoresis as a means of controlling bacterial, viral, and other types of infection. This potential treatment could be significant because of the critical need for adequate management of infection, especially in patients with a compromised immune system.

Treatment of Edema

Iontophoresis of the drug hyaluronidase has been reported to help reduce certain types of edema. Hyaluronidase is an enzyme that appears to increase permeability in connective tissue by hydrolyzing hyaluronic acid. Edema that is encapsulated by the connective tissue can then disperse into surrounding tissues and be carried away by the vascular and lymphatic systems. One study documented the ability of this technique to reduce edema in a large sample of patients with either acute injury (sprains) or chronic edema (postsurgical lymphedema) (22). No control or placebo group was used in this study, however, making it difficult to differentiate the drug effects from other factors (electrical current, spontaneous resolution). Furthermore, edema reduction was assessed using circumferential measurements rather than using a more exact and reliable measurement such as water displacement. In a different study, patients with soft-tissue and intra-articular hemorrhage secondary to hemophilia were treated with either hyaluronidase or a placebo (acetate buffer) (96). Circumferential measurements failed to reveal any difference in edema reduction between the two groups, suggesting that hyaluronidase iontophoresis may have limited value in treating this type of edema in patients with hemophilia.

Although hyaluronidase iontophoresis is often described as being helpful in reducing edema, no experimental evidence documents the clinical efficacy of this technique. It would be interesting to re-examine this technique using a valid and reliable measure of edema reduction (water displacement). Clinicians may then be able to make sound judgments about whether this technique has any real merit in treating certain types of edema.

Treatment of Hyperhidrosis

Iontophoresis has been successful in reducing sweating in the hands, feet, and armpits in many patients with hyperhidrosis (97–100). Electrodes containing tap water are typically placed over the affected areas, and cathodal current is applied for the first half of the treatment followed by anodal current. This simple technique appears to induce the formation of keratinous plugs in the sweat glands, thus blocking the flow of sweat to the skin's surface (99). A series of daily treatments lasting anywhere from 8 to 20 days is usually needed before an appreciable decrease in sweating is noted. Treatments must either be continued on a weekly or semiweekly basis, or the daily treatments must be repeated after about 6 weeks to maintain a relatively euhydrotic state.

Treatment of Scar Tissue and Adhesions

Iontophoresis may help reduce adhesions and scar tissue (45,46). Although iodine is usually applied for antimicrobial purposes, this substance is also reported to have sclerolytic effects. The exact cellular basis for the sclerolytic action of iodine has not been clearly defined. Iodine is typically administered from the negative pole in the form of 5% to 10 % ointment. A limited number of case reports have described the use of iodine iontophoresis in helping decrease joint restriction and tendon adhesions after surgical procedures (45,46). It would be interesting to see if these preliminary results are corroborated in the future by well-designed, placebo-controlled studies. Clinicians should be aware, however, that application of iontophoresis over scar tissue is sometimes contraindicated because of the decreased cutaneous sensation at the scar site. Hence, this technique should be used cautiously in any future clinical applications or research studies that study the effects of iontophoresis on cutaneous scarring or adhesions.

Iontophoresis has also been used to treat the localized penile adhesions associated with Peyronie disease (101,102). In one prospective study, a regimen of potassium iodide iontophoresis, infrared radiation, and continuous-wave ultrasound was used to treat 35 men with Peyronie disease (101). Results of this study suggested that this regimen was successful in eliminating pain and facilitating some degree of functional improvement in all patients (101). A different study used an iontophoresis regimen of dexamethasone, lidocaine, and a calcium channel blocker (verapamil) to treat 100 men with Peyronie disease. Improvements were seen in several outcomes, including resolution of pain (96% of the patients), plaque diminution (53%), reduced penile deviation (37%), and improved sexual function (44%) (102). Results from these studies suggest that iontophoresis might be an important component in the treatment of Peyronie disease. It is hoped that future research will clarify exactly which drugs offer the best treatment of this condition and whether other physical agents (e.g., ultrasound) can complement the iontophoresis effects.

Nontraditional and Newer Uses of Iontophoresis

Several other potential applications of iontophoresis techniques have been described as a means to deliver medications to a specific, localized site. Calcium iontophoresis, for example, has been reported to help reduce symptoms in a patient with suspected myopathy in the laryngeal musculature (20). Iontophoresis of vinca alkaloids, a technique discussed earlier in the treatment of PHN, has also been used to treat intractable pain in patients with advanced cancer (87), and this technique has been used to diminish the skin lesions associated with Kaposi sarcoma in people who have AIDS (103). Iontophoresis of the anticancer drug cisplatin has also been described in the treatment of a patient with basal cell carcinoma (104), and iontophoretic delivery of other agents such as 5-aminolevulinic acid might also be successful in treating localized skin lesions associated with skin cancer (105). Vitamin C iontophoresis has also been advocated for the treatment of localized skin discoloration (melasma) associated with excessive sun exposure (106).

As indicated at the beginning of this chapter, the idea that iontophoresis can be used to provide systemic delivery of many different medications has generated a great deal of interest in the medical literature. Studies, for example, using animal models and excised human skin suggest that iontophoresis could be used as a simple and predictable way to administer certain hormones, including insulin, parathyroid hormone, calcitonin, antidiuretic hormone, and luteinizing hormone releasing hormone (107–113). Iontophoresis might also be useful for administering drugs such as apomorphine to patients with Parkinson disease, thereby allowing the patient to control the amount of drug throughout the day by adjusting the current density/application (114). Likewise, iontophoretic administration of cardiovascular drugs might be feasible and offer a method to enhance the systemic administration and bioavailability of certain agents (115,116).

Clearly, the potential exists for using iontophoresis as a noninvasive method to deliver a drug either locally or into the systemic circulation. The use of iontophoresis in these newer/nontraditional situations might become more common as technological advancements are introduced, including miniaturized iontophoresis delivery systems, increased use of hydrogels or microemulsions as a method for delivering the medication, and incorporation of chemical enhancers that facilitate transdermal delivery of the medication (117–121). It remains to be seen, however, which iontophoresis techniques will be incorporated into widespread clinical use in the future.

CLINICAL CASE STUDIES

Case 1

Examination

History

A 16-year-old boy sustained a deep contusion of the anterior right thigh during a springboard diving accident (47). Over the course of 3 weeks, pain increased in the right anterior-lateral thigh, especially when he was running or descending stairs.

Systems Review

The patient was afebrile, and the right thigh was not visibly red and lacked any streaking around the site of the injury. The patient had not had any other recent injuries or impairments of the cardiovascular, neuromuscular, or musculoskeletal systems.

Tests and Measures

Pain was evident on palpation of the right vastus lateralis musculature. Palpation also revealed a well-defined mass in the right anterolateral thigh that was approximately 10 cm long and 6 cm wide. Passive knee flexion was limited to 80 degrees because of pain. The knee could be extended passively through a full range of motion, but active contraction of the right quadriceps caused pain, and strength of the right quadriceps could not be accurately evaluated because of pain. The right hip seemed unaffected by this injury.

Evaluation

The patient could not recall any other trauma to the thigh, and there was no history of recent injury or illness related to this condition. It appeared that the patient had developed a fairly large, localized mass in the thigh secondary to direct trauma to the thigh.

Diagnosis

The clinician suspected a diagnosis of myositis ossificans and referred the patient back to the physician. Radiographs confirmed that the mass was consistent with myositis ossificans in the right vastus lateralis musculature.

Prognosis

Although rest and relative inactivity of the right thigh should facilitate resorption of the lesion, complete reabsorption can take up to 2 years. To facilitate reabsorption, a program of acetic acid iontophoresis, ultrasound, and passive exercise was considered. The plan of care was to provide nine treatments over a 3-week period.

Intervention

Acetic acid iontophoresis was administered three times a week for 3 weeks. Before application of electrodes, the skin at each electrode site was cleansed using isopropyl alcohol. The active (delivery) electrode was a commercially available electrode (IOMED model EL5010) and was approximately 2.5 cm in diameter. Three milliliters of 2% acetic acid was added to the delivery electrode, and this electrode was fixed directly over the lesion. The dispersive (return) electrode was a 4.2-cm^2 karaya pad that was placed 8 cm distal to the delivery electrode. The active electrode was connected to the negative pole of the DC generator, and the dispersive electrode was connected to the generator's positive pole.

Current was applied using an iontophoresis-dedicated DC generator (IOMED model PM600 Phoresor Drug Delivery System). Current-dosage consisted of 4 mA applied for 20 minutes, for a total current-dosage of 80 mA•min.

Each treatment of acetic acid was followed by pulsed ultrasound (8 minutes of 1.5 W/cm^2, at 50% duty cycle), and 5 minutes of gentle, passive range of motion within the patient's pain-free range.

Assessment of Outcome

After the nine treatments, radiographs revealed a 99% reduction in the size of the lesion. The patient regained full active and passive range of motion, and he was able to resume regular activities, including running and playing soccer.

Case 2

Examination

History

Three weeks before referral, a 71-year-old woman experienced sudden pain in the left TMJ (17). She had previously had minor problems with her TMJ, but these problems were typically transient and resolved spontaneously. The recent problem, however, was severe enough to prevent her from fully opening her mouth and from chewing solid foods. She described her pain as a constant, dull ache in the area of her left TMJ, and this pain increased when chewing and at night. Her recent episode of TMJ pain did not seem to be initiated by any specific event or trauma.

Systems Review

The patient had a history of hypertension and degenerative joint disease affecting her hips and low back. Other aspects of her cardiovascular, neuromuscular, and musculoskeletal function seemed intact and functional.

Tests and Measures

The patient's left TMJ and surrounding musculature were tender to palpation. Jaw range of motion consisted of 27 mm of incisal opening, which is well below the normal range of 40 to 60 mm. Right lateral excursion was also reduced to 3 mm, and left lateral excursion was 10 mm (7 to 12 mm is considered normal).

Evaluation

The pain and limited range of motion suggested internal derangement of the left TMJ, perhaps involving displacement of the intra-articular disk. This derangement probably resulted from progressive degeneration of the TMJ that ultimately resulted in disk displacement during normal eating or opening and closing of the mouth.

Diagnosis

This patient appeared to have acute inflammation of the TMJ secondary to internal derangement and altered joint mechanics. These altered mechanics also impaired normal joint motion, resulting in decreased opening of the mouth and jaw.

Prognosis

It was determined that a reduction in inflammation and restoration of normal TMJ motion would decrease pain and allow the patient to resume chewing and eating. The plan of care was to provide symptomatic relief with iontophoresis using an anti-inflammatory steroid and a local anesthetic. To restore joint motion, the patient was instructed in a home exercise program designed to increase active jaw range of motion and stabilize the TMJ. Two iontophoresis treatments were provided initially, with a 2-day interval between these treatments. The home exercise program was reviewed at each of these sessions, 1 week after the second iontophoresis treatment, and at a final follow-up visit 6 weeks after the second iontophoresis treatment.

Intervention

Iontophoresis was applied over the left TMJ. The skin was first cleansed using alcohol, and the active (delivery) electrode was prepared by adding 1 mL of 0.4% dexamethasone sodium phosphate, and 2 mL of 4% lidocaine hydrochloride. The active electrode was adhered over the TMJ and connected to the positive pole of a DC generator. The dispersive (return) electrode was adhered over the left trapezius muscle and was connected to the generator's negative pole. Current was initiated at 1 mA for the first minute of treatment and then increased slowly to 4.0 mA when it was ascertained that the patient could tolerate this level of current. Current was maintained at 4.0 mA for the next 19 minutes to provide a total current-dosage of approximately 80 mA•min. Current was then slowly decreased to zero, the electrodes were removed, and the skin was inspected for any signs of irritation.

Two days later, a second iontophoresis treatment was applied in the identical manner. As indicated earlier, the patient was also instructed in a home exercise program, and this program was reviewed after each iontophoresis treatment and at each follow-up visit.

Assessment of Outcome

Incisal opening increased to 30 mm after the first iontophoresis treatment and to 34 mm after the second treatment. Right lateral excursion likewise increased to 10 mm after the second treatment. Incisal opening was within normal limits (45 mm) 1 week after the second iontophoresis treatment, and incisal opening was maintained at 43 mm 6 weeks after the second iontophoresis treatment. The patient likewise reported improvements in pain after the first treatment, and pain was progressively reduced until symptoms were absent at the 6 week follow-up visit.

Case 3

Examination

History

A 22-year-old man was injured in an automobile accident, sustaining bilateral open fractures of the tibia and fibula and several deep lacerations around the ankles. He was treated initially in the emergency room, where the fractures were immobilized and the wounds sutured. He was also started on antimicrobial therapy consisting of tetanus vaccine, antitetanus immunoglobulin, metamizole, penicillin, and streptomycin. Despite these antimicrobial medications and daily dressing changes, the wounds on both ankles developed extensive colonization of *Pseudomonas aeruginosa, Escherichia coli*, and *Staphylococcus aureus*. Over the next 7 months, the antimicrobial drug regimen was modified by adding or substituting other agents, until the wound on the right ankle was completely healed. The wounds on the medial and lateral aspects of the left ankle, however, were still purulent and heavily colonized by *Pseudomonas aeruginosa.* Radiographs of the left tibia and fibula likewise suggested osteomyelitis, which was presumed to be a result of the infected wound. The patient was referred to physical therapy for consideration of any possible interventions that might have antimicrobial effects and facilitate wound healing.

Systems Review

The patient did not have a history of diabetes mellitus, atherosclerosis, or other cardiovascular, neuromuscular, and musculoskeletal diseases. He did not smoke cigarettes and was not addicted to any medications.

Tests and Measures

The surface area of the wounds was measured by tracing the outline of each wound on sterile transparent paper. The surface area in square centimeters was calculated from the tracing before the first treatment, with the medial wound having a surface area of 4.06 cm^2 and the lateral wound having a surface area of 5.42 cm^2.

Evaluation

Physical examination revealed open wounds on the medial and lateral aspects of the left ankle. Both wounds were discharging yellowish green pus, and the wound border was tender to palpation. The wounds likewise appeared necrotic, and there was no indication of granulation tissue in either wound.

Diagnosis

This patient had two wounds infected with *Pseudomonas aeruginosa,* and osteomyelitis of the left tibia and fibula. This infection was inhibiting granulation tissue formation and thus preventing the wounds from healing.

Prognosis

The fact that these wounds were recalcitrant despite systemic antimicrobial therapy and dressing changes suggested that local antimicrobial treatment should be considered. The plan was to use iontophoresis to apply zinc oxide because this agent has broad-spectrum antimicrobial effects, and it is also reported to increase local blood flow. These effects should facilitate wound granulation and subsequent tissue healing. Treatments would be applied daily for 2 to 3 weeks to attempt to improve wound healing. Optimal improvement would occur when the wounds were completely closed and free of discharge or signs of infection.

Intervention

Before iontophoresis, the wounds were cleansed with hydrogen peroxide. Zinc oxide was then applied via a gel that was prepared by mixing 8.138 g zinc oxide powder, 10 g glycerol, 10 g bentonite, and 71.862 g water. A small amount of the gel was massaged into the skin proximal to the wound, and the gel was then covered with a layer of sterile moistened lint. The active (delivery) electrode was a 6 $\times$ 6 cm malleable sheet of metal. This electrode and two layers of towel pads soaked with water were placed over the lint and secured with an elastic bandage. The return (dispersive) electrode was a malleable sheet measuring 8 $\times$ 8 cm, and this electrode was sandwiched between two layers of water-soaked towel pads and strapped to the sole of the left foot by an elastic bandage.

The active (delivery) electrode was connected to the positive pole of a DC generator, and the return (dispersive) electrode was connected to the negative pole. Current was gradually increased until the patient reported a tingling sensation, and the current was then held at that amplitude throughout the treatment. Typically current amplitudes ranged between 3 and 6 mA. Treatment duration was 20 minutes during the first week of treatment, 25 minutes during the second week, and 30 minutes during the third and final week of treatment. Treatments were applied 7 days per week.

Assessment of Outcome

By the end of the first week, wound surface area on the medial and lateral aspects of the ankle had decreased to 1.20 cm^2 and 2.54 cm^2, respectively. After 2 weeks of treatment, wound surface area was 0.32 cm^2 and 0.44 cm^2 on the medial and lateral aspects, respectively. At the end of the third week, both wounds were healed and free of any signs of discharge or infection.

SUMMARY

Iontophoresis offers a means of introducing medications through the surface of the skin in a relatively safe, easy, and painless manner. This chapter presented some of the fundamental principles of using electric current as a means of enhancing transdermal drug delivery. Basic principles and clinical procedures for applying iontophoresis treatments were also described. Finally, this chapter described how iontophoresis can be used to administer specific medications to achieve specific clinical outcomes, including decreased inflammation, decreased pain, and several other beneficial effects.

Although iontophoresis techniques have been available to clinicians for several decades, iontophoresis appears to have rather limited acceptance as a primary therapeutic intervention. This is due at least in part to the relative lack of well-designed experimental studies documenting the clinical efficacy of these techniques. As with many electrotherapeutic interventions, there is a need for more studies that document the use and effects of iontophoresis in various clinical situations. Sufficient evidence supports consideration of iontophoresis, especially in certain conditions such as localized soft-tissue inflammation. Iontophoresis has the potential to provide substantial benefits when this intervention is applied in the appropriate manner to an appropriate patient population. More widespread clinical use combined with additional research may allow iontophoresis to assume a more prominent role in the armamentaria of contemporary clinical practice.

SELF-STUDY QUESTIONS

For answers, see Appendix B.

1. The basic principle of iontophoresis is electrostatic ________________ of charged particles, with positively charged ions being delivered from the ________________ and negatively charged ions being delivered from the ________________.
2. Iontophoresis uses ________________ current at amplitudes that typically range from ________________ to ________________ mA.
3. Current-dosage used during iontophoresis is determined by the product of current ________________ and current ________________, and current-dosages are expressed in units of ________________.
4. When iontophoresis is used to treat pain and inflammation, current-dosages typically range between ________________ and ________________.
5. An iontophoresis treatment is initiated at an amplitude of 2 mA, and this amplitude is maintained for 5 minutes. Amplitude is then increased to 4 mA. How much longer should the treatment be applied to achieve a total current-dosage of 50 mA•min?
6. With regard to polarity of the delivery electrode, administration of medications from the ________________ typically produces more skin irritation because this electrode causes the formation of ________________, which induces an ________________ reaction on the skin's surface.
7. List three advantages of commercial electrodes.
8. It has been recommended that current density should not exceed ________________ mA/cm^2 when the cathode is used for drug delivery, and ________________ mA/cm^2 when the anode is used for drug delivery.

9. True or False: doubling the recommended concentration of a medication will double the amount of drug administered during iontophoresis.

10. Current evidence indicates that dexamethasone carries a ________________ charge and lidocaine carries a ________________ charge when these drugs are used during iontophoresis.

11. The cathode is being used to deliver a drug that is a weak base. If pH increases at the cathode, this could ________________ the amount of drug delivered because ________________ of the drug exists in an ionized state.

12. List three contraindications or precautions to iontophoresis.

13. Glucocorticoids such as dexamethasone are used during iontophoresis for their powerful ________________ effects, but prolonged or extensive use of these drugs can produce a ________________ effect on collagenous tissues.

14. List three different types of medications that have been administered iontophoretically to specifically produce an analgesic effect.

15. Conditions involving soft-tissue calcification have been treated with iontophoretic application of ________________, and the polarity of this medication necessitates delivery from the ________________.

REFERENCES

1. Helmstadter A. The history of electrically assisted transdermal drug delivery ("iontophoresis"). *Pharmazie*. 2001;56:583–587.
2. LeDuc S. *Electric Ions and Their Use in Medicine*. Liverpool: Redman Ltd.; 1908
3. Pikal MJ. The role of electroosmotic flow in transdermal iontophoresis. *Adv Drug Deliv Rev*. 2001;46:281–305.
4. Banga AK, Bose S, Ghosh TK. . Iontophoresis and electroporation: comparisons and contrasts. *Int J Pharm*. 1999;179:1–19.
5. Jadoul A, Bouwstra J, Preat VV. Effects of iontophoresis and electroporation on the stratum corneum. Review of the biophysical studies. *Adv Drug Deliv Rev*, 1999;35:89–105.
6. Pliquett UF, Martin GT, Weaver JC. Kinetics of the temperature rise within human stratum corneum during electroporation and pulsed high-voltage iontophoresis. *Bioelectrochemistry*. 2002;57:65–72.
7. Fang JY, Sung KC, Wang JJ, et al. The effects of iontophoresis and electroporation on transdermal delivery of buprenorphine from solutions and hydrogels. *J Pharm Pharmacol*. 2002;54:1329–1337.
8. Hu Q, Liang W, Bao J, et al. Enhanced transdermal delivery of tetracaine by electroporation. *Int J Pharm*. 2000;202:121–124.
9. Manabe E, Numajiri S, Sugibayashi K, et al. Analysis of skin permeation-enhancing mechanism of iontophoresis using hydrodynamic pore theory. *J Control Release*. 2000;66:149–158.
10. Zhu H, Li SK, Peck KD, et al. Improvement on conventional constant current DC iontophoresis: a study using constant conductance AC iontophoresis. *J Control Release*. 2002;82:249–261.
11. Badkar AV, Banga AK. Electrically enhanced transdermal delivery of a macromolecule. *J Pharm Pharmacol*. 2002;54:907–912.
12. Kanikkannan N. Iontophoresis-based transdermal delivery systems. *Biodrugs*. 2002; 16:339–347.
13. Uitto OD, White HS. Electroosmotic pore transport in human skin. *Pharm Res*. 2003;20, 646–652.
14. Kochar C, Imanidis G. In vitro transdermal iontophoretic delivery of leuprolide—mechanisms under constant voltage application. *J Pharm Sci*. 2003;92, 84–96.

15. Guy RH, Delgado-Charro MB, Kalia YN. Iontophoretic transport across the skin. *Skin Pharmacol Appl Skin Physiol*. 2001;14(Suppl 1):35–40.
16. Marro D, Kalia YN, Delgado-Charro MB, et al. Contributions of electromigration and electroosmosis to iontophoretic drug delivery. *Pharm Res*. 2001;18:1701–1708.
17. Braun BL. Treatment of acute anterior disk displacement in the temporomandibular joint: a case report. *Phys Ther*. 1987;67:1234–1236.
18. Delacerda FG. A comparative study of three methods of treatment for shoulder girdle myofascial syndrome. *J Orthop Sports Phys Ther*. 1982;4:51–54.
19. Kahn J. Iontophoresis and ultrasound for postsurgical temporomandibular trismus and paresthesia: case report. *Phys Ther*. 1980;60:307–308.
20. Kahn J. Calcium iontophoresis in suspected myopathy. *Phys Ther*. 1975;55:376–377.
21. LaForest NT, Cofrancesco C. Antibiotic iontophoresis in the treatment of ear chondritis: clinical report. *Phys Ther*. 1978;58:32–34.
22. Magistro CM. Hyaluronidase by iontophoresis. *Phys Ther*. 1964;44:169–175.
23. Murray W, Lavine LS, Seifter E. The iontophoresis of C21 esterified glucocorticoids: preliminary report. *Phys Ther*. 1963;43:579–581.
24. Anderson CR, Morris RL, Boeh SD, et al. Effects of iontophoresis current magnitude and duration on dexamethasone deposition and localized drug retention. *Phys Ther*. 2003;83:161–170.
25. Ashburn MA, Stephen RL, Ackerman E, et al. Iontophoretic delivery of morphine for postoperative analgesia. *J Pain Symptom Manage*. 1992;7:27–33.
26. Rapperport AS, Larson DL, Henges DF, et al. Iontophoresis: a method of antibiotic adminstration in the burn patient. *Plast Reconstruct Surg*. 1965;36:547–552.
27. Shibaji T, Yasuhara Y, Oda N, et al. A mechanism of the high frequency AC iontophoresis. *J Control Release*. 2001;73:37–47.
28. Kinoshita T, Shibaji T, Umino M. Transdermal delivery of lidocaine in vitro by alternating current. *J Med Dent Sci*. 2003;50:71–77.
29. Meyer PF, Oddsson LI. Alternating-pulse iontophoresis for targeted cutaneous anesthesia. *J Neurosci Methods*. 2003;125:209–214.
30. Zhu H, Peck KD, Miller DJ, et al. Investigation of properties of human epidermal membrane under constant conductance alternating current iontophoresis. *J Control Release*. 2003;89:31–46.
31. Zhu H, Peck KD, Li SK, et al. Quantification of pore induction in human epidermal membrane during iontophoresis: the importance of background electrolyte solution. *J Pharm Sci*. 2001;90:932–942.
32. Backstrom KM. Mobilization with movement as an adjunct intervention in a patient with complicated de Quervain's tenosgnovitis: a case report. *J Orthop Sports Phys Ther.* 2002;32:86–97.
33. Gudeman SD, Eisele SA, Heidt RS, et al. Treatment of plantar fasciitis by iontophoresis of 0.4% dexamethasone. A randomized, double-blind, placebo controlled study. *Am J Sports Med*. 1997;25:312–316.
34. Nirschl RP, Rodin DM, Ochiai DH, et al. Iontophoretic administration of dexamethasone sodium phosphate for acute epicondylitis: a randomized, double-blinded, placebo-controlled study. *Am J Sports Med*. 2003;31:189–195.
35. Bertolucci LE. Introduction of antiinflammatory drugs by iontophoresis: double blind study. *J Orthop Sports Phys Ther*. 1982;4:103–108.
36. Harris PR. Iontophoresis: clinical research in musculoskeletal inflammatory conditions. *J Orthop Sports Phys Ther*. 1982;4:109–112.
37. Hasson SH, Henderson GH, Daniels JC, et al. Exercise training and dexamethasone iontophoresis in rheumatoid arthritis: a case study. *Physiother Can*. 1991;43:11–29.
38. Henley EJ. Transcutaneous drug delivery: iontophoresis and phonophoresis. *Crit Rev Phys Rehabil Med*. 1991;2:139–151.
39. Gangarosa LP, Mahan PE, Ciarlone AE. Pharmacologic management of temporomandibular joint disorders and chronic head and neck pain. *Cranio*. 1991;9:328–338.

40. Petelenz T, Axenti I, Petelenz TJ, et al. Mini set for iontophoresis for topical analgesia before injection. *Int J Clin Pharmacol Ther Toxicol*. 1984;22:152–155.
41. Guffey JS, Rutherford MJ, Payne W, et al. Skin changes associated with iontophoresis. *J Orthop Sports Phys Ther*. 1999;29:656–660.
42. Cummings J. Iontophoresis. In Nelson RM, Currier DP, eds. *Clinical Electrotherapy*. 2nd ed. – Norwalk, CT: Appleton and Lange; 1991:317–329.
43. Lark MR, Gangarosa LP. Iontophoresis: an effective modality for the treatment of inflammatory disorders of the temporomandibular joint and myofascial pain. *Cranio*. 1990;8:108–119.
44. Cornwall MW. Zinc iontophoresis to treat skin ulcers. *Phys Ther*. 1981;61:359–366.
45. Langley PL. Iontophoresis to aid in releasing tendon adhesions: suggestions from the field. *Phys Ther*. 1984;64:1395.
46. Tannenbaum M. Iodine iontophoresis in reduction of scar tissue. *Phys Ther*. 1980;60:792.
47. Weider DL. Treatment of traumatic myositis ossificans with acetic acid iontophoresis. *Phys Ther*. 1992;72:133–137.
48. Petelenz TJ, Buttke JA, Bonds C, et al. Iontophoresis of dexamethasone: laboratory studies. *J Control Release*. 1992;20:55–66.
49. Banta CA. A prospective, nonrandomized study of iontophoresis, wrist splinting, and antiinflammatory medication in the treatment of early-mild carpal tunnel syndrome. *J Occup Med*. 1994;36:166–168.
50. Hasson SM, English SE, Daniels JC, et al. Effect of iontophoretically delivered dexamethasone on muscle performance in a rheumatoid arthritic joint. *Arthritis Care Res*. 1988;1:177–182.
51. Li LC, Scudds RA, Heck CS, et al. The efficacy of dexamethasone iontophoresis for the treatment of rheumatoid arthritic knees: a pilot study. *Arthritis Care Res*. 1996;9:126–132.
52. Runeson L, Haker E. Iontophoresis with cortisone in the treatment of lateral epicondylalgia (tennis elbow)—a double-blind study. *Scand J Med Sci Sports*. 2002;12:136–142.
53. Smutok MA, Mayo MF, Gabaree CL, et al. Failure to detect dexamethasone phosphate in the local venous blood postcathodic iontophoresis in humans. *J Orthop Sports Phys Ther*. 2002;32:461–468.
54. De Bosscher K, Vanden Berghe W, Haegeman G. Mechanisms of anti-inflammatory action and of immunosuppression by glucocorticoids: negative interference of activated glucocorticoid receptor with transcription factors. *J Neuroimmunol*. 2000;109:16–22.
55. Neeck G, Renkawitz R, Eggert M. Molecular aspects of glucocorticoid action in rheumatoid arthritis. *Cytokines Cell Mol Ther*. 2002;7:61–69.
56. Saklavata J. Glucocorticoids: do we know how they work? *Arthritis Res*. 2002;4: 146–150.
57. McIlwain HH. Glucocorticoid-induced osteoporosis: pathogenesis, diagnosis, and management. *Prev Med*. 2003;36:243–249.
58. Schimmer BP, Parker KL. Adrenocorticotropic hormone; adrenocortical steroids and their synthetic analogs; inhibitors of the synthesis and actions of adrenocortical hormones. In Hardman JG Limbird LE, eds. *The Pharmacological Basis of Therapeutics*. 10th ed. New York: McGraw-Hill; 2001:1649–1677.
59. Levin C, Maibach HI. Topical corticosteroid-induced adrenocortical insufficiency: clinical implications. *Am J Clin Dermatol*. 2002;3:141–147.
60. Catterall WA. Molecular mechanisms of gating and drug block of sodium channels. *Novartis Found Symp*. 2002;241:206–218.
61. Strichartz GR, Zhou Z, Sinnott C, et al. Therapeutic concentrations of local anesthetics unveil the potential role of sodium channels in neuropathic pain. *Novartis Found Symp*. 2002; 241:189–201.
62. Bezzant JL, Stephen RL, Petelenz TJ, et al. Painless cauterization of spider veins with the use of iontophoretic local anesthesia. *J Am Acad Dermatol*. 1988;19:869–875.
63. Comeau M, Brummett R. Anesthesia of the human tympanic membrane by iontophoresis of a local anesthetic. *Laryngoscope*. 1978;88:277–285.
64. Gangarosa LP. Iontophoresis for surface local anesthesia. *J Am Dent Assoc*. 1974;88:125–128.
65. Sirimanna KS, Madden GJ, Miles S. Anaesthesia of the tympanic membrane: comparison of EMLA cream and iontophoresis. *J Laryngol Otol*. 1990;104:195–196.

66. Rose JB, Galinkin JL, Jantzen EC, et al. A study of lidocaine iontophoresis for pediatric venipuncture. *Anesth Analg*. 2002;94:867–871.

67. Schultz AA, Strout TD, Jordon P, et al. Safety, tolerability, and efficacy of iontophoresis with lidocaine for dermal anesthesia in ED pediatric patients. *J Emerg Nurs*. 2002;28:289–296.

68. Sherwin J, Awad IT, Sadler PJ, et al. Analgesia during radial artery cannulation: comparison of the effects of lidocaine applied by local injection or iontophoresis. *Anaesthesia*. 2003;58:474–476.

69. Bailey DC, Southern AP, Shamy TL, et al. A comparison of the use of iontophoresis and oral nonsteroidal anti-inflammatory medication in the pain management of acute soft tissue injuries in the emergency department setting. *Acad Emerg Med*. 2003;10:470.

70. Roberts LJ, Morrow JD. Analgesic-antipyretic and antiinflammatory agents and drugs employed in the treatment of gout. In: Hardman JG, Limbird LE, dds. *The Pharmacological Basis of Therapeutics*. 10th ed. New York: McGraw-Hill; 2001:687–731.

71. Vane JR, Botting RM. Mechanism of action of nonsteroidal anti-inflammatory drugs. *Am J Med*. 1998;30 (Suppl 3A):2S–8S.

72. Morrow JD, Roberts LJ. Lipid-derived autocoids: eicosanoids and platelet-activating factor. In: Hardman JG, Limbird LE, eds. *The Pharmacological Basis of Therapeutics*. 10th ed. New York: McGraw-Hill; 2001: 669–685.

73. Garzione JE. Salycilate iontophoresis as an alternative treatment for persistent thigh pain following hip surgery. *Phys Ther*. 1978;58:570–571.

74. Gordon AH, Weinstein MV. Sodium salicylate iontophoresis in the treatment of plantar warts: case report. *Phys Ther*. 1969;49:869–870.

75. Soroko YT, Repking MC, Clemment JA, et al. Treatment of plantar verrucae using 2% sodium salicylate iontophoresis. *Phys Ther*. 2002;82:1184–1191.

76. Baskurt F, Ozcan A, Algun C. Comparison of the effects of phonophoresis and iontophoresis of naproxen in the treatment of lateral epicondylitis. *Clin Rehabil*. 2003;17:96–100.

77. Panus PC, Ferslew KE, Tober-Meyer B, et al. Ketoprofen tissue permeation in swine following cathodic iontophoresis. *Phys Ther*. 1999;79:40–49.

78. Kanebako M, Inagi T, Takayama K. Transdermal delivery of indomethacin by iontophoresis. *Biol Pharm Bull*. 2002;25:779–782.

79. Curdy C, Kalia YN, Naik A, et al. Piroxicam delivery into human stratum corneum in vivo: iontophoresis versus passive diffusion. *J Control Release*. 2001;76:73–79.

80. Stein C. Peripheral mechanisms of opioid analgesia. *Anesth Analg*. 1993;76: 182–191.

81. Grond S, Radbruch L, Lehmann KA. Clinical pharmacokinetics of transdermal opioids: focus on transdermal fentanyl. *Clin Pharmacokinet*. 2000;38:59–89.

82. Conjeevaram R, Banga AK, Zhang L. Electrically modulated transdermal delivery of fentanyl. *Pharm Res*. 2002;19:440–444.

83. Csillik B, Knyihar-Csillik E, Szucs A. Treatment of chronic pain syndromes with iontophoresis of vinca alkaloids to the skin of patients. *Neurosci Lett*. 1982;31:87–90.

84. Layman PR, Argyras E, Glynn CJ. Iontophoresis of vincristine versus saline in post-herpetic neuralgia. A controlled trial. *Pain*. 1986;25:165–170.

85. Tajti J, Somogyi I, Szilard J. Treatment of chronic pain syndromes with transcutaneous iontophoresis of vinca alkaloids, with special regard to post-herpetic neuralgia. *Acta Med Hung*. 1989;46:3–12.

86. Chabner BA, Ryan DP, Paz-Ares L, et al. Antineoplastic agents. In Hardman JG Limbird LE, eds. *The Pharmacological Basis of Therapeutics*. 10th ed. New York: McGraw-Hill; 2001:1389–1459.

87. Szucs A, Csillik B, Knyihar-Csillik E. Treatment of terminal pain in cancer patients by means of iontophoresis of vinca alkaloids. *Recent Results Cancer Res*. 1984;89:185–189.

88. Dowd NP, Day F, Timon D, et al. Iontophoretic vincristine in the treatment of postherpetic neuralgia: a double-blind, randomized, controlled trial. *J Pain Symptom Manage*. 1999;17, 175–180.

89. Kahn J. A case report: lithium iontophoresis for gouty arthritis. *J Orthop Sports Phys Ther*. 1982;4:113–114.

90. Kahn J. Acetic acid iontophoresis for calcium deposits. *Phys Ther.* 1977;57:658–659.
91. Perron M, Malouin F. Acetic acid iontophoresis and ultrasound for the treatment of calcifying tendinitis of the shoulder: a randomized control trial. *Arch Phys Med Rehabil.* 1997;78: 379–384.
92. Balogun J, Abidoye AB, Akala EO. Zinc iontophoresis in the management of bacterial colonized wounds: a case report. *Physiother Can.* 1990;42:147–151.
93. Greminger RF, Elliott RA, Rapperport A. Antibiotic iontophoresis for the management of burned ear chondritis. *Plast Reconstruct Surg.* 1980;66:356–360.
94. Kwon BS, Hill JM, Wiggins C, et al. Iontophoretic application of adenine arabinoside monophosphate for the treatment of herpes simplex virus type 2 skin infections in hairless mice. *J Infect Dis.* 1979;140:1014.
95. Gangarosa LP, Payne LJ, Hayakawa K, et al. Iontophoretic treatment of herpetic whitlow. *Arch Phys Med Rehabil.* 1989;70:336–340.
96. Boone DC. Hyaluronidase iontophoresis. *Phys Ther.* 1969;49:139–145.
97. Akins DL, Meisenheimer JL, Dobson RL. Efficacy of the Drionic unit in the treatment of hyperhidrosis. *J Am Acad Dermatol.* 1987;16:828–833.
98. Karakoc Y, Aydemir EH, Kalkan MT, et al. Safe control of palmoplantar hyperhidrosis with direct electrical current. *Int J Dermatol.* 2002;41:602–605.
99. Stolman LP. Treatment of excess sweating of the palms by iontophoresis. *Arch Dermatol.* 1987;123:893–896.
100. Togel B, Greve B, Raulin C. Current therapeutic strategies for hyperhydrosis: a review. *Eur J Dermatol.* 2002;12:219–223.
101. Culibrk MS, Culibrk B. Physical treatment of Peyronie disease. *Am J Phys Med Rehabil.* 2001;80:583–585.
102. Riedl CR, Plas E, Engelhardt P, et al. Iontophoresis for treatment of Peyronie's disease. *J Urol.* 2000;163:95–99.
103. Smith KJ, Konzelman JL, Lombardo FA, et al. Iontophoresis of vinblastine into normal skin and for treatment of Kaposi's sarcoma in human immunodeficiency virus-positive patients. *Arch Dermatol.* 1992;128:1365–1370.
104. Bacro TR, Holladay EB, Stith MJ, et al. Iontophoresis treatment of basal cell carcinoma with cisplatin: a case report. *Cancer Detect Prev.* 2000;24: 610–619.
105. Rhodes LE, Tsoukas MM, Anderson RR, et al. Iontophoretic delivery of ALA provides a quantitative model for ALA pharmacokinetics and PpIX phototoxicity in human skin. *J Invest Dermatol.* 1997;108:87–91.
106. Huh CH, Seo KI, Park JY, et al. A randomized, double-blind, placebo-controlled trial of vitamin C iontophoresis in melasma. *Dermatology.* 2003;206:316–320.
107. Chang SL, Hofmann GA, Zhang L, et al. Transdermal iontophoretic delivery of salmon calcitonin. *Int J Pharm.* 2000;200:107–113.
108. Nair VB, Panchagnula R. Effect of iontophoresis and fatty acids on permeation of arginine vasopressin through rat skin. *Pharmacol Res.* 2003;47:563–569.
109. Smyth HD, Becket G, Mehta S. Effect of permeation enhancer pretreatment on the iontophoresis of luteinizing hormone releasing hormone (LHRH) through human epidermal membrane (HEM). *J Pharm Sci.* 2002;91:1296–1307.
110. Suzuki Y, Iga K, Yanai S, et al. Iontophoretic pulsatile transdermal delivery of human parathyroid hormone (1-34). *J Pharm Pharmacol.* 2001;53:1227–1234.
111. Suzuki Y, Nagase Y, Iga K, et al. Prevention of bone loss in ovariectomized rats by pulsatile transdermal iontophoretic administration of human PTH (1-34). *J Pharm Sci.* 2002;91:350–361.
112. Pillai O, Borkute SD, Sivaprasad N, et al. Transdermal iontophoresis of insulin. II. Physiochemical considerations. *Int J Pharm.* 2003;254:271–280.

113. Pillai O, Panchagnula R. Transdermal delivery of insulin from poloxamer gel: ex vivo and in vivo skin permeation studies in rat using iontophoresis and chemical enhancers. *J Control Release*. 2003;89:127–140.

114. Junginger HE. Iontophoretic delivery of apomorphine: from in-vitro modeling to the Parkinson patient. *Adv Drug Deliv Rev*. 2002;54 (Suppl 1):S57–S75.

115. Sanderson JE, Caldwell RW, Hsiao et al. Noninvasive delivery of a novel inotropic catecholamine: iontophoretic versus intravenous infusion in dogs. *J Pharm Sci*. 1987;76:215–218.

116. Wang H, Hou HM. Improvement of transdermal permeation of captopril by iontophoresis. *Acta Pharmacol Sinica*. 2000;21:591–595.

117. Alvarez-Figueroa MJ, Blanco-Mendez J. Transdermal delivery of methotrexate: iontophoretic delivery from hydrogels and passive delivery from microemulsion. *Int J Pharm*. 2001;215:57–65.

118. Barry BW. Novel mechanisms and devices to enable successful transdermal drug delivery. *Eur J Pharm Sci*. 2001;14:101–114.

119. Kanikkannan N, Kandimalla K, Lamba SS, et al. Structure-activity relationship of chemical penetration enhancers in transdermal drug delivery. *Curr Med Chem*. 2000;7:593–608.

120. Mitragotri S. Synergistic effect of enhancers for transdermal drug delivery. *Pharm Res*. 2000;17:1354–1359.

121. Pillai O, Panchagnula R. Transdermal iontophoresis of insulin. V. Effect of terpenes. *J Control Release*. 2003;88:287–296.

CHAPTER 11

Electromyographic Biofeedback for Improvement of Voluntary Motor Control

Stuart A. Binder-Macleod and Jennifer A. Bushey

Biofeedback training is the use of electronic instrumentation to provide objective information (feedback) to an individual about a physiological function or response so that the individual becomes aware of his or her response. The individual then attempts to alter the feedback signal to modify the physiological response (1). Though the clinical application of biofeedback includes monitoring the electrical activity of muscles (electromyogram; EMG) or the brain (electroencephalogram; EEG), blood pressure, heart rate, and visceral and vasomotor responses, the present chapter addresses only the application most widely used in physical rehabilitation, EMG biofeedback. EMG biofeedback is the use of electronic instrumentation to detect and feed back the electric signals from skeletal muscle to allow the patient to gain better volitional control over the muscle. EMG biofeedback is used either to train patients to relax hyperactive muscles or to increase the level of recruitment in hypoactive muscles.

This chapter discusses the relationship between the EMG and muscle activation, technical considerations related to the clinical application of EMG biofeedback, advantages of using biofeedback, current clinical applications of EMG biofeedback, guidelines for the selection of appropriate patients for the application of EMG biofeedback, and development of training strategies during the use of EMG biofeedback.

EMG AND MUSCLE ACTIVATION

The electromyogram is a recording of the voltage changes associated with the activation of skeletal muscle fibers. In normal muscle at rest (not contracting), skeletal muscle exhibits no significant electrical activity. Voluntary activation of skeletal muscle results from the activation of alpha motoneurons innervating skeletal muscle fibers. The motoneuron axons then excite skeletal muscle fibers at the neuromuscular junctions. Each of the muscle fibers excited undergoes a marked increase in the permeability of their membranes to sodium and potassium ions. Due to the electrochemical forces acting on these two ions, they move into and out of muscle fibers, effectively changing the concentrations of ions in the extracellular fluid. These changes in ion concentration can be detected by surface electrodes connected to a very sensitive voltage measuring device placed over the muscle. It is the voltage changes monitored in this manner that constitute the EMG.

During voluntary muscle contractions, the force of contraction is regulated by the central nervous system in two primary ways. First, descending motor control pathways activate a varying number of alpha motoneurons. This is the process of recruitment. The greater the number of motoneurons, and hence motor units activated, the greater the force of contraction and the greater the electrical activity recorded from muscle fibers. The second way that the central nervous system controls the force of contraction is by controlling the frequency of activation of motoneurons and motor units, a process called rate coding. The higher the frequency of activation, the greater the force of contraction, and the higher the amount of electrical activity recorded from skeletal muscle.

This section reviews the factors that determine the amplitude of the EMG, outlines the rationale for specific electrode selection and placement, discusses the method and purpose of each step in the processing of the EMG feedback signal, presents the various methods of displaying the biofeedback signal, and the advantages and indications for each.

The EMG is the recording of the electrical activity of the muscle in response to the physiological activation of skeletal muscles. The amplitude of the EMG reflects the size and number of active motor units, as well as the distance of the active muscle fibers from the recording electrodes. Although no direct information is contained within the EMG regarding the force or torque that a muscle produces, a nearly linear relationship exists between the EMG and the force that a muscle produces under carefully controlled isometric conditions (2,3). Clinicians should be aware, however, that this linear relationship no longer holds when contractions change from isometric to nonisometric or as the muscle fatigues. Similarly, because the EMG only records from a limited area of a muscle, the EMG cannot be used to compare the strength of contraction across muscle groups or even within the same muscle if different electrode placements or types of electrodes are used (see below). To illustrate this concept, recording electrodes may be applied over the abductor digiti minimi muscle of one person and over the quadriceps femoris muscle of another. Depending on the electrode size and spacing, the electrical activity from the abductor of one subject's little finger may approximate the activity from the other subject's knee extensor during volitional activation, despite the marked differences in force output between the two muscles.

In addition to physiological factors, such as the size and number of active motor units, the size of the recording area and the interelectrode distance of the recording electrodes also affect the amplitude of the EMG. The larger the recording area, the greater the volume of muscle that is monitored, and hence the greater the EMG recorded. Similarly, the larger the interelectrode distance, the larger the volume of the muscle that is monitored, and the larger the EMG. Thus, to increase the specificity of the EMG recording electrodes, small recording areas and close interelectrode spacing could be used. The use of close spacing minimizes the recording of electrical activity from muscles other than the targeted muscle. This may be particularly helpful if the EMG from the targeted muscle is being contaminated by input from a muscle that is an antagonist of the targeted muscle. This phenomenon is termed *cross-talk*. Subcutaneous recording electrodes, such as fine wire electrodes, are examples of small, closely spaced electrodes that allow precise localization from within the muscle. Subcutaneous electrodes also offer the advantage of being able to record from deep muscles without interference from more superficial muscles, and they show greater sensitivity than surface electrodes due to their proximity to the active muscle fibers. Skin, subcutaneous fat, and fascia all serve to attenuate the EMG recorded by surface electrodes. Nevertheless, inserted electrodes are rarely used with EMG biofeedback (4). Surface electrodes are much more convenient for the clinician, more acceptable to the patient, and produce much less movement artifact than subcutaneous electrodes. Movement artifact is the high-voltage, nonphysiological contamination of the EMG due to the physical perturbation of the electrodes, input cables, and wires. The spacing between the recording electrodes should be as small as is practicably possible to minimize the recording from unwanted muscle groups. Interelectrode spacing of 1 to 2 cm is generally adequate.

TECHNICAL CONSIDERATIONS

Essentially, five steps are involved in the processing of the EMG feedback signal: amplification, filtering, rectification, integration, and level detection. The processes of amplification, filtering, and integration are discussed in Chapter 2. A schematic representation of the changes in the EMG biofeedback signal is shown in Figure 11.1. Most feedback devices allow the clinician to modify many of these processes. The *amplification*, *gain*, or *sensitivity* are all terms used to describe the relationship between the input and output voltages of the amplifier. The greater the amplification, the more sensitive the device. That is, with a high amplification, even very small EMG signals produce discernible changes in the output displayed to the patient. In general, the greatest sensitivity that does not produce an output signal that exceeds the limits of the output display is used. When training a patient to increase recruitment, and given a choice of sensitivities from an output meter of 10, 100, or 1000-μV to produce full-scale deflection, if the client has a maximum recruitment of 80-μV, then the best choice would be the 100-μV sensitivity.

Differential amplification is used by virtually all biofeedback devices. As described in Chapter 2, differential amplification requires the use of two recording electrodes and a reference

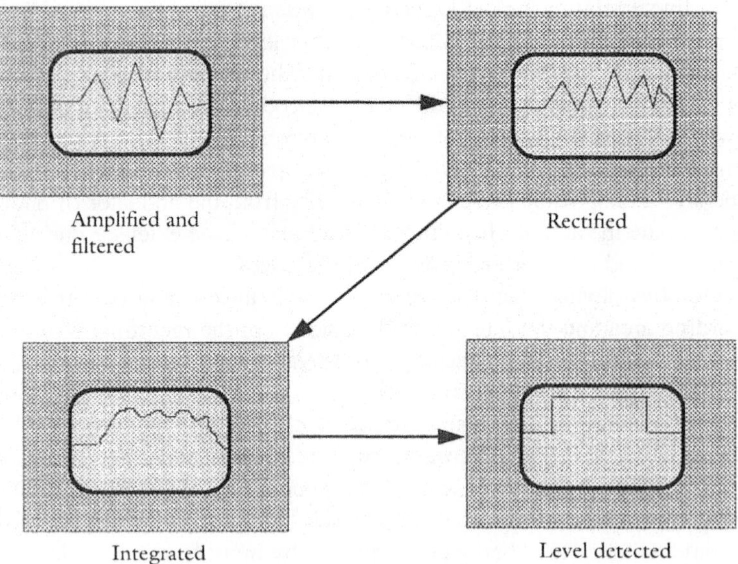

Figure 11.1. Schematic representation of the changes in the EMG biofeedback signal.

electrode. Also, the use of close spacing between the recording electrodes helps minimize the noise recorded and give the cleanest signal possible. Thus, particularly when attempting to record low levels of electrical activity, close spacing is used to minimize the noise that would be amplified.

The *filtering* characteristics of most feedback devices can be modified. By restricting the frequency range of the signal that is passed through the amplifier, we can attempt to reduce noise and make the recording more selective. Movement artifact tends to be low frequency (<100 Hz), and much of the electronic noise is high frequency (>1,000 Hz). Because most of the EMG signal falls within the 100 to 1,000 Hz range, this is the range most often used. However, if high-frequency noise is a problem, a narrower frequency range may be required to eliminate more of the high-frequency signal (e.g., only pass a signal between 100 and 500 Hz). Because the EMG actually includes a fairly wide frequency range, the disadvantage of using a narrower frequency band is that some of the EMG is lost when a narrower range is used. There are times, however, when some of the EMG is purposely eliminated. Because muscle attenuates high-frequency signals more than lower frequencies, the EMG signals from distant motor units are lower frequency than nearby motor units (5). Eliminating more of the low-frequency signal allows the amplifier to reduce the contribution made by distant motor units to the EMG. Surface electrodes therefore become more selective (record from a narrower area) if the lower limit of the frequency band passed is raised.

If the filtered output from a differential amplifier is fed into an audio speaker or oscilloscope, a *raw EMG* is displayed. This is the signal used to see the actual EMG or to listen for a 60-Hz interference. Having access to the raw EMG is particularly helpful if there is a question about whether the processed feedback signal is of physiological origin. With modern amplifiers, even with surface electrodes, single motor units potentials can easily be identified.

The next steps in the processing of the EMG are the *rectification* and *integration* of the signal. The signal needs to be full-wave rectified to be integrated. The integration of the signal involves summing the signal over some period of time. If a leaky capacitor is used to accomplish this task, what is seen is a smoothing of the signal. Other integrators can be made to sum over a period of time or until some preset maximum voltage is reached before the integrator is reset to zero. The rate at which the EMG sums and declines is a function of the time constant of the integrator. A short time constant will allow the integrated EMG to follow the peaks and valleys of the rectified signal closely. A longer time constant will produce much greater smoothing of the signal and require a longer time for the integrated signal to reach its peak, and a longer time to relax back to baseline. An integrated signal is required to display anything other than the raw EMG.

Setting an appropriate time constant is important in producing an appropriate feedback signal. If the time constant is too short, the display (e.g., a digital or analog voltage meter) will fluctuate too rapidly (display jitter); little sense can be made from such an output. In contrast, a time constant that is too long will cause the display to lag behind the actual activity of the muscle. As an example, even if the subject relaxes, it may take several seconds for the display to return to zero. Neither of these situations is acceptable. An appropriate time constant will help accurately reflect the overall state of activation of a muscle, but will not show the wide and rapid fluctuations seen within the raw or rectified EMG. A time constant of approximately one-third of a second works well for most muscle training applications. Longer time constants are often used for general relaxation training in which the activity of a specific muscle (e.g., frontalis muscle) is being used to reflect the overall state of relaxation of the patient.

The last step in signal processing is the use of a *threshold detector* to determine whether a preset level of integrated EMG activity has been met. The output of a threshold detector is a binary function (i.e., "on" or "off"). The logic of the output can be set to be on or off when the threshold is exceeded. For example, when training a young child with cerebral palsy to relax his plantar flexor muscle while standing at a table, the feedback can be set to allow an electric train to run as long as the EMG is below a preset threshold. Whenever the EMG exceeds this threshold, the train can be made to stop. The logic would thus have been set to give an "on" signal whenever the EMG voltage was below threshold, and an "off" signal whenever the voltage exceeded the threshold.

Many devices allow a combination of feedback signals. For instance, the output of the integrator may simultaneously be sent to a light meter display (i.e., a series of lights is turned on) and a threshold detector. The meter can provide continuous visual feedback, and the output of the threshold detector can be used to trigger an audio signal. Thus the audio signal can be turned on when the threshold is exceeded.

As already noted, *feedback signals* can be raw or processed, auditory or visual, continuous or threshold-triggered. Within the limits of the available equipment, the clinician and patient must decide on the most appropriate signal. The raw output (i.e., amplified and filtered only) can give the experienced clinician considerable information regarding the source of the signal. That is, is the source truly physiological, or is it primarily noise that is being recorded? Other than identifying the peak voltages from an oscilloscope screen, the raw signal cannot be quantified. This is a limitation when attempting to document progress objectively or when trying to identify targeted levels of recruitment for the patient. When deciding to use an auditory (e.g., raw EMG, tone, or beep) or a visual (e.g., digital meter or light bar) display, patient preference and other practical factors need to be considered. If a lower extremity muscle is being monitored in preparation for ambulation training, auditory feedback may be preferred because visual feedback is not practical during ambulation (the patient needs to watch where he or she is going). Similarly, during relaxation training, most clients prefer auditory feedback because they may want to close their eyes to help them relax.

The use of a threshold is necessary whenever EMG levels are used to turn on or off another device, such as a radio or CD player. The use of an audio threshold during relaxation is also generally preferred. Most patients find the audio signal annoying and unnecessary if they are able to relax below the target. Only when the activity exceeds that target does the patients need to be alerted.

As previously noted, more than one feedback signal can be used simultaneously, especially if more than one muscle group is monitored. When two muscle groups are monitored simultaneously (dual-channel monitoring), continuous feedback is generally provided from one channel, whereas the other channel uses a threshold detector to "sound an alarm" only if the second muscle exceeds the threshold. This technique is commonly used when training for recruitment of one muscle and relaxation of its antagonist. As an example, to train for increased active finger extension from a patient who shows spasticity as the result of cerebral vascular accident (CVA), the finger flexor and extensor muscles may be simultaneously monitored. Continuous auditory and visual feedback to train for recruitment of the extensors could be provided while using a threshold detector to provide a separate auditory signal from the flexors. Only when the flexor activity exceeds a level that is believed to be interfering with finger extension would feedback from the flexors be provided to the client.

ADVANTAGES OF USING EMG BIOFEEDBACK

EMG biofeedback is a tool that clinicians can use to help their patients learn new tasks or modify existing motor patterns by providing useful information both to the clinician and patient (see Fig. 11.2). The actual treatment is the activities or exercises that patients perform. To illustrate this point, parallels may be drawn between the use of a mirror during posture training and the use of biofeedback. One would never say that the mirror is being used to treat a patient. Rather, the mirror is merely a tool that is used to provide feedback to the patient. Similarly, in EMG biofeedback, the electromyographic signal is a tool that clinicians and patients use to provide information about the electrical activity of specific muscles.

One advantage of EMG biofeedback is the *speed* and *continuity* with which information is provided to the clinician and patient. Without biofeedback, clinicians must rely on palpation or visual inspection to determine if the appropriate muscles are being recruited or relaxed during an exercise. At best, the detection, processing, and formulation of a response by the health care

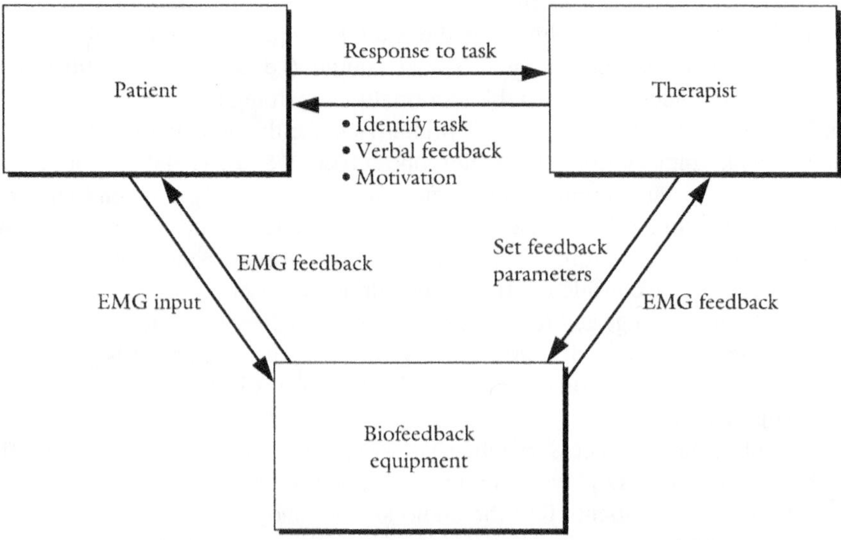

Figure 11.2. EMG feedback signal is used by both patient and therapist.

worker takes several hundred milliseconds. Given the ephemeral nature of most motor responses, by the time the patient receives and processes verbal or manual feedback from the clinician, the patient may be performing at a very different level than was originally perceived by the clinician. For feedback to be effective, it must be coincidental with the task that is to be modified. EMG biofeedback can be nearly instantaneous, thus reflecting the existing state of muscle contraction.

Related to the speed of processing information is the ability of the EMG biofeedback to provide continuous feedback. If verbal feedback requires several hundred milliseconds to be processed and presented to the patient, the fastest rate that verbal feedback could be updated and presented to the patient would be one to two times per second. In contrast, most biofeedback machines can inform patients of their responses in a nearly continuous manner.

The *sensitivity, objectivity, accuracy*, and *quantitative nature* of the feedback signal are also major advantages of EMG biofeedback. Only with biofeedback can relatively subtle changes in the recruitment of muscles be detected. Small changes in motor unit recruitment are particularly difficult to detect with palpation or visual inspection when patients are contracting at either high or low force levels. Knowledge of these subtle changes, however, may be necessary to allow patients to make appropriate changes in recruitment. For example, if a muscle contains relatively few active motor units, due to either a peripheral or central nervous system problem, the recruitment may not be sufficient to produce any joint displacement. The activity in the muscle would thus be very difficult to detect or quantify by the clinician without EMG biofeedback. The use of manual detection and verbal feedback to train motor unit recruitment may not reflect the true changes in the recruitment. Even if small increases in motor unit recruitment are produced, the clinician may not detect the change, and appropriate positive feedback may not be provided. Positive verbal reinforcement in the absence of additional recruitment during maximal effort is also ineffective in recruitment training. In contrast, EMG biofeedback is sensitive enough to detect small changes in the level of recruitment, and it accurately reflects the actual level of recruitment. EMG biofeedback is also not biased by the subject's effort. The quantitative nature of EMG feedback clearly shows which efforts increase recruitment and which efforts show less recruitment. The clinician can objectively observe which techniques or activities really help recruitment, and when the patient is beginning to fatigue.

Modern feedback devices can provide a variety of novel feedback signals that can motivate the patient. These signals range from the "raw" or unprocessed visual and auditory EMG signal, to tones whose frequencies increase or decrease in proportion to the level of EMG activity, to computer-controlled images on a video display terminal. In addition, biofeedback devices can be used to turn on or off other electronic devices, such as radios or tape recorders, which can be used as positive reinforcements for young children.

Despite the many applications of this tool, one common concern of clinicians is the perceived amount of time required to prepare the patient (e.g., prepare the skin and apply the electrodes) and perform the biofeedback training. Because of the time element, many clinicians who would agree that their patients would benefit from the information provided by EMG biofeedback are reluctant to use the modality. Given the present quality of amplifiers and filters used in most biofeedback devices, and the availability of disposable self-adhering electrodes, the time required for skin preparation and electrode application is minimal. In fact, recording an EMG from a subject may begin in as little as 1 minute after the individual is seated at a table. Furthermore, specific training objectives can generally be reached faster with biofeedback than without. Admittedly, some initial patient training is required to explain the purpose of the equipment. However, the information provided by most feedback signals is so intuitive to most patients that long explanations are usually not necessary. A simple demonstration using an uninvolved muscle of the patient is usually sufficient.

CURRENT CLINICAL APPLICATIONS

EMG biofeedback is one of the best researched tools currently used in rehabilitation. Publications began appearing in the early 1960s supporting the use of EMG biofeedback in physical rehabilitation. The rate of publication reached its peak in the late 1970s and began to decline by the mid-1980s (6–8). Although the most thoroughly investigated application of EMG biofeedback involves the treatment of patients after CVAs (8,9), numerous reports exist for the treatment of a plethora of conditions, including spinal cord injuries, cerebral palsy, spastic torticollis, peripheral nerve injuries, musculoskeletal pain, and incontinence. There is a range of evidence to support the clinical efficacy of EMG biofeedback. We will discuss the evidence for those applications that have been most rigorously studied; however, a thorough review of each of the above noted applications is beyond the scope of this chapter. Instead, the interested reader is referred to a number of related textbooks or review articles (1,10–15).

The most commonly studied applications of EMG biofeedback are in the treatment of patients with motor impairments resulting from central nervous system dysfunction. Several recent meta-analyses using randomized, controlled or matched group trials found improvement in measures such as muscle strength, gait, and functional outcome scores (11,13,14) when using EMG biofeedback following a CVA. In contrast, other than showing an increase in the ability of patients to increase motor unit recruitment, there is little evidence currently available showing any advantage in using EMG biofeedback versus conventional therapy in improving function in patients with partial paralysis resulting from spinal cord injuries (16–20).

Another problem for which EMG biofeedback has been often studied is training patients to relax hyperactive muscles that are producing pain. The effectiveness of EMG biofeedback was recently evaluated in a meta-analysis using controlled and uncontrolled trials for the treatment of patients with temporomandibular pain (10). The authors concluded that the available data support the efficacy of EMG biofeedback treatments for temporomandibular dysfunction; 69% of patients who received EMG biofeedback treatments became symptom-free or significantly improved versus 35% of patients treated with a variety of placebo interventions. In addition, the patients receiving EMG biofeedback showed no deterioration from post-treatment levels at follow-up. Relaxation training with the help of EMG biofeedback has also been used in the treatment of patients with chronic pain. Studies evaluating the efficacy of EMG biofeedback relaxation training demonstrate the short-term efficacy of EMG biofeedback relaxation strategies (21,22); however, the evidence is less conclusive with respect to the long-term benefits (22). A meta-analysis comparing treatment options for people with recurrent tension headache found that EMG biofeedback relaxation training was superior to no treatment (23). However, Bogaards and ter Kuile (23) noted that subject characteristics such as duration of symptoms and age were negatively related to treatment outcome (23).

The use of EMG biofeedback to increase recruitment of the quadriceps femoris muscles of patients that have recently had knee surgery has also been evaluated (24,25). Biofeedback can be very helpful in quickly training a patient to perform an isometric contraction of the quadriceps femoris muscle with the knee in full extension and produce greater quadriceps femoris muscle recruitment during dynamic exercise. Additionally, investigators have also used EMG biofeedback to promote relaxation of the quadriceps femoris during anterior tibial translation testing following ligamentous injury (26).

Finally, EMG biofeedback has been studied as an adjunct to the rehabilitation of patients with urinary incontinence. A recent meta-analysis concluded that biofeedback may be a useful adjunct to the treatment of patients with incontinence (15). In addition, several nonrandomized, controlled trials have suggested that this modality may be clinically useful, and it has been shown to improve pelvic floor strength, incontinence, and performance on cough stress tests (27–33).

GUIDELINES FOR SELECTION OF APPROPRIATE PATIENTS

There are several considerations that each clinician must take into account before using EMG biofeedback. The first question that should be answered is whether the patient's motor impairment would benefit from biofeedback. Furthermore, the patient must demonstrate the ability for voluntary control (e.g., a palpable contraction). For biofeedback training to be appropriate, the patient must have the ability to control the targeted muscle. The inappropriateness of the use of biofeedback training with patients with complete spinal cord injuries or complete peripheral nerve impairment before reinnervation by the peripheral nerve is obvious. Other conditions may not make the selection of appropriate patients so apparent. Wolf and Binder-Macleod (34) demonstrated that in a group of patients who had sustained CVAs at least 1 year before treatment, only patients who demonstrated voluntary finger extension before the initiation of therapy showed any improvement in hand function as a result of 60 sessions using EMG biofeedback. That is, none of the patients who were unable to perform active finger extension before commencement of training demonstrated any improvement as a result of treatment. This suggests that at least a minimum amount of voluntary control must be present for patients to use biofeedback to improve their function. However, several of these patients who lacked even minimum finger extension did show improvement in shoulder, elbow, and wrist function.

Typically, the advantages of this "faster learning" with the use of EMG biofeedback is most easily demonstrated in patients who have intact nervous systems, yet, due to a prior injury or trauma, are having a difficult time either recruiting or relaxing a specific muscle. As previously discussed, the use of EMG biofeedback with patients with impaired motor control due to central nervous system pathology is much more difficult to demonstrate (11–14,16,17).

In addition to having the ability to volitionally control a muscle, the patient must be motivated and have sufficient cognitive ability to learn to use the feedback signal. Training with the use of feedback is generally not a passive process; it requires the active participation of the patient. For example, a person who has sustained a traumatic brain injury and is not oriented to person, place, or time would not be able to sufficiently use any information provided by EMG biofeedback. However, one exception is when the clinician uses the EMG for his or her own feedback to determine the effectiveness of a particular intervention. For instance, a clinician may use a Swiss ball to help reduce the tone in a young child with cerebral palsy. EMG biofeedback could be used to provide quantitative information to the clinician about whether the specific techniques being used are actually producing the desired responses.

Thus far, only the appropriateness of EMG biofeedback has been discussed. Recently, other forms of feedback relevant to physical rehabilitation have been developed. Positional, force feedback, as well as EMG-activated functional electrical stimulation systems have also been included in the clinician's plan of care. In general, EMG biofeedback should be used when information regarding the activity of a specific muscle or muscle group is desired, such as the anterior tibialis muscle in a person exhibiting drop foot following a CVA. Additionally, if patients are very weak and little force or joint displacement is produced, position or force feedback would not be sufficiently sensitive to provide any meaningful information for these patients. EMG biofeedback is also generally most appropriate in situations where training specific muscles to relax while patients perform a particular task is desired. In contrast, the training of a specific muscle or muscle group may not be appropriate when the patient is trying to perform a task that requires the coordination of multiple muscle groups. For instance, when training a child with cerebral palsy to maintain proper head position, head position feedback would be much more helpful than EMG feedback from any specific muscle group. Similarly, in training patients to shift their weight either onto or off of an involved lower extremity, force feedback, providing the exact amount of weight bearing by the involved extremity, is most appropriate.

DEVELOPMENT OF TRAINING STRATEGIES

Although the information provided through the use of EMG biofeedback generally motivates patients, because of its objective nature this information can be a source of frustration. Clinicians are therefore encouraged to consider all factors related to learning theory when developing their training strategies. Positive reinforcement is better than negative reinforcement when training patients. Obtainable short- and long-term goals must be clearly communicated to patients. Clinicians should listen to each patient to be certain that the established goals are important to him or her. Experience has shown that if patients are told to simply try their best, no matter how well they perform, they are always disappointed that they did not do better. In contrast, if specific tasks or goals are identified within and across sessions, then a real sense of accomplishment can be achieved. Tasks that demonstrate achievement of each goal must be specific enough so that the patient knows all of the relevant conditions, and the criteria must be specific enough so that the patient knows when the task is accomplished. One of the skills that the clinician must acquire is setting goals that are sufficiently difficult to challenge and motivate patients, but that are attainable within a specified time.

Several considerations need to be made regarding the *sequencing* or *progression* of any treatment program. As an example, when treating a patient who has sustained a CVA, clinicians must decide if it is better to train for relaxation of spastic muscles before training recruitment of a weak antagonist, or if training should begin directly with weak or poorly recruited muscles. Without the use of EMG biofeedback, exercises to train spastic muscles to relax are difficult to design and evaluate. As previously noted, the addition of EMG biofeedback makes monitoring and training spastic muscles much more objective and straightforward. For this reason, when using EMG biofeedback to train patients with disturbances in muscle tone, treatments have traditionally begun with training for relaxation of spastic muscles before working on recruitment of weak antagonist muscles (35–39). However, the need for targeted relaxation training has been questioned (40,41). Similar decisions regarding the progression of training need to be made concerning the choices to train (i) proximal muscles first and to then progress distally or to begin distally and progress proximally; (ii) stability first and then progress to mobility training or reverse this order; or (iii) component movements first and then integrate the components into a functional movement pattern, or to commence training with functional movement patterns. These, as well as other choices, need to be made by clinicians based on their own treatment philosophy and on objective research findings supporting various approaches to treatment.

The use of biofeedback requires several additional considerations regarding the progression of training. Should only one muscle group be monitored, or should a dual-channel system be used? When should the patient be weaned from using the feedback signal? After all, the goal of training is the performance of functional tasks without the use of biofeedback. Thus, the benefits of training with feedback need to be weighed against the long-term need to perform without feedback. One option would be to begin with a continuous feedback signal and progress to the use of some form of threshold feedback in an attempt to wean the patient from the need for any feedback.

What level of success should the patient demonstrate before increasing the level of difficulty? That is, does a patient have to reach a targeted level of recruitment 100% or 50% of the time before we raise the targeted microvolt level that the patient is to achieve? These questions must be answered during each training session. Unfortunately, little objective information is currently available to help clinicians answer these and other relevant questions.

The final strategy that will be considered is the *selection of appropriate sites for electrode placement.* To record an EMG, the recording electrodes must be placed over or near the belly of the relevant muscle. In contrast, the placement of the reference electrode is not as critical.

Some workers in this field have suggested that the reference electrode be placed equidistant from the two recording electrodes; however, the exact placement is not critical as long as good contact between the skin and electrode is maintained (4). Nevertheless, a number of factors, including goals of training, level of control, available muscle mass, subcutaneous fat, movement artifact, and cross-talk, must be considered when selecting the electrode sites. All of these factors interact, so it is impossible to determine the optimal electrode sites without considering all of them. As previously noted, the smaller the distance between the recording electrodes, the greater the specificity of the recording, and the less noise that is recorded. Also, the greater the distance of the recording electrodes to the active muscle, the greater the attenuation of the EMG. Thus, when placing electrodes over a muscle, the following requirements must be met:

1. Areas that have a thickened layer of adipose tissue must be avoided.
2. The distance between the recording electrodes and any muscles that are producing unwanted electrical activity (i.e., cross-talk) must be maximized.
3. The smallest interelectrode distance that is practical must be used.

As an example, if the clinician wants to record from the anterior tibialis muscle, it may be best to place the recording electrodes <1 cm apart and over the most medial aspect of the muscle (Fig. 11.3). This placement puts the recording electrodes over the targeted muscle, while still being as far away as possible from other active muscles that may contaminate the intended feedback signal.

Also, the electrodes should be placed over the muscle when the limb is in the position that it will assume when the patient is performing the exercise. If a patient supinates his or her forearm while electrodes are placed over the forearm flexor muscle mass, but then pronates his or her forearm during training, the electrodes may no longer be lying over the flexors; rather, the electrodes may now be over the brachioradialis muscle. In addition, electrodes and unshielded lead wires should be placed in a position so that they will not be jostled during training. This prevents movement artifact from contaminating the feedback signal.

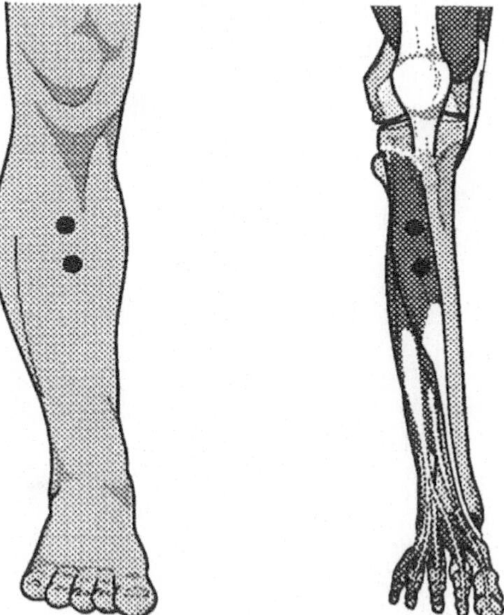

Figure 11.3. Placement of electrodes for recording anterior tibialis muscle.

Within limits, if a patient has poor control over a muscle, the interelectrode distance can be used to advantage by sampling a larger or smaller area of the muscle. If a patient has difficulty recruiting from any of the heads of the quadriceps femoris muscle, training may begin using a relatively wide spacing to sample from a large portion of the muscle. However, care should be taken that the spacing is not so wide that activity from the hip adductor or hamstring muscles is erroneously fed back to the patient. As the patient's control increases, closer spacing may be used to monitor individual heads of the quadriceps femoris muscle. In contrast, if a patient displays spasticity and the goal is to train for relaxation of finger and wrist flexors during passive stretch of the muscle to maintain range of motion, training should begin with electrodes relatively closely spaced, so as to limit the recording area. As the patient gains better control, a slightly wider spacing could be used to sample more of the forearm flexor muscle mass.

CLINICAL CASE STUDIES

Case 1

History, Tests, and Measures

The patient is a 35-year-old male from India who contracted poliomyelitis at age 7. He has never received physical therapy. He now has severe foot-drop on the right side and wears a short leg brace (SLB). He is highly motivated and would like to strengthen his ankle dorsiflexors to shed his brace. Electrodiagnostic testing reveals several small motor units present in his anterior tibialis and extensor digitorum longus muscles. No visible contraction of any of his ankle dorsiflexors can be observed. Passive range of motion is intact.

Guide to Physical Therapist Practice

Preferred practice pattern: 5A, "Impaired Motor Function and Sensory Integrity Associated with Congenital or Acquired Disorders of the Central Nervous System in Infancy, Childhood, and Adolescence."

Assessment

This patient has impaired ankle dorsiflexor strength and a gait deviation. According to *Guide to Physical Therapist Practice*, biofeedback may be implemented to address strength and gait.

Plan

1. Initial treatment in the clinic using EMG biofeedback to work on increased motor unit recruitment.
2. Assess progress and evaluate the patient for use of portable EMG biofeedback for independent home training.
3. After visible contractions can be produced, begin a resistive strengthening program.

Detailed Treatment Plan

Mode of feedback: initially provide both auditory and visual EMG biofeedback. Make the transition to auditory feedback before gait training with the feedback.

Short-term goal of training: increase EMG from targeted muscles. Will set specific targeted levels of recruitment to encourage an increase in the discharge rate of already active motor units and to attempt the recruitment of additional motor units.

Electrode placement: over the ankle dorsiflexor muscles, placed anteriorly about 5 cm distal to the lateral joint line. Second electrode placed 15–20 cm superior to the lateral malleolus. Could monitor the plantiflexors for cross-talk.

Duration of each treatment session: to patient tolerance. When EMG recruitment levels begin to decline, the patient is fatiguing. Allow the patient to rest. When recovery from fatigue is incomplete, terminate treatment.

Case 2

The patient is a 56-year-old female who has been referred to physical therapy for range-of-motion exercises for her right upper extremity. The patient sustained a Colle fracture of her right wrist approximately 6 months ago and maintained her entire right arm nearly totally immobilized for the first 6 weeks while in her cast. After removal of her cast, the patient presented with marked limitation in all active movements of her right shoulder, elbow, forearm, and wrist. The patient was then briefly instructed in an exercise program and followed by her surgeon. Due to a lack of progress in range of motion, the patient underwent a closed manipulation under anesthesia 2 weeks ago. The surgeon's report indicates that the patient was able to achieve nearly full passive range of motion in all joints.

The patient is alert, pleasant, and cooperative, though obviously quite apprehensive. As you begin your evaluation, you note marked splinting at all joints during all active or passive movements. Both active and passive range of motion of the finger joints, wrist, elbow, and shoulder are markedly reduced.

Guide to Physical Therapist Practice

Preferred practice pattern 4E, "Impaired Joint Mobility, Muscle Performance, and Range of Motion Associated with Ligament or Other Connective Tissue Disorders."

Assessment

This patient's lack of both active and passive range of motion are likely due to her inability to relax and to splinting of the upper extremity. She is a good candidate for EMG biofeedback for targeted muscle training.

Plan

1. EMG biofeedback to promote relaxation and decrease splinting during passive range of motion to all affected joints.
2. Compare EMG from involved and uninvolved upper extremities during active range of motion exercises to assess recruitment pattern
3. Train appropriate muscle groups to produce more "normal" recruitment levels during active range of motion.
4. Progress to functional training using EMG biofeedback to help normalize movement.

Detailed Treatment Plan

Mode of feedback: initially provide both auditory and visual EMG biofeedback. Then have the patient use the signal that is most effective.

Short-term goal of training: to have the patient display similar recruitment patterns from comparable involved and uninvolved muscle groups during passive and active movements. Will set specific targeted levels of recruitment to train for either relaxation or recruitment.

Electrode placement: over the targeted muscles. Narrow interelectrode distance to increase recording specificity.

Duration of each treatment session: use EMG to indicate tolerance. When the patient begins to show decreasing ability to recruit or relax muscles, terminate treatment to prevent patient frustration.

Case 3

The patient is a 24-year-old graduate student referred by her dentist for pain due to temporomandibular joint dysfunction. She reported that her pain begins after working on her computer for more than 30 minutes and worsens with prolonged computer use. She has no pain upon waking in the morning. The dentist also indicated that the patient has significant wear on her teeth for someone her age. Upon examination, the patient reports tenderness to palpation bilaterally at the temporomandibular joint and over the masseter and temporalis muscles. Joint mobility is unrestricted bilaterally. The patient is concerned her pain will continue to worsen and is eager to begin treatment.

Guide to Physical Therapist Practice

Preferred practice pattern 4E, "Impaired Joint Mobility, Muscle Performance, and Range of Motion Associated with Ligament or Other Connective Tissue Disorders."

Assessment

This patient's pain is likely due to hyperactivity of the muscles of mastication at rest. She is a good candidate for targeted EMG biofeedback relaxation training and re-education.

Plan

1. EMG biofeedback to demonstrate relaxation of the masseter and temporalis muscles at rest.
2. Train appropriate muscle activation during active range of motion.
3. Progress to relaxation training during functional training (e.g., computer use).

Detailed Plan

Mode of feedback: initially provide both auditory and visual EMG biofeedback. Then have the patient use the signal that is most effective.

Short-term goal of training: patient will demonstrate relaxation of the masseter and temporalis muscles bilaterally at rest, and appropriate recruitment during functional activities. The patient will also demonstrate decreased pain levels when using her computer.

Electrode placement: directly over the muscle bellies of the masseter and temporarilis bilaterally. Will need to target one muscle group at a time.

Duration of each treatment session: use the EMG to indicate tolerance, initially 15–20 minutes in the physical therapy clinic. If the patient demonstrates decreasing ability to recruit or relax muscles or begins to report pain, terminate the session. Progress to training at home while using the computer.

Case 4

The patient is a 78-year-old female who sustained a right CVA 2 months ago and has been referred to the outpatient physical therapy clinic for residual left-upper-extremity weakness. She is alert and oriented to person, place, time, and situation. Upon examination, it is determined she has full passive range of motion of her wrist, elbow, and shoulder, with no evidence of shoulder subluxation. However, wrist extension active range of motion is limited to 20 degrees. Finger-extension active range of motion is also lacking, being 50 degrees at the metacarpal phalangeal (MP) and interphalangeal (IP) joints. When electrical stimulation is applied to the wrist and finger extensors, full active range of motion is achieved. Although the patient is right-hand dominant, her goal is to be able to cook dinner for herself using her involved upper extremity and she is very motivated to begin treatment.

Guide to Physical Therapist Practice

Preferred practice pattern 5B, "Impaired Motor Function and Sensory Integrity Associated with Acquired Nonprogressive Disorders of the Central Nervous System in Adulthood."

Assessment

The patient's inability to actively extend her wrist and fingers is not due to strength deficits alone, because she demonstrates full active range of motion with electrical stimulation. Her inability to perform full active wrist and finger extension is the result of decreased recruitment of the wrist and finger extensors. She would benefit from EMG biofeedback for targeted recruitment of these muscles.

Plan

1. Initial treatment in the clinic using EMG biofeedback to work on increased motor recruitment.
2. Assess and evaluate the patient for use of portable EMG biofeedback for home use.
3. Incorporate the EMG biofeedback into functional activities (e.g., cooking).
4. Once the patient demonstrates full active range of motion, begin resistive exercises.

Detailed Treatment Plan

Mode of feedback: initially provide both auditory and visual EMG biofeedback. Make the transition to auditory feedback during use with functional activities.

Short-term goal of training: increase the EMG from targeted muscles. Will set specific targeted levels of recruitment to encourage an increase in the discharge rate of already active motor units and to attempt the recruitment of additional motor units.

Electrode placement: superior electrode placed 3 to 5 cm distal to the lateral epicondyle on the dorsal forearm. Distal electrode placed on the dorsal mid forearm (10 to 12 cm proximal to the wrist). Narrow the interelectrode distance to increase specificity.

Duration of each treatment session: to patient tolerance. When EMG recruitment levels begin to decline, the patient is fatiguing; allow time for rest. Treatment should be terminated when recovery from fatigue is not complete.

SUMMARY

The EMG can be used by both clinicians and patients to help provide information regarding the activation state of a muscle. EMG biofeedback is a valuable tool that should be considered by clinicians whenever a patient displays poor volitional motor control. Although a number of technical and practical considerations need to be taken into account when using EMG biofeedback, this tool can easily be incorporated into most traditional treatment approaches.

SELF-STUDY QUESTIONS

For answers, see Appendix B.

1. Define EMG biofeedback training.
2. Discuss the advantages of EMG biofeedback over simple verbal feedback.
3. Identify the specific characteristics of a patient that would suggest an appropriate use of EMG biofeedback
4. How might the use of EMG biofeedback be helpful to the clinician if a patient does not demonstrate the ability to cognitively process the information obtained during the task?
5. Review the physiological factors that determine the amplitude of the raw EMG.
6. Identify the relationship between both the size and interelectrode distance of the recording electrodes to the amplitude and specificity of the EMG.
7. Define cross-talk.
8. Discuss the advantages and disadvantages of the use of subcutaneous electrodes during EMG biofeedback.
9. Define movement artifact.
10. During filtering of the EMG, why is it necessary to restrict the frequency range of the signal that has passed through the amplifier?
11. List each step in the processing of the EMG feedback signal.
12. What are the types of feedback signals the clinician can choose from when using EMG biofeedback?
13. Discuss the advantages and limitations of using the raw EMG during biofeedback training.
14. Identify the factors that need to be considered in selecting appropriate sites for electrode placement.
15. What requirements should be met when determining electrode placement?
16. What limitation does EMG biofeedback training present when used with a patient who has sustained neurological impairment?
17. During the performance of a task by a patient, should positive or negative feedback be used?
18. The clinician determines that a patient would benefit from improving knee extension during the stance phase of gait. What factors related to goal setting need to be made clear to the patient before starting EMG biofeedback training?

19. What advantages does EMG biofeedback have over devices that monitor position of the desired extremity?

20. What is the desired goal upon completion of EMG biofeedback training?

REFERENCES

1. Basmajian JV. Introduction. Principles and background. In: Basmajian JV, ed. *Biofeedback: Principles and Practices for Clinicians.* 3rd ed. Baltimore, Md: Williams & Wilkins; 1989:1–4.
2. Lippold OCJ. The relationship between integrated action potential in a human muscle and its isometric tension. *J Physiol.* 1952;117:492–499.
3. Bigland B, Lippold OCJ. The relation between force, velocity and integrated electrical activity in human muscles. *J Physiol.* 1954;123:214–224.
4. Basmajian JV, Blumenstein R. Electrode placement in electromyographic biofeedback. In: Basmajian JV, ed. *Biofeedback: Principles and Practices for Clinicians.* 3rd ed. Baltimore, Md: Williams & Wilkins; 1989:369–382.
5. Clamann HP, Lamp RL. A simple circuit for filtering single motor unit action potentials for electrograms. *Physiol Behav.* 1976;17:149–151.
6. Hatch JP, Saito I. Growth and development of biofeedback: a bibliographic update. *Biofeedback Self Regul.* 1990;15:37–46.
7. Hatch JP, Saito I. Declining rates of publications within the field of biofeedback continue: 1988–1991. *Biofeedback Self Regul.* 1993;18:174.
8. Wolf SL. Electromyographic biofeedback applications to stroke patients: a critical review. *Phys Ther.* 1983;63:1448–1459.
9. Basmajian JV. Research foundations of EMG biofeedback in rehabilitation. *Biofeedback Self Regul.* 1988;13:275–298.
10. Crider AB, Glaros AG. A meta-analysis of EMG biofeedback treatment of temporomandibular disorders. *J Orofacial Pain.* 1999;13:29–37.
11. Glanz M, Klawansky S, Stason W, et al. Biofeedback therapy in poststroke rehabilitation: a meta-analysis of the randomized controlled trials. *Arch Phys Med Rehabil.* 1995;76:508–515.
12. Glanz M. Biofeedback therapy in stroke rehabilitation: a review. *J R Soc Med.* 1997;90:33–39.
13. Moreland JD, Thomson MA, Fuoco AR. Electromyographic biofeedback to improve lower extremity function after stroke: a meta-analysis. *Arch Phys Med Rehabil.* 1998;79:134–140.
14. Schleenbaker RE, Mainous AG. Electromyographic biofeedback for neuromuscular reeducation in the hemiplegic stroke patient: a meta-analysis. *Arch Phys Med Rehabil.* 1993;74:1301–1304.
15. Weatherall M. Biofeedback or pelvic floor muscle exercises for female genuine stress incontinence: a meta-analysis of trials identified in a systematic review. *Br J Urol Int.* 1999;83:1015–1016.
16. Brucker BS, Bulaeva NV. Biofeedback effect on electromyography responses in patients with spinal cord injury. *Arch Phys Med Rehabil.* 1996;77:133–137.
17. Kohlmeyer KM, Hill JP, Yarkony GM, et al. Electrical stimulation and biofeedback effect on recovery of tenodesis grasp: a controlled study. *Arch Phys Med Rehabil.* 1996;77:702–706.
18. Klose KJ, Needham BM, Schmidt D, et al. An assessment of the contribution of electromyographic biofeedback as an adjunct therapy in the physical training of spinal cord injured persons. *Arch Phys Med Rehabil.* 1993;74:453–456.
19. Klose KJ, Schmidt D, Needham BM, et al. Rehabilitation therapy for patients with long-term spinal cord injuries. *Arch Phys Med Rehabil.* 1990;71:659–662.
20. Petrofsky JS. The use of electromyogram biofeedback to reduce Trendelenburg gait. *Eur J Appl Physiol.* 2001;85:491–495.

21. Flor H, Birbaumer N. Comparison of the efficacy of electromyographic biofeedback, cognitive-behavioral therapy, and conservative medical interventions in the treatment of chronic musculoskeletal pain. *J Consult Clin Psychol.* 1993;61:653–658.

22. Spence SH, Sharpe L, Newton-John T, et al. Effect of EMG biofeedback compared to applied relaxation training with chronic, upper extremity cumulative trauma disorders. *Pain.* 1995;63:199–206.

23. Bogaards MC, ter Kuile MM. Treatment of recurrent tension headache: a meta-analytic review. *Clin J Pain.* 1994;10:174–190.

24. Draper V. Electromyographic biofeedback and recovery of quadriceps femoris muscle function following anterior cruciate ligament reconstruction. *Phys Ther.* 1990;70:11–17.

25. Krebs DE. Clinical electromyographic feedback following menisectomy. A multiple regression experimental analysis. *Phys Ther.* 1981;61:1017–1021.

26. Feller J, Hoser C, Webster K. EMG biofeedback assisted KT-1000 evaluation of anterior tibial displacement. *Knee Surg Sports Traumatol Arthrosc.* 2000;8:132–136.

27. Dattilo J. A long-term study of patient outcomes with pelvic muscle re-education for urinary incontinence. *J Wound Ostomy Continence Nurs* 28(4):199–205.

28. Hirsch A, Weirauch G, Steimer B, et al. Treatment of female urinary incontinence with EMG-controlled biofeedback home training. *Int Urogynecol J.* 1999;10:7–10.

29. Jundt K, Peschers UM, Dimpfl T. Long-term efficacy of pelvic floor re-education with EMG-controlled biofeedback. *Eur J Obstet Gynecol Reprod Biol.* 2002;105:181–185.

30. Berghmans, LM, Frederiks de Bie RA, Weil EJ, et al. Efficacy of biofeedback, when included with pelvic floor muscle exercise treatment, for genuine stress incontinence. *Neurourol Urodynam.* 1996;15:37–52.

31. Burns PA, Pranikoff K, Nochajski TH, et al. A comparison of effectiveness of biofeedback and pelvic muscle exercise treatment of stress incontinence in older community-dwelling women. *J Gerontol.* 1993;48:M167–M174.

32. Glavind K, Nohr SB, Walter S. Biofeedback and physiotherapy versus physiotherapy alone in the treatment of genuine stress urinary incontinence. *Int Urogynecol J Pelvic Floor Dysfunct.* 1996;7:339–343.

33. Morkved S, Bo K, Fjortoft T. Effect of adding biofeedback to pelvic floor muscle training to treat urodynamic stress incontinence. *Am J Obstet Gynecol.* 2002;100:730–738.

34. Wolf SL, Binder-Macleod SA. Electromyographic biofeedback applications to the hemiplegic patient: changes in upper extremity neuromuscular and functional status. *Phys Ther.* 1983;63:1393–1403.

35. Wolf SL, Binder-Macleod SA. Electromyographic biofeedback applications to the hemiplegic patient: changes in lower extremity neuromuscular and functional status. *Phys Ther.* 1983;63:1404–1413.

36. Baker MP, Regenos E, Wolf SL. Developing strategies for biofeedback: applications in neurologically handicapped clients. *Phys Ther.* 1977;57:402–408.

37. Binder SA, Moll CB, Wolf SL. Evaluation of EMG biofeedback as an adjunct to therapeutic exercise in treating the lower extremities of hemiplegic patients. *Phys Ther.* 1981;61:886–893.

38. Brudny J, Korein J, Grynbaum BB, et al. Sensory feedback therapy in clients with brain insult. *Scand J Rehabil Med.* 1977;9:155–163.

39. Kelly JL, Baker MP, Wolf SL. Procedures for EMG biofeedback training in involved upper extremities of hemiplegic patients. *Phys Ther.* 1979;59:1501–1507.

40. Gowland C, de Bruin H, Basmajian JV, et al. Agonist and antagonist activity during voluntary upper-limb movement in patients with stroke. *Phys Ther.* 1992;72:624–633.

41. Wolf SL, Catlin PA, Blanton S, et al. Overcoming limitations in elbow movement in the presence of antagonist hyperactivity. *Phys Ther.* 1994;74:826–835.

CHAPTER 12

Clinical Electrophysiologic Examination and Evaluation: Principles, Procedures, and Interpretation of Findings

Andrew J. Robinson, with Case Studies Provided by Robert M. Kellogg

Clinical electrophysiological examination and evaluation consists of the recording, analysis, and interpretation of bioelectrical activity of muscle and nerve in response to volitional activation or electrical stimulation. Clinical electrophysiologic evaluation is also called *electroneuromyography* (ENMG). The process of electrophysiologic evaluation includes the performance of a wide array of tests. The results of ENMG tests are integrated with clinical measurements, laboratory findings, imaging studies, and symptomatology to establish a diagnosis and to make plans for subsequent care. Electrophysiologic test results viewed in isolation are not characteristic or indicative of specific diseases or disorders. That is, ENMG findings alone will not establish the diagnosis associated with existing pathology, but will supplement findings from other clinical and laboratory tests used in differential diagnosis.

The main purpose of ENMG is to determine the functional integrity of nerve or muscle. Special testing procedures are available for examining alpha motoneurons and their axons, neuromuscular junctions, skeletal muscles, motor units, peripheral sensory nerve fibers, stretch reflex pathways, and selected central nervous system pathways. Electroneuromyographic examination of these structures and pathways may help the practitioner determine the location, magnitude, distribution, and duration of neuromuscular compromise.

The objectives of this chapter are to (i) discuss the instrumentation and recording procedures used in electrophysiologic examination procedures; (ii) describe specific modern and traditional approaches of ENMG testing; (iii) discuss the normal and abnormal results of ENMG tests; (iv) briefly describe supplemental clinical tests of neuromuscular function; and (v) present clinical case studies to illustrate the usefulness of understanding ENMG procedures and findings in establishing a diagnosis. Emphasis is placed on illustrating how the electrophysiologic tests results can be interpreted to establish the location and nature of the neuromuscular disorder. This chapter is intended to provide enough information for readers to develop an understanding of how ENMG is performed, to understand what components of the neuromuscular system can be examined by different tests, and to appreciate the significance and limitations of test results. The chapter explains how to read and understand an ENMG report derived from testing and how to integrate the findings of the report with those from tests within a particular area of clinical expertise. Competence in the actual performance of ENMG procedures cannot be achieved by a rudimentary understanding of the information presented in this chapter. Readers familiar with the instrumentation and concepts of stimulation and recording nerve and muscle activity may wish to proceed immediately to the section of this chapter on procedures of electrophysiologic evaluation.

EXTRACELLULAR RECORDING VERSUS INTRACELLULAR RECORDING TECHNIQUES

Bioelectrical responses of excitable tissue during volitional or electrical activation are nerve and muscle action potentials. When muscle or nerve fibers are depolarized to threshold, action potentials (characteristic changes in transmembrane voltage) are propagated along their membranes. The action potentials result from sodium ions moving into these cells while potassium ions flow out of the cells. This process sweeps along the membrane from the point of initiation in a process called propagation. As a result of the transmembrane ionic fluxes associated with the action potential, changes occur in the concentration of ions in the fluids surrounding these tissues. These ionic movements and resultant transmembrane potential changes that occur in single nerve cells are monitored in research laboratory experiments on very large axons by actually penetrating the excitable cell membrane with a glass microelectrode and placing a second recording (reference) electrode outside the cell. Such a system to monitor action potentials with one intracellular and one extracellular recording electrode (Fig. 12.1A) monitors the transmembrane electrical potential differences produced when ions move through the membrane. This *intracellular recording technique* cannot be used on the nerve and muscle cells of humans in clinical electrophysiologic examination because these cells are too small and cannot be stabilized sufficiently.

Clinical ENMG requires the use of extracellular as opposed to intracellular recording techniques to monitor the electrical activity in nerve and/or muscle fibers. In the *extracellular recording technique*, two small conductors (called recording electrodes) are placed near but outside nerve or muscle cells (Fig. 12.1B). The electrodes are then connected by wires to an electronic device that amplifies and displays the relative voltage (electrical potential difference) between the two electrodes. When no action potentials are transmitted along excitable cells, the concentration of ions beneath each of the electrodes is approximately equal, and the voltage difference between the electrodes is zero. However, when action potential currents are propagated along nerve or muscle membranes, the relative concentration of ions beneath each of the electrodes changes over time, and electrical potential differences are recorded.

To understand the origin of extracellular voltage changes recorded during nerve or muscle excitation, consider a situation where action potentials are activated simultaneously and propagated

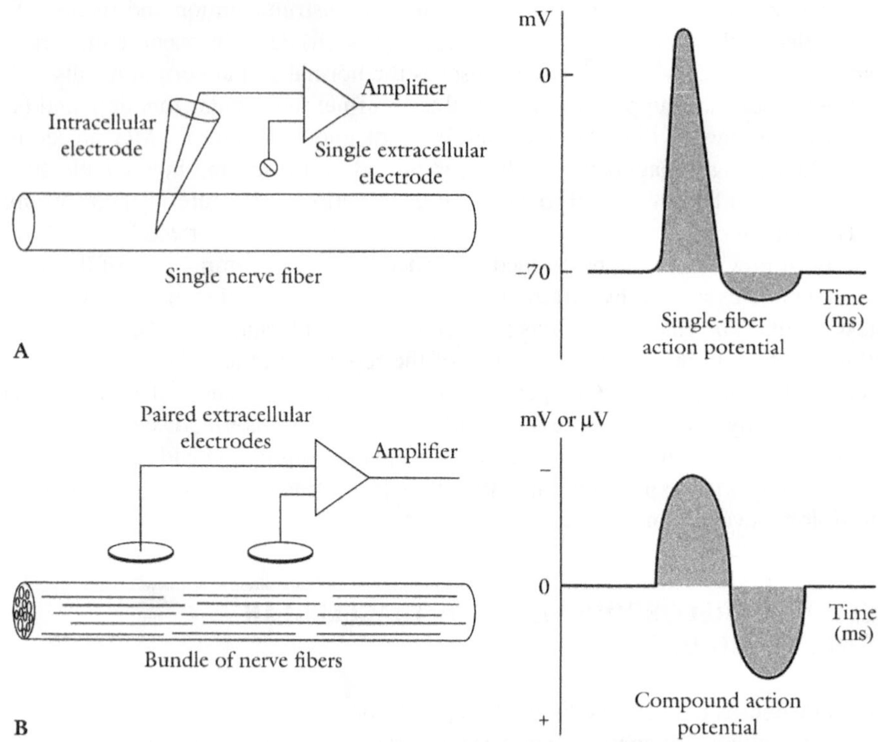

Figure 12.1. A: Illustration of intracellular recording technique showing one electrode inside a nerve or muscle cell and a second electrode outside the cell and the changes in transmembrane potential associated with a single nerve fiber action potential. **B:** Illustration of the extracellular recording technique showing both recording electrodes outside of the nerve or muscle fibers and the compound action potential recorded as action potentials sweep along the bundle of nerve or muscle fibers.

along a bundle of nerve fibers. As positively charged sodium rushes into the nerve fibers away from the first of the recording electrodes, the region beneath the electrode becomes more negative (less positive) than the area beneath the second recording electrode (Fig. 12.2A). An instant later, the potassium leaves the fibers beneath the first electrode while sodium is rushing into the fibers between the two electrodes. At this instant, the concentration of ions beneath each electrode is about the same, and the electrical potential difference between the electrodes falls to zero (Fig. 12.2B). An instant later, as the inward sodium currents sweep beneath the region of the second electrode, the relative difference in voltage between the two electrodes becomes reversed. That is, the first electrode "sees" a higher concentration of positive ions than the second electrode because sodium is now rushing into the cell at the second electrode. Hence the relative voltage difference between electrodes is positive (Fig. 12.2C). This characteristic set of voltage changes recorded near bundles of nerve fibers is called a *compound nerve action potential* (CNAP). When this response is initiated by synchronous activation of alpha motoneuron axons and recorded from a group of muscle fibers, the response is called a *compound muscle action potential* (CMAP).

The extracellular recording technique differs from the intracellular approach in that extracellular electrodes are used to monitor the electrical activity in many nerve axons or muscle fibers, whereas the intracellular technique only monitors the electrical activity in a single fiber. Hence, the electrical signals recorded are referred to as compound nerve or muscle action potentials. Compound nerve and muscle action potentials can be characterized by their shape,

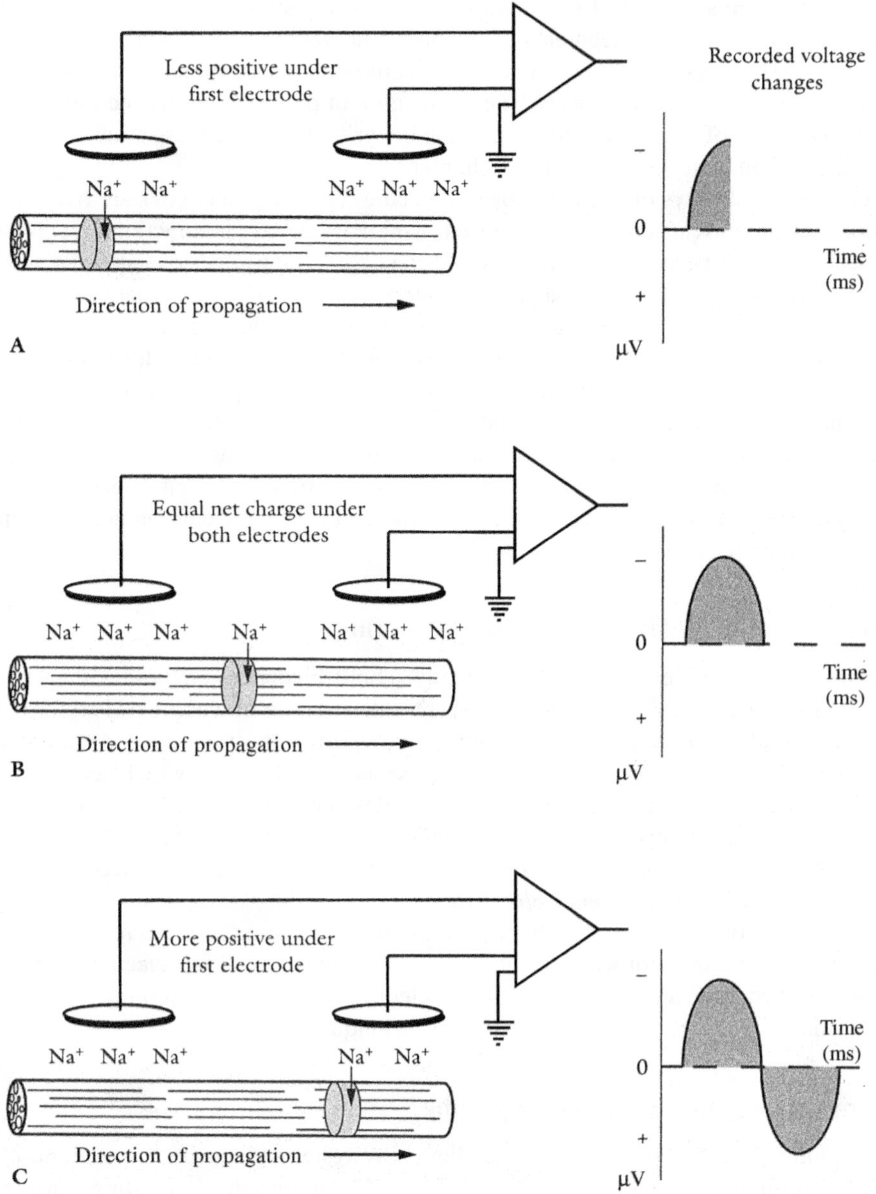

Figure 12.2. Extracellular voltage changes (compound nerve or muscle action potentials). **A:** Sodium ions rush into nerve fibers beneath the first electrode, leaving the area more negative (fewer positive sodium ions) than the area beneath the second electrode. **B:** Sodium ions move into nerve fibers between the two electrodes and concentrations of ions beneath each electrode are the same. **C:** Sodium ions rush into nerve fibers beneath the second electrode, leaving the area beneath the first electrode more positive (more sodium ions) than the area beneath the second electrode.

amplitude, and duration. Also, the time delay (latency) between the electrical stimulus applied at one point along a nerve and the appearance of the compound evoked potential in nerve or muscle can be measured. Measurements of these parameters obtained during electrophysiologic examination can be compared with established normal values to differentiate among conditions including denervation, demyelination, conduction block, and/or axonal loss.

With appropriate selection of stimulation and recording sites, information can be obtained about the function of different segments of peripheral nerves, neuromuscular junctions, skeletal muscles, reflex pathways, anterior horn cells (alpha motoneurons), spinal nerve roots, and even some central nervous system pathways. The application of the extracellular recording technique and selected patterns of stimulation for testing the integrity of each of these structures in humans are detailed in subsequent segments of this chapter.

In clinical electrophysiologic examination, needle recording electrodes are frequently used to monitor skeletal muscle activity in response to voluntary muscle contraction. In contrast, routine clinical testing of peripheral nerves is performed by placing surface electrodes on the skin over a nerve or muscle innervated by a particular nerve. In spite of the fact that needle electrodes are actually inserted into skeletal muscle, the tips of these needles are actually between rather than within muscle fibers, and hence are extracellular. At times, needle electrodes are used to record the electrical activity in peripheral nerves or stimulate peripheral nerves, but these electrodes are placed near peripheral nerve bundles rather than penetrating the nerve bundle.

In all extracellular recording procedures, a third surface electrode is attached to the skin and is connected to the testing unit's electrical ground. This electrode, referred to as the *ground electrode*, is required to reduce electrical artifact generated in tissues by environmental electromagnetic fields.

Monopolar versus Bipolar Extracellular Recording

When using the extracellular recording technique, both recording electrodes may be placed either over or in the excitable tissue monitored. This positioning of electrodes is referred to as a *bipolar recording electrode placement*. Alternatively, only one recording electrode may be placed near the excitable tissue examined, and the second electrode may be placed at some distance from the excitable tissue. Electrode positioning in this manner is referred to as *monopolar recording electrode placement.* In monopolar electrodes setups, the electrode directly over or within the tissue of interest is called the *active electrode*, and the electrode placed away from the excitable tissue is called the *reference electrode*.

The closer the two recording electrodes are to each other and to the nerve or muscle examined, the smaller the area from which electrical potential change will be detected. Consequently, the bipolar electrode arrangements will sense electrical activity in excitable tissues from a smaller volume of tissue than will the monopolar technique.

Electromyography and Electroneurography

Compound muscle action potentials may be elicited by voluntary activation of the muscle or by electrically stimulating motor nerve axons to a particular muscle. Recording muscle action potentials that occur spontaneously or as the result of volitional or stimulated activation using an extracellular recording technique is called *electromyography*. An individual record of CMAPs generally recorded during volitional contraction or electrically elicited contraction of muscle is called an *electromyogram* (EMG).

Compound nerve action potentials may be elicited by electrical stimulation. For example, in electrophysiological examination, nerve action potentials may be evoked by electrical stimulation in the cutaneous distribution of the sensory nerve, and the evoked peripheral sensory potentials are monitored using the extracellular surface recording technique over peripheral nerves at some point remote to the site of stimulation. In more sophisticated procedures, extracellular recordings of compound nerve action potentials are made by placing electrodes over the surface of the brain or spinal cord. Recording nerve action potentials is called *electroneurography*, and the record of the nerve action potentials is called an *electroneurogram*.

INSTRUMENTATION FOR ELECTROPHYSIOLOGIC EXAMINATION AND EVALUATION

A basic understanding of the equipment and materials used in ENMG provides a clearer understanding of what is actually done in electrophysiologic examination in order to gain insight into the integrity of the neuromuscular system. For those interested in developing expertise in the clinical application of ENMG procedures, an understanding of the characteristics of electrodes and controls of ENMG instrument components is essential for the safe and effective implementation of testing procedures, as well as accurate interpretation of test findings.

Types of Recording Electrodes in Electrophysiological Examination

In monitoring the responses of excitable tissues to voluntary or evoked activation, compound nerve and muscle action potentials are recorded via recording electrodes. The physiologic response to stimulation is recorded as a voltage change by the recording electrodes. The placement of the recording electrodes, their orientation, contact area, shape, and composition may influence the size and shape of the recorded responses.

Surface Recording Electrodes

Surface recording electrodes are placed on the skin overlying nerve or muscle. One of the most common types of surface electrodes is a flattened or concave round disc 10 mm in diameter made of bare metals such as tin, silver, gold, or platinum that conducts electricity well (Fig. 12.3A, B). These metal electrodes are more effective conductors if the skin is properly prepared by cleaning, mild abrasion, and an electrolytic coupling medium is placed between the electrode and the skin. Coupling media such as electrolytic pastes or creams decrease the impedance at the interface between the recording electrode and the skin. The use of coupling media allows surface electrodes to record smaller signals more accurately, improving the quality of the recorded signal. Concave metal recording discs retain the electrode paste or gel, increasing the time the electrode can be used. Disc electrodes must be secured firmly in place with adhesive pads, tape, or straps to obtain consistent recordings of nerve or muscle activity. Some manufacturers provide a "bar electrode," which consists of two disk electrodes embedded in plastic with about 3 cm between the centers of the disks.

A third type of surface recording electrode is the self-adhesive, flexible tab-type silver/silver chloride electrode (Fig. 12.3C). One style of self-adhesive electrodes has a conductive surface area similar to that of a standard metal disc electrode. Self-adhesive electrodes do not require the application of electrode paste because the adhesive gel is electrically conductive. The self-adhesive electrodes are connected to recording apparatus by alligator clip connectors attached to metal wires. The use of these disposable electrodes is becoming more common because their use speeds the set up for recording procedures. Self-adhesive electrodes are used primarily to record CMAPs from muscle, such as during motor nerve conduction tests, or when the reference electrode is placed over muscle during needle electromyography. At times, a larger self-adhesive electrode is used as the ground electrode.

Another type of surface recording electrode is called the ring or loop electrode. This type of electrode is made from flexible stainless-steel wire tightly coiled and formed into a loop. These electrodes are designed to be applied to the fingers or toes and are secured to the digits by sliding a rubber collar along the loop. As with metal disc electrodes, electrically conductive paste or gel must be used as a coupling agent between the ring electrodes and the skin to enhance electrical conduction. In more recent years, disposable, self-adhesive, silver/silver chloride loop electrodes have been developed as an alternative to stainless-steel loop electrodes. These long, thin strip electrodes (~8 mm wide and 10 cm long), like loop electrodes, are typically used when performing

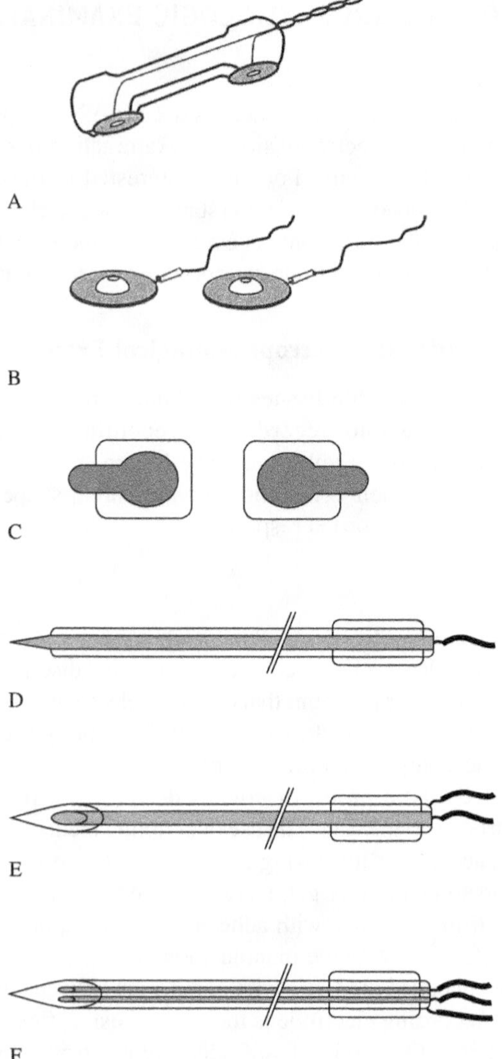

Figure 12.3. Recording electrodes in clinical ENMG. **A:** bar electrode. **B:** disk electrodes. **C:** self-adhesive electrodes. **D:** monopolar needle electrode. **E:** concentric needle electrode. **F:** bipolar needle electrode.

routine sensory nerve conduction studies. The self-adhesive loop electrodes do not require the application of conductive gel and hence are easier and faster to use during routine clinical electrophysiological examination.

Surface recording electrodes are generally used when the excitable tissues encompass a fairly large area. For example, surface electrodes are used to record CMAPs elicited from skeletal muscle and CNAPs monitored from a superficial bundle of nerve fibers.

Needle Electrodes

Needle or other types of subcutaneous recording electrodes are placed beneath the skin either near or directly in the excitable tissue to be examined. Such indwelling electrodes used for recordings are often made of platinum, silver, or stainless steel. Platinum tolerates sterilization well, and tissue reactance to platinum is small. Stiff wire electrodes of platinum or silver may be used for recording from deep muscles. These electrodes are insulated with substances such as Teflon or nylon, except at the tip. Subcutaneous electrodes do not require an electrolyte because they come in direct contact with conductive body fluids. Typical applications include the use of needle electrodes in EMG and ENG, and fine needle electrodes for recording potentials from the scalp in somatosensory evoked potential. Fine wire electrodes are used to record EMG signals from deeper muscles, whose potentials would be masked by overlying muscles when recording with surface electrodes. Fine-wire electrodes are also used to record nerve signals (ENG) from small and deep nerves. Fine-wire electrodes are preferred over rigid-needle electrodes in kinesiologic studies to minimize tissue damage during movement. Fine-wire electrodes are not generally used in routine clinical electrophysiological examination.

Needle electrodes are preferred for recording from small areas. For example, needles are chosen to monitor motor unit recruitment patterns in skeletal muscle during voluntary contraction. Because the electrodes are in direct contact with body fluids, the impedance at the recording site is low. Unfortunately, however, insertion of needle electrodes can occasionally cause some discomfort and possibly tissue damage if movement of the electrode is not minimized.

Several types of needle electrodes are available for clinical electrophysiologic examination procedures. The simplest of the needle electrodes is the *monopolar needle electrode* (Fig. 12.3D). Monopolar electrodes consist of a central stainless-steel core conductor surrounded by a thin coating of Teflon. Only the pointed tip of the central core is exposed for approximately 0.4 mm. The final gauge of the available electrodes varies between 24 and 30 depending on the overall length of the electrode; the longer the electrode the thicker the gauge. Monopolar needle electrodes are available in lengths ranging from 25 mm to 75 mm. Monopolar electrodes are placed into or near the excitable tissue of interest and serve as the active electrode in the recording circuit. Monopolar needle electrodes must be used in conjunction with either an additional monopolar needle electrode, or a small surface recording electrode that functions as the reference electrode and a third surface electrode that serves as the ground electrode. Monopolar needle electrodes are commonly used in EMG studies. They are inexpensive, disposable, and are generally the most comfortable for patients because of their small diameter.

Another common type of needle electrode is the *concentric needle electrode* (Fig 12.3E). One of the commercially available types of concentric needle electrodes consists of a central platinum or stainless-steel core surrounded by a polyimide insulator contained within a stainless-steel cannula. These electrodes are ground to a very fine point at an angle of 15 degrees. The central conductive core is exposed only at the tip and acts as the active recording electrode, and the stainless-steel housing acts as the reference electrode of the recording circuit. As always, a separate surface ground electrode must also be used.

A third type of electrode available for use in electrophysiologic examination procedures is the *bipolar needle electrode* (Fig 12.3F). This electrode consists of two very fine platinum conductors insulated from each other by polyimide and from the stainless-steel cannula in which they are housed. Like the concentric needle electrodes, the tips of bipolar electrodes are ground to a point so that both central conductors are exposed to the tissues only at the tip of the electrode. Electrical potential differences are recorded between the two core electrodes, one serving as the active electrode and the second acting as reference. The shaft of the needle serves as the ground electrode. Bipolar needle electrodes are used to record electrical activity in a very small area. Concentric and bipolar needle electrodes may be sterilized and reused. They are more expensive than monopolar needle electrodes and are not routinely used in clinical electrophysiological examination.

Signal Processing Components in Electroneuromyography Examination

When electrical potential differences (e.g., compound nerve or muscle action potentials, motor unit potentials) are recorded in response to activating excitable tissue, the voltage changes are generally too small to be immediately visualized on common display devices (e.g., oscilloscope or strip chart recorder). The amplitudes of biological electrical signals recorded from nerve and muscle are in the range of several microvolts (millionths of a volt) to a few millivolts (thousandths of a volt). Furthermore, the frequency components of signals may range from DC to several thousand Hertz. Adequate display of the responses requires some signal processing by other electronic devices such as amplifiers, filters, signal averages, integrators, and analog-to-digital converters.

Amplifiers

An amplifier is an electronic device that increases the amplitude of electrical voltages monitored in electrophysiological examination. Such devices are used to make small electrical signals larger on signal display instruments such as oscilloscopes, computer screens, or strip chart recorders. In some cases when low-voltage signals are being monitored, the amplifier built into the display device increases the signal size enough for accurate measurements. In other cases, amplifiers with special features may be required to create an adequate display of the electrical potentials.

A feature characteristic of all amplifiers is the device's *gain*. The gain of an amplifier describes the relationship between the input voltage amplitude of the actual, recorded signal and the output voltage amplitude from the amplifier (Fig 12.4A). If the peak voltage of a monophasic input signal is doubled from 1 mV to 2 mV, the gain of the amplifier is two. If the same input signal's peak amplitude is increased by the amplifier to 10 mV, the gain of the amplifier is ten. Most amplifiers are constructed so that the user may set the amplifier gain to a level appropriate to clearly visualize the electrical activity of interest. The amplifier control for such an adjustment is often labeled "sensitivity." The typical range of sensitivity settings on modern instruments for electrophysiologic testing is from about 2 μV per vertical division to 10 mV per vertical division.

Amplifiers used in electrophysiological examination should uniformly increase signal size for all signals within a specified frequency range (or bandwidth) from 2 to 10 Hz to 10,000 Hz (10 kHz). The *frequency response* of an amplifier (Fig. 12.4B) is determined by applying sinusoidal alternating voltages at various frequencies and known amplitude to the inputs of the amplifier. The ratio of the peak-to-peak voltages (V out/V in) should remain constant over the normal frequency spectrum of the recorded signals (2 Hz to 10 KHz) to ensure that recorded potentials are faithfully reproduced by the amplification process. Any signals composed of frequencies falling above or below the bandwidth of the particular amplifier will be attenuated (decreased) in relative amplitude or not displayed at all.

Electrophysiological testing amplifiers should have a *high input impedance* (>1 megaohm) relative to the impedance of the recording electrodes used. A high input impedance will not allow the amplifier to draw much current from the biological tissue so the voltage changes recorded will more accurately reflect the ionic movements actually occurring in the tissue.

SIMPLE VERSUS DIFFERENTIAL AMPLIFICATION

A *simple* (or *single-ended*) *amplifier* is a device that enhances all voltage differences between recording electrodes. At times, the ionic movements beneath each of the recording electrodes will be similar. When 60 Hz line current is sensed by each electrode or wire leading to the amplifier, this electrical "interference" is amplified along with any biological signal. Because biological potentials are often several orders of magnitude lower in amplitude than 60 Hz interference, the use of simple amplification in electrophysiological testing may not allow the examiner to adequately visualize the bioelectric potentials of interest.

To overcome this problem, the signals recorded from test electrodes are generally fed to a *differential amplifier*. A differential amplifier is in fact two simple amplifiers linked together. The differential amplifier increases the difference of two input signals monitored from the active and reference electrodes. In the case of bipolar electrodes, the differential amplifier enhances the

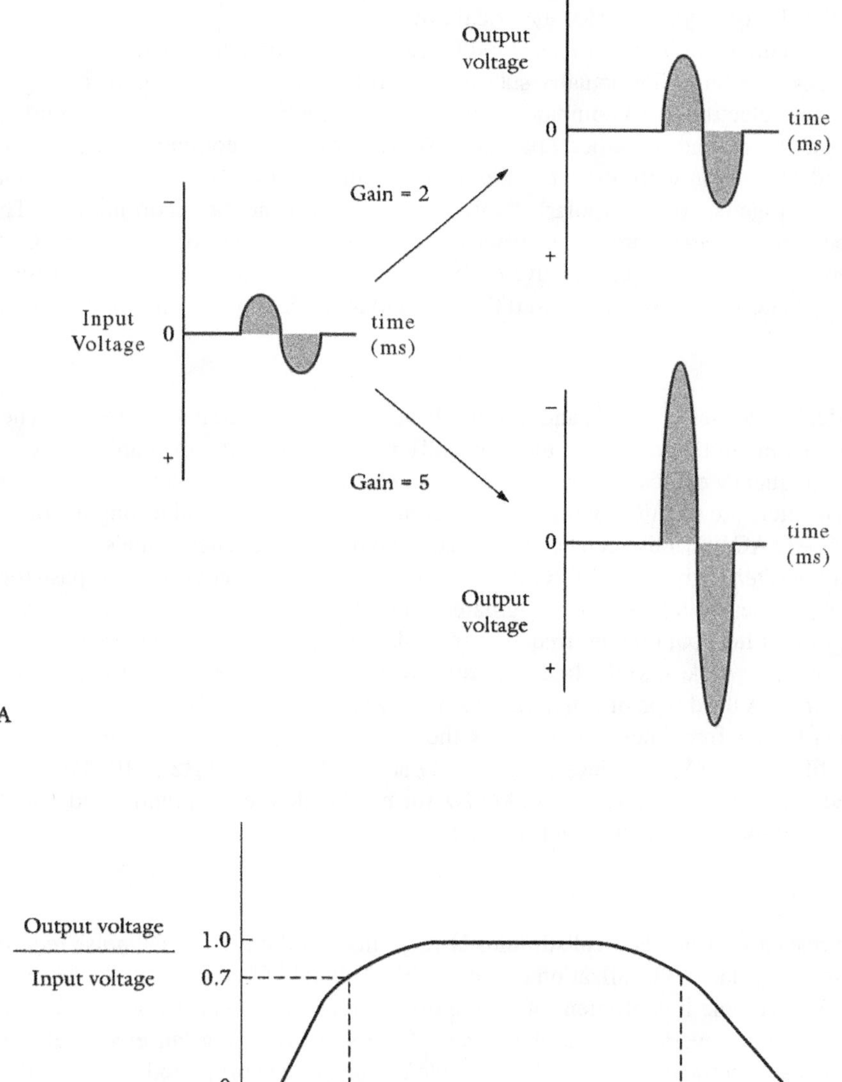

Figure 12.4. A: Effects of increasing amplifier gain ("sensitivity") on the display of a compound action potential. **B:** Graph of the frequency–response characteristics of an amplifier showing the attenuation of frequency components <10 Hz and >10,000 Hz.

differences of the signals from the two closely spaced recording electrodes. In monopolar electrode placement, the differential amplifier increases the differences between the signals from the active recording electrode and a more distant reference electrode. The differential amplification technique rejects signals that are common to both electrodes and enhances signals that are different. This is called *common-mode rejection*. Two recording surfaces tend to see different potentials for a given localized electrochemical event (e.g., a nerve or muscle potential). These signals are passed through the amplifier and recorded. Any signals common to the two recording electrodes, such as 60-Hz noise from the power supply and DC noise, are blocked by the amplifier.

In this way, the amplifier takes the signals recorded from electrodes, filters out noise, and improves the clarity of the recorded electrical event.

The differential amplifier uses a ground electrode to compare the signals of the two recording electrodes. The amplifier actually subtracts the difference between one recording electrode and the ground electrode and compares that with the difference between the second recording electrode and the ground. Whether a particular source of noise is common mode depends on its location and orientation with respect to the recording electrodes. Thus, for recording electrodes that are close together (e.g., bipolar), "noise" sources are near the recording site. This noise appears the same at both recording electrodes and will be rejected as common mode. Conversely, with electrodes that are far apart relative to the noise, the noise may appear to be different at the two recording sites, and it will be passed through and amplified by the differential amplifier.

Filters

Physiological responses of nerves and muscles have characteristic frequency ranges. The "noise" of the external environment can be electronically removed from the excitable tissue signal (as long as the frequency ranges do not overlap) by an electronic device called a *filter*. Several types of bandpass filters are commonly found on modern electrophysiological testing instruments. For example, 60-Hz AC line noise can be eliminated from higher frequency signals by using a device called a *notch filter*. This type of filter can be set to reject signals at 60 Hz and pass (or keep) a band of frequencies both less than and greater than 60 Hz. A second type of filter, called a *low frequency filter*, filters out the low-frequency signals (like those associated with movement of the electrode) and passes (keeps) the higher frequency signals (this type of filter is also known as a *high pass filter*). A third type of filter, called a *high-frequency filter* (also known as a *low pass filter*), rejects higher frequencies and passes the lower frequency signals. The low- and high-frequency filters of ENMG devices are generally adjusted to 2 to 10 Hz to 10,000 Hz for motor nerve conduction studies, 10 Hz to 10,000 Hz for needle electromyography, and 2 to 30 Hz to 2000 Hz for sensory nerve conduction studies.

Signal Averagers

If a single response to an electrical stimulus is very small, and the electrical noise recorded from the environment is large, visualization of the electrical signal of interest may not be immediately possible. To overcome this problem of an important electrical signal being buried in noise, the technique of signal averaging was developed. In signal averaging, an electrical stimulus is applied to evoke electrical activity in an excitable tissue. For a short period of time following the stimulus, all electrical activity (voltage changes) from the tissue is recorded and stored. When a second stimulus is applied, the electrical response is again stored and electronically added to the record from the first stimulus. This process is repeated, with each successive record being added to the sum of all previous records. Because the elicited potentials are time locked to the stimulus and reoccur at a fixed time after the stimulus, signal averaging will enhance these signals. Electrical interference (noise) is not time locked to the stimulus, and the averaged noise voltage transients will be eliminated by the averager. In other words, the effect of signal averaging is that all voltage changes that occur at the same time after the stimulus are enhanced, while all randomly occurring voltage fluctuations characteristic of random interference are reduced or eliminated.

The signal averaging technique is used to record sensory nerve action potentials and somatosensory evoked potentials. Sensory NCAPs can be on the order of a few microvolts in peak amplitude, whereas electrical noise may be larger in amplitude. This is especially true when conduction in sensory pathways has been compromised. Signal averaging allows the clinician to separate the sensory signal from the background noise, as shown in Figure 12.5. Signal

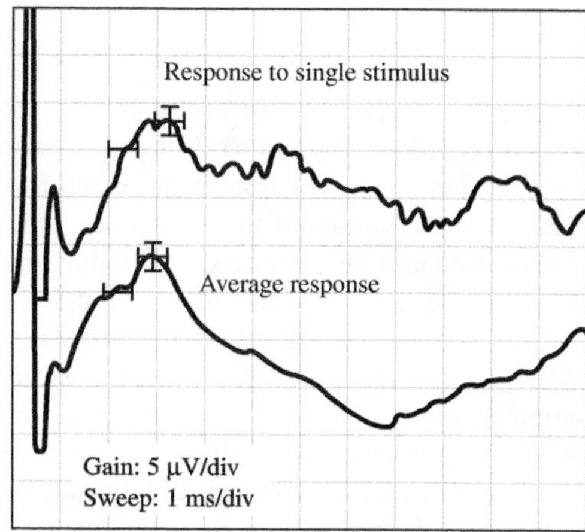

Figure 12.5. Effects of signal averaging on evoked potentials showing the enhancement of the evoked potential and the reduction in random electrical activity ("noise"). *Upper trace*: medial antebrachial cutaneous sensory nerve compound action potential evoked in response to a single stimulus. Note difficulty in determining the onset latency and amplitude. *Lower trace*: medial antebrachial cutaneous compound sensory nerve action potential average of 10 successive responses. Latency to peak and amplitude from takeoff to peak can be clearly identified.

averaging is also used in monitoring brain and spinal cord electrical activity in response to peripheral sensory stimulation. The somatosensory evoked potentials recorded in electrophysiological techniques are normally about 1 to 10 μV (10^{-6} volts) in amplitude, but the background EEG size is about 0.1 to 1.0 mV (10^{-3} volts). The somatosensory evoked potential is distinguished from the noise of the EEG by averaging the response to 100 to 2,000 stimuli. Once again, the signal of interest is separated from the background or interference activity through the use of the signal averaging procedure.

Integrators

Integration of an electrical signal is the calculation of the area under a signal waveform or curve. The units of the output of an electronic integrator are volts-seconds. An observed signal which has an average value of zero has a total integrated value of zero. Therefore, integration is used on a full-wave rectified signal; the rectified value is always positive. The integrated value of a rectified signal increases as a function of time.

Analog-to-Digital Converters

For many clinical applications, the physiologic electrical responses from nerve or muscle are recorded, processed (e.g., amplified and filtered), and displayed as an *analog output.* This is the form of the output signal displayed on strip charts and many oscilloscopes and stored on FM tape recorders. However, for modern microprocessor-based digital instruments, the analog signal must be converted into a digital signal for precise data acquisition, storage, and later retrieval for analysis. The data are digitized by an electronic device called an *analog-to-digital* (A/D) *converter*, whose sampling rates and signal processing times are specified. The characteristics of the A/D converter are dictated by the frequency of the recorded signal and the number of channels of data being simultaneously sampled. A/D converters used in electrophysiological testing should have sampling rates high enough to faithfully digitize even the highest frequency components of the EMG signal.

Display and Storage Devices

An electrical response of excitable tissue can be displayed in analog (continuous) or digital form (discrete or digitized measurements). An entire waveform may be displayed on an oscilloscope, computer screen, or a strip chart recorder (polygraph). Although a photograph may be taken of the waveform on an oscilloscope display and measurements made from this or from the waveform displayed on a strip chart recorder, neither of these methods allows further automated data processing. That is to say, the data cannot be reprocessed (filtered, amplified) or redisplayed in any other manner. In addition, some older strip chart recorders using electromechanically controlled ink pens cannot accurately reproduce the highest frequency EMG signals. Modern microprocessor-based ENMG systems typically provide automated signal analysis or recorded nerve or muscle action potentials. For example, in nerve conduction studies, values for onset latency, peak latency of the initial phase, peak amplitude of the first phase, or peak-to-peak amplitude of the entire signal are automatically detected, and the values (milliseconds for latency or microvolts or millivolts for amplitude) are displayed.

An entire event or series of events may be preserved for future analysis on an FM tape recorder (analog data) or in computer memory (digitized data). Both of these data storage methods allow further analysis.

Neuromuscular Stimulators in Electroneuromyography

The electrical stimulators used in activation of peripheral nerve or muscle in ENMG are similar, yet simpler in many respects, to neuromuscular electrical stimulators used in therapeutic stimulation applications. Both constant-current and constant-voltage stimulators have been used in electrophysiologic examination procedures, and either appears to be satisfactory for clinical testing, although the constant-current type has been recommended for some applications (1). In general, these stimulators produce a rectangular, monophasic pulsed current. Control over the stimulation parameters is usually limited to pulse amplitude, pulse duration, and pulse frequency. Amplitude and timing modulations are not required for routine evaluation applications and are thus not included. Pulse durations may generally be selected from 0.05 ms to 1.0 ms. Maximum amplitudes of stimulation may reach 600 V for constant-voltage devices or about 100 mA for constant-current stimulators. Frequencies of stimulation may be selected through a range of 1 pulse per second (pps) to 50 pps.

Stimulating Electrodes in Electrophysiological Assessment

A hand-held bipolar electrode or stimulator probe (Fig. 12.6A) is used to activate peripheral nerve and/or muscle in many commonly applied electrophysiological examination techniques. In this probe, the two stainless-steel electrodes (anode and cathode) of the stimulating circuit are fixed at a distance of approximately 3 cm apart. The cathode (negative) and anode (positive) are commonly color-coded black and red, respectively. In the application of stimuli to evoke nerve or muscle action potentials, this pair of electrodes is placed longitudinally along the particular peripheral nerve of interest with the cathode and anode orientation determined by the specific ENMG procedure performed.

Other types of stimulating electrodes used in electrophysiological testing include flexible, stainless-steel ring or loop electrode (Fig. 12.6B) and bar electrodes described earlier in this chapter. Loop electrodes are most often used to stimulate the sensory nerves in the fingers, whereas bar electrodes are used in general to stimulate peripheral nerve bundles at points where they travel close to the skin.

For these three types of stimulating electrodes, electrolytic pastes or gels must be applied to the electrodes to ensure sufficient electrical conduction of the stimulus to the body tissues.

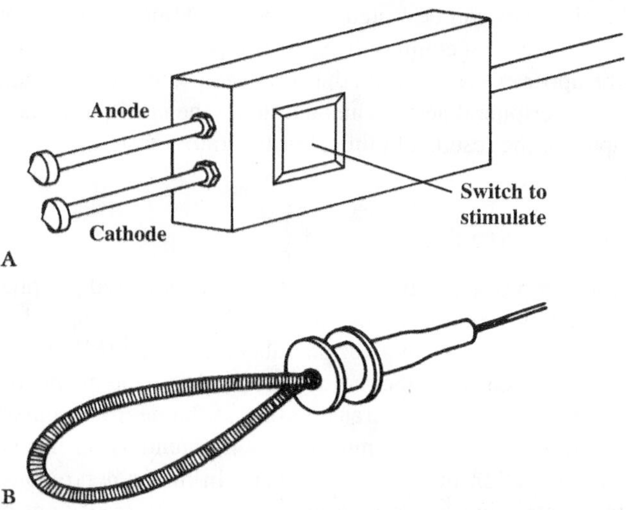

Figure 12.6. Stimulating electrodes used to activate peripheral nerves. **A:** bipolar probe electrode. **B:** metal ring (loop) electrode.

In some cases, needle electrodes like those described previously may be connected to a stimulator and used as stimulating electrodes to obtain localized activation of electrically excitable tissues. One more common use of needle electrodes for stimulation in ENMG is in the activation of individual spinal nerve roots, a technique that cannot be achieved using surface stimulation.

PROCEDURES OF ELECTROPHYSIOLOGICAL EXAMINATION

Nerve Conduction Studies

Nerve conduction studies examine peripheral motor and sensory nerve function (action potential propagation) by recording the evoked potential generated in nerve or muscle in response to electrical stimulation of a peripheral nerve. Studies of action potential conduction in peripheral nerve fibers are used clinically to answer the numerous important clinical questions that are of value in determining a diagnosis. These questions include:

1. Are peripheral nerve fibers compromised?
2. Are sensory fibers, motor fibers, or both involved?
3. What are the locations of the peripheral lesions?
4. How many peripheral nerves are involved?
5. Is the nerve involvement limited to one limb, or is involvement bilateral? Are both upper extremity and lower extremity nerves involved?
6. What is the magnitude of peripheral nerve involvement? Is the lesion partial or complete?
7. Is the peripheral nerve impairment increasing or decreasing over time? Is there evidence for recovery or further degeneration?
8. Is there evidence for localized nerve block, axonal degeneration, or segmental demyelination?
9. Does the pattern of nerve involvement suggest a localized (e.g., single nerve) or a widespread (e.g., polyneuropathy) disorder?

In theory, all peripheral nerves can be tested electrophysiologically, but some nerves are much easier to test than others. The most commonly examined peripheral nerves are the median, radial, and ulnar nerves in the upper extremities and the peroneal, posterior tibial, and sural nerves in the lower extremities. Other peripheral nerves can be tested if the need for further information is dictated by patient symptoms, the results of clinical or laboratory tests, or the results of initial electrophysiologic tests.

Motor Nerve Conduction Studies

To examine the conduction properties of motor nerve fibers, a mixed peripheral nerve is electrically stimulated with a single, short duration (0.1 to 0.2 ms) stimulus, and action potentials are generated in alpha motoneuron axons of a peripheral nerve bundle (Fig. 12.7). The evoked nerve action potentials are propagated along the motor fibers and activate the neuromuscular junctions of the stimulated motor axons. Synaptic transmission at the neuromuscular junctions between motor axons and muscle fibers produces muscle action potentials on innervated muscle fibers and triggers a twitch contraction in the muscle fibers. In motor nerve conduction studies, the actual force of twitch contraction is not measured. Rather, electrodes are placed either over a muscle or into a muscle to record the biphasic (or triphasic) CMAP (also called the *M wave*) that precedes the actual muscle contraction. The amplitude of the evoked CMAP is proportional to the number of muscle fibers depolarized, and hence is a reflection of the extent of activation of muscle fibers produced as a result of motor nerve stimulation.

As the current amplitude is increased during motor nerve stimulation, more motor axons are progressively recruited, and a maximum twitch contraction is produced. At this level of stimulation, further increases in stimulus amplitude will not increase the amplitude of the recorded response. At this point, all of the motor axons directly beneath the stimulator have been excited, the maximum number of neuromuscular junctions is triggered, and action potentials are generated on the membranes of all innervated muscle fibers. Stimulation of peripheral motor fibers at amplitudes greater than those required to recruit all motor axons near the electrodes and subsequently all innervated muscle fibers is called *supramaximal stimulation.* By ensuring

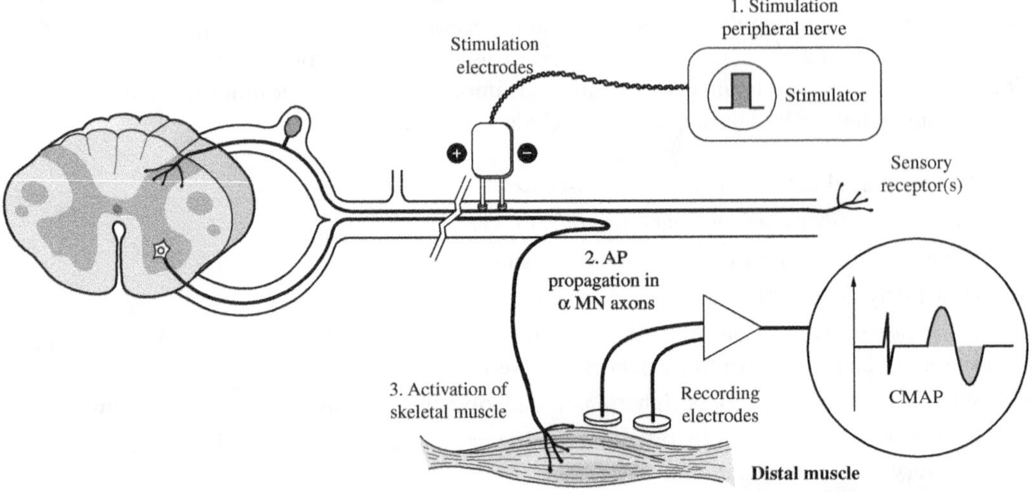

Figure 12.7. Illustration of pathways and stimulation and recording sites associated with performing motor nerve conduction studies. Supramaximal stimulation is applied to the peripheral nerve innervating a muscle, and compound muscle action potentials are recorded with surface electrodes from the muscle activated by stimulation.

maximal activation of all innervated muscle fibers, supramaximal stimulation results in the recording of maximal amplitude CMAPs.

Care must be taken during motor conduction testing to use both the appropriate magnitude of stimulation that activates all axons conducting to the muscle, and the optimal location of the stimulating electrodes over the peripheral nerve. Submaximal amplitudes of stimulation or poor placement of the stimulating electrodes fails to activate all axons capable of propagating action potentials to muscle and hence would produce M-waves that would be lower in amplitude. Low-amplitude M-waves are associated with conditions such as conduction block at some point between the stimulation and recording electrodes or, alternatively, degeneration of motor axons. Excessive stimulation amplitudes may result in the inadvertent stimulation of other nearby nerves innervating other muscles. Such inappropriately high levels of stimulation may produce activation in nearby muscles that contaminates the M-wave response in the muscle of interest. The artificially large-amplitude response could result in a normal interpretation when, in fact, conduction block, axonal degeneration, or muscle fiber loss may actually be present.

Example Application: Median Nerve Motor Conduction Study

To examine motor nerve axon conduction in the median nerve (Fig. 12.8) (2), surface recording electrodes (either disc or self-adhesive) are placed over one of the most distal muscles innervated by the nerve, such as the abductor pollicis brevis (APB). One recording electrode (called active or G1) is placed over the APB motor point, and the second electrode (called reference or G2) is placed 3 or 4 cm distally over the tendinous insertion area of the muscle. A third electrode, the ground electrode, is placed between the stimulating electrodes and the recording electrodes on a bony area such as the dorsum of the wrist. Electrical stimulation is provided by use of a hand-held bipolar probe electrode connected to a stimulator that produces a rectangular, monophasic pulsed current with 0.1 to 1.0 ms pulse duration and an adjustable amplitude. Frequency of stimulation may be controlled manually or preset at 1 pps. The cathode of the bipolar probe is placed distal to the anode over the median nerve, closest to the most proximal recording electrode over the muscle. Stimuli of increasing magnitude are applied to the median nerve until the amplitude of the CMAP of APB reaches a maximum. The CMAP response is amplified, filtered (10 Hz to 10 kHz), displayed, and recorded by the microprocessor-based system.

Testing is begun by increasing the current amplitude until the maximal amplitude of the recorded CMAP is reached. This signal is the evoked CMAP (or M-wave) and represents the summated electrical activity of all of the muscle fibers in the region of the recording electrodes that are innervated by the nerve axons being stimulated (Fig. 12.9). To ensure that the maximal response is recorded, a supramaximal stimulus must be delivered to the nerve. Supramaximal stimulation is technically defined as stimulus amplitude 20% greater than that required to obtain the maximal CMAP. The characteristics of the CMAP (onset latency, peak amplitude of first phase, or peak-to-peak amplitude) may then be measured to provide a quantitative indication of functioning nerve and muscle fibers.

The CMAPs shown in Figure 12.9 represent the summed electrical signals from muscle fibers innervated by large, intermediate, and small myelinated motor fibers. The amplitude of the CMAP (peak amplitude of negative phase or peak-to-peak amplitude) increases as more motor units are recruited. Because the action potential conduction speed of these nerve fibers depends on their size, the initial deflection from the baseline represents the beginning of activation of the largest diameter muscle fibers innervated by the largest diameter motor axons. The beginning of activation of intermediate-size fibers contributes to the middle of the response, and the slower conducting fibers contribute to the end of the negative portion of the waveform.

The display of the CMAP appears in a consistent position on the face of the display device, because the display sweep is triggered at the beginning of each applied stimulus. The time elapsed between onset of the stimulus and the beginning of the CMAP represents the time taken for motor nerve action potentials to propagate from the point of stimulation to the neuromuscular

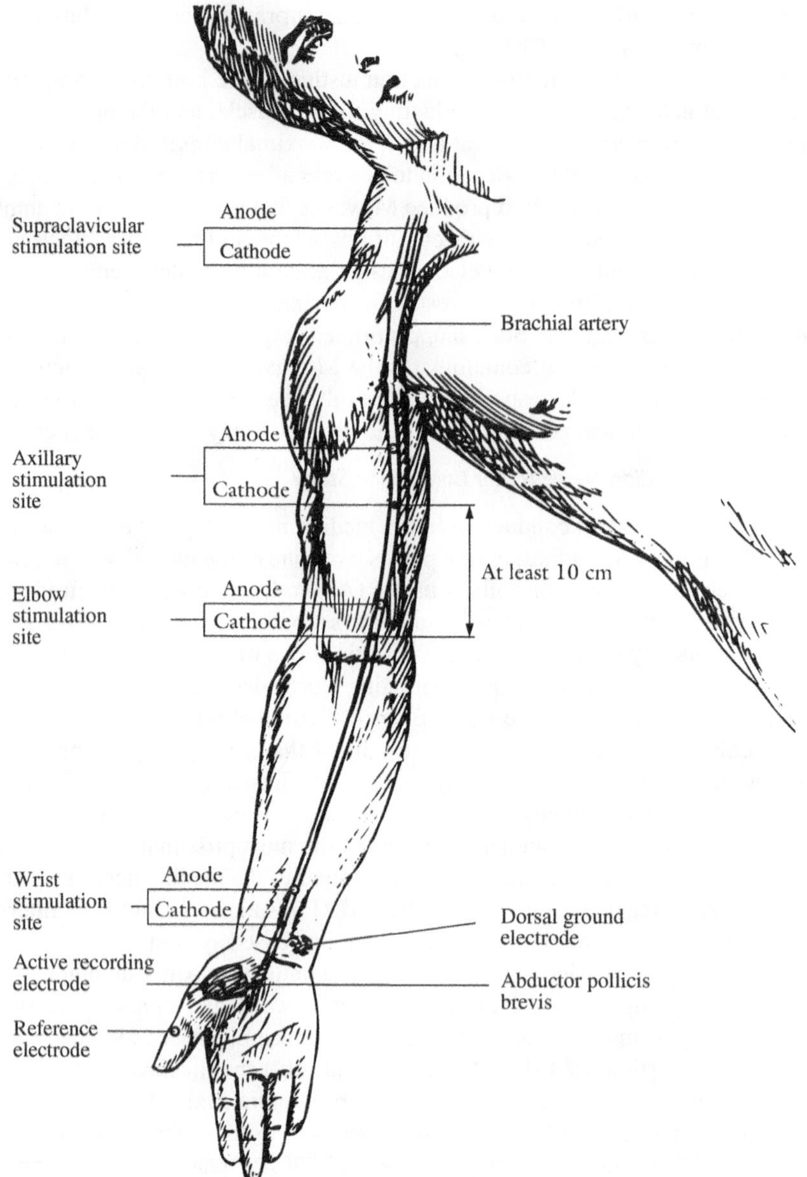

Figure 12.8. Stimulation and recording sites for conducting motor nerve axon conduction studies in the median nerve. (Modified from reference 7.)

junction, plus the neuromuscular junction transmission time, plus the time required for muscle action potentials to sweep by the first recording electrode. The time between the onset of the stimulus and the beginning (initial negative deflection) of the CMAP is called the *latency* of the response. Latency values (measured in milliseconds) are one of the primary measurements taken in motor nerve conduction studies. The recorded latency is proportional to the distance between stimulating and recording electrodes. The further the stimulating electrodes are from the recording electrodes, the longer the time delay before the appearance of the CMAP. The latency is inversely proportional to the motor axon conduction velocity between the stimulation site over the nerve and the recording site over the muscle. Latency measurements to the initial takeoff from the baseline are a reflection of conduction for the largest diameter and fastest conducting fibers.

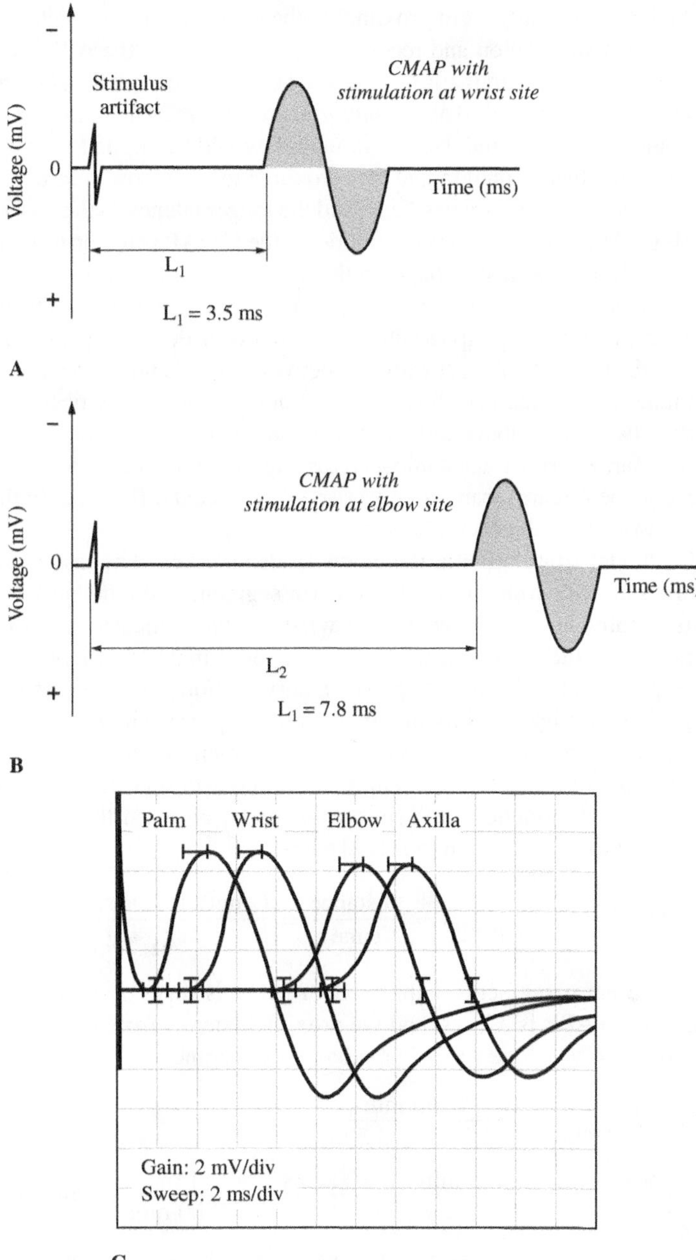

Figure 12.9. Compound muscle action potentials (CMAPs; M-waves) recorded from the abductor pollicis brevis (APB) evoked during median stimulation at the wrist **(A),** and with stimulation at the elbow **(B).** (Note: the latency of these responses is measured from the beginning of the trace to the onset of the CMAP.) Actual APB CMAPs recorded during motor nerve conduction testing **(C)** with stimulation at the palm, wrist, elbow, and axilla.

By applying bipolar stimulation to the median nerve at several sites (palm, wrist, elbow, axilla, and supraclavicular fossa), several latency values may be recorded and used to calculate motor nerve conduction velocity for various segments of the median nerve. Say, for example, that you are interested in determining the motor nerve conduction velocity in the segment of the median nerve lying between the elbow and the wrist. First, stimulation as described above would be applied to the median nerve at the wrist, normally 8 cm proximal to the active recording electrode over the APB. The latency (L_1) between stimulation and recording the CMAP from the APB would be recorded (Fig 12.9A). Since median nerve stimulation at the wrist is often the most distal point of stimulation of this nerve, this latency is referred to as the *motor distal latency*. The point of cathodal stimulation at the wrist would also be marked. Next, stimulation would be applied over the median nerve at the elbow medial to the biceps tendon and just proximal to the elbow crease. A CMAP evoked from the APB appears later on the display screen, and the longer latency to the onset of this M-wave is recorded as L_2 (Fig 12.9B). Under normal conditions, the CMAP waveform should be similar in configuration (amplitude, duration, and shape) to that elicited by stimulation at the wrist. This similarity in configuration ensures that the same group of nerve fibers is being activated by the stimulus at each site, and hence that one is assessing conduction over the same group of nerve fibers. If the configurations of the CMAPs are very different between the two points of stimulation, this may mean that the examiner is stimulating different populations of motor nerve fibers or that significant compromise exists between the elbow and wrist stimulation sites. In the median nerve, anatomic anomalies such as a Martin-Gruber anastomosis (crossing of median nerve fibers from the median nerve to ulnar nerve in the forearm) can also give rise to significant differences in the configuration of the M-wave after wrist and elbow stimulation.

The point of cathodal stimulation at the elbow is also marked. The last measurement made to calculate motor conduction velocity in the forearm segment is the distance between the two cathodal stimulation points at the elbow and the wrist. Distance measurement is performed by laying a tape measure on the skin in a manner that approximates the anatomic course of the nerve. This value represents the distance over which nerve action potentials are propagated in the elbow to wrist segment. Because velocity of conduction is expressed in units of length divided by units of time (e.g., meters per second), the conduction velocity of the forearm segment of the median nerve is calculated by dividing the length of the forearm segment (measured in millimeters) by the difference in conduction time (in milliseconds) between the elbow and the thenar eminence, and the wrist to the thenar eminence. That is,

$$\text{Conduction velocity}_{\text{elbow to wrist}} = \frac{\text{Distance}}{\text{Time}} = \frac{\text{Length forearm segment (mm)}}{L_2 - L_1\ \text{(ms)}}$$

If the length of the forearm segment of the median nerve is measured as 235 mm, the distal latency (L_1) from wrist to APB is 3.5 ms, and the proximal latency from elbow to APB is 7.8 ms, the conduction velocity (CV) of the forearm median nerve segment is 54.7 m per second:

$$\begin{aligned} CV_{\text{elbow to wrist}} &= \frac{235\ \text{mm}}{(7.8\ \text{ms} - 3.5\ \text{ms})} \\ &= \frac{235\ \text{mm}}{4.3\ \text{ms}} \times \frac{1000\ \text{ms}}{1\ \text{s}} \times \frac{1\ \text{m}}{1000\ \text{mm}} = 54.7\ \text{m/s} \end{aligned}$$

Note that a conversion is shown to obtain the CV value in meters per second. In fact, if distances and latencies are measured in millimeters and milliseconds, respectively, the numerical value of the division of millimeters by milliseconds is the same as that obtained by performing the measurement unit conversions. Conduction velocities may also be calculated for the axilla-to-elbow segment and the supraclavicular fossa-to-axilla segment by using the appropriate latencies of the responses for each site and an estimation of the length of each respective segment. In the measurement of the transaxillary segment length, calipers are often used to measure the length of the segment.

The motor nerve conduction technique described here can be applied at recommended points to determine CV values for segments of a variety of other peripheral nerves. Figure 12.8 shows stimulation points for the median nerve at locations (axilla and supraclavicular fossa/Erb's point) proximal to the elbow that can be stimulated to determine the motor conduction velocities of nerve axons in the upper arm and transaxillary regions. Figure 12.10 shows examples of

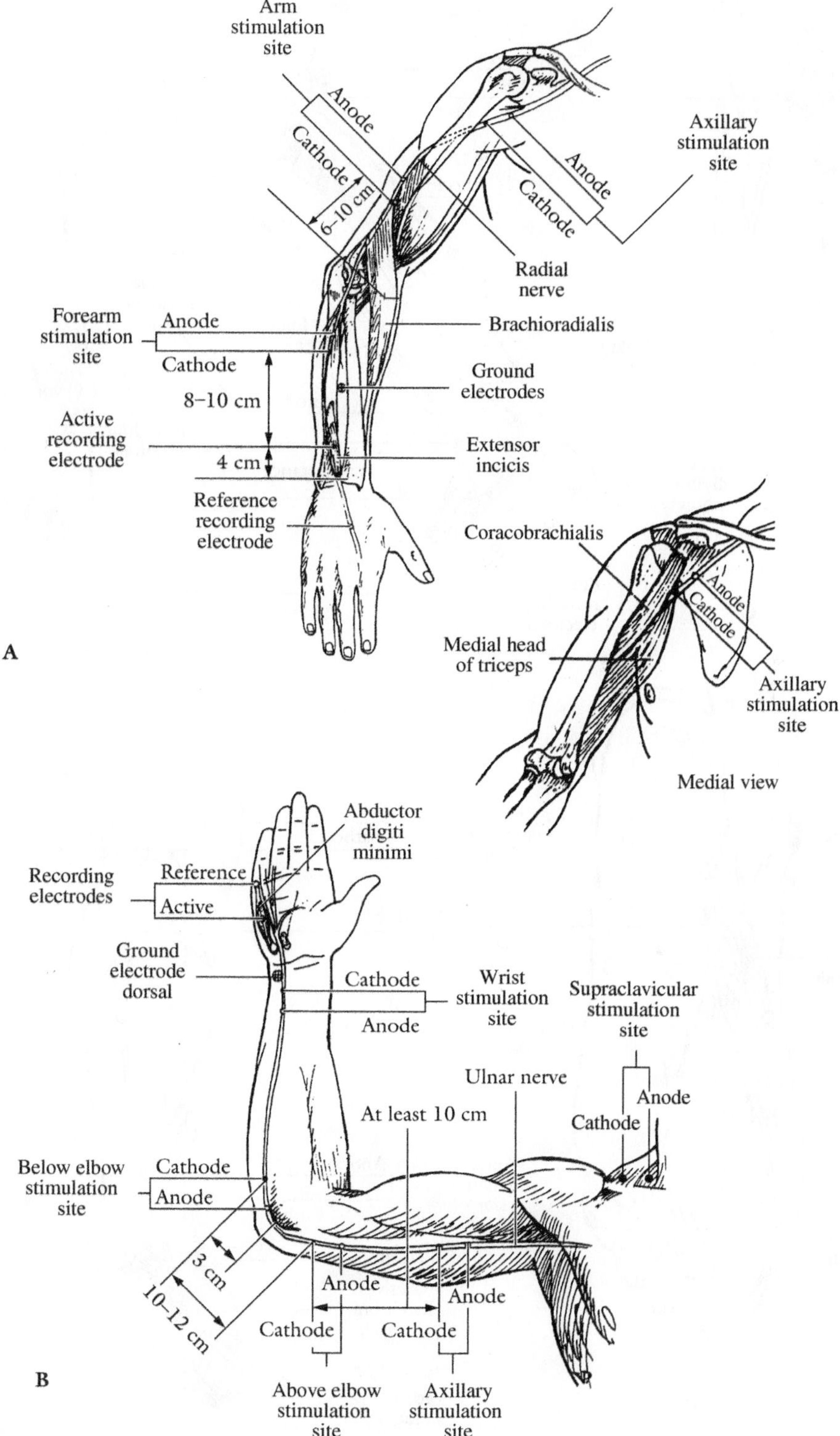

Figure 12.10. Illustration of stimulation and recording sites for performing motor conduction velocity studies from **(A)** radial nerve, **(B)** ulnar nerve, **(C)** deep fibular nerve, and **(D)** tibial nerve. (Modified from reference 7.)

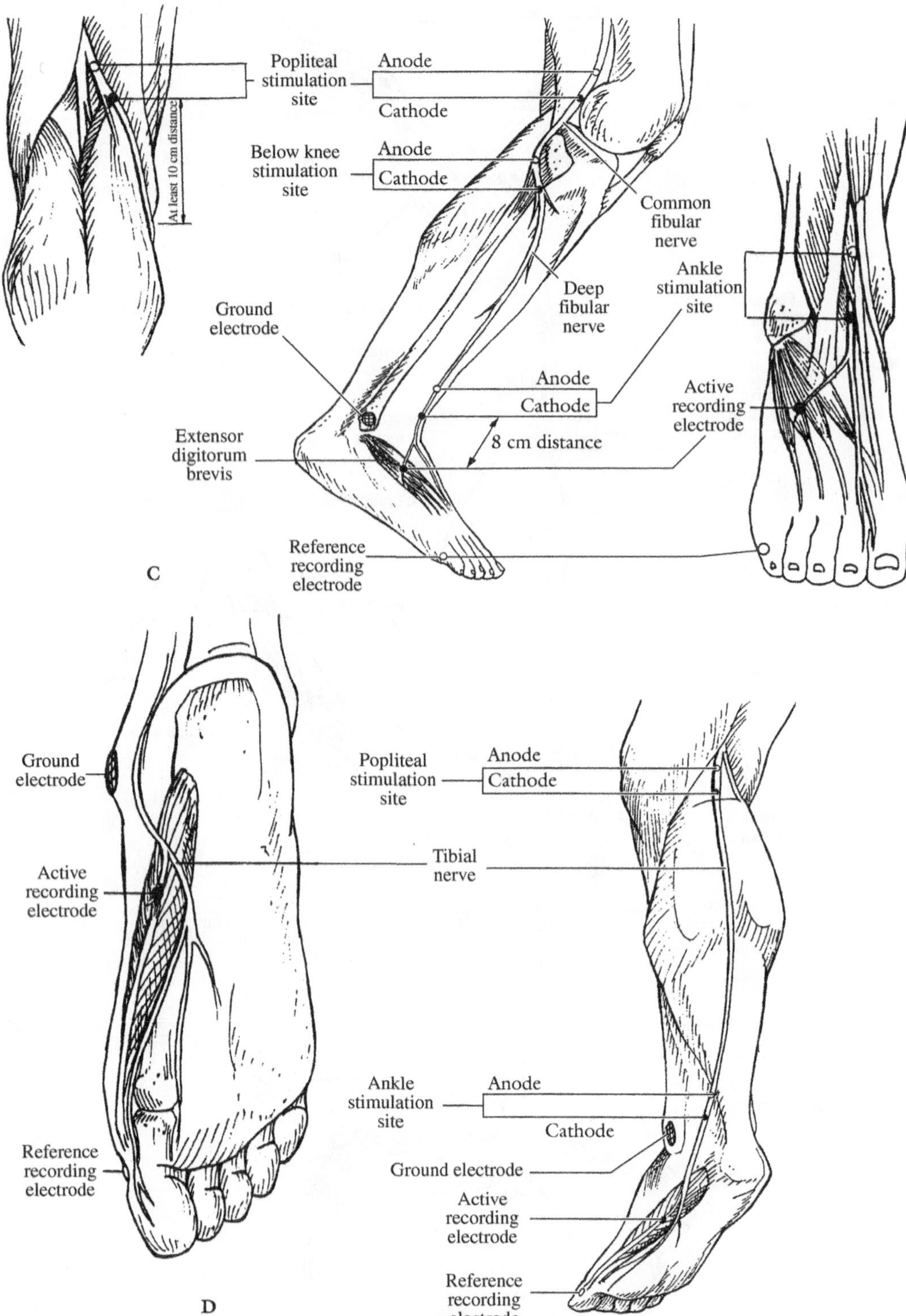

Figure 12.10. *Continued*

stimulation and recording sites for obtaining motor conduction velocities from segments of several other commonly tested upper and lower extremity peripheral nerves. Table 12.1 shows ranges of normal values for motor distal latencies and motor conduction velocities of various segments of several major peripheral nerves. Normal values for distal latencies and segment conduction velocities may be used for comparison purposes only if the testing procedure used to assess a patient is identical to that used to establish the normal values. Each electrophysiologic testing laboratory should develop its own normative values, because variations in the techniques of the motor conduction velocity procedures may alter the results. The differences in normal values from a variety of sources highlight the variation that may occur with slight differences in the particular procedure of testing used in clinical electrophysiologic examination (3). In addition, the inter-rater reliability of nerve conduction studies is not as high as the intrarater reliability of the test results (4).

Table 12.1. Normal Values for Motor Conduction Studies of Several Commonly Tested Peripheral Nerves

Nerve/Segment	***Distal Latency (over 8 cm) (ms)***	***Conduction Velocity (m/s)***	***CMAP Amplitude (Onset to Negative Peak) (mV)***
Median nerve			
Wrist to APB	<4.0		>4
Elbow to wrist		>48	>4
Axilla to elbow		>48	>4
Erb's point to axilla		>50	>4
Ulnar nerve			
Wrist to ADM	<3.7		>4
Wrist to FDI	<5.8		>4
Below elbow to wrist		>48	>4
Above to below elbow		>45	>4
Axilla to above elbow		>50	>4
Erb's point to axilla		>50	>4
Radial nerve			
Forearm to EI	<3.5		>3.5
Above elbow to forearm		>52	>3.5
Axilla to above elbow		>58	>3.5
Erb's point to axilla		>58	>3.5
Deep fibular nerve			
Ankle to EDB	<6.0		>2.0
Fibular head to ankle		>40	>2.0
Popliteal fossa-fibular head		>40	>2.0
Tibial nerve			
Ankle to AH	<6.2		>3.5
Popliteal fossa to ankle		>40	>3.5

APB , abductor pollicis brevis; ADM , abductor digiti minimi; FDI, first dorsal interosseus; EI, extensor indicis; EDB, extensor digitorum brevis; AH, abductor hallucis.
Note: Values in table may differ from those determined for different testing laboratories or from those derived from different testing procedures.

Meaning of Measured Variables in Motor Nerve Conduction Studies

Motor nerve conduction velocities may decrease and distal motor latencies may increase with peripheral nerve pathology. Conditions such as nerve compression and demyelination, as well as other disorders, may slow axonal conduction and/or prolong distal latencies. Environmental factors such as cold may dramatically reduce CV, and examiners must be careful to control limb temperature while performing nerve conduction tests to avoid obtaining reduced CVs and/or prolonged distal latencies that do not represent the existence of underlying pathology. No pathology is known that increases CV in peripheral fibers above normal values. Only vigorous heating of peripheral nerve may result in CV increases, and this effect is not as dramatic as the influence of cold on slowing CV.

Motor conduction velocities cannot be accurately determined for the segments of peripheral nerves lying between the most distal stimulation points and the innervated muscle for two reasons. First, the length of the most distal segment is difficult to accurately measure. Second, the distal latency measurement includes not only the actual conduction time along the distal segment, but also a significant synaptic delay time at the neuromuscular junction, and conduction time along the innervated muscle fibers. For these reasons, the distal latency values for peripheral nerves are simply compared to the normal range of established values or to those of normal contralateral nerves to gain a sense of whether conduction in the distal segment is normal or slowed. A longer than normal distal motor latency may reflect a slowing of distal segment conduction, a neuromuscular junction delay, or a muscle action potential conduction slowing.

Several other measurements are made to characterize the evoked CMAP (Fig. 12.11). They include (i) peak amplitude of each phase; (ii) duration of each phase (in milliseconds); and (iii) configuration (biphasic, triphasic, etc.).

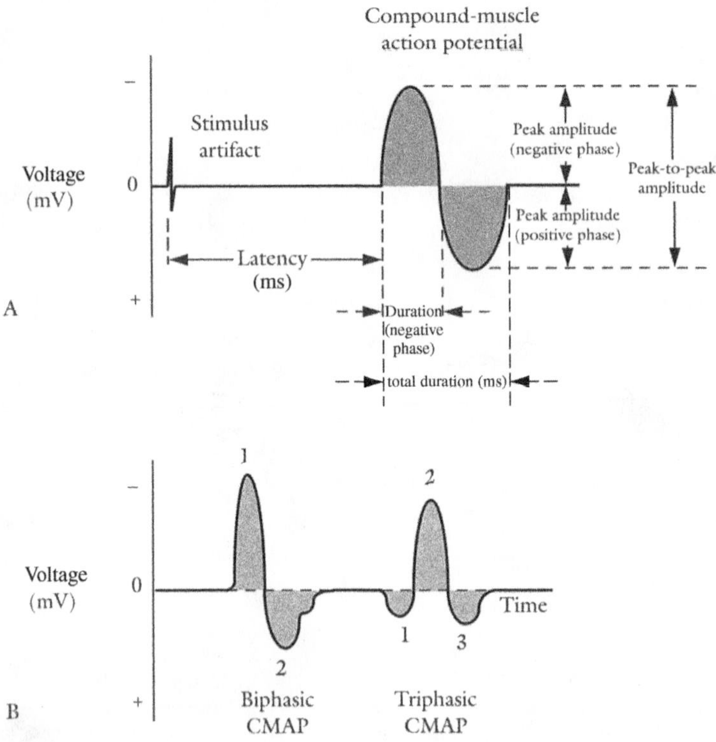

Figure 12.11. A: Parameters measured from compound muscle action potentials (CMAPs) during motor nerve conduction studies to characterize the CMAP, including peak amplitude of each phase, duration (in milliseconds). **B:** configuration (biphasic, triphasic,etc.).

The *amplitude of the CMAP* is measured in microvolts or millivolts from the baseline (isoelectric or zero voltage line) to the negative peak of the CMAP, or alternatively from the negative peak to the positive peak. The CMAP amplitude is a function of (i) the total number of motor axons propagating action potentials to the innervated muscle; (ii) the number of muscle fibers responding in the particular muscle being monitored; (iii) the size of the muscle monitored; and (iv) the placement of the recording electrodes. The CMAP amplitude should not change significantly with stimulation at different points along the peripheral nerve. Occasionally, the CMAP amplitude may be slightly attenuated at proximal stimulation sites due to differing rates of conduction within the motor axon dispersing their action potential arrival times at the muscle. Nerve pathology such as axonal degeneration that reduces the number of motor axons activated would result in a reduction of the CMAP amplitude. In localized conduction block of motor nerve axons, stimulation distal to the block produces a normal amplitude CMAP, while stimulation proximal to the block results in a reduced CMAP amplitude. In individuals without pathology, the amplitude of the CMAP evoked by stimulation of a nerve in one limb will be similar to that evoked in the contralateral limb. Side-to-side differences in CMAP amplitude of 50% (one side amplitude half of the opposite side) are considered to be clinically significant. Some laboratories consider differences in CMAP amplitude of 20% to 30% to be clinically significant.

The *duration of the CMAP* is measured from the initial negative deflection to the point where the CMAP again crosses the baseline. The duration is a function of the different speeds of the motor axons, the degree of synchronous activation of their muscle fibers, and the distance between the stimulating and recording electrodes. Any pathological process such as demyelination that slows the conduction velocity of a portion of the axons may cause the CMAP duration to increase.

Some laboratories are beginning to calculate the *area of the negative phase of the CMAP*. The area depends on both the amplitude and duration characteristics of the CMAP. The area of the CMAP appears to be related to the number of nerve and muscle fibers activated, but does not yet appear to be a more sensitive indicator of recruitment than does the amplitude alone.

The normal *configuration of the CMAP* is biphasic when the recording electrode has been properly placed over the motor point or motor endplate region, and triphasic when not optimally placed. Triphasic CMAPs may also represent a disease state or may result from volume conduction from a nearby muscle. When this occurs, the three measurements above are less reliable because one cannot always reproduce the CMAP. Stimulating at proximal sites should not significantly change the configuration of the CMAP of the same muscle recorded distally.

Sensory Nerve Conduction Studies

In performing sensory nerve conduction studies, peripheral sensory fibers are electrically stimulated with single short-duration shocks at levels sufficient to produce action potentials simultaneously in all sensory axons beneath the stimulator probe. The evoked sensory nerve action potentials are propagated along the sensory fibers, and the summed effect of these sensory action potentials propagated along the nerve can be monitored using surface or needle electrodes as the *compound sensory nerve action potential* (CSNAP).

The CSNAP is either biphasic or triphasic in shape. When the CSNAP is triphasic, an initial positive deflection is followed by a much larger amplitude negative deflection. The positive deflection may represent local current flow before depolarization occurs under the recording electrodes. The amplitude of the negative phase is proportional to the number of sensory nerve fibers activated in response to the applied stimulus. The normal sensory response (CSNAP) is much smaller (microvolts) in amplitude than the CMAP (millivolts), and may require the use of signal averaging to obtain a clear display of this response, especially in cases of neuropathy involving sensory peripheral axons. Stimulating with small needle electrodes placed near the nerve or recording with needle electrodes placed near the nerve may enhance the sensory response considerably and mitigate the need for signal averaging.

When a peripheral nerve is electrically stimulated, nerve action potentials are propagated in both directions (proximally and distally) from the point of stimulation. The action potentials propagated in the same direction as the normal physiologic propagation are referred to as *orthodromically* transmitted. Those action potentials traveling opposite to the normal, physiologic direction are said to be propagated *antidromically*. Orthodromic conduction in sensory fibers is from the periphery toward the central nervous system. Antidromic conduction in sensory fibers is toward the periphery.

Sensory nerve conduction may be studied by stimulation at some point and recording either the orthodromically propagated potentials or antidromically transmitted potentials (Fig 12.12). Sensory compound action potentials are usually larger in amplitude when monitoring antidromically propagated potentials as opposed to monitoring orthodromically conducted signals. This difference in amplitude is generally the result of the recording electrodes being closer to the signal's source (sensory axons) in the antidromic procedure. In contrast, the chance of producing interference from activation of muscle fibers is reduced using the orthodromic technique. Clinical measurements of sensory conduction are performed using several approaches including (i) stimulating and recording from a pure sensory cutaneous nerve; (ii) recording from a mixed nerve (containing both sensory and motor components) while stimulating a sensory cutaneous nerve (orthodromic technique); or (iii) recording from a sensory cutaneous nerve while stimulating a mixed nerve (antidromic technique).

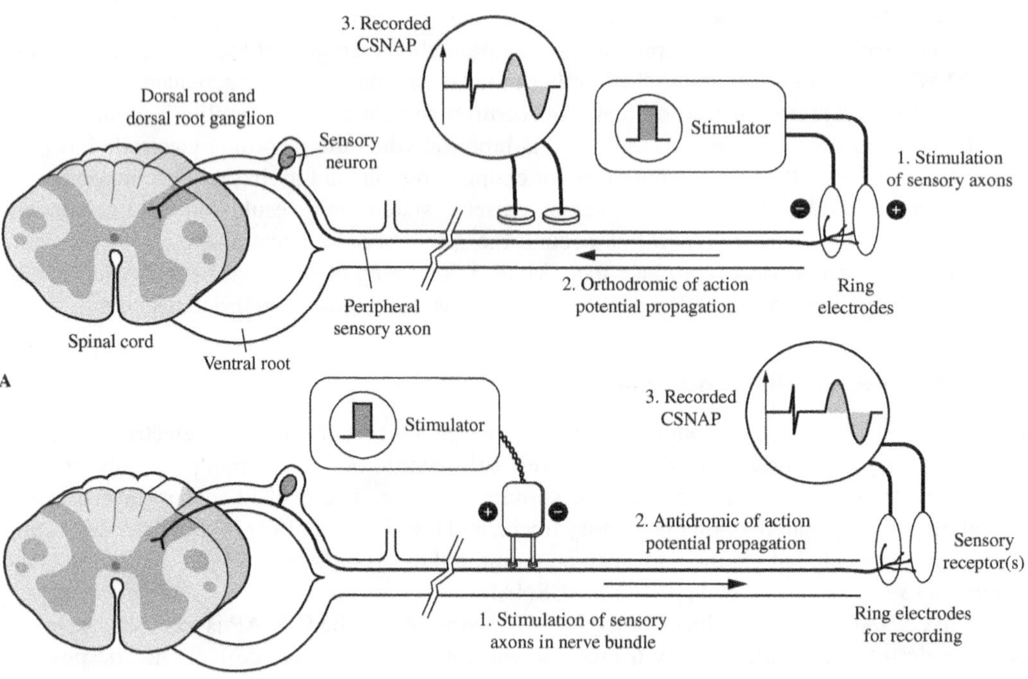

Figure 12.12. Illustration of the pathways, stimulation sites, and recording sites for performing sensory nerve conduction studies. **A:** orthodromic sensory conduction technique. **B:** antidromic sensory conduction technique.

Example Application: Median Nerve Sensory Conduction

Figure 12.13 shows the stimulation and recording electrode arrangement for performing the antidromic sensory nerve conduction study in the median nerve (7). In this procedure, ring electrodes connected to a recording apparatus are placed over a finger (usually the index or long fingers) innervated exclusively on the volar surface by digital sensory branches of the median nerve. For consistency in implementation of the technique from trial to trial and patient to patient, the more proximal ring electrode (active recording) is placed over the midpoint of the proximal phalanx, while the distal ring electrode (reference recording) is placed over the distal interphalangeal crease. A ground electrode is placed on the dorsum of the hand or over the styloid process of the ulna. Stimulation to the median nerve is provided with a bipolar surface electrode placed over the median nerve at the wrist and over branches of this nerve in the palm leading to the particular digit.

Stimulation is applied at a frequency of 1 pps, pulse duration of 0.1 ms, and stimulus amplitude that is increased to supramaximal levels. Action potentials are elicited in both sensory and motor nerve axons at the cathodal points of stimulation. The sensory potentials and motor potentials are transmitted distally. The summed effect of these sensory potentials passing along the median nerve axons can be monitored as the CSNAP using the ring or loop recording electrodes placed over the fingers.

The time between the application of the stimulus and the peak of the negative phase of the CSNAP is called the *sensory latency* and is measured in milliseconds. The sensory latency is most often measured to this negative peak as opposed to the onset of the potential, because the precise point at which the potential begins (leaves the isoelectric baseline) may not be accurately determined in some cases. More modern microprocessor-based testing systems may allow the

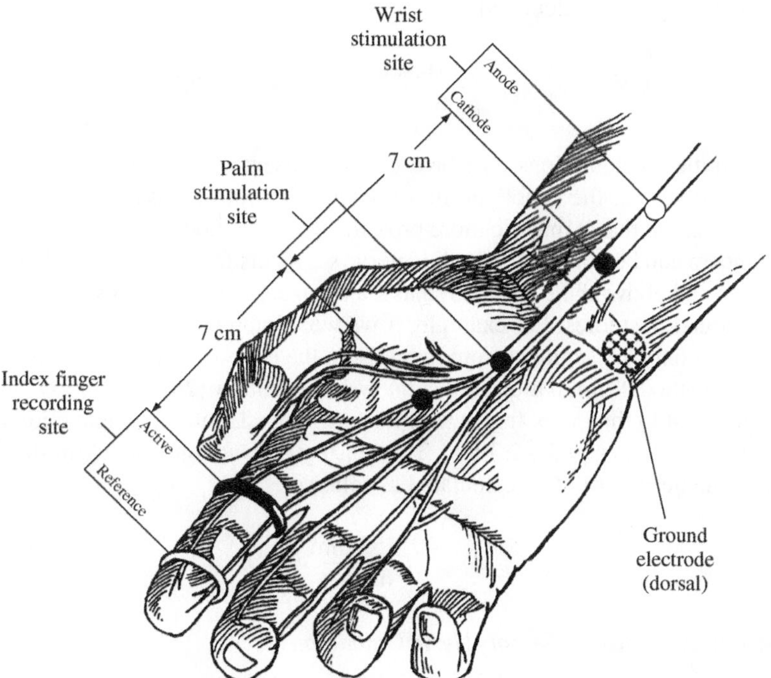

Figure 12.13. Stimulation and recording electrode sites for performing the antidromic sensory nerve conduction study in the median nerve from the wrist to the index finger. (Modified from reference 7.)

examiner to measure the sensory response latency to the beginning of the CSNAP. Regardless of the method of latency measurement chosen, the latency value represents the time of conduction of sensory potential between the stimulator cathode and the most proximal (active) recording electrode. The longer the distance between the stimulating cathode and the proximal recording electrode, the greater the latency value measured. Each position of the cathodal stimulating electrode should be clearly marked so that the distance between the stimulating sites and recording electrode (conduction distance) can be measured using a metal tape. The latency between the wrist stimulation site and the recording site on the finger is often called the distal sensory latency. Historically, this wrist stimulation site was the most distal location at which one could stimulate the median nerve and then record a clear, uncontaminated CSNAP. Today, with improvements in amplifiers and recording instruments, stimulation may be provided much closer to the finger (e.g., the palm) and still record a clear CSNAP. The ability to stimulate the median nerve both proximal and distal to the wrist allows one to calculate a transcarpal conduction time that reflects the speed of conduction through the carpal tunnel segment of the median nerve. Over a 7-cm distance, this "transcarpal" latency should not exceed 1.7 ms.

Knowledge of the conduction distances and conduction latencies for various segments of the nerve allows one to calculate conduction velocities. For example, if the distance between the stimulating cathode at the wrist and the proximal recording electrode on the index finger is 120 mm and the latency of the CSNAP is 2.8 ms, the conduction velocity along this segment would be calculated as:

$$CV_{\text{wrist to digit}} = \frac{\text{distance}}{\text{time}} = \frac{120\text{ mm}}{2.8\text{ ms}} = 42.9\text{ m/s}$$

If the conduction distance between the digit and stimulating electrode placed over the median nerve at the elbow is 375 mm and the sensory conduction latency is 9.3 ms, the conduction along this entire segment would be calculated as:

$$CV_{\text{elbow to digit}} = \frac{\text{distance}}{\text{time}} = \frac{375\text{ mm}}{9.3\text{ ms}} = 40.3\text{ m/s}$$

Even though these calculations may be a good representation of the conduction over these segments, some argue that the exact site of stimulation is not necessarily directly beneath the stimulating cathode, but that it may lie more proximal to the cathode or between the cathode and anode. This concern can be allayed for median nerve segments from the wrist to below the elbow, across the elbow, and above the elbow to the axilla by using a calculation similar to that used in motor nerve conduction studies. For example, if we were interested in learning the sensory conduction velocity for only the segment from the wrist to the elbow, we would first measure the distance between the cathodal stimulation sites at the wrist and elbow (255 mm). Next, the conduction latency from the wrist to the index finger would be subtracted from the conduction latency from the elbow to the index finger (9.3 – 2.3 ms). The sensory conduction velocity of the forearm segment of the median nerve would be calculated as follows:

$$CV_{\text{wrist to elbow}} = \frac{255\text{ mm}}{6.5\text{ ms}} = 39.2\text{ m/s}$$

Meaning of Measured Variables in Sensory Nerve Conduction Studies

CSNAP latencies and sensory segmental conduction velocities are a function of the speed of propagation of action potentials along sensory fibers. Increases in distal latencies or decreases in segmental conduction are commonly thought to be associated with sensory axon demyelination.

Sensory conduction may also be slowed with axonal compression without demyelination. Such changes may or may not be accompanied by axonal loss.

When performing sensory conduction studies using stimulation at several locations along a nerve, the evoked CSNAPs are often reduced in amplitude and prolonged in duration (8). The longer the distance of the stimulating electrode from the recording electrode, the smaller (lower amplitude) and more dispersed (longer duration) will be the response. The attenuation and dispersion is due to the difference in the CV of the axons and the difference in time to reach the recording electrodes. Because of the dispersion of the CSNAP, durations are not generally reported. Amplitudes of CSNAPs are measured from either (i) the peak of the largest negative deflection to the peak of the largest positive deflection (peak-to-peak amplitude); or (ii) baseline to peak of the major negative deflection (peak amplitude). The amplitude of the CSNAP is a function of the number of conducting sensory axons and the relative CVs of the sensory axons activated by the stimulation. Marked reductions in the amplitude of elicited CSNAPs may represent conduction block distal to the stimulation site in some of the axons or actual loss (degeneration) of sensory axons as might occur in certain types of polyneuropathy or chronic compression neuropathies. Amplitudes of CSNAPs may be reduced in cases of sensory axon degeneration associated with localized brachial plexopathies (9). Caution must be exercised in interpreting the meaning of CSNAP amplitudes in peripheral nerves, because these amplitudes vary substantially between subjects and significantly between the same nerves in opposite limbs in an asymptomatic population (5). Sensory nerve conduction studies are an important part of clinical electrophysiologic examination because sensory fiber disorders commonly precede motor fiber dysfunction in entrapment lesions, and in certain diseases, neuropathy is limited to sensory components of peripheral nerve.

Table 12.2 shows the ranges of normal values for sensory distal latencies, sensory nerve conduction velocities, and CSNAP amplitudes for a variety of upper and lower extremity peripheral nerves. Electrode placements for determining sensory conduction velocities in other commonly tested nerves are shown in Figure 12.14.

Mixed Nerve Conduction Studies

Several mixed nerve conduction studies are being routinely used and reported in clinical practice. Mixed nerve conduction studies are those in which stimulation activates both sensory and motor axons, and recording electrodes are positioned to monitor the summed effect of action potential propagation along both types of these axons. More simply put, stimulation is applied to a nerve bundle (usually distally) containing both sensory and motor axons, and recording electrodes are placed over the nerve (usually proximally) at another location to monitor the evoked summed, mixed nerve action potential (MNAP). Stimulation is ordinarily applied with a surface hand-held bipolar electrode or a bar electrode. The MNAP is recorded using a bar electrode over a nerve bundle where it lies close to the skin. The most common mixed nerve study is performed on the median nerve. Stimulation is applied in the palm of the hand over branches of the median nerve. Recording electrodes are positioned over the median nerve at the wrist approximately 7 cm proximal to the cathodal stimulation point. The latency to the peak of the negative phase of the MNAP is determined and reflects the speed of conduction of the nerve fibers through the carpal tunnel. In normal individuals, the transcarpal median MNAP latency over 7 cm should not exceed 1.7 ms. This test of median nerve function at the wrist may be among the most sensitive to detect median nerve compromise at the wrist as may be seen in carpal tunnel syndrome. Another more commonly performed mixed nerve conduction test is performed by stimulation of the medial and lateral plantar nerves on the sole of the foot while recording from the tibial nerve proximal to the posterior tarsal tunnel on the medial side of the ankle.

Table 12.2. Normal Values for Sensory Conduction Studies of Several Commonly Tested Peripheral Nerves

Nerve/Segment	Distal Latency (ms) (Segment Length; cm)	Conduction Velocity (m/s)	CSNAP Amplitude (to Peak Negative Phase) (μV)
Median			
Palm to fingers 2–3	<1.9 (7)	>40	>10
Wrist to fingers 2–3	<3.5 (14)	>40	>10
Elbow to wrist		>40	>10
Ulnar			
Palm to little finger	<1.9 (7)	>40	>10
Wrist to little finger	<3.5 (14)	>40	>10
Elbow to wrist		>40	>10
Radial			
Forearm to thumb	<3.2 (14)	>45	>5
Forearm to webspace	<3.2 (14)	>45	>10
Medial antebrachial cutaneous			
Elbow to forearm	<3.5 (14)	>40	>3
Lateral antebrachial cutaneous			
Elbow to forearm	<3.5 (14)	>40	>5
Sural cutaneous			
Calf to malleolus	<4.0 (14)	>35	>5
Medial or lateral plantar (tibial)			
Foot to above malleolus	<3.7 (14)	>37	>3
Superficial fibular (peroneal)			
Calf to dorsum of foot	<4.2 (14)	>33	>2

CSNAP, compound sensory nerve action potential. Note: normal values for distal sensory latencies differ between references according to the distance between the stimulating cathode and the active recording electrode. Amplitudes of responses referenced here are measured from onset to peak of the first negative phase of the CSNAP. Other references may report peak-to-peak amplitudes that are significantly greater than those reported here.

Factors Affecting Motor, Sensory, and Mixed Conduction Parameters

Besides injury or disease, many different factors may influence the results of nerve conduction studies (5). Tissue temperature has long been known to alter nerve conduction. Increases in temperature increase CV by about 5% per degree Celsius and reduce distal latencies. Conversely, cooling of peripheral nerves reduces CV and increases distal latencies. Decreases in temperature also increase the amplitude of M-waves by 1.7% for every degree Celsius decrease (10). For these reasons, it is important to perform nerve conduction tests in a temperature-controlled environment (21° to 23°C) with skin temperatures of the feet >31°C and of the hand >33°C.

Upper extremity nerves generally have CVs that range from 7 to 10 m per second faster than lower extremity nerves. More proximal segments of peripheral nerves usually conduct faster than more distal segments, but are generally within 5 to 10 m per seconds of the most distal segment. Failure to monitor and control temperature might reduce the speed of axonal conduction and result in an erroneous interpretation of the study findings.

Age is another factor that effects nerve conduction. Infants and children younger than 3 to 5 years of age have conduction velocities as low as 50% of normal adult levels due to incomplete myelination. Conduction velocities comparable to those of normal young to middle-aged adults

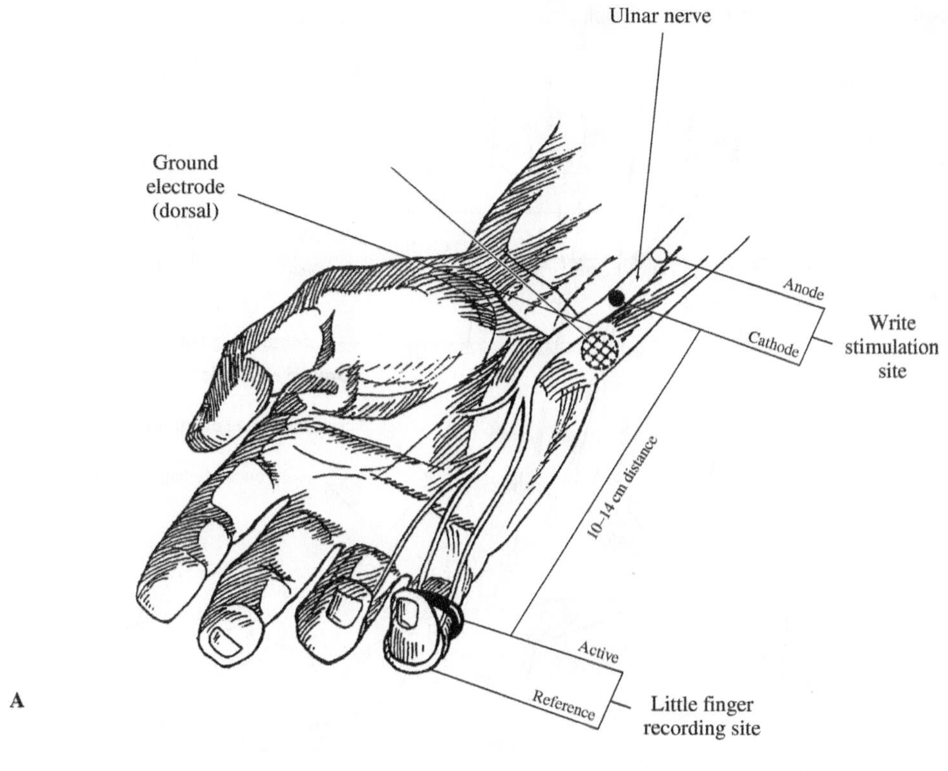

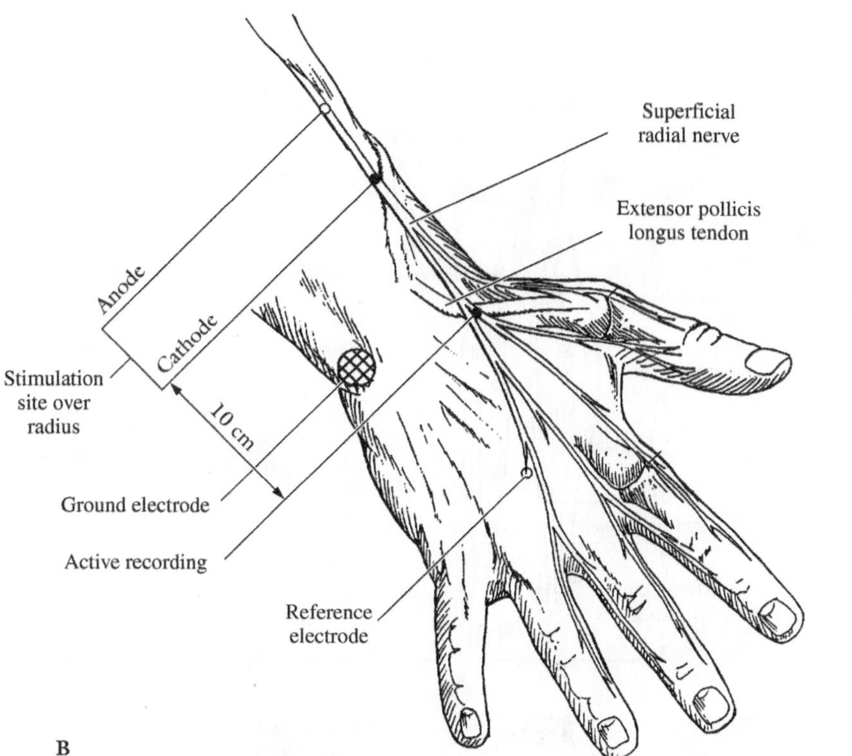

Figure 12.14. Stimulation and recording sites for performing sensory conduction velocity studies on **(A)** ulnar nerve, **(B)** superficial radial nerve, **(C)** sural nerve, and **(D)** superficial fibular (superficial peroneal) nerve. (Modified from reference 7.)

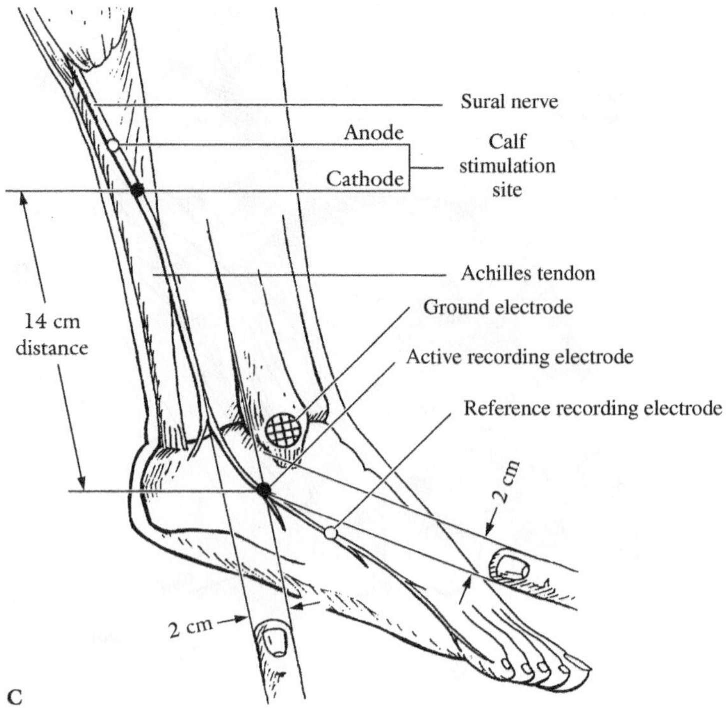

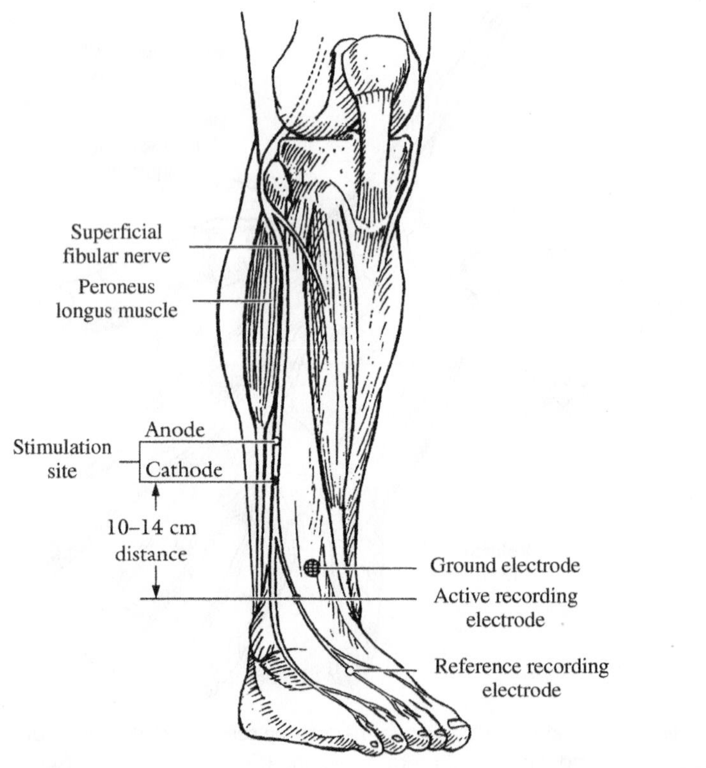

Figure 12.14. *Continued*

are reached in the mid-teens. Gradual slowing of conduction may appear after age 40. Conduction velocities in persons in their 60s or 70s are approximately 10 m per second lower than those of healthy middle-aged individuals.

Gender has been demonstrated to influence amplitudes of sensory nerve action potentials in the upper extremities. Asymptomatic women generally have larger digital CSNAPs than do men for both median and ulnar nerves. In addition, women generally have slightly higher segmental nerve conduction velocities in upper and lower limb nerves than men of comparable ages.

General Principles of Nerve Conduction Testing

Whenever nerve conduction velocity testing is selected as an evaluation procedure, several important testing principles should be observed. These include:

1. Both motor and sensory conduction studies should be performed when possible. Rationale: certain diseases or disorders may preferentially affect sensory or motor axons, and staging of compression neuropathies requires knowledge of the relative degree of compromise in sensory and motor axons.
2. Several segments of the nerves that are suspected to be involved should be examined. Rationale: an objective of nerve conduction testing is to determine if the underlying pathology in peripheral nerve is localized to a single segment or is spread over long nerve segments.
3. Nerves contralateral to those suspected of being involved should be tested. Rationale: side-to-side comparison of distal latencies and segmental conduction velocities may enhance the sensitivity of testing and often reveal the presence of conduction compromise in the absence of significant clinical symptoms.
4. Nerves in both upper and lower limbs should be examined if symptoms exist in both areas or if polyneuropathy is suspected. Rationale: polyneuropathic diseases often produce symmetric, bilateral compromise in the distal segments of both upper extremity and lower extremity nerves.
5. Testing should be performed at the appropriate time in the context of the suspected disorder.

Types of Nerve Lesions and Interpretation of the Results of Motor and Sensory Nerve Conduction Studies

Abnormal Findings in Different Types of Nerve Lesions

Nerve conduction studies are used to examine the ability of peripheral nerves to propagate action potentials, to assess the relative involvement of sensory and motor peripheral axons in individual nerves, and to determine the number of nerves involved in a particular disorder. In disease or injury, the ability of nerve fibers to conduct action potentials may be decreased or abolished depending on the extent of involvement of the tissues. Three levels of nerve injury have been defined (11). The most mild disturbance of peripheral nerve function is called *neuropraxia* (also known as type I lesion, transient neuropraxia, or delayed reversible neuropraxia). Neuropraxia is characterized by localized conduction slowing with or without conduction block. Neuropraxic lesions are not associated with an interruption of axon continuity and hence do not produce axonal degeneration. Conduction block in cutaneous sensory axons may result in reduced tactile sensitivity (e.g., numbness) as revealed by monofilament testing. Conduction block in motor axons may produce measurable weakness (paresis), if some of the motoneuron axons are blocked, or absence of voluntary muscle contraction (paralysis), if all of the motor axons have conduction block. Conduction slowing in sensory axons without conduction block is often associated with the presence of paresthesia (tingling or pins-and-needles sensation).

Neuropraxias are often caused by excessive nerve compression (e.g., crutch palsy, stretching, or inflammation) that is thought to produce changes in axon membrane function due to localized demyelination, compression of membrane channel proteins, or closing of nodes of Ranvier due to pressure on myelin. In neuropraxic disorders, peripheral nerve axons and the connective tissues in nerve remain intact. Regardless of the underlying nature of the disturbance in neuropraxia, the most common effect is reduced nerve conduction in the involved segment as reflected by either increased distal latencies or reduced segmental conduction velocities, depending on the site of the neuropraxic lesion. If conduction is actually blocked in a significant number of sensory or motor axons, the amplitudes of evoked compound action potentials may also be reduced below normal values. Because the nature of the lesion is generally mild and often temporary, over time, the speed of conduction and compound action potential amplitudes will frequently return to normal values. Figure 12.15 illustrates the types of electrophysiologic findings that may be detected in localized partial neuropraxic lesion of the motor axons innervating a muscle.

The second level of nerve injury is called *axonotmesis* (also known as a type II lesion). Axonotmetic lesions are those caused by more severe injury or disease and are characterized by partial or complete disruption in axon continuity without significant damage to the connective tissue layers in peripheral nerves. In axonotmesis, the endoneurial tubes remain intact. The axonal disruption associated with this type of lesion subsequently results in degeneration of the distal axonal segments. If sensory axons are involved, diminished or altered cutaneous sensation arises, or, if motor axons are involved, muscle weakness may be apparent. The sensory receptors or muscle fibers normally innervated by the disrupted axons are referred to as denervated. If significant numbers of nerve axons are disrupted while remaining axons are intact (partial denervation), amplitudes of evoked compound action potentials (with stimulation above the level of the lesion) are reduced once degeneration of the distal segments has occurred. Incomplete disruption of all axons in a peripheral nerve may not produce detectable changes in the conduction velocity of nerves distal to the site of pathology because conduction remains normal in uninvolved fibers. Depending on the nature of the injury or disorder producing the axonal disruption, conduction slowing may occur at the site of the injury in the axons whose continuity remains intact. Complete disruption of all axons in an axonotmetic injury followed by degeneration of distal axon segments (complete denervation) will be apparent by the absence of compound action potentials in the distal distribution of the nerve. Figure 12.16 illustrates the types of electrophysiologic findings that may be detected in localized partial and complete axonotmetic lesions of the motor axons innervating a muscle.

Numbness in the distribution of cutaneous sensory axons and weakness in the associated peripheral nerve myotome distal to the site of the lesion are suggestive of an axonotmetic lesion. If nerve conduction velocity testing is performed before degeneration has taken place in distal nerve segments (within 3 to 5 days after injury), nerve CVs and amplitudes of evoked motor and sensory responses may be normal with stimulation below the level of the lesion, because distal segments may retain conduction capacity until the axon membranes undergo significant degeneration. However, stimulation proximal to the lesion will not elicit sensory and/or motor responses at sites distal to the complete (100%) axonotmetic lesion.

The third and most severe type of nerve injury is called *neurotmesis* (also known as a type III, IV, or V lesion). This type of nerve lesion is characterized by axonal disruption accompanied by damage to one or more of the connective tissue layers within the peripheral nerve. Neurotmetic lesions are often associated with trauma to peripheral nerve (lacerations, tearing the nerve, etc.). The effects of neurotmetic lesions on the conduction characteristics of peripheral nerves are the same as those noted above for axonotmetic lesions.

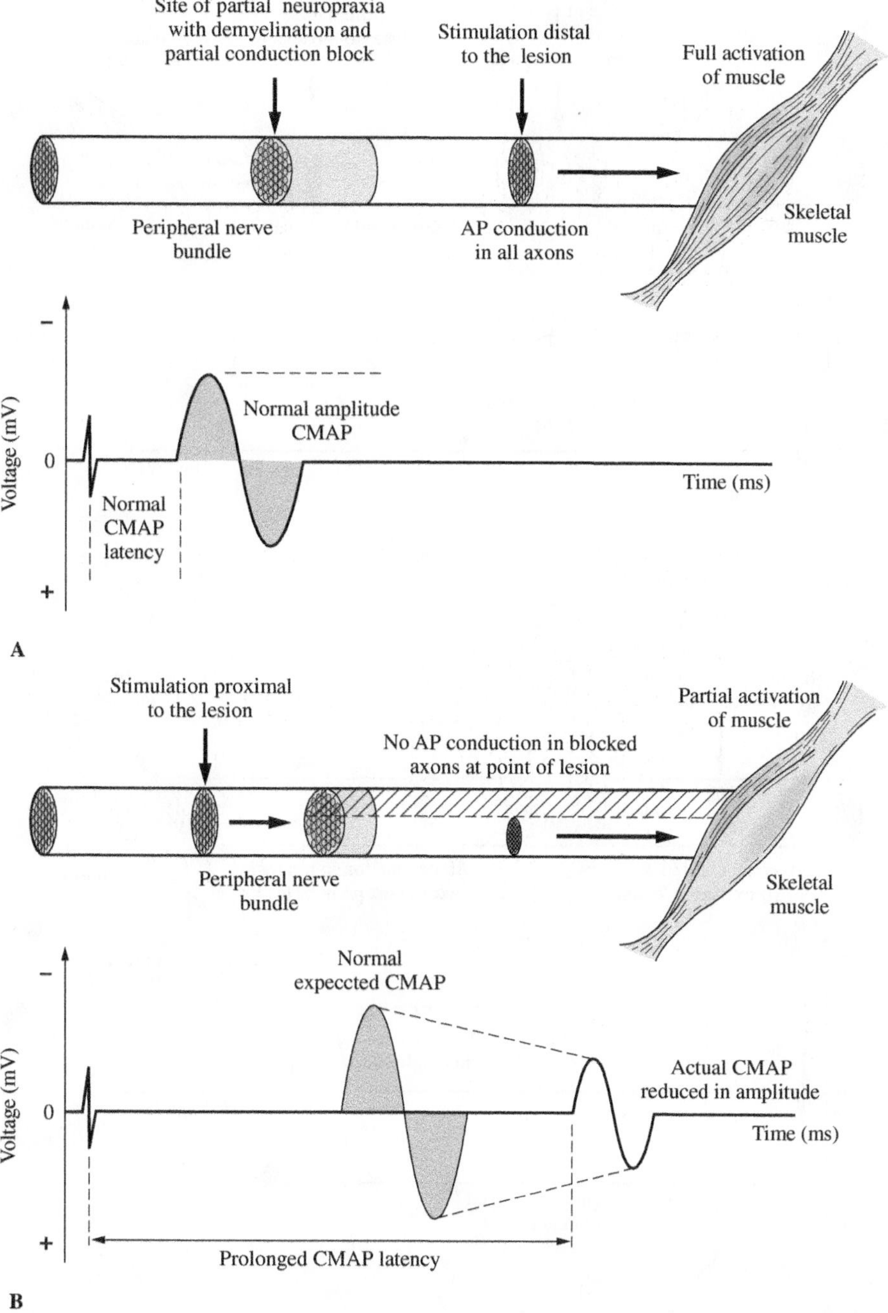

Figure 12.15. Illustration of findings from motor nerve conduction studies in partial neuropraxia with partial conduction block and conduction slowing at the site of the lesion. **(A)** Stimulation below the level of the lesion evokes a normal CMAP at a normal latency. **(B)** Stimulation proximal to the lesion evokes a reduced amplitude CMAP (due to the partial conduction block) and at a prolonged latency (due to the conduction slowing at the site of the lesion. CMAP: compound muscle action potential

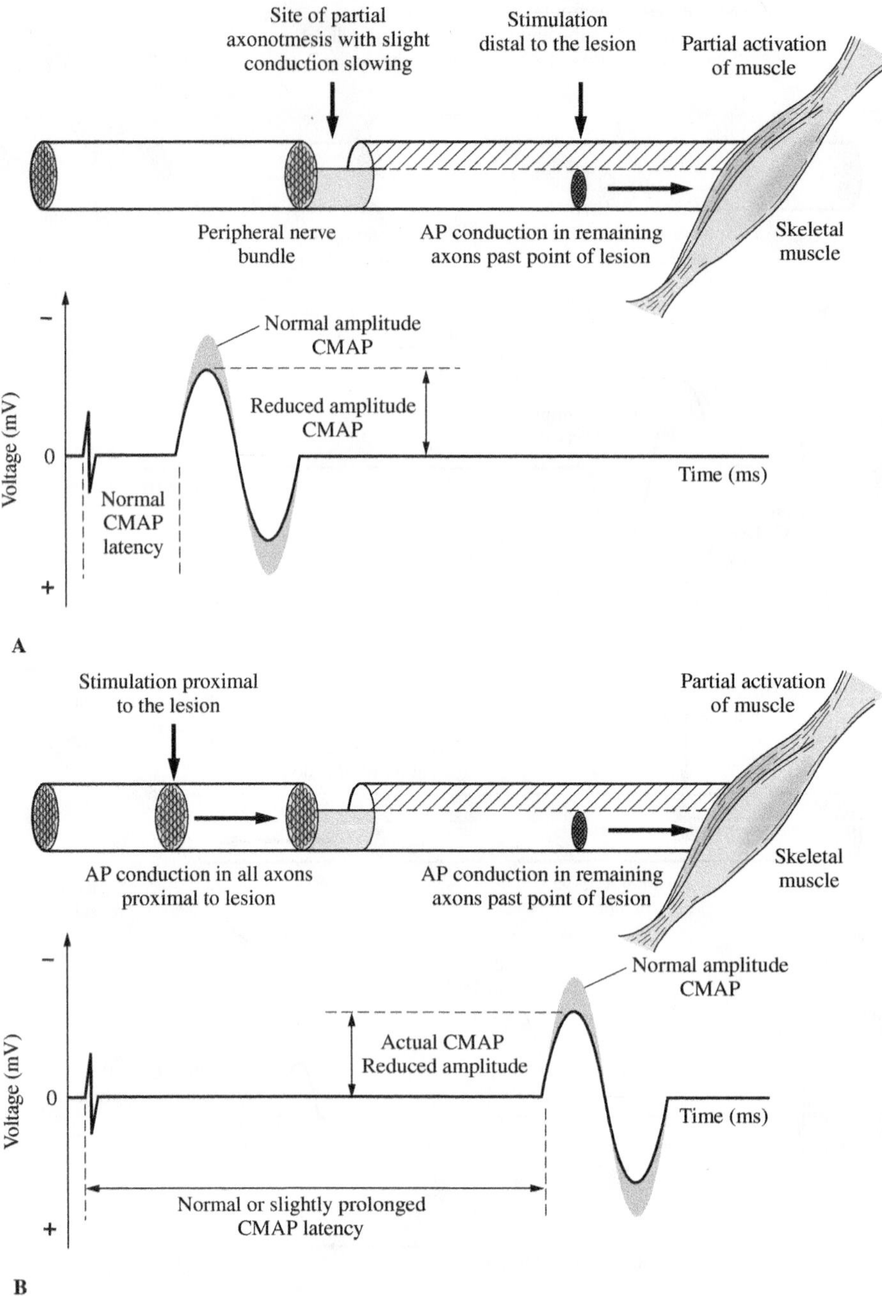

Figure 12.16. A and B. Illustration of findings from motor nerve conduction studies in a partial (50%) axonotmetic lesion (21 days duration) without conduction slowing in remaining functional motor axons. **(A)** Stimulation distal to the lesion evokes a reduced amplitude CMAP (due to partial axonal degeneration) at a normal latency (because no significant conduction slowing in the remaining motor axons). **(B)** Stimulation proximal to the lesion evokes a reduced amplitude CMAP (due to partial axonal degeneration distal to the lesion) at a normal latency (because no significant conduction slowing in the remaining motor axons at or distal to the site of the lesion).*(continued)*

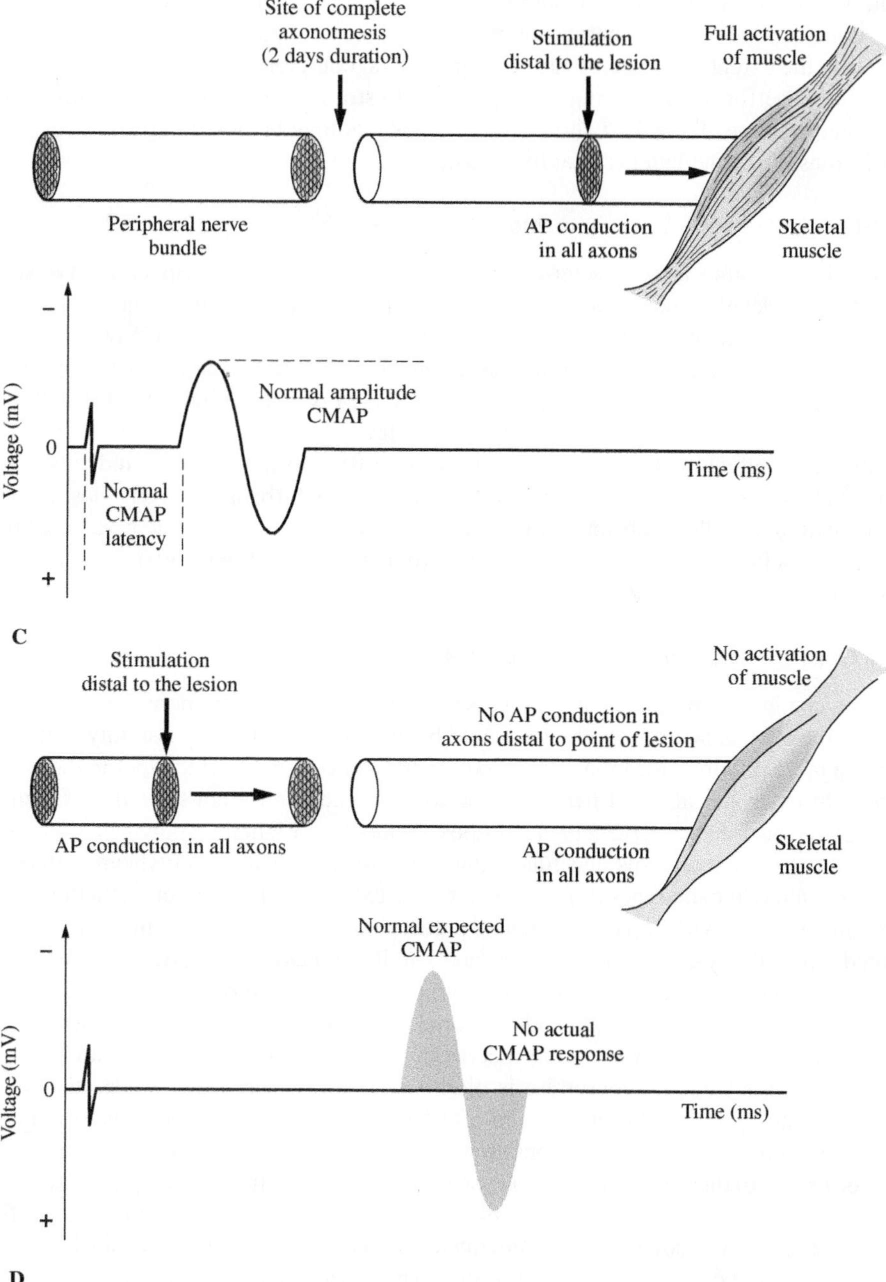

Figure 12.16. C and D. Illustration of findings from motor nerve conduction studies in a complete (100%) axonotmetic lesion (1 day duration) without conduction slowing in remaining functional motor axons. **(C)** Stimulation distal to the lesion evokes a normal amplitude CMAP (because axons have not yet axonal degenerated) at a normal latency. **(D)** Stimulation proximal to the lesion evokes no CMAP (due to complete disruption of axonal continuity at the site of the lesion).

From the previous discussion, it should be apparent that interpretation of nerve conduction velocity data depends on the nature of the nerve lesion (neuropraxia vs. axonotmesis or neurotmesis), the extent of the nerve damage (partial vs. complete involvement), and the time at which testing is performed following the injury. To illustrate the significance of these factors on CV data interpretation, Table 12.3 shows the changes that may be noted in response to different types of lesions of the median nerve at the mid-forearm level.

Abnormal Findings in Double Crush Syndrome

Double crush syndromes are characterized by pathology in proximal peripheral nerve segments giving rise to the development of a secondary site of peripheral nerve function compromise at a more distal location along the peripheral nerve pathway. Examples include C6 or C7 radiculopathy giving rising to median nerve function at the level of the carpal tunnel, or C8 or T1 radiculopathy giving rise to ulnar nerve compromise in the area of the cubital tunnel. Routine motor nerve conduction studies extending from the supraclavicular fossa to the hand may detect the compromise to conduction at the distal location, but often do not give any indication such as reduced CMAPs that the origin of the distal conduction disturbance actually lies at the more proximal location. Needle electromyographic examination of the appropriate paraspinal muscles and limb muscles innervated by the suspect nerve root are essential in localizing the lesion to the nerve-root level.

Abnormal Conduction Study Findings in Multiple Nerves

When nerve conduction studies reveal the presence of abnormalities in more than one nerve in a single limb, the clinical neurophysiologist should begin to investigate the possibility of nerve compromise at a more proximal location (e.g., plexus, nerve root) through which motor and/or sensory axons pass to reach the affected nerves. Alternatively, one should consider the existence of a polyneuropathic disorder (e.g., diabetic, infectious, metabolic, or inherited polyneuropathies) as the cause of the patient's symptoms and functional limitations. In general, polyneuropathies can be characterized into two main types differentiated by the existence of either demyelination or axonal degeneration. Some polyneuropathies produce predominantly sensory nerve impairment, whereas others predominantly affect the motor nerve function. Regardless of the specific disease or condition giving rise to the polyneuropathy, nerve conduction studies will provide valuable information regarding the extent of demyelination and/or axonal loss and the extent of the involvement of various upper extremity and lower extremity nerves. In more advanced polyneuropathic conditions, peripheral nerve conduction compromise is often symmetrical from side to side, and frequently nerves in both the upper and lower limb are affected. Early in some polyneuropathic conditions, however, electrophysiologic findings consistent with focal mononeuropathy are not uncommon. Findings of nerve conduction studies are important in the differential diagnosis because they may identify the distribution of nerve compromise and the nature of the compromise. Such findings from electrophysiologic studies must be integrated with the patient's history, physical examination, imaging findings, and other laboratory test results to establish a definitive diagnosis.

F-Wave Testing

When a peripheral nerve is stimulated along its course, action potentials are generated in nerve fibers and propagated in both directions from the site of stimulation. If motoneuron axons are activated by the stimulation, a motor response, the CMAP (the M-wave), may be recorded in distally innervated muscles. In some muscles stimulated in this manner, along with the M-wave, one may observe a second muscle action potential that appears on the record at a point much later in time (Fig.12.17B). This second late potential is called the *F-wave*. It is called the F-wave because

Table 12.3. NCV Results for Median Nerve with Different Types of Lesions at the Mid-Forearm Level

		Extent of lesion	Nature of lesion	Day 1	Day 7
Stimulation at wrist	*Amplitude*	Partial	Neuropraxia	Normal	Normal
			Axonotmesis	Normal	Decreased
		Complete	Neuropraxia	Normal	Normal
			Axonotmesis	Normal	Absent
	Latency	Partial	Neuropraxia	Normal	Normal
			Axonotmesis	Normal	Normal
		Complete	Neuropraxia	Normal	Normal
			Axonotmesis	Normal	Absent
Stimulation at elbow	*Amplitude*	Partial	Neuropraxia	Decreased	Decreased
			Axonotmesis	Decreased	Decreased
		Complete	Neuropraxia	Absent	Absent
			Axonotmesis	Absent	Absent
	Latency	Partial	Neuropraxia	Delayed	Delayed
			Axonotmesis	Slight delay	Slight delay
		Complete	Neuropraxia	Absent	Absent
			Axonotmesis	Absent	Absent
	Velocity	Partial	Neuropraxia	Slowed	Slowed
			Axonotmesis	Slightly slow	Slightly slow
		Complete	Neuropraxia	Absent	Absent
			Axonotmesis	Absent	Absent
Stimulation at upper arm	*Amplitude*	Partial	Neuropraxia	Decreased	Decreased
			Axonotmesis	Decreased	Decreased
		Complete	Neuropraxia	Absent	Absent
			Axonotmesis	Absent	Absent
	Latency	Partial	Neuropraxia	Delayed	Delayed
			Axonotmesis	Slight delay	Slight delay
		Complete	Neuropraxia	Absent	Absent
			Axonotmesis	Absent	Absent
	Velocity	Partial	Neuropraxia	Slowed	Slowed
			Axonotmesis	Slightly slow	Slightly slow
		Complete	Neuropraxia	Absent	Absent
			Axonotmesis	Absent	Absent

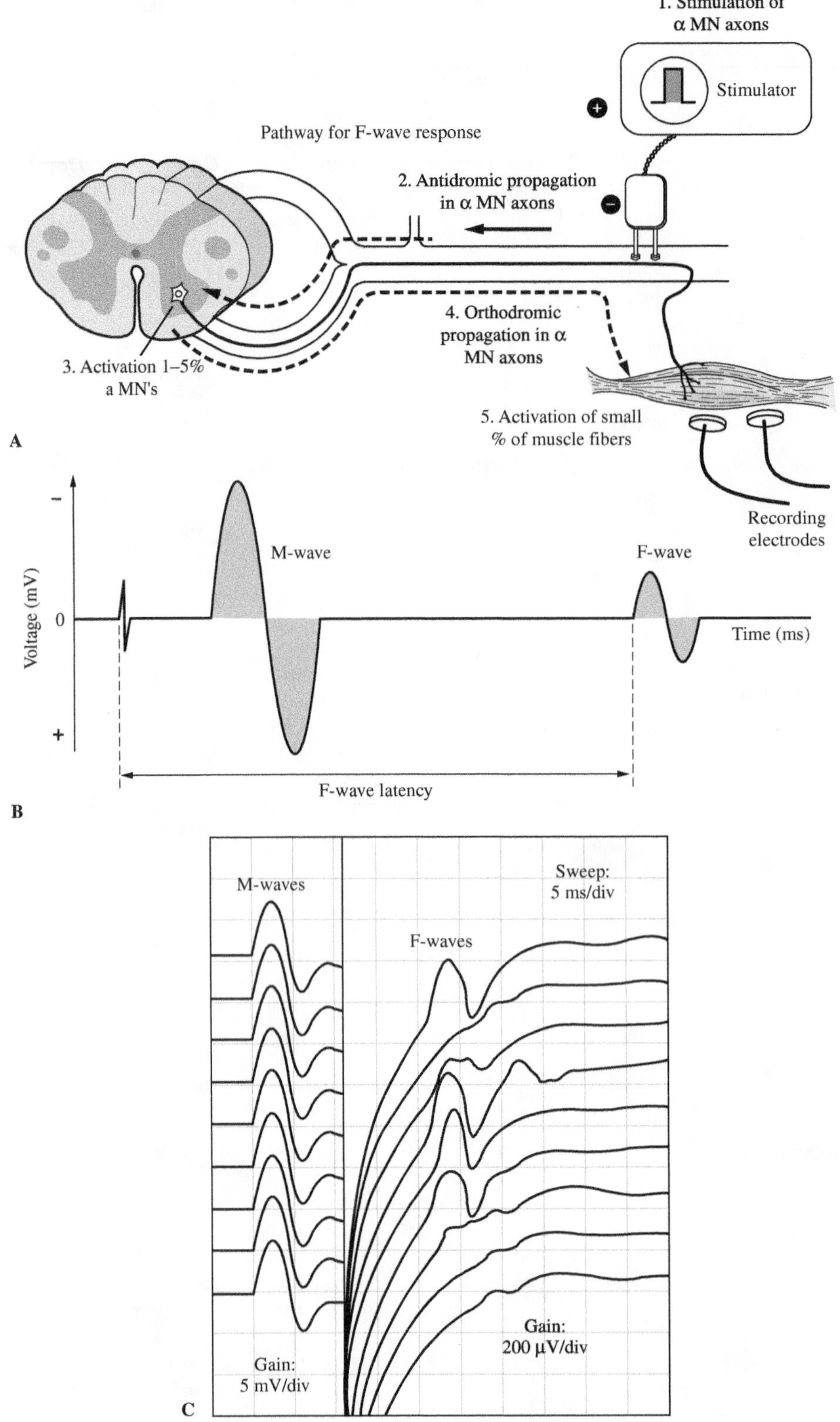

Figure 12.17. **A:** Illustration of pathways, stimulation sites, and recording sites for conducting the F-wave test. **B:** Illustration of M-waves and F-waves recorded during median F-wave test. **C:** Actual record of F-wave test results showing M-waves (left) and F-waves (right) recorded from the abductor pollicis brevis.

it was first recorded from foot muscles in response to tibial nerve stimulation. F-waves are very low in amplitude (<500 μV) and represent the activation of just a few motor units in muscle. In addition, F-waves are normally variable in both configuration and latency to onset. Whereas the M-wave results from the orthodromic propagation of action potentials in the motoneuron axons, the F-wave is produced as the result of antidromically propagated action potentials transmitted to the cell bodies (alpha motoneurons) or the initial segments (axon hillocks) of the alpha motoneuron axons located in the anterior (ventral) horn of the spinal cord. This antidromic invasion of action potentials in turn produces action potentials at the axon hillock of a small number (1% to 5%) of motoneurons. These antidromically activated action potentials then propagate orthodromically back along the motor fibers to the muscle monitored with surface or needle recording electrodes (Fig. 12.17A). This second set of action potentials reactivates the muscle, initiating a second CMAP, the F-wave. Support for the contention that F-waves are produced via purely motor pathways is derived from the finding that F-waves persist in deafferented animal models. The exact physiologic mechanism underlying the antidromic activation of spinal motoneurons has not been established.

Although the F-wave response may be produced during routine motor nerve conduction studies, the MNCV procedure is generally modified in F-wave testing by reversing the stimulation electrodes (placing the cathode proximal to the anode). Stimulation is applied distally to the peripheral nerve with rectangular, monophasic pulsed current with pulse durations at 0.1 ms and a frequency of 1 pps. The amplitude of stimulation is then increased until the amplitude of the M-wave response is at its maximum. In routine clinical practice, 10 to 20 stimuli are applied at this level, and the response to each stimulus is recorded. Recording electrodes are placed in a manner identical to that for performing motor conduction studies over a muscle located distal to the point of stimulation. The most common muscles used in F-wave testing are those of the hands, feet, and lower portions of the legs. F-waves are more difficult to clearly record from muscles that are in the more proximal musculature of the arms and legs because M-wave responses may overlap with F-wave responses. F-waves are not consistently evoked in response to each stimulus applied to the peripheral nerve. F-waves are more consistently produced in response to stimulation of nerves to antigravity muscles (upper limb flexors and lower limb extensors). Mild volitional contraction during testing of a muscle will enhance the frequency of appearance of F-waves during electrophysiological testing.

The most common variable measured is the time elapsed between stimulation and recording the onset of the F-wave, called the *F-wave latency*. In contrast to the M-wave latency, the F-waves recorded during motor nerve conduction studies have variable latencies. In routine clinical practice, only the shortest or minimal F-wave latency of all the evoked responses is measured and reported (Table 12.4). In some laboratories, the mean F-wave latency (average latency

Table 12.4. Normal Values for F-wave Latencies

Nerve	Muscle	Minimum F-wave Latency (ms)	Mean F-wave Latency (ms)	Mean F-wave Latency Difference (Side-to-Side) (ms)
Median	APB	26.8 ± 2.4	28.3 ± 2.6	0.2 ± 1.2
Ulnar	ADM	26.5 ± 2.5	27.7 ± 2.5	0.2 ± 1.1
Peroneal (fibular)	EDB	50.2 ± 5.5	52.0 ± 5.6	0.7 ± 2.4
Tibial	AH	50.8 ± 5.3	53.0 ± 5.6	0.6 ± 2.3

APB, abductor pollicis brevis; ADM, abductor digiti minimi; EDB, extensor digitorum brevis; AH,: abductor hallucis.

for the number of elicited F-waves) is calculated and recorded. The mean F-wave latency may be more reflective of the motoneuron conduction delay in the overall population of motor axons stimulated during the test, and may be preferable over the minimum F-wave latency on a statistical basis. F-wave latencies depend on the distance from the point of stimulation to the spinal cord and back to the muscle, as well as on the conduction velocity of the motoneurons axons along the pathway. The longer the limb in which testing is performed, the longer the latency of the F-wave response. The F-wave latency also increases with increasing age. The upper limit of normal minimal F-wave latency in the hand muscles is approximately 32 ms, in calf muscles 36 ms, and in the foot muscles 61 ms. Mean latencies are 2 to 3 msec longer on average (12). Comparison of F-wave latencies between limbs is sometimes useful in identification of pathology. Side-to-side differences in minimal F-wave latencies should not be >2 ms for F-waves recorded in hand muscles, 3 ms for F-waves in calf muscle, and 4 ms for F-waves recorded in foot muscles (13). One recent study on healthy adults concluded that the minimum F-wave latency for the ulnar nerve to abductor digiti minimi had only moderate test–retest reliability, and hence interpretation of minimum F-wave latency in the clinical setting may be of questionable value (14).

An alternative method that evaluates F-latency values is the calculation of F-chronodispersion. In this method, 100 or more F-wave responses are elicited, and the difference between the shortest and the longest F-wave latency is calculated. Normal values for F-chronodispersion for several muscles are shown in Table 12.5. The major limitation to determination of F-chronodispersion is patient intolerance of the 100 or more supramaximal stimuli used to evoke the F-wave response. In patients with radiculopathies, polyneuropathies, and mononeuropathies, the F-wave chronodispersion has been found to be abnormal more often than minimum, mean, and maximum F-wave latencies or F-wave persistence (15).

F-waves do not have a consistent configuration (waveform size and shape). F-waves are much smaller in amplitude (<5%) than the M-waves produced by the direct activation of the motor fibers at the point of stimulation. Because F-waves are smaller in amplitude (usually <500 μV), this signal reflects the activation of a smaller population (1% to 5%) of the motor units in the muscle. F-wave amplitude is sometimes expressed as a percentage of the associated M-wave amplitude. F-wave amplitude and persistence are indicative of the relative excitability of alpha motoneuron axons. The F-wave amplitudes and frequency of appearance (F-wave persistence) increase as motoneuron pool excitability increases.

What do the findings derived from F-wave testing mean? The F-wave testing is commonly performed for the assessment of conduction in the proximal nerve segments. In all cases, F-wave data interpretation must be made in conjunction with the interpretation of conventional motor nerve conduction testing. F-waves are routinely evoked by ulnar, median, peroneal, and tibial nerve stimulation recording from abductor digiti minimi, APB, extensor digitorum brevis and soleus, or abductor hallucis respectively. F-wave studies via stimulation of these nerves may

Table 12.5. F-wave Chronodispersion Values

Nerve	*Muscle*	*Chronodispersion Average ± SD (ms)*
Median nerve	Abductor pollicis brevis	3.6 ± 1.2
Ulnar nerve	Abductor digiti minimi	3.3 ± 1.1
Peroneal nerve	Extensor digitorum brevis	6.4 ± 0.8
Tibial nerve	Soleus	2.8 ± 1.1

provide insight into the integrity of C8, T1, L5, and S1 nerve roots (16). Techniques have also been developed to measure F-wave latencies for the median nerve to the flexor carpi radialis (17), and for the radial nerve to the extensor indicis (18).

F-wave latencies are often abnormally long in polyneuropathies, even when conduction in distal nerve segments is normal (19,20). F-chronodispersion may be increased in demyelinating polyneuropathies as well. For example, some have suggested that minimal F-wave latency is an extremely sensitive measure for the detection of diabetic polyneuropathy (21). Prolonged F-wave latencies in the presence of normal amplitude M-waves are suggestive of motoneuron axonal demyelination (22,23). In the most common form of acute inflammatory demyelinating polyneuropathy (e.g., Guillain-Barré syndrome), F-wave latency increases may be the only nerve conduction abnormality detected (24). F-wave latencies may also be significantly increased in amyotrophic lateral sclerosis and myotonic dystrophy (13). F-wave testing is controversial in the assessment of suspected compromise of brachial or lumbosacral plexus structures. When F-wave latency increases are found in sacral plexopathy, such latency increases are of little value in localization of any plexus compromise. F-wave testing may well yield findings within normal limits in the presence of a well-localized significant axonal lesion in the brachial plexus. One investigation in patients with clinical cervical radiculopathy found less than 10% of patients had F-wave latency increases (16).

F-wave testing has low sensitivity to detect isolated nerve-root lesions. In fact, mild focal lesions of motor axons, regardless of the location, may not produce significant increase in the F-wave latency. Central nervous system lesions or disease may influence F-wave test findings. Hypotonia and hyporeflexia are generally accompanied by decreased F-wave amplitudes and decreased persistence. In contrast, central nervous system lesions that result in spasticity (hypertonia and hyperreflexia) increase F-wave amplitudes and persistence. In myopathic disorders, F-wave latencies are normal, but amplitudes of F-waves may be markedly reduced due to a loss of muscle fibers. Finally, the clinician must remember that F-wave testing provides no information regarding the functional integrity of sensory axons in the peripheral nervous system, and F-waves will not be abnormal in disorders that primarily affect sensory axons.

Reflex Testing

Axon Reflex

Another voltage response that may be seen during motor nerve conduction studies is the axon reflex. These small, time-locked potentials are often seen in peripheral nerve diseases that produce chronic partial denervation and subsequently produce proximal nerve collateral branching. Axon reflex potentials usually appear following the M-wave but preceding F-waves or H-reflexes (Fig. 12.18B). Axon reflexes may be differentiated from F-waves because they have a persistent shape after each stimulus. Axon reflexes do not usually appear when supramaximal levels of stimulation are applied to peripheral nerves. This response is poorly named, in that the pathway for the response does not involve the spinal cord or reflex mechanisms. Rather, stimulation evokes antidromically propagated action potentials in motor axons that make a "U-turn" at a point where the axons branch (Figure 12.18A). The action potentials then travel orthodromically down the axon branches and reactivate the innervated muscle fibers.

With each submaximal stimulus, the amplitude and latency of the axon reflex waveform remain stable. These small, time-locked potentials occur infrequently, but may be seen in peripheral nerve diseases or injury where proximal nerve branching has occurred. The axon reflex is of little value in electrophysiologic assessment and simply reflects reinnervation of previously denervated muscle fibers. The axon reflex appears rarely in normal, healthy individuals. Observation of axons reflexes during electrophysiologic examination is generally interpreted as a finding consistent with chronic neuropathies or chronic nerve entrapment.

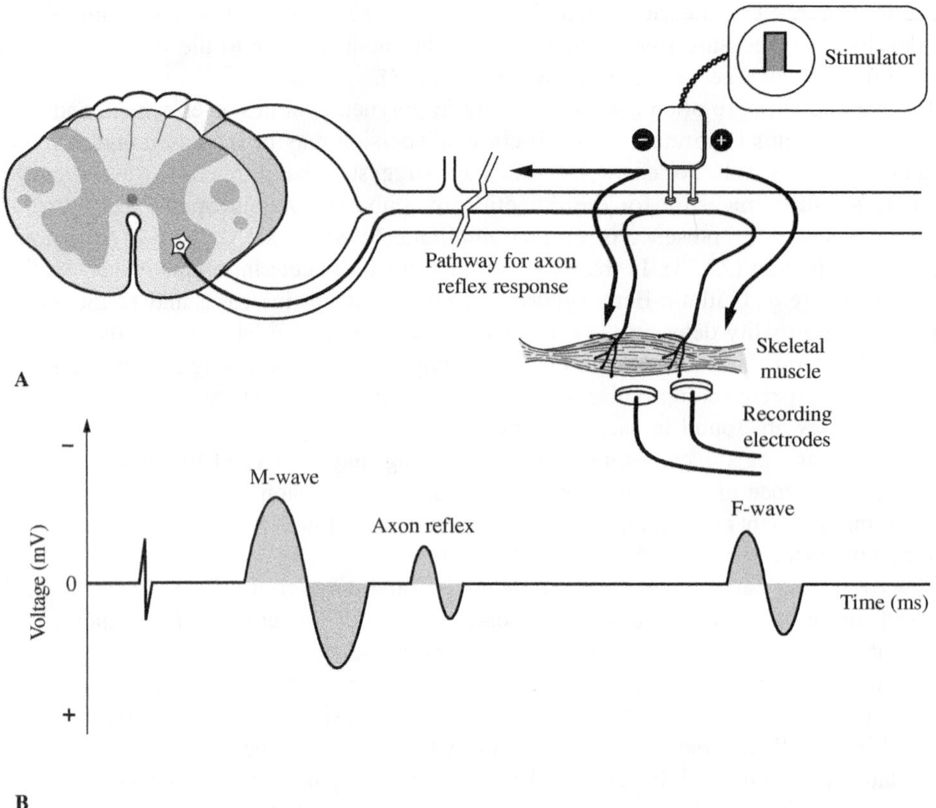

Figure 12.18. A: Illustration of the pathways, stimulation sites, and recording sites for eliciting the axon reflex. **B:** Diagram of M-wave, axon reflex potential, and F-wave that may be elicited during motor nerve conduction testing.

H-Reflex

In routine neurological testing, the phasic stretch reflex (myotatic reflex, deep tendon reflex, monosynaptic reflex) is elicited by providing a quick stretch to a muscle. Phasic stretch reflex testing is performed by tapping a muscle tendon or muscle belly using a reflex hammer (e.g., patellar tendon reflex, Achilles tendon reflex). The quick stretch activates stretch receptors in the muscle called muscle spindles. One particular class of muscle spindle afferent (sensory) fibers, the Ia afferents, produces a burst of action potentials that are propagated toward the central nervous system. The central processes of Ia afferent axons synapse directly on the alpha motoneurons that innervate the muscle stretched. In normal individuals, the quick stretch produces enough Ia afferent activation to excite some of the alpha motoneurons to the stretched muscle. Action potentials produced in the alpha motoneurons then pass along the alpha motoneuron axons to the muscle, resulting in a brief twitchlike contraction, the characteristic reflex response. The contraction response to tendon tapping is subjectively graded by the examiner as being either normal, less than expected (hypoactive, +1 or absent), or greater than expected (hyperactive, +3 or +4). The reliability of routine neurological stretch reflex testing depends on the skill of the examiner, and test results may not be particularly sensitive in identification of abnormalities in the reflex pathway. Inexperienced examiners may fail to apply sufficient muscle stretch or may not ensure that the patient's muscles are relaxed during stretch reflex testing and hence may not gain a valid indication of the integrity of the reflex pathway.

As an alternative approach, the integrity of phasic stretch reflex pathways may be examined using electrophysiologic evaluation techniques. For example, the pathway associated with the Achilles tendon reflex may be examined by placing recording electrodes over the soleus muscle and stimulating the tibial nerve at the popliteal fossa with progressively larger amplitude stimuli. In response to relatively low-amplitude stimuli, the first observed response recorded is usually a CMAP that appears at a latency considerably longer than that anticipated for the M-wave evoked during motor nerve conduction studies. This long latency CMAP is called an *H-wave*, *Hoffman response*, or *H-reflex*. The H-wave results from stimulation of Ia muscle spindle afferents that reflexively activate soleus motoneurons within the spinal cord (Figs. 12.19 and 12.20A). This reflex activation of soleus motoneurons sends action potentials to the soleus, resulting in the excitation of soleus muscle fibers and hence the CMAP that is the H-wave response.

If the amplitude of stimulation is increased, the M-wave response appears simultaneously on the display preceding the H-wave (Fig.12.20B). The M-wave occurs when the alpha motoneuron axons (slightly smaller in diameter than Ia afferents) are activated directly at the site of stimulation and subsequently activate innervated muscles fibers. As the amplitude of stimulation is increased even more, the amplitudes of both the M-wave and H-wave increase. The M-wave size increases as more motor axons to the muscle are recruited directly at the stimulation site. The H-wave increases in size as greater numbers of soleus muscle spindle afferents are activated, resulting in greater reflex

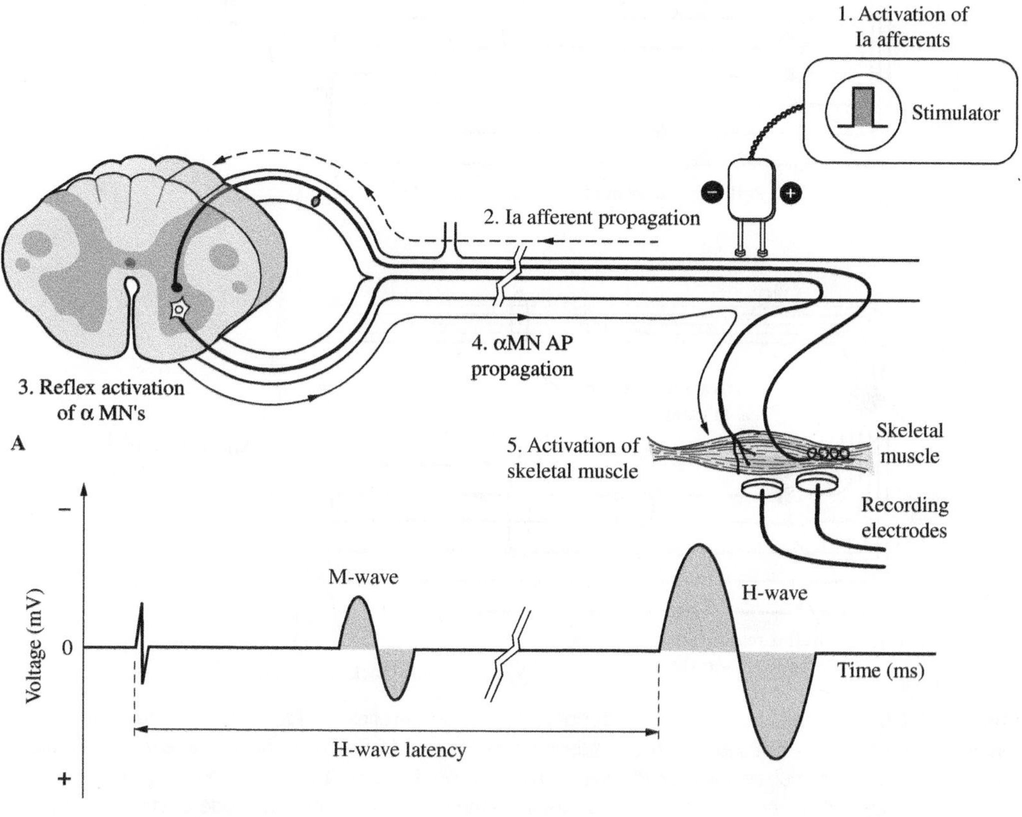

Figure 12.19. A: Illustrations of the pathways, stimulation sites, and recording sites for conducting the H-reflex test. **B:** Recording of M-wave and H-wave responses during H-reflex test.

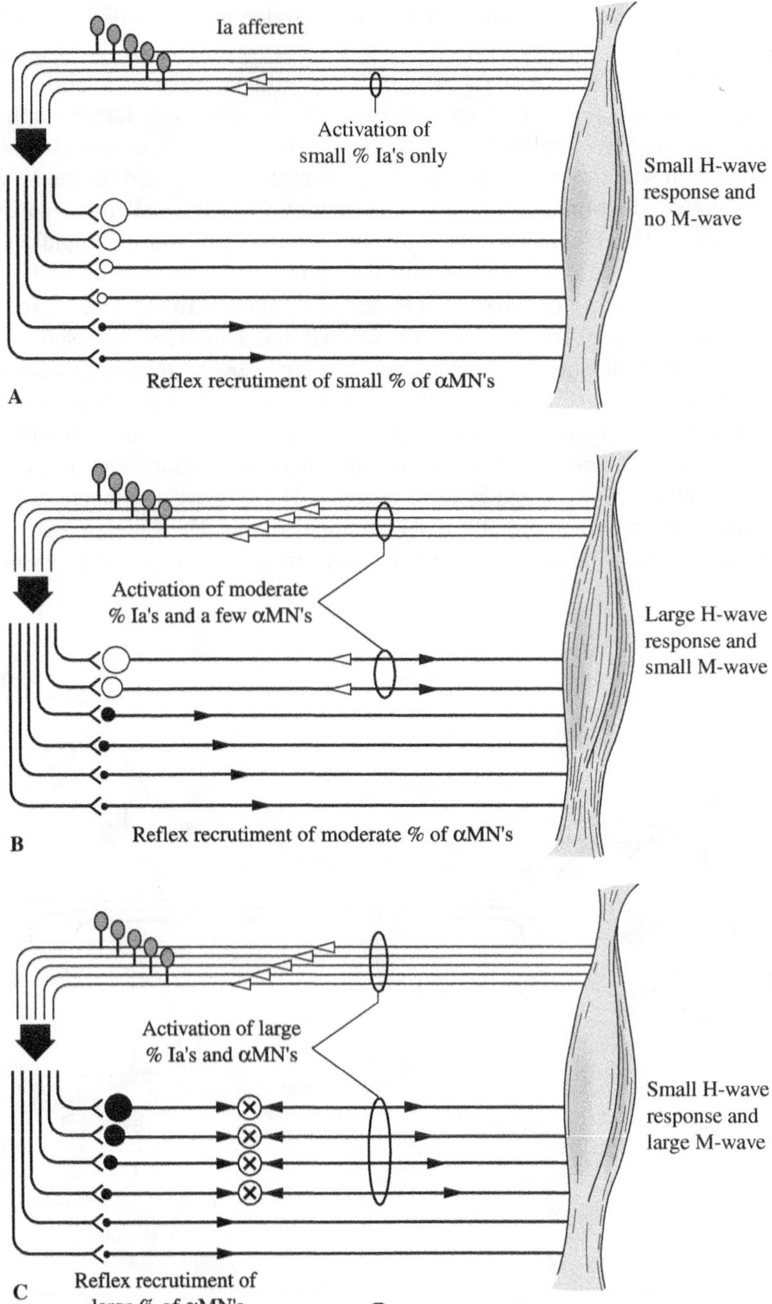

Figure 12.20. Differential recruitment of peripheral axons in H-reflex testing as the amplitude of stimulation is increased from submaximal to supramaximal levels. **A:** Recruitment of Ia afferent axons alone using low-amplitude stimulation and producing a small H-wave. **B:** Recruitment of more Ia afferents and some of the larger diameter alpha motoneuron axons using an intermediate amplitude of stimulation and producing both an M-wave and a larger H-wave. **C:** Excessive stimulation activating all Ia afferents and all alpha motoneurons producing a maximal M-wave but partial blocking the H-reflex response.

recruitment of soleus motoneurons. During this procedure, the direct activation of muscle producing the M-wave tends to activate axons of larger diameter first and hence the largest motor units (e.g., type FF). In contrast, the reflex activation of the soleus motoneurons that produces the H-wave tends to activate the smallest of the motoneurons first and hence the smallest motor units (e.g., type S).

As the amplitude of stimulation is increased to even higher levels, the amplitude of the H-wave begins to diminish. This reduction in H-wave size results when the reflexively activated soleus motoneuron action potentials traveling orthodromically collide with antidromically activated action potentials in the same axons initiated at the site of stimulation (Fig. 12.20C). Reflexively produced action potentials elicited by spindle afferent feedback that may have initially contributed to the H-wave are blocked and hence no longer contribute to the H-wave response. If stimulation amplitudes are high, the reflex activation of the soleus may be completely blocked, and the H-wave may disappear. An inexperienced examiner may unknowingly apply stimuli at inappropriately high levels that block the production of the H-reflex response. This error by the examiner could lead to an inappropriate interpretation of the absent H reflex.

Because the H-reflex test employs similar neural pathways as the stretch reflex, this procedure is also referred to as the *electrically elicited stretch reflex.* H-reflex testing allows one to obtain quantitative, objective information regarding the integrity of the stretch reflex pathway. In contrast, the evaluation of the standard deep tendon reflex using a reflex hammer is highly subjective in nature.

The latency to onset of the H-wave depends on the integrity of the sensory afferent neurons, the synapses between Ia afferents and motoneurons, the alpha motoneuron cell bodies and axons, the neuromuscular junctions, and the muscle fibers themselves. Delays in conduction or transmission at any of these sites may increase the H-reflex latency. The H-wave can be tested in muscles of both lower (e.g., triceps surae, quadriceps, and tibialis anterior) and upper limbs (e.g., flexor carpi radialis). H-reflexes are difficult to elicit in other muscles in normal subjects unless the subject voluntarily contracts simultaneously with the testing stimulation. The latency of the soleus H-response normally ranges from 24 to 32 ms and is dependent on leg length, height, and age. Soleus H-reflex latencies should not differ by more than 1.5 to 2.0 ms between opposite limbs. H-reflex latencies recorded from flexor carpi radialis should not normally differ by more than 1 ms between limbs. Peak-to-peak amplitudes of H-reflex responses vary considerably between individuals and even from side to side in healthy individuals. Consequently, H-wave amplitudes are rarely reported in documentation of electrophysiologic test results.

Abnormal findings in H-reflex testing are commonly associated with disorders in the proximal segments of peripheral nerves. The soleus reflex response is useful for determining pathology of the S1 nerve root, while the H-reflex test of flexor carpi radialis is implemented in suspected brachial plexopathy or C6 to C7 nerve root compromise. Both upper and lower limb H-reflex latencies may be abnormally long in cases of demyelinating peripheral polyneuropathy (e.g., Guillian-Barré syndrome) (12). H-reflex findings may also be abnormal with central nervous system disorders. After cerebrovascular accident, amplitudes of H-responses may be larger than normal (>70% of M-wave maximum amplitude) and may not be augmented by voluntary contraction. Central nervous system lesions or disease may also result in H-reflex appearance in the intrinsic hand muscles or tibialis anterior where such responses are normally not readily observed.

Blink Reflex Tests

The *blink reflex test* is used to assess the functional integrity of both the trigeminal nerve (CN V) and the facial nerve (CN VII) (6), as well as the central nervous system connections between these two cranial nerves in the principle sensory nucleus of V and the facial motor nucleus. The afferent limb of the reflex is the trigeminal nerve, and the efferent limb is the facial nerve (Figure 12.21A). The central relay nuclei of the reflex are located in the sensory trigeminal nucleus and facial motor nucleus.

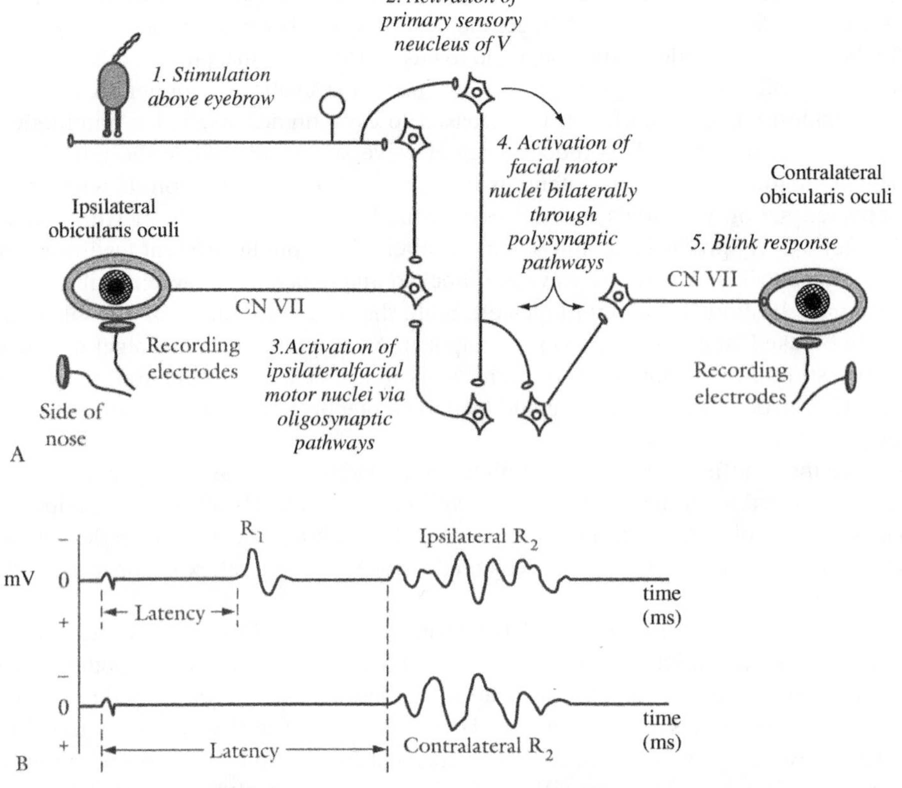

Figure 12.21. A: Illustration of pathways associated with the blink reflex test. **B:** Diagram of R_1 and R_2 responses recorded from the obicularis oculi ipsilateral and contralateral to the side of stimulation.

To perform this test, recording electrodes are placed bilaterally over the obicularis oculi muscles, and stimulating electrodes are positioned over the supraorbital branch of the trigeminal nerve. Electrical stimulation of the supraorbital branch of the trigeminal nerve evokes two separate CMAP responses of the ipsilateral obicularis oculi (Fig. 12.21B). The earliest CMAP response is called R_1, and the latter response is called R_2. In the contralateral obicularis oculi, only R_2 will be recorded. The latency of R_1 is a reflection of the conduction over the reflex pathway that includes the time associated with cranial nerve V (trigeminal) afferent conduction, brainstem pontine nuclei synaptic delays and conduction between nuclei, and cranial nerve VII (facial) efferent conduction to blink muscles.

Prolongation or absence of R_1 suggests compromise of any or all of the components that make up the reflex pathway. R_2 latencies reflect the afferent conduction in the trigeminal nerve, synaptic delays in both pontine and medullary relay nuclei, internuclear conduction, and efferent conduction in the facial nerve. With trigeminal neuropathy on one side, R_2 latencies both ipsilaterally and contralaterally will be prolonged. With a facial neuropathy on one side, R_2 latency will be abnormal on the involved side but within normal limits on the opposite, uninvolved side.

In normal individuals the R_1 latency should not exceed 13 ms and usually falls in the 9- to 12-ms range. Side-to-side differences for R_1 should not exceed 1.2 ms. R_2 latencies ipsilaterally should not be greater than 41 ms, and R_2 contralaterally should not be greater than 44 ms. By determining the respective response latencies, a lesion of either the facial or trigeminal nerve in the reflex loop can be detected. The function of the distal segment of the facial nerve can be assessed by direct stimulation distal to the stylomastoid foramen and measuring the latency of the M-wave response in the obicularis oculi. In most cases of facial neuropathy (e.g., Bell palsy), the site of pathology is proximal to the stimulation site producing the facial motor response. Testing the blink reflex in cases of facial neuropathy will result in diminished and/or delayed ipsilateral R_1 and R_2, while the contralateral R_2 will be unaffected. A lesion of the trigeminal nerve may delay and/or reduce both the ipsilateral R_1 and R_2 and the contralateral R_2 component. This test is useful in identifying pathologies affecting the cranial nerves that include but are not limited to Bell palsy, cerebellar-pontine angle tumors, brainstem aneurysms, acoustic neuromas, Guillain-Barré syndrome, and central demyelinating processes such as multiple sclerosis.

Central Evoked Potential Testing

Evoked potentials are voltage changes monitored from the electrically excitable tissue of the cerebral cortex, brainstem, and spinal cord in response to various applied sensory stimuli. The function of pathways leading to three different central nervous system sensory areas, the somatosensory cortex, the visual cortex, and the auditory region of the brainstem, can be evaluated using electrophysiologic tests. In general, to test the integrity of the pathways to these areas, appropriate sensory stimuli are applied consistent with the sensory modality examined. Under normal circumstances, the adequate amplitude sensory stimuli activate respective sensory receptors. Action potentials are initiated at receptors and propagated along peripheral and/or central nervous system pathways. Action potentials reaching destinations in the central nervous system subsequently alter the electrical activity of the central nervous system cells associated with processing incoming sensory information. The change in electrical activity of the cortical or brainstem area is monitored by surface recording electrodes placed on the skin over the appropriate regions of the cortex or brainstem.

Somatosensory Evoked Potential Testing

The integrity of the ascending somatosensory pathways can be assessed using electrophysiological procedures. These procedures are characterized by electrical activation of sensory fibers in skin and peripheral mixed nerves while simultaneously monitoring the propagation of synchronous volleys of sensory action potentials at sites along these pathways. Stimulation of peripheral sensory fibers is applied at amplitudes sufficient to activate sensory action potentials in large-diameter sensory afferents, including Ia muscle spindle afferents and group II cutaneous touch-pressure afferents. In mixed nerves (e.g., median, ulnar, peroneal or tibial; Fig. 12.22A) containing both motor and sensory axons, stimulation during testing is sufficient in amplitude to produce a simultaneous twitchlike contraction of muscles innervated by the motor fibers of these nerves. This ensures that a substantial number of the sensory fibers within the nerve bundle are adequately stimulated. Frequencies of stimulation are normally in the 1 to 5 pps range, and monophasic pulsed currents of 0.1 to 0.2 ms pulse duration are used. In general, stimuli are applied with surface electrodes, although use of needle electrodes to stimulate near nerve trunks is not uncommon. Stimulation is provided first unilaterally near a particular nerve, and later bilaterally. The sensory action potentials elicited by such stimulation are monitored by placing an active surface recording electrode over Erb's point (lower inner angle of the supraclavicular fossa), the spinal cord (C5 for upper extremity, T12 for lower extremity) and/or cortex (Fig. 12.22B). Different recording site combinations are used in evoked potential testing; refer to more detailed texts on this topic for further information on recording electrode placement (1,25).

The evoked sensory potentials, called *somatosensory evoked potentials* (SSEP), are so small that, in some cases, up to 2,000 responses must be evoked and averaged to clearly visualize the responses on a display device. Once SSEP are clearly visualized from recording sites, measurements are made of latencies to the onset of the potentials, latencies to the peaks of the potentials,

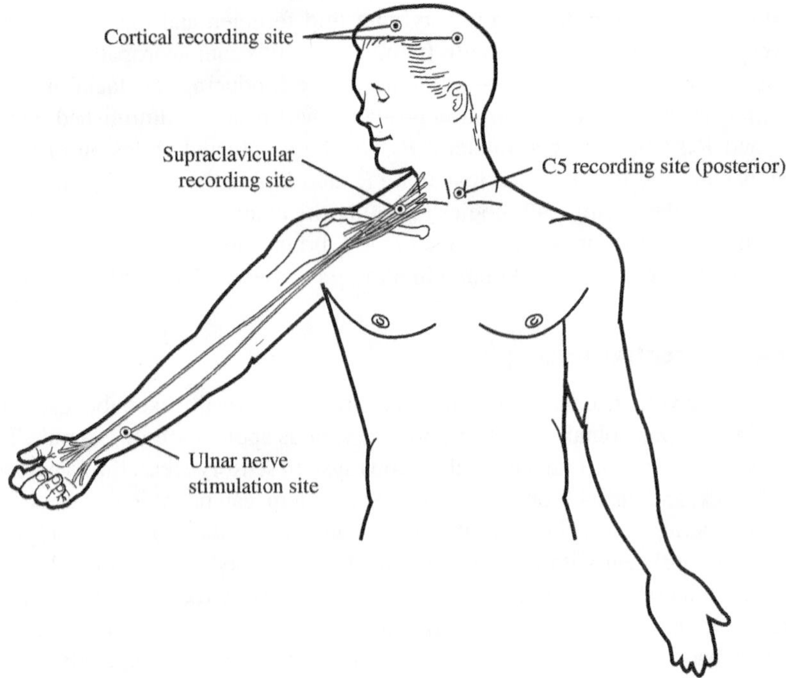

Figure 12.22. Illustration of the stimulation and recording electrode placement in somatosensory evoked potential testing using the ulnar nerve.

and the time between peaks recorded at several different sites. Peak-to-peak amplitude of each recorded potential is also measured. The latency values measured using cortical electrodes reflect both the peripheral and central conduction times for sensory action potential transmission. To gain insight into the central pathway conduction, the peripheral conduction latency measured with C5 or T12 electrodes is subtracted from the total conduction latency measured from cortical electrode recordings. This test is useful for identifying demyelinating diseases and spinal cord, cortical, and brainstem dysfunction.

The waveforms of SSEPs are often complex and characterized by combinations of positive and negative peaks. The latency to each positive and negative peak is measured to the nearest millisecond. Each peak is then labeled according to the polarity of the deflection (P for positive, N for negative) and the measured latency. For example, a peak labeled P13 would apply to a positive deflection peak occurring at a latency of 13 ms. Figure 12.23 illustrates SSEPs evoked by ulnar nerve stimulation and recorded over Erb's point, C5 spinous process, and two scalp locations associated with sensation of the hand. The latencies of the somatosensory potentials recorded at various locations are compared with normal latencies limits to determine the location of sensory nerve compromise. For example, if the latency of the SSEP between the wrist and Erb's point is normal, but the latency between wrist and C5 is prolonged, a spinal nerve-root lesion might be the underlying problem. In contrast, if the latency to Erb's point was prolonged (given normal distal segmental conduction), but the latency between Erb's point and C5 (wrist to C5 minus wrist to Erb's point) was normal, a brachial plexus lesion may be the source of compromise. The important point is that somatosensory evoked potential testing provides a means to examine nerve conduction in proximal segments of peripheral sensory axons analogous to the F-wave testing procedure used to examine proximal conduction in motor nerve axons. See other texts (25) for a more detailed description of the clinical applications and analysis of somatosensory evoked potential testing.

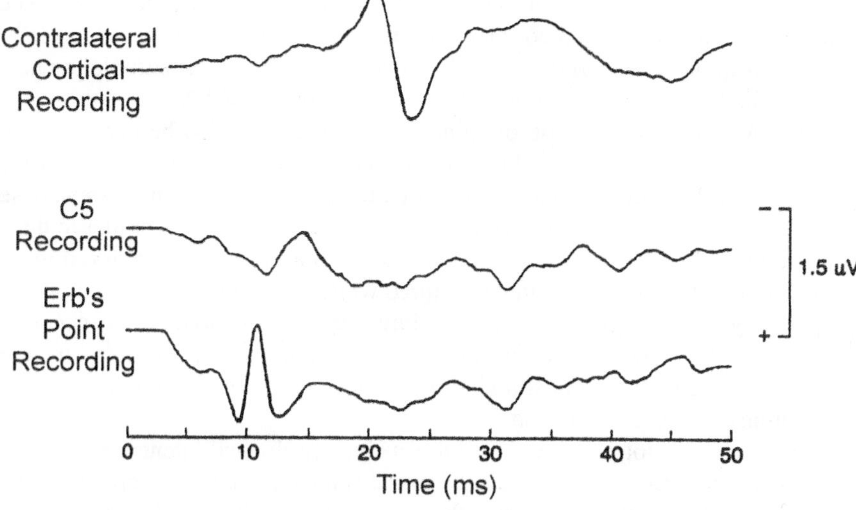

Figure 12.23. Somatosensory evoked potentials evoked by ulnar nerve stimulation at the wrist and recorded at Erb's point, at the C5 level, and over the cortex.

Brainstem Auditory Evoked Potential Testing

Brainstem auditory evoked potentials (BAEPs) are electric waveforms recorded from the brain elicited in responses to sound. To produce BAEPs, a clicklike sound is applied through one ear. Surface scalp electrodes are applied over the vertex on the same side as stimulation. Individual evoked potentials are very small in amplitude; therefore up to 2,000 responses to stimuli may need to be averaged to visualize the evoked waveform. Subjects must remain very still during the test because small movements such as neck movement or swallowing may contaminate the recording. A detailed presentation of the interpretation of BAEPs is beyond the scope of this text. The test is applied to assess the integrity of the auditory pathway from the cochlea to the auditory cortex. BAEP testing is applied in cases where demyelinization, neuromas, tumors, or other disorders of auditory pathways are suspected. Brainstem evoked potential testing is generally considered a primary assessment tool of the clinical audiologist.

Visual Evoked Potential Testing

Visual evoked potentials are bioelectric signals recorded during electrical activity in occipital lobe cortex in response to light stimuli. Compared to the other cortical evoked potentials, visual evoked potentials are technically easier to record. Surface electrodes are placed on the scalp overlying the occipital cortex. A controlled light pattern generator is used to stimulate either one eye or both eyes simultaneously. The stimuli are presented from 100 to 200 times with signal averaging of successive cortical responses. The test is clinically useful in determining the integrity and conduction characteristics of the visual pathways. Changes in the waveform or latency provide information concerning disruption of the visual system. Performance of visual evoked potential testing is primarily the domain of the ophthalmologist.

Motor Evoked Potential Testing

The integrity of the descending motor pathways (e.g., corticospinal tract) may be assessed using electrophysiological procedures that activate the motor cortex or central motor pathways while monitoring the propagation of a synchronous volley of motor action potentials at sites along these pathways, including the spinal cord and skeletal muscle. Although transcutaneous electrical stimulation was initially used to stimulate the motor cortex, magnetic stimulation has become the preferred method to activate neurons in the cerebral cortex, which give rise to descending motor pathways. Magnetic stimulation of spinal nerve roots may also be performed by placement of the magnetic coil over the vertebral column. The amplitude of stimulation is adjusted to a level approximately 20% greater than that required to evoke a minimal motor response. Motor evoked potentials are recorded with surface electrodes placed in a manner similar to that used for conventional peripheral motor nerve conduction studies. Subjects are often asked to perform a voluntary contraction of the muscle being monitored while stimulation is being applied at proximal motor pathway sites. Amplitudes and absolute latencies of motor evoked potentials are recorded in response to stimulation. Central motor conduction time is calculated by subtracting the latency between spinal nerve root stimulation and muscle response from the latency between cortical stimulation and muscle response.

Abnormalities in the motor evoked response include prolonged latency, reduced or absent response, or abnormal response configuration. Central conduction latencies are prolonged in diseases that demyelinate descending motor pathways, such as multiple sclerosis, or in disorders that destroy upper motoneurons, such as amyotrophic lateral sclerosis. Loss of upper motoneurons may also be reflected by reduced amplitude or absent motor evoked potentials in response to cortical stimulation.

Repetitive Nerve Stimulation Testing

The *repetitive nerve stimulation test* or Jolly test has been used for more than 90 years to assess the function of the neuromuscular junction. In this procedure, supramaximal stimuli are applied to peripheral nerves, and the CMAPs evoked are recorded from innervated muscles. Stimulation frequencies used range from 2 to 3 pps. The evoked CMAP's peak-to-peak amplitude or peak negative amplitude is observed while stimulation is applied. In subjects with normal neuromuscular

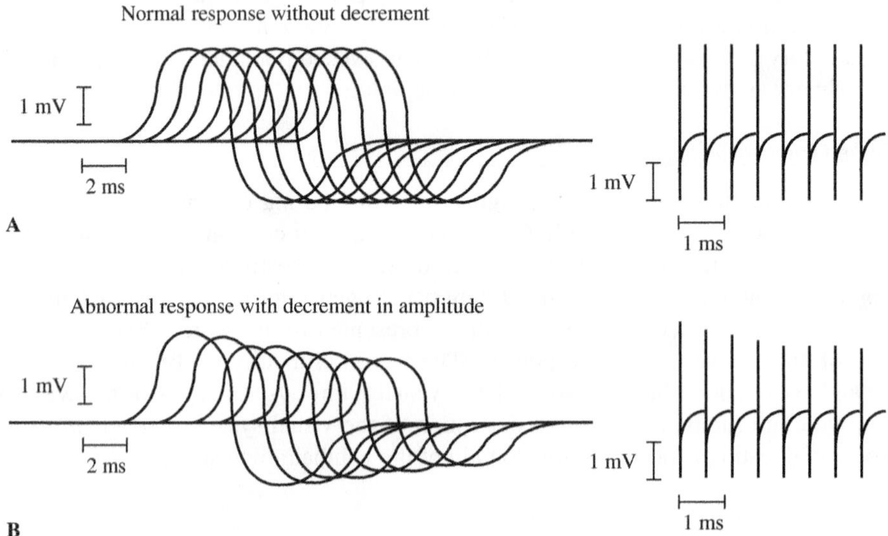

Figure 12.24. Compound muscle action potential produced during the repetitive nerve stimulation test; **A:** normal response. **B:** abnormal response with decrement in the amplitude.

junctions, repeated stimulation (2 to 3 pps) will slightly deplete the junction of acetylcholine, resulting in a small drop in muscle fiber recruitment and a small drop (5% to 8%) in the amplitude of the recorded CMAPs. In diseases where neuromuscular junction transmission is impaired, the drop in CMAP amplitude is more marked (>10% drop in amplitude between first CMAP and fourth through sixth CMAP). Figure 12.24 shows the responses of both normal and abnormal neuromuscular junction function on the amplitude of CMAPs during repetitive stimulation. The test is generally repeated several times and on several muscles to establish the consistency of the response and improve its sensitivity. Significant reductions in the amplitude of the CMAPs during repetitive nerve stimulation are most frequently associated with either myasthenia gravis, an autoimmune disorder that reduces the number of acetylcholine receptors at the neuromuscular junction, or Lambert–Eaton myasthenic syndrome, another autoimmune disorder that impairs calcium ion entry into presynaptic motor axon terminals and hence interferes with neurotransmitter release.

Like many of the more sophisticated electrophysiologic testing procedures, repetitive nerve stimulation testing procedures are technically difficult to perform accurately. For example, false positive results may be obtained when either electrode or limb stabilization is inadequate. For further details on repetitive nerve stimulation testing, see Oh's extensive dissertation on the topic (26).

CLINICAL ELECTROMYOGRAPHIC EXAMINATION

All the procedures that examine the conduction in nerve pathways employ the activation of excitable tissues by electrical or magnetic stimulation. These techniques produce electrical activity in nerve and muscle in a manner that is not typical of normal physiological activation. In contrast, the procedure of electromyography examines the electrical activity of skeletal muscle fibers at rest and during normal physiological voluntary activation of muscle. Electromyography is used clinically to answer the following types of questions:

1. Is the muscle normally innervated, partially innervated, or denervated?
2. Does evidence of reinnervation exist?
3. Are EMG findings consistent with neuropathic or myopathic disease?
4. Is the pattern of EMG abnormalities in muscles examined consistent with a nerve root, plexus, anterior horn cell, or peripheral nerve lesion?
5. In neuropathy, what are the specific locations of the nerve lesion?
6. Does the problem involve muscle in the extremities (anterior primary rami innervation), paraspinal musculature (posterior primary rami innervation), or head/neck musculature (cranial nerve innervation)?

Needle electromyographic studies, like nerve conduction studies, are an extension of the routine clinical neurological examination. The advantages of needle electromyography over clinical examination alone include greater sensitivity to mild levels of denervation, better selectivity for the distribution of denervation, and more insight into the possible pathologic mechanism underlying the patient's problems (27).

Electromyographic recording technique employs three electrodes connected to the recording instruments. These electrodes are connected to three inputs of the recording instrument labeled active (also known as negative), reference (also known as positive), and ground, respectively. The three most common types of EMG needle electrodes are defined by the number of conductors contained within the needle. Generally, the greater the number of electrodes, the larger the diameter of the needle. Bipolar needle electrodes contain electrodes that can be connected to the active, reference, and ground inputs of the recording system. Concentric needle electrodes contain wires for active and reference inputs and require an additional surface electrode that is connected to ground. Monopolar electrodes, the most commonly used, contain one conductor connected to the active input and require not only a second surface electrode connected to external ground, but also another surface or needle electrode connected to the reference input. The reference electrode is placed within 2 cm of the active monopolar needle electrode. Reusable, sterilizable concentric electrodes were the most widely used until recently because of their clean signal and relatively large gauge (small diameter). Currently, disposable monopolar and concentric electrodes have become more common because of concerns about the transmission of infectious diseases and because of their smaller size.

The EMG examination is divided into four segments per area of muscle studied: (i) insertional activity, (ii) activity at rest or spontaneous activity, (ii) activity upon minimal voluntary activation and recruitment patterns, and (iv) activity during voluntary maximal activation.

Normal and Abnormal Electrical Activity in Skeletal Muscle at Rest

Insertional Activity

As the EMG needle electrode is inserted into muscle, a brief electrical discharge can be seen on a visual display and heard on an audio amplifier. The discharge is characterized as a high-frequency burst of positive and negative spikes associated with a "crisp static sound" from the audioamplifier (28). This is normal *insertional activity* (Fig. 12.25). Insertional activity can be reproduced by tapping the muscle or any time the needle electrode is repositioned or moved within the muscle. This electrical activity is thought to be associated with mechanical stimulation of muscle fiber membranes that may or may not cause minor membrane damage. Insertional activity in healthy muscle normally lasts 50 to 200 ms and slightly outlasts the movement of the electrode (28).

A *reduction in normal insertional activity* (fewer than expected voltage fluctuations) is commonly associated with a loss of muscle fibers and is often seen in fibrotic or severely atrophied, chronically denervated muscles. When reduced insertional activity is observed, the clinician may notice an increase in the mechanical resistance to advancement of the needle

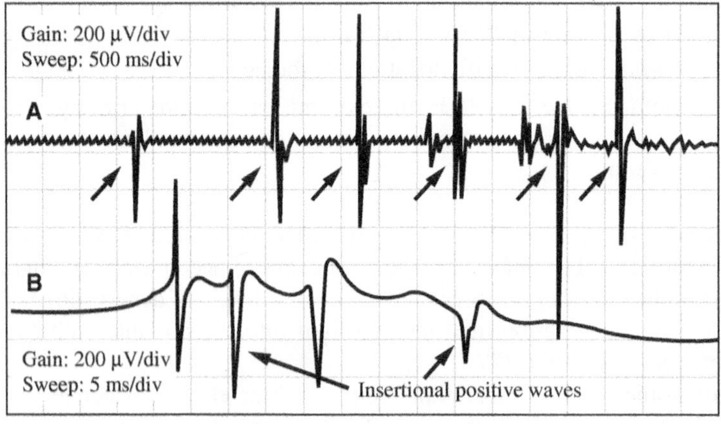

Figure 12.25. A: Insertional activity (indicated by arrows) during advancement of needle electrode during an electromyographic examination. **B:** Insertional positive waves.

electrode. Reduced insertional activity has also been noted in metabolic disorders such as hypokalemic periodic paralysis. An *increase in insertional activity* is another change that may occur with pathology and generally refers to electrical activity that persists for more than 500 ms after the needle electrode movement has stopped. This prolongation of insertional activity is indicative of muscle membrane hyperexcitability associated with either neuropathic and myopathic disorders. *Prolonged insertional activity* is commonly seen after acute denervation, in inflammatory muscle disorders such as polymyositis, and in diseases such as muscular dystrophy. Within 3 days to 3 weeks after denervation of muscle, insertional activity may be followed by a series of positive spikelike waveforms that persist for up to several minutes after needle movement in the muscle is stopped. These *insertional positive waves* (Fig. 12.25) discharge at rates ranging from 3 to 30 spikes per second (29). Such prolonged discharges may also be found in cases of acute polymyositis or in muscles that have been denervated for extended periods of time.

Normal and Abnormal Spontaneous Activity in Muscle at Rest

Healthy muscle at rest is generally electrically silent when the needle electrode is not moving. If the recording electrodes are positioned at the motor endplate (neuromuscular junction), however, very small electrical potentials may be observed. These very low amplitude (usually 10 to 40 μV) potentials with initial negative deflection are called *miniature end-plate potentials* (MEPPs) and are thought to be produced by localized, transient depolarization of the muscle membrane near the neuromuscular junction (9). MEPPs are a normal electrophysiologic finding. Passing such signals through an audio amplifier produces a sound described as that heard when a seashell is held to the ear (28). Often a subject reports a dull, aching pain at the electrode site when MEPPs are recorded, and this pain generally disappears if the electrode is withdrawn slightly and repositioned within the muscle. Other normal electrical potentials that may be occasionally noted when the electrode is near the motor end-plate include *end-plate potentials* (EPP) and *end-plate spikes* (EPS) (Fig.12.26). Both of these potentials have amplitudes generally ranging from 100 to 300 μV with 2 to 4 ms durations, and generally discharge at 5 to 50 per second. The EPSs and EPPs are thought to occur when the needle electrode activates single muscle fibers. Like MEPPs, EPPs and EPSs disappear when the electrode is moved away from the neuromuscular junction. Care

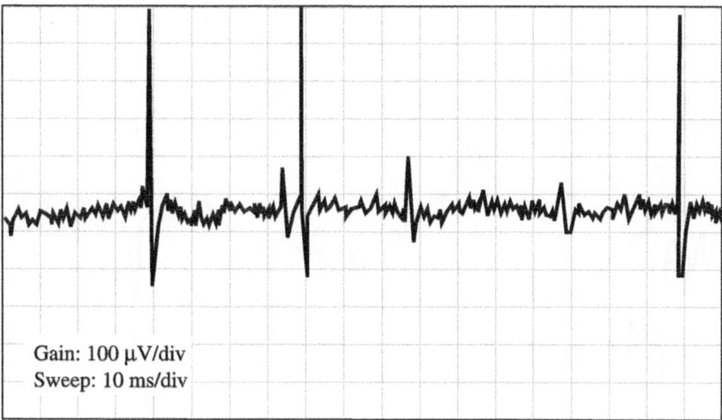

Figure 12.26. End-plate spikes.

must be taken during the electromyographic examination not to confuse EPPs, a normal finding, with fibrillation potentials (discussed below), which are indicative of pathology. Both of these potentials are biphasic and may be of similar amplitudes. EPPs, however are characterized by an initial negative deflection, whereas fibrillation potentials have an initial positive deflection.

MEPPs and EPPs do have diagnostic relevance, and the identification of these potentials during an examination should not be dismissed. End-plate activity does indicate that some axons are intact up to the neuromuscular junction and suggests that at least a portion of the muscle examined is innervated. This finding may be useful in cases of hysterical paralysis or in uncooperative clients who are either unable or unwilling to volitionally activate muscle, and suggests that the failure to contract muscle is not the result of muscle denervation.

Electrical activity other than MEPPs and EPPs in muscle at rest is indicative of neuropathy or myopathy (29). One such type of electrical potential seen at rest in patients with suspected neuropathy or myopathy is *fibrillation potentials* (Fig. 12.27A). Fibrillation potentials have amplitudes usually ranging from 20 to 300 μV and durations in the 1 to 5 ms range. Amplitudes are usually larger in the acute phase of disorders and have been reported as high as 1000 μV (30). These biphasic (sometimes triphasic) potentials with an initial positive deflection generally discharge regularly at rates between 1 and 30 per second but may discharge irregularly. Fibrillation potentials reflect the spontaneous discharge of one or a few muscle fibers and may arise in

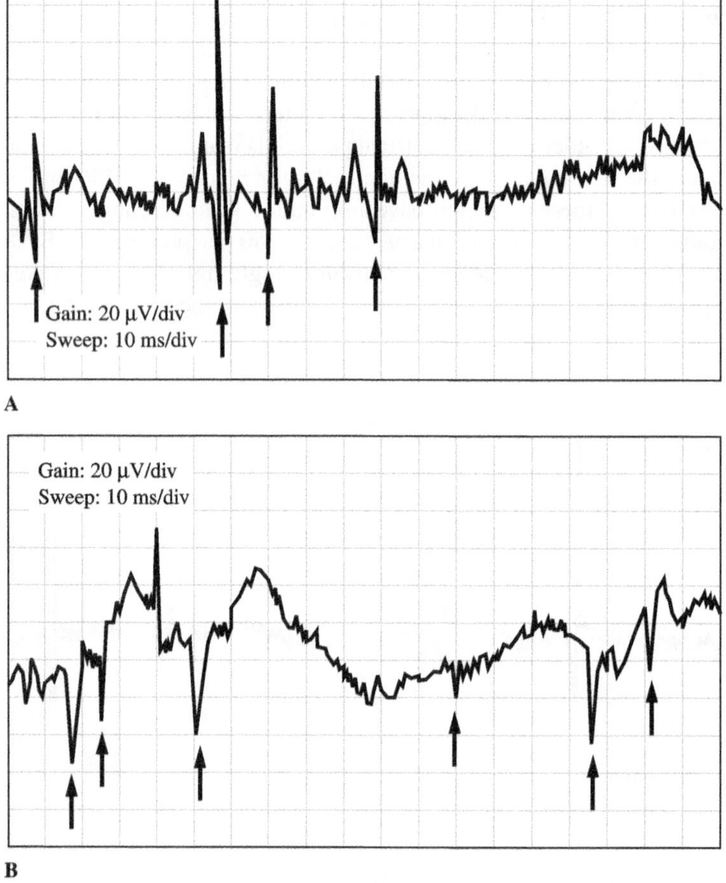

Figure 12.27. A: Fibrillation potentials. **B:** Positive sharp waves.

muscles for a number of reasons. The appearance of fibrillations is thought to represent the existence of unstable muscle fiber membranes. Fibrillation potentials may result from the generalized spread of acetylcholine receptors over the muscle membrane after denervation, making the denervated muscle fibers hypersensitive to acetylcholine. The presence of acetylcholine near the muscle binds to these receptors and produces depolarization of single muscle fiber membranes that results in the generation of this type of short-duration, low-amplitude potential observed in the absence of volitional contraction. Alternatively, fibrillations may represent spontaneous depolarization of muscle fibers resulting from alterations in muscle fiber membrane sodium conductance or decreases in intracellular potassium concentration (31).

Fibrillation activity is most commonly interpreted as a manifestation of motor nerve disruption to skeletal muscle fibers. Indeed, within 14 to 21 days after denervation, fibrillation potentials are usually found within the denervated muscle, and these potentials are generally of relatively high amplitude (>500 μV). Very low-amplitude fibrillation potentials (50 to 100 μV) are commonly associated with long-standing denervation. Fibrillation potentials may not be present in some areas of partially denervated muscles and may disappear as reinnervation takes place. Fibrillation potentials may also be present in patients with myopathy (e.g., muscular dystrophy, polymyositis, hyperkalemic periodic paralysis) or with dysfunction of neuromuscular junction transmission (e.g., myasthenia gravis). The frequency of fibrillation potentials is reduced in muscles that are ischemic or in limbs that are cold. When observed in muscle during a needle examination, the frequency and location of fibrillation potentials is rated on a scale of +1 to +4. Transient fibrillation potentials found at two or more locations is graded as +1. Persistent fibrillation in three or more locations is rated at +2. When fibrillations are observed in all locations, a +3 score is assigned, and when fibrillations are so profuse that they fill the display screen, a +4 score is made. The fibrillation scores do not appear to be related to any particular type of underlying pathology, nor do they necessarily relate to the relative severity of the disorder. For those who read reports of EMG findings, it is important to note that several different variations of the grading scale for fibrillations exist in the literature, and so the meaning of the +1 to +4 scores may vary between laboratories.

Positive sharp waves are another spontaneously occurring electromyographic finding associated with either neuropathy or myopathy (29). These potentials are characterized as sawtooth in appearance, with an initial marked positive deflection followed by a low-amplitude, long-duration negative phase (Fig. 12.27B). The amplitude of positive sharp waves usually increases and decreases within the range of 10 μV to 1 mV, with discharge rates usually in the 5 to 10 per second range, but may discharge at rates as high as 100 per second. Discharge rates are generally regular but may be irregular.

The clinical significance attributed to the presence of positive sharp waves is similar to that of fibrillation potentials, and often these two spontaneous potentials will appear simultaneously in the same record during needle EMG examination. Grading of positive sharp waves is performed using a +1 to +4 scale like that used for fibrillation potentials.

At times during electrophysiologic examination, spontaneous, repetitive, twitchlike contractions of the examined muscle at rest called fasciculations may be observed. Such contractions reflect the discharge of either the fibers of a single motor unit or groups of fibers within a muscle fascicle. When these spontaneous twitches arise, they are accompanied by the production of electrical potentials called *fasciculation potentials* (29). Characterization of fasciculation potentials is difficult due to the broad variation in their parameters. In general, however, fasciculation potentials have characteristics of normal motor unit potentials. The discharge rate of fasciculation potentials is low compared to fibrillation potentials and positive sharp waves. Fasciculation potentials often appear from about once per second to once every 4 or 5 seconds.

Fasciculation potentials are commonly associated with neuropathic diseases or disorders that affect the alpha motoneuron either centrally or peripherally. They appear in diseases like poliomyelitis, syringomyelia, and more commonly in amyotrophic lateral sclerosis. They may also be encountered in disorders such as radiculopathies and entrapment neuropathies, as well as selected myopathies. Fasciculation potentials may be present for a few days after denervation of a muscle, but after 3 or 4 days these potentials may no longer be recorded in a totally denervated muscle. The appearance of a few isolated fasciculations in muscles of healthy individuals (especially the elderly) is not considered abnormal unless accompanied by other abnormal electromyographic findings (32).

Myotonic discharges are rhythmic electrical discharges often initiated by muscle tapping or needle electrode insertion that continue in spite of no further needle movement (29). They arise from spontaneous, repeated activation of muscle fibers. The amplitudes of myotonic potentials range from 10 μV to 1 mV and spontaneously rise or fall. Discharge frequency may initially be as high as 50 pps and may drop to 20 to 30 pps. Characteristically, both amplitude and discharge frequency of myotonic discharges increase and decrease (wax and wane) spontaneously (Fig 12.28A). In cases where the frequency drops rapidly, the sound from an audio amplifier has been described as like that associated with a WWII dive-bomber, hence the description of these discharges as "dive-bomber potentials." When discharge amplitude and frequency waxes and wanes, the sound produced by myotonic potentials has been described as similar to that heard when revving a motorcycle. Individual discharges may be made up of waveforms similar to fibrillation potentials or positive sharp waves. For myotonic discharges to be considered clinically significant, they should persist for >0.5 seconds and be observed in several different locations within the muscles examined (33).

Myotonic discharges are thought to arise from muscle fibers with membrane dysfunction that alters muscle fiber resting membrane potentials and/or permeability to ions associated with the muscle action potential. The existence of myotonic discharges is commonly associated with myotonic diseases (e.g., myotonia congenita, myotonic dystrophy, paramyotonia) or hyperkalemic periodic paralysis, although they may appear in muscles of patients with chronic polyneuropathy and other disorders (34).

In diseases such a polymyositis or anterior horn cell disease, needle EMG examination may reveal the presence of polyphasic waveforms of fixed amplitude and relatively high, stable discharge rates (5 to 100 pps) (Fig 10.28B) (29). Such findings commonly encountered in chronic diseases are referred to as *complex repetitive discharges* (CRDs) or *bizarre, high-frequency discharges*. Like myotonic discharges, CRDs are often initiated by EMG needle electrode movement. Usually discharges start and stop abruptly without marked change in discharge frequency. Passing such signals through an audio amplifier often results in a sound described as "machine-gun fire."

CRDs are thought to represent the spontaneous discharge of several muscle fibers that fire asynchronously yet in the same sequence each time. The asynchronous discharge gives rise to the polyphasic appearance, while the fixed order of discharge accounts for the consistency of shape between potentials. CRDs are found most commonly in chronic or long-standing pathologies. The pathologies that give rise to CRDs may be either myopathic or neuropathic in origin. Neuropathies associated with CRDs include chronic polyneuropathies, chronic nerve entrapment (e.g., radiculopathies, carpal tunnel syndrome), and hereditary neuropathies (e.g., Charcot-Marie-Tooth disease). Diseases that affect motoneurons such a amyotrophic lateral sclerosis and spinal muscular atrophy, as well as muscle diseases such as muscular dystrophy and polymyositis, may manifest CRDs as well.

Myokymia is a muscle disorder characterized by wormlike or undulating spontaneous contractions of long-strip segments of muscle. Such muscular contractions are associated with spontaneous electrical activity in the muscle followed by electrical silence called *myokymic discharges* (Fig. 10.28C) (29). These bursts of electrical activity are like those occurring when several motor units (2 to 10) discharge at nearly the same moment in time and at rates of 30 to

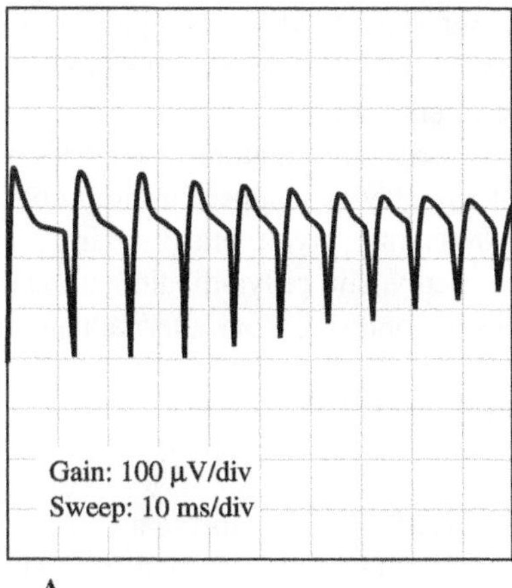

A

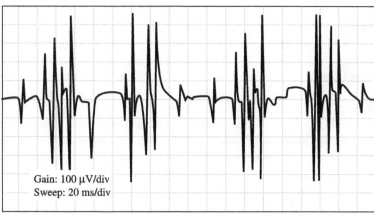

Gain: 100 µV/div
Sweep: 20 ms/div

B

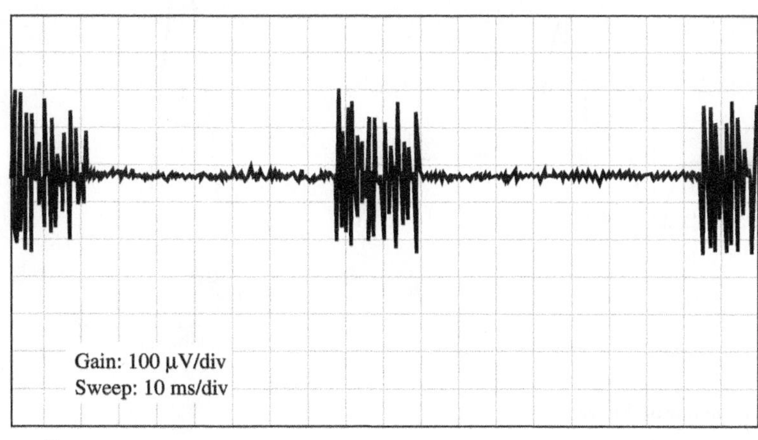

C

Figure 12.28. A: Myotonic discharge, **B:** Complex re-petitive discharge, and **C:** Myokymic discharge.

40 impulses per burst. Volitional activation does not alter the discharge pattern, which persists even during sleep. Unlike myotonic discharge, myokymic discharge may be reduced or stopped by chemical block of the innervating motor nerve fibers.

Myokymic discharges are commonly found in facial musculature in patients with disorders such as multiple sclerosis and brainstem tumors. They may also appear in limb musculature after radiation-induced plexopathy or myelopathy. Less frequently, myokymic discharges may arise subsequent to chronic radiculopathy, entrapment neuropathy, and polyradiculoneuropathy. Electrical myokymia is also a frequent finding in plexopathies 6 months or more after radiation therapy (35).

Normal and Abnormal Electrical Activity in Skeletal Muscle During Volitional Contraction

When a monopolar needle recording electrode is placed within a muscle and a person voluntarily contracts the muscle, a series of electrical waveforms can be recorded from skeletal muscle fibers on a display device. In normal, innervated muscle, these electrical representations of the activation of the muscle fibers of individual motor units during contraction are called *motor unit potentials* (MUPs). MUPs are generally thought to reflect the electrical activity of from 5 to 12 muscle fibers of the motor unit that lie in close proximity to the tip of the active recording electrode. Characteristics of the motor units (Fig. 12.29A) are measured in clinical electrophysiologic examination to gain insight into muscle function. These motor unit characteristics include the number of phases and turns in the MUPs (configuration), the amplitude and duration of the MUPs, and the motor units' firing rates or discharge frequencies.

The majority of MUPs recorded from healthy muscle are triphasic in configuration, with an initial relatively small positive deflection from the baseline, followed by a larger amplitude negative deflection when recorded with concentric or monopolar needle electrodes. Some MUPs

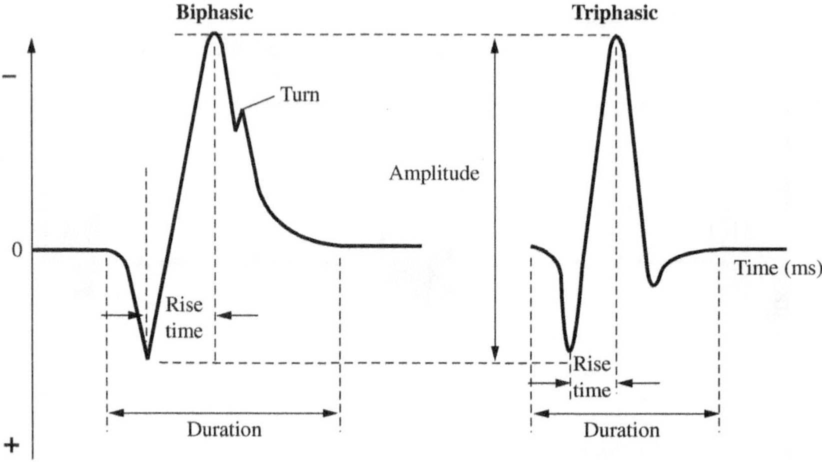

Normal motor unit parameters

Amplitude: 200 μV-5 mV

Duration: 5–15 ms

Rise time: 100–200 μs (<500 μs)

Frequency: 5–15/s (<60/s)

*Measured from initial positive peak to negative peak for triphasic potenntials

Figure 12.29. Motor unit potential characteristics measured during electrophysiological examination.

in normal muscle may have two phases (biphasic) or four phases. Motor units with five or more phases are called polyphasic and may be associated with nerve or muscle pathology. Discovery of a few (<15%) polyphasic MUPs during needle EMG examination is not necessarily indicative of pathology. The existence of polyphasic MUPs in excess of 15% of the analyzed population in a muscle is considered abnormal.

In a single phase of some MUPs, a change in voltage will occur that is not great enough to cross the baseline and that produces the appearance of serrations in the waveform. Such voltage changes within a single phase are called *turns*. The typical MUP in muscle of a young, healthy adult does not contain any turns. Therefore, the presence of turns in many MUPs is considered an abnormal finding. The presence of MUP turns in older individuals without any other abnormal findings is not considered clinically significant.

Motor unit potential *amplitude* is measured from the greatest positive deflection to the largest negative deflection. The peak-to-peak amplitudes of the main spike of motor unit potentials range from 300 μV to 5000 μV and vary among proximal and distal muscles. MUP *duration* is measured from the beginning of the initial positive deflection from the baseline to the point at which the potential returns to baseline after all phases. Durations of MUPs normally vary from 2 to 15 ms. The *rise time* of the MUP is measured from the first positive peak to the top of the first negative peak. Normal rise times should not exceed 500 μs, and most should fall in the 100 to 200 μs range. Motor units usually begin to discharge at a frequency of about 5 to 7 per second. With increasing levels of mild to moderate volitional contraction, the discharge rate normally increases to 10 to 12 per second and may rise to 20 to 30 per second.

MUP characteristics vary between the different types of motor units. The variations in amplitude, duration, and configuration are due to differences in muscle fiber size, the number of fibers in each motor unit, and the spatial distribution of the motor unit fibers within the muscle. For example, the MUP duration is thought to be representative of the spatial distribution of muscle fibers of the motor unit within the muscle, with larger units having longer durations than smaller units. As the needle recording electrode is passed through the muscle, these motor unit characteristics will change. Each muscle has a different mix of the types of motor units, so each has unique characteristics.

In a volitional muscle contraction, the first motor units activated by the central nervous system are those with the lowest threshold (Fig 12.30A). These are generally thought to be type S motor units consisting of a relatively few number of slowly contracting, very fatigue-resistant muscle fibers (type I or type SO) and innervated by relatively small alpha motoneurons. These motor units have amplitudes that vary between 300 μV and 1,000 μV. When a higher level of volitional contraction is required, the type S motor units increase their discharge frequency (rate coding), and the central motor pathways simultaneously activate more motor units (recruitment). In general, as moderate levels of contraction force are required, the somewhat larger (>1,000–1,500 μV) fast-twitch, fatigue-resistant (FR) motor units, consisting of type IIA muscle fibers and slightly larger alpha motoneurons, are the next to be activated. When very strong voluntary contractions are needed, type S and FR units may discharge at even higher rates, and, finally, the third motor unit class, fast-twitch, readily-fatigable (FF), consisting of type IIb fibers and the largest alpha motoneurons, are recruited. The type II motor units routinely have amplitudes ranging from 1,000 μV to 5,000 μV.

Changes in the distribution of motor unit amplitudes, duration, configuration, and discharge frequencies during needle examination may be associated with either myopathic or neuropathic disorders. Small-amplitude MUPs of short duration are often noted in muscle disease or inflammation. Smaller-than-normal MUPs with longer-than-normal durations are also consistent with early reinnervation of muscle following peripheral nerve lesions or neuromuscular junction failure. In either case, smaller-than-normal MUPs are believed to reflect a reduction in the number of activated muscle fibers in the motor units. Commonly this reduction in amplitude of MUPs is accompanied by a reduction in the average duration of the potentials.

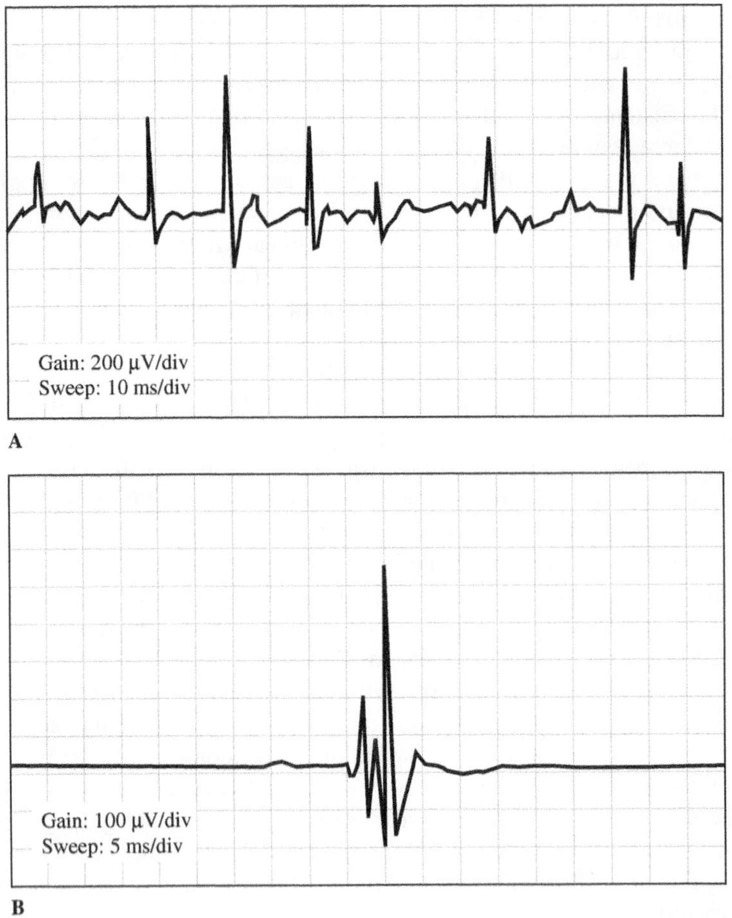

Figure 12.30. A: Motor unit potentials recorded during mild voluntary, isometric contraction. **B:** Polyphasic motor unit potential.

Larger-than-normal amplitude motor units may also be observed in disorders of nerve or muscle. MUPs that are very large in amplitude and often prolonged in duration are associated with chronic partial denervation with subsequent reinnervation and with the later stages of polymyositis and muscular dystrophies. The increase in amplitude results from axons that either regenerate or undergo collateral sprouting. In either case, axons reattach to a larger-than-normal number of muscle fibers or a group of muscle fibers that are closer together (higher density) than muscle fibers in a normal motor unit (29).

Polyphasic motor unit potentials (Fig 12.30B) are found in disorders of either neurogenic or myogenic origin. Polyphasic potentials are believed to indicate the presence of either deteriorating or regenerating motor units. The polyphasic appearance is believed to result from desynchronization of distal conduction of the terminal branches of the axon that innervates the muscle fibers of the motor unit (30), or from differences in conduction time over the muscle fiber membranes within the motor unit. Such desynchronization disrupts the normally simultaneous activation of the motor unit's muscle fibers that gives rise to the characteristic triphasic or biphasic motor unit potential. Polyphasic MUPs of low amplitude and short duration are regularly observed in the early stages of reinnervation subsequent to nerve laceration. As reinnervation progresses, polyphasic MUPs of increased amplitude and longer duration are observed. In diseases of muscle where the number of muscle fibers innervated by a single axon may decrease, polyphasic MUPs of small amplitude and short duration are typical. Some muscle diseases such as polymyositis or Duchenne muscular dystrophy are associated with small-amplitude, long-duration polyphasic potentials (36).

In electrophysiological examination, after observation of a muscle's electrical activity during needle insertion and at rest, electrical activity in the muscle is observed during mild to moderate volitional contraction of the muscle. Normally, MUPs with smaller amplitude potentials (<1,000 μV) are observed first, followed by progressively larger amplitude potentials as the force of contraction is increased (Figure 12.31A). The observation that a few larger amplitude potentials (>1,000 to 1,500 μV) are recruited before some smaller amplitude potentials is not uncommon and may merely represent relative differences in the distance of the recording electrodes from activated motor unit fibers rather than a true reversal in the recruitment order of motor units.

When the number of normal motor units in a muscle is decreased, or if the force produced by the muscle fibers in motor units is reduced, discharge rates of motor units may exceed those observed in normal muscle during voluntary contraction. Under normal conditions, the force of muscle contraction is determined by the number of motor units activated and the frequency of activation of motor units. If the desired force of a volitional contraction is not achieved by recruitment of motor units discharging at low rates, the central nervous system drive of motor units increases the frequency of discharge of the motor units already recruited. This mechanism

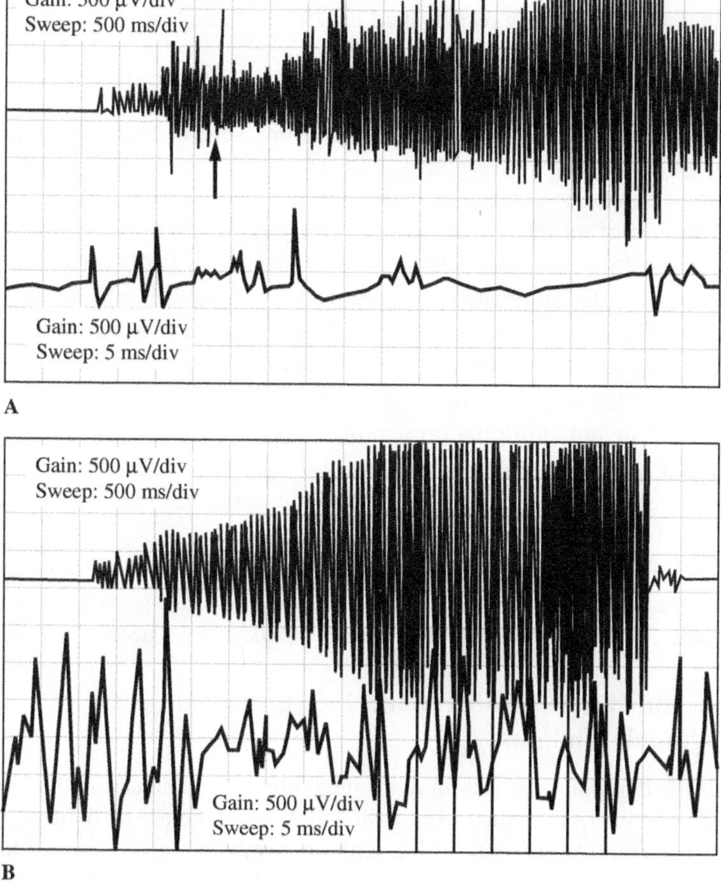

Figure 12.31. Recruitment patterns of motor unit potentials during **(A)** mild voluntary contraction (*lower trace*), and **(B)** strong voluntary isometric contraction (*lower trace*; full interference pattern).

to increase the contraction force is used in cases of neuropathy (reduced number of functional motor units) or myopathy (weak contraction of muscle fibers within units), and may increase motor unit discharge to rates as high as 50 per second.

With vigorous, strong contraction of normal muscle, so many motor units are recruited that an *interference pattern* is observed on the display device (Figure 12.31B) (30). The discharge of many motor units required to produce strong contraction obliterates the baseline and does not allow one to accurately distinguish individual motor unit characteristics. The obliteration of the display baseline and filling of the display screen with MUPs is described as a "full" or "complete" interference pattern.

Interpretation of recruitment and interference patterns in clinical electromyography must be performed with an awareness of the relative force of contraction produced by the muscle examined. Interference patterns are often reduced in cases of peripheral nerve injury with axonal conduction block, in spite of maximum volitional contraction efforts by the patient. Reduced recruitment in the presence of lost (degenerated) motoneuron axons results from loss of the ability to activate denervated muscle fibers. Reduced interference patterns may also be produced by individuals who do not fully cooperate, as might occur with either pain during contraction or malingering. Full interference patterns during strong volitional contraction are a normal finding. Observation of a full interference pattern without an awareness of the level of contraction, however, may not reflect normal function of muscle. For example, full interference patterns are generated with only weak or moderate contraction forces in subjects with myopathic disease. This full interference pattern results from premature or early recruitment of motor units at low contraction forces that would normally be activated only at much higher contraction forces.

General Principles of Electromyographic Testing

When electromyography is selected as a testing procedure, several general principles apply:

1. Examination of a number of muscles both above and below the suspected site of the nerve pathology. Rationale: muscles distal to the site of the lesion may exhibit abnormal EMG activity, but those proximal to the lesion should have normal EMG activity.
2. Examination of muscles innervated by nerves other than those implicated by clinical symptoms. Rationale: EMG abnormalities may be detected in muscles before there are clinically measurable changes (e.g., weakness) in these muscles.
3. Sampling of EMG activity of the full cross-section of each muscle tested. Rationale: abnormalities in EMG are not uniformly present in all areas of every muscle.
4. Examination of muscles in contralateral limbs or both upper and lower limbs in suspected systemic disease or disorders. Rationale: EMG abnormalities may be present before these muscles present with clinical symptoms.
5. Examination should be performed at the appropriate time in the context of the suspected disorders. Rationale: EMG changes associated with conditions such as denervation may take 10 days to 2 weeks to develop after axons to muscle have been disrupted.

Types of Nerve and Muscle Disorders and Interpretation of Electromyographic Findings

Abnormal electromyographic findings may be indicative of either myopathic, neuropathic, or combined muscle and nerve disorders (33). EMG findings alone are difficult to interpret, however, unless they are examined in conjunction with the results of nerve conduction studies.

The presence of abnormal EMG potentials in the absence of abnormal nerve conduction velocity findings suggests that the disorder is confined to the skeletal muscle (i.e., it is a myopathic disorder). However, neuropathic disorders that result in partial axonal degeneration may also give rise to similar findings (abnormal EMG and normal nerve conduction). Numerous muscle diseases and disorders (e.g., muscular dystrophy, polymyositis, myotubular myopathy) can give rise to spontaneous activity at rest, such as fibrillation potentials, positive sharp waves, and complex repetitive discharges. Early in the course of myopathies, motor unit amplitudes may appear normal. As the disease progresses and the number of functional muscle fibers in motor units decreases, motor unit amplitudes on average are reduced. In the late stages of myopathies such as muscular dystrophy, larger-than-normal MUPs may be found. In general, MUP duration is shorter than normal and decreases further with disease progression. Myopathic disorders are also associated with an increase in the number of polyphasic MUPs and an increase in the number of turns within MUPs. In some myopathic diseases, recruitment of single MUPs during voluntary contraction may be difficult for the patient.

Mild to moderate neuropathic problems, such as nerve compression and associated partial or complete neuropraxia, will often give rise to changes in evoked compound action potential latencies, amplitudes, or durations without any apparent abnormal EMG findings. These changes in nerve conduction parameters may frequently involve sensory axons and evoked CSNAPs before any changes are noted in motor fibers or evoked CMAPs. In more severe neuropathic lesions where motor axons degenerate distal to the site of the problem, abnormal nerve conduction findings are generally accompanied by abnormal EMG findings. Whether abnormal EMG potentials are noted upon examination after peripheral nerve damage depends, however, on the time at which the EMG examination is performed. If, for instance, electromyography is performed within 2 days after a lesion (e.g., partial or complete axonotmesis) to the innervating nerve, fibrillations and positive sharp waves suggestive of denervation will not generally be detected, and insertional activity will appear normal. In contrast, EMG testing of the same muscles 14 to 21 days after partial or complete axonotmesis will usually reveal the presence of these abnormal potentials indicative of muscle fiber denervation, as well as increased insertional activity associated with the hyperexcitable membranes of denervated muscle fibers.

Observation of MUPs during volitional activation of muscle may allow the examiner to differentiate whether nerve lesions to muscles involve all the motor axons or only some of the motor axons. In partial neuropraxic and partial axonotmetic lesions, MUPs recorded from associated muscles will appear normal, but recruitment and interference patterns with strong volitional effort will generally be decreased. Partial axonotmetic lesions may also be accompanied by the presence of polyphasic motor units. These results occur because some motor units remain normally innervated in partial nerve lesions and still produce normal-appearing action potentials, while other motor axons branch to reinnervate higher-than-normal numbers of muscle fibers. Interference patterns are often reduced in partial nerve lesions because conduction block (neuropraxic lesion) or disruptions in axon continuity (axonotmetic lesion) do not allow action potentials produced at the alpha motoneuron cell bodies to reach the muscle through the damaged or degenerating axons distal to the lesion. As such, some of the muscle's motor units cannot be volitionally activated.

With partial motor nerve lesions, large-amplitude MUPs appear earlier in the recruitment pattern, and initial discharge frequency of MUPs may be higher than normal (>5 to 7 per second). Larger-than-normal MUPs appear during volitional contraction if (i) sufficient time has passed to allow reinnervation due to collateral sprouting of unaffected motor axons; or (ii) axons to many type I motor units have been compromised, requiring type II units to be activated in order to produce sufficient contraction force. In partial neuropraxic lesions, MUP durations will usually appear normal. In most axonotmetic neuropathies, MUP durations will be increased, reflecting a more asynchronous activation of muscle fibers associated with collateral sprouting reinnervation. Complete neuropraxia (100% conduction block) or complete axonotmesis (100% axonal disruption) is present if volitional effort does not produce any motor unit activity. In these

Table 12.6. EMG Findings for Various Lesions

	Extent of lesion	Nature of lesion	Day 1	Day 21
Insertional activity	Partial	Neuropraxia	Normal	Normal
		Axonotmesis	Normal	Increased
	Complete	Neuropraxia	Normal	Normal
		Axonotmesis	Normal	Increased
Spontaneous activity	Partial	Neuropraxia	None	None
		Axonotmesis	None	Fibs., +sharps
	Complete	Neuropraxia	None	None
		Axonotmesis	None	Fibs., +sharps
Volitional activity	Partial	Neuropraxia	Normal	Normal
		Axonotmesis	Normal	Normal
	Complete	Neuropraxia	None	None
		Axonotmesis	None	None
Interference patterns	Partial	Neuropraxia	Decreased	Decreased
		Axonotmesis	Decreased	Decreased
	Complete	Neuropraxia	Absent	Absent
		Axonotmesis	Absent	Absent

instances, MUPs and interference patterns are absent because the pathways (axons) for activating muscle fibers are completely blocked or broken, and therefore no signals are transferred to muscle to initiate excitation.

Table 12.6 summarizes the EMG findings discussed above that allow one to differentiate between neuropraxic and axonotmetic lesions, and to determine whether these nerve lesions involve all of the motor nerve fibers (complete lesions) or only a portion of the motor nerve fibers (partial lesions). Findings from electromyography may suggest the presence of motor nerve lesions, but give no indication of the integrity or level of involvement of sensory or autonomic fibers contained within the peripheral nerve.

Electromyographic Findings in Mononeuropathies

Electromyographic examination of muscles in disorders where only one peripheral nerve is compromised generally leads to the discovery of abnormal findings in muscles distal to the location of the nerve lesion. For this reason the examiner must know the order of innervation of muscles by individual peripheral nerves from proximal to distal along the course of the nerve. In neuropraxic lesions that produce conduction slowing in some motor axons without conduction block in axons, the EMG findings are often normal but may, on occasion, be associated with spontaneous activity in innervated muscles at rest, such as fasciculation potentials. In neuropraxic lesions with partial conduction block in a significant number of axons, the interference pattern generated by motor unit recruitment may be reduced. With axonotmetic or neurotmetic lesions that have resulted in degeneration of motor axons, examination commonly reveals increased insertional activity, abnormal spontaneous potential (e.g., fibrillation potentials and positive sharp waves) at rest accompanied by a reduced interference pattern in muscles distal to the site of the axonal lesion. In early denervation, fibrillation potentials and positive sharp waves tend to be of relatively large amplitude, while in long-term denervation such spontaneous activity is generally much lower in amplitude. If reinnervation of previously denervated muscle fibers has begun, polyphasic and/or larger-than-normal MUPs may be observed in muscles distal to the lesion. Regardless of the type of localized nerve lesion, EMG activity at rest and during voluntary contraction is normal in muscles innervated by the involved nerve if they are above the level of the lesion. Muscles innervated by other peripheral nerves should also exhibit normal findings during EMG examination.

Electromyographic Findings in Brachial Plexopathies

Lesions of the brachial plexus often require a more extensive EMG examination. Abnormalities in EMG findings in brachial plexopathies are often detected in several muscles whose motor axons pass through the damaged component of the plexus. For this reason, examiners must have an understanding of the pathways of motor axons from their origin at the nerve roots through the plexus and ending in either the five terminal branches of the plexus (median, ulnar, musculocutaneous, radial, or axillary nerves) or the supraclavicular or infraclavicular branches extending directly from the plexus components. Like peripheral mononeuropathies, brachial plexopathies may be neuropraxic, axonotmetic, or neurotmetic in nature. Hence, the specific EMG findings in each of these types of lesions will be similar to those described previously. The localization of nerve injury to a component of the brachial plexus differs from that of a mononeuropathy in terms of the muscles where the abnormal findings are detected. For example, an isolated ulnar nerve lesion at the cubital tunnel may be associated with EMG abnormalities in ulnar innervated muscles distal to the lesion, including both the intrinsic muscles of the hand, as well as the medial portion of the flexor digitorum profundus with sparing of the flexor carpi ulnaris that is innervated from above the level of the lesion. In contrast, lower trunk lesions may affect all ulnar innervated muscles as well as some of the median and radial innervated muscles associated with either the C8 or T1 nerve roots.

Electromyographic Findings in Isolated Nerve-Root Lesions

Electromyographic examination findings in isolated nerve-root lesions are generally detected in many of the muscles than receive innervation originating from the particular nerve-root level. For example, in a C7 nerve-root lesion, muscles receiving C7 fibers in the arm (e.g., triceps) and forearm (e.g., wrist/finger flexors and extensors, pronator teres, and supinator) may yield abnormal findings. In contrast, other muscles of the shoulder (e.g., C5/C6 innervated deltoid and supraspinatus), arm (e.g., C5/C6 innervated biceps and brachioradialis), and hand (e.g., C8/T1 innervated abductor digiti minimi or interossei) should appear normal during EMG examination.

CLASSICAL ELECTROPHYSIOLOGICAL TESTS

Before the development of the modern nerve conduction studies and electromyography, a number of electrophysiologic testing procedures were routinely used to evaluate neuromuscular disorders. Although these tests have largely been replaced by modern electrophysiologic examination procedures, a fundamental understanding of how to perform and interpret these classical tests may allow the clinician to gain some insight into the nature of a neuromuscular disorder in situations where modern examination procedures are not readily available. The three tests discussed here are the strength–duration test, the reaction to degeneration test, and the galvanic twitch/tetanus ratio test.

Strength–Duration Test

When the electrically excitable tissues, nerve and muscle, are activated by pulsatile electrical currents, the type of fibers stimulated depends on the amplitude ("strength") and duration characteristics of the applied waveforms. When a monophasic pulse of a fixed amplitude and duration is applied near normal excitable tissues, the amount of activation is fairly consistent from one stimulus to the next. For example, if a few alpha motoneuron axons are activated in response to a single stimulus, the twitch contraction (response) elicited will remain constant in amplitude. By varying stimulus amplitudes and durations in a systematic manner, one may determine the set of amplitude and duration combinations necessary to evoke twitch contraction of the same magnitude. Plotting the stimulus amplitude and duration combinations sufficient to evoke twitches generates a strength–duration curve, as shown in Figure 12.32. The curve represents all the stimulus amplitude and duration combinations that will evoke the same response, in this case a small twitch contraction. The data reveal that to activate a particular set of excitable fibers, one may use stimuli that range from those with high amplitudes and short durations to those with low amplitudes and long durations to activate the same subset of fibers. The product of the amplitude and duration (the phase charge) of all applied pulses that fall on the curve are equal. Any stimulus that falls below the curve will not be sufficient in phase charge to activate the same subset of motoneuron axons, and hence the size of the evoked contraction will disappear. Any stimulus that lies above the curve will activate more alpha motoneuron axons (recruitment) and generally results in larger contractions.

In traditional strength–duration testing procedures, the cathode of a pulsed monophasic stimulator is applied to the motor point of muscles, and the anode of the circuit is placed over the muscle a few centimeters away from the motor point of the same muscle (37). Recall that the motor point is the location over muscle where the nerve innervating the muscle is most easily excited. Stimuli with initial pulse durations >100 ms and an amplitude sufficient to produce a minimally detectable (e.g., palpable) twitch contraction are delivered. The duration of the stimuli

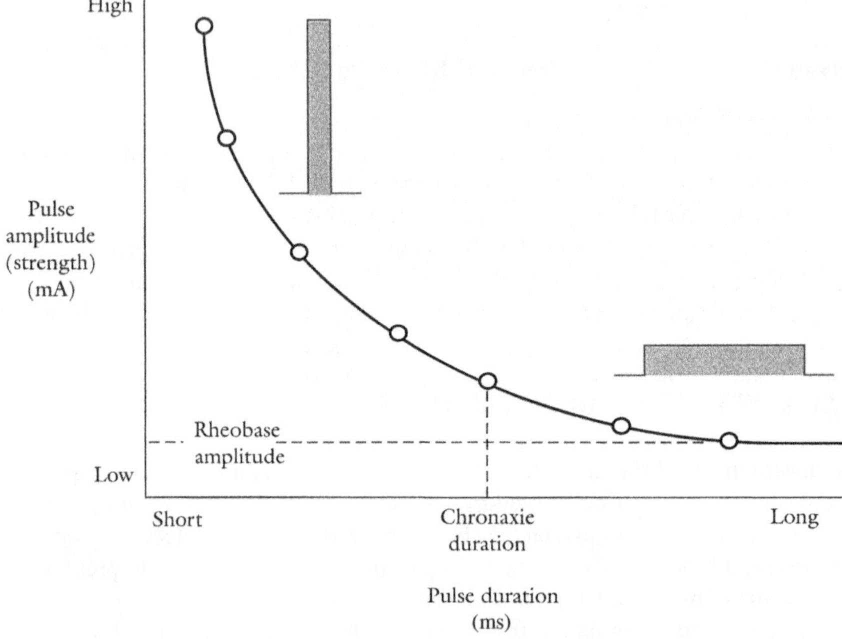

Figure 12.32. Strength–duration curve for a normally innervated muscle showing the rheobase amplitude and the chronaxie duration.

is then systematically reduced in a stepwise manner, and the amplitudes required to produce the same response are noted. The combinations of stimulus amplitude and duration sufficient to produce the just-palpable response are then plotted to produce the strength–duration curve. The minimum amplitude required to produce the response at the very long pulse durations (100 to 300 ms) is called the *rheobase* strength stimulus (Fig. 10.27). The minimum duration required to produce the twitch when the amplitude is set at twice the rheobase level is called the *chronaxie.* Normal chronaxie durations depend in part on the type of stimulator used in the assessment. For constant voltage stimulators, Ritchie (38) found that 90% of normal chronaxie values fell between 0.03 and 0.08 ms. For constant-current stimulators, normal chronaxie values ranged from 0.15 to 0.80 ms for 90% of the muscles examined. In contrast, completely denervated muscle may exhibit chronaxie values of more than 30 ms.

Figure 12.33 shows the strength–duration curve for a normally innervated muscle, a denervated muscle, and a partially reinnervated (or partially denervated) muscle. The strength–duration curve for the denervated muscle is shifted markedly up and to the right because denervated muscle fibers are inherently less excitable than motor nerve fibers and hence require higher levels of stimulation to reach threshold excitation. In denervated muscle, no contraction will be elicited by stimuli with very short pulse durations, regardless of the amplitudes applied. This finding is represented by the steep rise at the left of the strength–duration curve that appears between 1- to 10-ms pulse duration. If reinnervation begins to take place, the strength–duration curve for the partially reinnervated muscle appears to shift down and to the left and is frequently characterized by discontinuities or kinks in the curve. These kinks most commonly occur in the 3- to 10-ms pulse duration range.

The purpose of strength–duration testing is to determine the level of innervation of skeletal muscle by alpha motoneuron fibers after nerve injury or disease. That is, the test results are thought to reflect the ratio of innervated to denervated muscle fibers. The test may reveal normal innervation, partial innervation, or complete denervation. Strength–duration testing is of primary value in assessing progress or deterioration of motor innervation; thus serial testing is recommended. Testing is generally not performed more often than every 2 to 3 weeks to allow time for

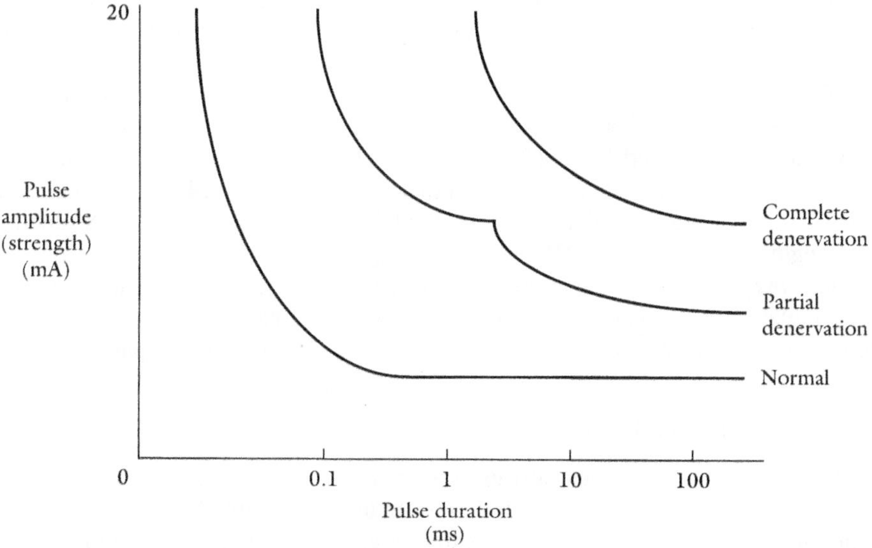

Figure 12.33. Graph of strength–duration curves for normally innervated muscle, partially denervated muscle, and completely denervated muscle.

significant reinnervation (or further denervation) to occur. The test may reveal which nerves are compromised, but it does not reveal the precise location of the nerve lesion (37).

A number of factors may influence the results of strength–duration tests. These include temperature, blood supply, edema, and electrode position. Excitation thresholds are elevated with decreased temperature, decreased blood supply, increased edema, or poor localization of the motor point.

Strength duration testing was used in patient populations as early as 1916 to assess the extent of nerve injury (39). Widespread clinical use of strength–duration testing continued through the 1960s. However, with the development of nerve conduction studies and electromyographic techniques, the use of this test today is rare. For the clinician who does not have ready access to nerve conduction and electromyographic testing services, strength–duration testing may provide some insight into the extent of innervation of relevant superficial muscles.

Reaction of Degeneration Test

The reaction of degeneration (RD) test is used to assess the level of innervation of skeletal muscles. Like strength–duration testing, RD tests provide information on the integrity of alpha motoneurons innervating skeletal muscle.

To perform this test, either monophasic or biphasic pulsed currents are used to electrically stimulate the normal motor point of a muscle suspected of having impaired innervation. The current waveforms applied have pulse durations of 1 ms and are delivered initially at frequencies in excess of 20 pps. In normal muscle, such a pattern of stimulation will, with sufficient amplitude of stimulation, evoke a smooth tetanic contraction. In a totally denervated muscle, this form of stimulation will not evoke a muscle contraction, and this result is reported as a *reaction of degeneration*. The presence of the RD simply reflects the loss of innervation to the muscle. The current described above does not activate the denervated muscle directly because the charge of applied pulses is not sufficient to bring muscle fiber membranes to a threshold level of depolarization.

In clinical cases with partial denervation, some but not all of the motor nerve fibers innervating skeletal muscle are lost. In such situations, the stimulation used in RD testing may elicit a contraction, but the magnitude of the response (force of contraction) is dramatically reduced. This type of result in RD testing is called a *partial reaction of degeneration*. When a partial RD is elicited, the percentage of remaining motor axons innervating the muscle cannot be determined from the results of this test.

One of the more common uses of RD tests was in the evaluation of individuals with Bell palsy, the unilateral degeneration of facial nerve fibers and associated atrophy of the muscles of facial expression. Oester and Licht (40) wrote that motor degeneration is nearly complete 2 weeks from the onset of the nerve lesion and that no RD after day 14, even in the presence of clinical palsy, represents a favorable prognosis for full recovery of facial muscle function. Like classical strength–duration testing, RD tests are no longer commonly used in electrophysiological examination. This test, however, may provide the clinician who is considering neuromuscular electrical stimulation as a possible therapeutic intervention with a quick and easy means to determine the feasibility of neuromuscular electrical stimulation for a particular patient.

Galvanic Twitch–Tetanus Ratio Test

Another classical electrophysiologic test used to examine whether skeletal muscle is normally innervated is the galvanic twitch–tetanus ratio test. In this procedure, direct current (monophasic pulsed current with long duration) is intermittently applied over the motor point of a muscle suspected to be denervated using the cathode of the stimulator circuit. The duration of DC stimulation is controlled manually by use of a hand-held electrode with a manual switch. The amplitude of stimulation is gradually increased until a twitch contraction is produced, and this minimum (rheobase) level of stimulation is recorded. Next, the current amplitude is increased to the point where a sustained tetaniclike contraction is evoked. and this amplitude is recorded.

In normally innervated muscle, the ratio of the amplitude that elicited the twitch to the amplitude that produced the tetaniclike response ranges from 1: 3.5 to 1: 6.5 (40). In a completely denervated muscle, this ratio ranges from 1:1 to 1: 1.5 (40).

Because this procedure can be extremely uncomfortable to the subject and modern assessment procedures are safer and more reliable, the galvanic twitch–tetanus ratio test, like many other classical tests, is rarely used.

CONTRAINDICATIONS/PRECAUTIONS IN ELECTROPHYSIOLOGIC TESTING

As with any clinical procedure, a variety of conditions or situations may limit or preclude the use of clinical electrophysiologic examination procedures. Other conditions may simply call for additional caution during testing. These conditions include (28)

- Abnormal blood clotting factors/anticoagulant therapy
- Extreme swelling
- Dermatitis
- Uncooperative or confused patient
- Recent myocardial infarction
- Blood transmittable disease (Creutzfeldt–Jakob disease, HIV, hepatitis, etc.)
- Immunosuppression
- Central going lines
- Pacemakers or other implanted medical devices
- Hypersensitivity to stimulation (open wounds, burns).

In performing needle electromyography, latex gloves and eye protection should be worn to protect the examiner from possible blood-borne transmission of infectious agents. In cases where transmittable diseases are known to exist, additional measures such as gowns may be required for all ENMG procedures.

ROUTINE CLINICAL EXAMINATION OF NEUROMUSCULAR FUNCTION

Interview

Practicing clinicians are well aware that the thoroughness of the patient interview is of paramount importance when attempting to determine the nature and location of neuromuscular disorders. Typically the examiner clarifies with the individual the type of symptoms they are experiencing, the location or distribution of those symptoms, duration of symptoms, and the nature of symptom onset. The clinician then correlates those symptoms to known neuromuscular disorders. Clients should also be asked what activities either aggravate or relieve the symptoms. These initial questions should be followed by a detailed medical history including but not limited to diagnosed medical conditions, current medications, surgical or trauma history, family medical history, vocational and avocational activities, and potential exposure to toxic substances. The responses to these other questions are essential in making the most appropriate choices for ENMG testing procedures.

Observational and Functional Assessment

The experienced clinician will attest to the fact that no clinical testing procedure may be more valuable than observation of patient's posture and movement during the functional activities of daily living. Observation begins as soon as a patient enters the clinic during the initial visit. Functional assessment may proceed with a variety of specific tests that are becoming more commonplace in clinical practice. The observation of function may include a visit to the home or workplace as soon as possible to determine which postures and movement are prerequisite to the individual's occupation, and to identify those factors that may predispose the individual to additional or repeated injury.

In cases of partial or complete loss of innervation, the skin may undergo changes including dryness, scaly appearance, or variations in color or temperature. In other instances the skin may sweat excessively. Swelling, especially of the hands and feet, is not uncommon in peripheral neurological disorders. Swelling may also be observed in overlying structures such as tendons or synovial sheaths that lie in close proximity to nerves.

Cutaneous Somatosensory Tests

The procedures of electrophysiologic examination are of greatest value in the establishment of a diagnosis when findings are integrated with those of other clinical tests and the clinical signs and symptoms. The clinician involved in the use of these procedures should be aware of a variety of other tests of neuromuscular function to select the ENMG procedures most appropriate for the patient.

In ENMG, only the sensory nerve conduction studies provide insight into whether the sensory systems are involved. In the routine neurological exam, qualitative and rather crude tests are often used to assess sensory function. These tests include the use of pinwheels, brushes, or pins to examine tactile acuity. Today, more sensitive and reliable clinical tests are available to evaluate touch–pressure sensibility, especially in the skin of the hands and feet. For example, use of Semmes–Weinstein monofilaments (the modern version of the VonFrey hair) allows the clinician to accurately determine cutaneous touch-pressure psychophysical thresholds in injured or diseased areas and compare these thresholds with those in uninvolved areas or with the established normal values (41). Similarly, two-point discrimination testing that assesses one's ability to differentiate between two points separated by different distances provides another index of sensory function. The repeated use of such tests of sensory function help the clinician determine whether sensory function is improving, deteriorating, or whether it remains unchanged. In some cases, these tests may provide the earliest indication of dysfunction in the somatosensory system. A detailed discussion of the correct application of these procedures is beyond the scope of this text, and the reader is referred to other references for more specific information on the clinical application of these tests (41,42).

Reports of the results of Semmes–Weinstein monofilament testing and two-point discrimination testing are best reported on diagrammatic representations of the regions tested. Such cutaneous sensibility diagrams are often color coded to give a clear picture of the nature and extent of sensory nerve involvement. The pattern of sensory deficits revealed by monofilament and/or two-point discrimination tests is then compared to standard sensory dermatome diagrams (see Appendix A) for either peripheral nerve cutaneous innervation or spinal nerve root cutaneous innervation. The results may allow the examiner to determine whether the pattern of cutaneous deficit is consistent with a disorder that involves a single peripheral nerve, multiple peripheral nerves, or possibly a single spinal nerve root. Changes in the color patterns over time as sensory function either improves or deteriorates provide a clear picture of the progress or decline, respectively, in sensory function and allow the clinician to make adjustments in the treatment program or in functional activities to help the patient better accommodate to the sensory loss. Sensory deficits discovered with cutaneous tactile threshold testing may help the clinician make decisions regarding the selection of sensory nerve conduction tests that are appropriate during electrophysiologic examination.

Cutaneous Tests of Autonomic Function

Electrophysiologic tests are not commonly used to assess the function of autonomic nerve fibers in peripheral nerves. Several simple clinical tests are available to provide some insight into the involvement of autonomic fibers in injury or disease (43). These tests use staining techniques to examine sweating, an activity controlled by the sympathetic division of the autonomic nervous system. One of the more common of these tests is the *ninhydrin sweat test.* To perform the test, sweating is induced by heating the area, performing exercise, or some other technique. The area of sweating is then carefully covered with filter paper. Acidified 1% ninhydrin in acetone is then sprayed on the paper, which is then dried and heated. If the record is to be preserved for long periods of time, the tester may choose to fix the test with acidified copper nitrate in acetone. The test will reveal those areas in which sweat production remains and those areas where sweating is absent. The test is valuable in following the recovery of nerve after laceration and repair to monitor the extent of reinnervation of sweat glands.

Muscle Tests

Although EMG provides information regarding motor nerve fiber and muscle fiber function, the results of EMG testing should be integrated with a variety of other clinical tests of muscle function. Specific manual muscle tests (44) should be performed by a trained practitioner for each muscle or muscle group suspected to be involved. A significant limitation to manual muscle testing is the lack of sensitivity in the detection of mild muscle weakness. Clinical dynamometry (hand dynamometers, pinch meters, isometric and isokinetic dynamometers, etc.) may also be useful for identifying mild to moderate deficits in voluntary muscle force production.

Provocative Tests

Provocative tests consist of specific procedures performed by an examiner or a patient in order to reproduce or provoke the symptoms of a nerve compression syndrome. These tests are useful in initial evaluation to localize peripheral nerve lesions to guide the planning of an electrophysiologic examination. Table 12.7 lists some examples of the more commonly applied provocative tests used in initial evaluations and the disorders with which they are linked. Clinicians should be aware that individual provocative tests may have limited sensitivity and specificity. For example, Tinel testing and Phalen sign testing for the presence of median nerve compromise at the wrist are only about 33% sensitive and specific for the presence of this disorder.

Although detailed descriptions of the clinical examination of neuromuscular function are beyond the scope of this text, this process must be performed along with electrophysiological examination to obtain a complete picture of the effects of injury and disease on neuromuscular function. Reference has been made to these additional procedures to emphasize their importance in establishing a diagnosis and in developing a comprehensive plan of care.

PROBLEM SOLVING AND THE ELECTRONEUROMYOGRAPHIC EVALUATION

The previous sections have detailed the various procedures used to examine motor and somatosensory function electrophysiologically. How does one decide which tests are appropriate to perform in order to establish a diagnosis? What tests of which nerves and muscles must be performed to help determine the site, extent, and severity of the problem? What clues from the

Table 12.7. Common Clinical Provocative Tests

Name	Test for	Manuever	Provocative Response
Phalens test	Median nerve compression at carpal tunnel	Full wrist flexion held for 60 s.	Tingling sensation (paresthesia) in the median distribution
2-minute compression test	Nerve entrapment at compression site	Digital pressure over peripheral nerve distribution	Paresthesia in compressed
Tinel's or percussion Test	Nerve regeneration or compression site	Tapping along course of nerve	Tingling sensation at site of compression or regeneration
EAST (elevated arm Stress test)	Nerve compression in thoracic outlet	Arm's abducted to 90° Elbows flexed to 90° Open/close hands	Symptom reproduction before 3 min.
Adson's test	Nerve compression in thoracic outlet	Rotate neck to affected side Brace shoulder inhale deeply and hold	Radial pulse reduced symptom reproduction
Wright's test	Nerve compression in thoracic outlet	Arms abducted to 90° Full shoulder external rotation	Radial pulse reduced Symptom reproduction
Costoclavicular test	Nerve compression in thoracic outlet	Shoulder retraction and depression	Radial pulse reduced Symptom reproduction
Spurling's test	Cervical nerve root compression	Downward pressure on head in neutral position	Symptom reproduction

clinical evaluation are used to electrophysiologically evaluate the patient's problem? How do ENMG results correlate with other tests, and how can ENMG data be used in planning appropriate comprehensive plans of care?

The next section of this chapter deals with the problem solving that an examiner performs in the ENMG examination and evaluation. Knowledge of the anatomy of the peripheral nerves, plexuses, nerve roots, skeletal muscle actions, and the dermatomal, sclerotomal, and myotomal innervations is extremely important. Before proceeding, a review of the neuroanatomy of the peripheral nervous system may be appropriate for some readers. For a brief overview of the sensory and motor innervation of the upper and lower extremities, see Appendix A. Appendix A provides several figures illustrating the muscles innervated by major peripheral nerves in the extremities, as well as common sites where these nerves may be injured or compressed. In addition, peripheral nerve sensory dermatome charts and spinal nerve root dermatome charts are provided. Charts covering the peripheral nerve and spinal nerve-root innervation of muscles of the upper and lower extremity are provided in Figures 12.34 and 12.35.

The *patient interview* is an essential component of the comprehensive evaluation process and should always precede any form of electrophysiologic testing. Questions typically asked during the patient interview include

1. What are your complaints? (e.g., pain, tingling sensation, functional deficit, anesthesia, fatigue, weakness, etc.)
2. Are the symptoms/signs diffuse, or are they localized to one area or extremity?
3. Is an entire extremity involved or only one area?

Spinal Nerve and Muscle Chart
neck, diaphragm and upper extremity

Name

PERIPHERAL NERVES

KEY→ D. = Dorsal Prim. Ramus
V. = Vent. Prim. Ramus
P.R. = Plexus Root
S.T. = Superior Trunk
P. = Posterior Cord
L. = Lateral Cord
M. = Medial Cord

		MUSCLE STRENGTH GRADE	MUSCLE	Cervical	Cervical	Cervical	Phrenic	Long Thor.	Dor. Scap	N. to Subcl.	Suprascap	U. Subscap.	Thoracodor	L. Subscap.	Lat. Pect.	Med. Pect.	Axillary	Musculocu.	Radial	Median	Ulnar	SPINAL SEGMENT C1	C2	C3	C4	C5	C6	C7	C8	T1
				D.	V.	V.	V.	P.R.	P.R.	S.T.	S.T.	P.	P.	P.	L.	M.	P.	L.	P.	L.M.	M.									
			Cervical	1-8	1-8	1-4	3, 4, 5	5, 6, 7, (8)	4, 5	5, 6	4, 5, 6	(4), 5, 6, (7)	(5), 6, 7, 8	5, 6, (7)	5, 6, 7	(6), 7, 8	5, 6	(4), 5, 6, 7	5, 6, 7, 8	5, 6, 7, 8	7, 8									
			T.	1												1			1	1	1									
			HEAD & NECK EXTENSORS	•																		1	2	3	4	5	6	7	8	1
Cervical nerves			INFRAHYOID MUSCLES			•																1	2	3						
Cervical nerves			RECTUS CAP ANT. & LAT.			•																1	2							
Cervical nerves			LONGUS CAPITIS			•																1	2	3	(4)					
Cervical nerves			LONGUS COLLI		•																		2	3	4	5	6	(7)		
Cervical nerves			LEVATOR SCAPULAE			•			•															3	4	5				
Cervical nerves			SCALENI (A. M. P.)		•																			3	4	5	6	7	8	
Cervical nerves			STERNOCLEIDOMASTOID			•																(1)	2	3						
Cervical nerves			TRAPEZIUS (U. M. L.)			•																	2	3	4					
Cervical nerves			DIAPHRAGM				•																	3	4	5				
Brachial Plexus	Root		SERRATUS ANTERIOR					•																		5	6	7	8	
Brachial Plexus	Root		RHOMBOIDS MAJ & MIN						•																4	5				
Brachial Plexus	Trunk		SUBCLAVIUS							•																5	6			
Brachial Plexus	Trunk		SUPRASPINATUS								•														4	5	6			
Brachial Plexus	Trunk		INFRASINATUS								•														(4)	5	6			
Brachial Plexus	P Cord		SUBSCAPULARIS									•		•												5	6	7		
Brachial Plexus	P Cord		LATISSIMUS DORSI										•														6	7	8	
Brachial Plexus	P Cord		TERES MAJOR											•												5	6	7		
Brachial Plexus	L		PECTORALIS MAJ (UPPER)												•											5	6	7		
Brachial Plexus	M&L		PECTORALIS MAJ (LOWER)												•	•											6	7	8	1
Brachial Plexus	M&L		PECTORALIS MINOR													•											(6)	7	8	1
Axil.			TERES MINOR														•									5	6			
Axil.			DELTOID														•									5	6			
Musculo-cutan			CORACOBRACHIALIS															•									6	7		
Musculo-cutan			BICEPS															•								5	6			
Musculo-cutan			BRACHIALIS															•								5	6			
Radial			TRICEPS																•								6	7	8	1
Radial			ANCONEUS																•									7	8	
Radial	Lat. M		BRACHIALIS (SMALL PART)																•							5	6			
Radial	Lat. M		BRACHIORADIALIS																•							5	6			
Radial	Lat. M		EXT CARPI RAD L																•							5	6	7	8	
Radial	Post Inter		EXT CARPI RAD B																•								6	7	8	
Radial	Post Inter		SUPINATOR																•							5	6	(7)		
Radial	Post Inter		EXT DIGITORUM																•								6	7	8	
Radial	Post Inter		EXT DIGITI MINIMI																•								6	7	8	
Radial	Post Inter		EXT CARPIULNARIS																•								6	7	8	
Radial	Post Inter		ABD POLLICIS LONGUS																•								6	7	8	
Radial	Post Inter		EXT POLLICIS BREVIS																•								6	7	8	
Radial	Post Inter		EXT POLLICIS LONGUS																•								6	7	8	
Radial	Post Inter		EXT INDICIS																•								6	7	8	
Median			PRONATOR TERES																	•							6	7		
Median			FLEX CARPI RADIALIS																	•							6	7	8	
Median			PALMARIS LONGUS																	•							(6)	7	8	1
Median			FLEX DIGIT SUPERFICIALIS																	•								7	8	1
Median			FLEX DIGIT PROF I & II																	•								7	8	1
Median	A Inter		FLEX POLLICIS LONGUS																	•							(6)	7	8	1
Median	A Inter		PRONATOR QUADRATUS																	•								7	8	1
Median			ABD POLLICIS BREVIS																	•							6	7	8	1
Median			OPPONENS POLLICIS																	•							6	7	8	1
Median			FLEX POLL BREV (SUP. H)																	•							6	7	8	1
Median			LUMBRICALES I & II																	•							(6)	7	8	1
Ulnar			FLEX CARPI ULNARIS																		•							7	8	1
Ulnar			FLEX DIGIT. PROF. III & IV																		•							7	8	1
Ulnar			PALMARIS BREVIS																		•							(7)	8	1
Ulnar			ABD DIGITI MINIMI																		•							(7)	8	1
Ulnar			OPPONENS DIGITI MINIMI																		•							(7)	8	1
Ulnar			FLEX DIGITI MINIMI																		•							(7)	8	1
Ulnar			PALMAR INTEROSSEI																		•								8	1
Ulnar			DORSAL INTEROSSEI																		•								8	1
Ulnar			LUMBRICALES III & IV																		•							(7)	8	1
Ulnar			ADDUCTOR POLLICIS																		•								8	1
Ulnar			FLEX POLL BREV. (DEEP H.)																		•								8	1

Figure 12.34. Upper extremity muscle innervation chart showing both the peripheral nerve innervation and the spinal nerve-root innervation of individual muscles. (From reference 44.)

Spinal Nerve and Muscle Chart
trunk and lower extremity

Name

		MUSCLE STRENGTH GRADE	MUSCLE	D. T1-12, L1-5, S1-3	V. T1, 2, 3, 4	V. T5, 6	V. T7, 8	V. T9, 10, 11, 12	V. Iliohypogastric T12 L1	V. Ilioinguinal T(12) L1	V. Lumb. Plex. T(12) L1, 2, 3, 4	P. Femoral L(1) 2, 3, 4	A. Obturator L(1) 2, 3, 4	P. Sup. Glut. L4, 5, S1	P. Inf. Glut. L5, S1, 2	V. Sac. Plex. L4, 5, S1, 2, 3	P. Sciatic L4, 5, S1, 2	A. Sciatic L4, 5, S1, 2, 3	P. Fibular L4, 5, S1, 2	A. Tibial L4, 5, S1, 2, 3	L1	L2	L3	L4	L5	S1	S2	S3
			ERECTOR SPINAE	•																	1	2	3	4	5	1	2	3
Thoracic Nerves			SERRATUS POST SUP		•																							
			TRANS THORACIS		•	•	•																					
			INT INTERCOSTALS		•	•	•	•																				
			EXT INTERCOSTALS		•	•	•	•																				
			SUBCOSTALES		•	•	•	•																				
			LEVATOR COSTARUM		•	•	•	•																				
			OBLIQUUS EXT ABD			(•)	•	•																				
			RECTUS ABDOMINIS			•	•	•																				
			OBLIQUUS INT ABD				•	•	•	(•)											1							
			TRANSVERSUS ABD				•	•	•	(•)											1							
			SERRATUS POST INF					•																				
Lumbar Plexus			QUAD LUMBORUM								•										1	2	3					
			PSOAS MINOR								•										1	2						
			PSOAS MAJOR								•										1	2	3	4				
Femoral			ILIACUS									•									(1)	2	3	4				
			PECTINEUS									•	(•)									2	3	4				
			SARTORIUS									•										2	3	(4)				
			QUADRICEPS									•										2	3	4				
Obturator	Ant.		ADDUCTOR BREVIS										•									2	3	4				
			ADDUCTOR LONGUS										•									2	3	4				
			GRACILIS										•									2	3	4				
	Post.		OBTURATOR EXT										•										3	4				
			ADDUCTOR MAGNUS										•					•				2	3	4	5	1		
Gluteal	Sup.		GLUTEUS MEDIUS											•										4	5	1		
			GLUTEUS MINIMUS											•										4	5	1		
			TENSOR FAS LAT											•										4	5	1		
	In.		GLUTEUS MAXIMUS												•										5	1	2	
Sacral Plexus			PIRIFORMIS													•									(5)	1	2	
			GEMELLUS SUP													•									5	1	2	
			OBTURATOR INT													•									5	1	2	
			GEMELLUS INF													•								4	5	1	(2)	
			QUADRATUS FEM													•								4	5	1	(2)	
Sciatic	P.		BICEPS (SHORT H)														•								5	1	2	
	Tibial		BICEPS (LONG H)															•							5	1	2	3
			SEMITENDINOSUS															•						4	5	1	2	
			SEMIMEMBRANOSUS															•						4	5	1	2	
Fibular	Deep		TIBIALIS ANTERIOR																•					4	5	1		
			EXT HALL LONG																•					4	5	1		
			EXT DIGIT LONG																•					4	5	1		
			PERONEUS TERTIUS																•					4	5	1		
			EXT DIGIT BREVIS																•					4	5	1		
	Sup.		PERONEUS LONGUS																•					4	5	1		
			PRONEUS BREVIS																•					4	5	1		
Tibial	Tibial		PLANTARIS																	•				4	5	1	(2)	
			GASTROCNEMIUS																	•						1	2	
			POPLITEUS																	•				4	5	1		
			SOLEUS																	•					5	1	2	
			TIBIALIS POSTERIOR																	•				(4)	5	1		
			FLEX DIGIT LONG																	•					5	1	(2)	
			FLEX HALL LONG																	•					5	1	2	
	Med Pl		FLEX DIGIT BREVIS																	•				4	5	1		
			ABDUCTOR HALL																	•				4	5	1		
			FLEX HALL BREVIS																	•				4	5	1		
			LUMBRICALIS I																	•				4	5	1		
	Lat Plant		ADB DIGITI MIN																	•						1	2	
			QUAD PLANTAE																	•						1	2	
			FLEX DIGITI MIN																	•						1	2	
			OPP. DIGITI MIN																	•						1	2	
			ADDUCTORS HALL																	•						1	2	
			PLANT INTEROSSEI																	•						1	2	
			DORSAL INTEROSSEI																	•						1	2	
			LUMB II, III, IV																	•				(4)	(5)	1	2	

KEY

D Dorsal Prim. Ramus
V Vent. Prim. Ramus
A Anterior Division
P Posterior Division

Figure 12.35. Lower extremity muscle innervation chart showing both the peripheral nerve innervation and the spinal nerve-root innervation of individual muscles. (From reference 44.)

4. Does the problem occur continuously or at certain times of the day or night?
5. Do any activities change the symptoms?
6. When did the symptoms/problems begin?
7. Did the symptoms occur suddenly or gradually?
8. Did an accident or injury precipitate the problem?
9. Has the problem worsened or improved over time?
10. Do any family members or coworkers have similar problems?
11. What medications are you currently taking? Do any of these medications have neuropathic or myopathic side effects?
12. What is your working environment? Are you exposed to any chemicals which might give rise to neuropathy or myopathy?

The *clinical neuromuscular evaluation* is also important in clinical problem solving and routinely also precedes ENMG procedures. The examiner commonly looks for signs of neuromuscular dysfunction such as

- Atrophy (localized vs. diffuse)
- Trophic or temperature changes in the skin
- Differences in appearance of the extremities (e.g., skin color, skin texture, girth)
- Joint deformities or limitations in joint movement
- Functional abnormalities or limitations (e.g., gait deviations, balance disorders, asymmetry of upper extremity/lower extremity movement)
- Muscle weakness (unilateral vs. bilateral; upper vs. lower limbs vs. trunk)
- Reflex changes (decreased, increased, or asymmetric)
- Sensory disturbances (nerve root dermatome vs. peripheral nerve dermatome distribution).

Answers to interview questions and findings from the neuromuscular examination dictate the types of ENMG testing procedures to be used and the specific nerves and muscle to be tested.

Most patients referred for ENMG have some type of peripheral nerve pathology. Primary muscle diseases, neuromuscular junction pathology, and anterior-horn-cell diseases do not occur as frequently. Case studies of patients are presented below to illustrate how the patient interview and the clinical neuromuscular evaluation guide the choice of ENMG testing, and to show how the results of ENMG testing assist in identification of the problem.

In interpreting ENMG findings, one important question to be addressed is, what do the interview, clinical neuromuscular results, and ENMG findings have in common?

CLINICAL CASE STUDIES

Case 1: Carpal Tunnel Syndrome Referral

History from Patient Interview

The patient is a 42-year-old female with a 1-year history of progressively worsening right-hand paresthesias. She reports no history of trauma. Her symptoms are worse at night and with prolonged driving. She states that it feels like "my hand goes to sleep" and that symptoms ease with changing her hand position or shaking her hand. She reports a prior episode of similar, but less severe, symptoms 12 years ago while pregnant. She has not noticed any change in her daily functional abilities. She has recently had a regular physical exam and has no history of chronic orthopedic, neurological, or metabolic disease. She is taking no medication at this time.

Clinical Exam

The patient ambulates independently with a normal gait. Her posture is good, without visible abnormality. She has full cervical spine range of motion without pain or reproduction of symptoms and full upper extremity range of motion without pain. Manual muscle testing reveals that strength is normal in both upper extremities. Deep tendon reflexes (biceps, triceps, brachioradialis, wrist extensors, quadriceps, and triceps surae) are intact and equal bilaterally for upper and lower extremities. Cutaneous sensation to light touch and two-point discrimination appear normal in both upper extremities. Tinel sign is negative over median and ulnar nerves at the wrists and elbows bilaterally. Phalen sign is positive on right after 2 minutes.

Results

Nerve Conduction Velocity Studies

	Latency (ms)		**Distance (mm)**		**Conduction Velocity (m/s)**		**Amplitude (μV)**	
Nerve Study	Right	Left	Right	Left	Right	Left	Right	Left
Median motor								
Wrist—APB	3.8	3.8	80	80			7,000	9,000
Elbow	8.0	7.8	220	220	52	55	7,000	9,000
Upper arm	10.2	9.8	120	120	54	60	6,800	9,000
F-wave	27.8	28.0						
Median sensory								
Wrist—index	**3.7**[a]	3.2	140	140			30	42
Wrist—long	**3.7**[a]	3.2	140	140			28	40
Transcarpal	**2.2**[a]	1.7	80	80			68	90
Ulnar motor								
Wrist—ADM	3.0		80				6,000	
Below elbow	6.8		210		55		6,000	
Above elbow	8.6		100		55		5,800	
Upper arm	10.6		125		56		5,600	
F-wave	27.6							
Ulnar sensory								
Wrist—little	2.8		120				30	
Radial sensory								
Forearm—web	2.4		120				30	

APB, abductor pollicis brevis; ADM, abductor digiti minimi.
[a]Indicated abnormal value.

EMG Studies

Muscle	Insertional Activity	Spontaneous Activity	Motor Units	Interference Pattern
Right APB	Normal	None	Normal	Full
Right OP	Normal	None	Normal	Full
Right FPL	Normal	None	Normal	Full
Right PT	Normal	None	Normal	Full
Right first DI	Normal	None	Normal	Full
Right ADM	Normal	None	Normal	Full
Right ECR	Normal	None	Normal	Full

APB, abductor pollicis brevis; OP, opponens pollicis; PT, pronator teres; DI, 1st dorsal interosseus; ADM, abductor digiti minimi; ECR, extensor carpi radialis longus; FPL, flexor pollicis longus.

Summary of ENMG Findings

Prolonged distal sensory latencies of the right median nerve to the index and long fingers, with normal sensory response amplitudes. Also, the right median transcarpal sensory response latency is prolonged but of normal amplitude. All other motor and sensory conductions were normal. EMG study of the right upper extremity showed no signs of denervation. Motor units were of normal amplitude, duration, and form, with complete interference patterns.

Impression of ENMG Findings

EMG/nerve conduction velocity findings as listed above are consistent with mild involvement of the median nerve at or about the right wrist, primarily neuropraxic in nature, without signs of axonal degeneration or conduction block.

Discussion

This is a fairly typical electrophysiological study that shows a mild or early carpal tunnel syndrome. In referring to prior discussions of peripheral nerve injury, note that the only abnormalities associated with this case are the prolonged distal sensory latencies for the right median nerve. All calculated conduction velocities were within normal limits, as were the evoked motor and sensory response amplitudes. These normal amplitudes and the absence of spontaneous activity noted during the EMG needle exam are all consistent with peripheral nerve compression and/or a demyelinating process. Also note how the summary describes the neurological lesion in anatomical perspective (location) and avoids the diagnostic label of carpal tunnel syndrome.

Case 2: Carpal Tunnel Syndrome Referral

History from Patient Interview

The patient is a 39-year-old white male referred for EMG/nerve conduction velocity study of the right upper extremity to rule out carpal tunnel syndrome. The patient reports a several month history of paresthesias, cramping, and pain in his right hand. Patient is a surgeon and notes symptoms are worse during long operative procedures. He denies any history of trauma, but does complain of episodic neck and back pain without frank radicular symptoms. He indicates that his general state of health is good and that he takes no medication at this time.

Clinical Exam

The patient is a healthy-appearing male, ambulating independently, in no apparent distress. His posture shows a mild forward head, but otherwise posture is unremarkable. Neck range of motion is mildly restricted in right rotation but pain free. Spurling test was negative. The upper extremity range of motion is normal and without pain. Strength in the upper extremities was also found to be normal. Deep tendon reflexes were absent in the upper and lower extremities, even with facilitatory techniques. Cutaneous sensation to light touch was grossly intact. Tinel sign over median and ulnar nerves was negative, while Phalen sign was positive.

Results

Nerve Conduction Velocity Studies

	Latency (ms)		Distance (mm)		Conduction Velocity (m/s)		Amplitude (μV)	
Nerve Study	Right	Left	Right	Left	Right	Left	Right	Left
Median motor								
Wrist—APB	5.6[a]	5.2[a]	80	80			3,900[a]	5,000
Elbow	11.6[a]	11.0[a]	250	250	42[a]	43[a]	3,000[a]	4,600[a]
Upper arm	14.1[a]	13.5[a]	120	120	48[a]	49[a]	2,600[a]	4,400[a]
F-wave	34.0[a]	32.2[a]						
Median sensory								
Wrist—index	5.0[a]	4.6[a]	140	140			10[a]	14[a]
Ulnar motor								
Wrist—ADM	5.0[a]	4.8[a]	80	80			3,000[a]	4,000[a]
Below elbow	10.4[a]	10.0[a]	220	220	41[a]	42[a]	3,000[a]	3,800[a]
Above elbow	**13.2[a]**	12.2[a]	110	120	39[a]	50	2,200[a]	3,400[a]
F-wave	34.8[a]	32.0[a]						
Ulnar sensory								
Wrist—little	4.2[a]	3.8[a]	120	120			8[a]	12[a]
Radial sensory								
Forearm—web	3.6[a]	3.4[a]	120	120			10[a]	12[a]
Tibial motor								
Ankle—AH	8.2[a]	8.0[a]	100	100			800[a]	1200[a]
Popliteal	22.0[a]	21.8[a]	410	400	30[a]	29[a]	200[a]	400[a]
H-reflex	Absent	Absent						
Sural sensory								
Calf-foot	Absent	Absent						

APB, abductor pollicis brevis; ADM, abductor digiti minimi; AH, abductor hallucis.
[a]Indicated abnormal value.

EMG Studies

Muscle	Insertional Activity	Spontaneous Activity	Motor Units	Interference Pattern
Right APB	Slight Decrease	Occasional sharp waves	Large amplitude	Decreased
Left APB	Slight Decrease	Occasional sharp waves	Large amplitude	Decreased
Right first DI	Decreased	Occasional sharp waves	Large amplitude	Decreased
Left first DI	Decreased	Occasional sharp waves	Large amplitude	Decreased
Right PT	Normal	None	Occasional polyphasic	Decreased
Left PT	Normal	None	Occasional polyphasic	Decreased
Right ECR	Normal	None	Normal	Decreased
Right deltoids	Normal	None	Normal	Slight decrease
Right VM	Decreased	None	Large amplitude, polyphasic	Decreased
Right gastrocnemius	Decreased	Occasional sharp waves	Large amplitude, polyphasic	Decreased
Right AH	Absent	Occasional sharp waves	Increased duration	Severely decreased
Left AH	Absent	Occasional sharp waves	Increased duration	Severely decreased
Left TA	Increased	Sharp waves, fibrillations	Large amplitude, polyphasic	Decreased

APB, abductor pollicis brevis; DI, dorsal interosseus; PT, pronator teres; ECR, extensor carpi radialis longus; VM, vastus medialis; AH, abductor hallucis; TA, tibialis anterior.

Summary of ENMG Findings

Nerve conduction studies of both upper and lower extremities show diffuse widespread abnormalities of conduction and amplitude. H-reflexes were absent bilaterally. The changes in amplitude and conduction values indicated a mixed axonal degeneration and demyelinating process. EMG study shows chronic changes more pronounced in a distal distribution, with lower extremities worse than the upper extremities.

Impression of ENMG Findings

EMG/nerve conduction velocity study as listed above is consistent with a peripheral polyneuropathy involving both the motor and sensory nerve fibers. These findings are more severe in a distal distribution, involving the lower more than the upper extremities. The chronic changes noted during the needle EMG study would indicate that this process has been present for a long period of time.

Discussion

This case is a good example of a patient presenting with what appears to be a simple peripheral nerve compression syndrome, when in fact the underlying pathology is anything but simple. This patient was ultimately diagnosed as having a hereditary motor sensory neuropathy. Of particular interest is the manner in which he had adapted to his level of decreased capabilities. On clinical exam, he presented as essentially normal except for the absent deep tendon reflexes. This was in part a result of decreased thoroughness during the initial clinical interview and exam, in that we focused upon his complaints and the most likely probable causes. Because we did not examine his lower extremities, we missed the exceptionally high arched feet and obvious loss of lower leg muscle mass. During the electrophysiological exam, it became obvious that there was a diffuse process occurring. The widespread abnormal findings in the upper extremities dictated that the lower extremities be examined, subsequently leading to the impression of a peripheral polyneuropathic process.

Case 3: Fibular Nerve Palsy Referral

History from Patient Interview

A 19-year old male is referred with a three day history of weakness in the right ankle and numbness over the dorsal right foot. He does not complain of pain. The patient reports that he awoke with the above symptoms. He reports no history of trauma, but indicates that four days ago he was on a long hike in rough terrain sustaining multiple falls. His general state of health is good and he has no prior history of similar symptoms.

Clinical Examination

Patient ambulates independently with a high steppage gait on right with obvious inability to dorsiflex his right ankle. He has full active range of motion of the trunk, hips, knees, and left ankle. Right ankle shows full passive range of motion, but the patient is unable to actively dorsiflex or evert the ankle, or extend the toes. Right manual muscle testing shows 5/5 hip groups, 5/5 quads/hamstrings, 5/5 gastroc/soleus, 5/5 posterior tibialis, 5/5 toe flexors, 1/5 peroneus longus, 0/5 anterior tibialis, 0/5 extensor digitorum longus and brevis. Left lower extremity was 5/5 throughout. Sensation was severely diminished over the dorsal right foot and between the great and long toe. DTR's were intact and equal bilaterally for quadriceps and triceps surae. No specific point tenderness was noted, and no Tinel's about the ankle or around the knee could be elicited.

Results of Nerve Conduction Velocity Studies

	Latency (ms)		***Distance (mm)***		***Conduction Velocity (m/s)***		***Amplitude (μV)***	
Nerve	Right	Left	Left	Right	Right	Left	Right	Left
Fibullar motor								
Ankle-EDB	4.1	4.0	80	80			4900	5200
Fibular neck	10.1	10.2	340	340	57	55	4700	5000
Popliteal fossa	Absent*	12.4	120	120	None*	55	None*	5000
Superficial fibullar sensory								
Lat. fibula	3.7	3.6	120	120			24	22
Tibial motor								
Ankle-ABD HAL.	4.6		100				10600	
Popliteal	13.8		480		52		9400	
H-reflex	28.4							
Sural sensory								
Calf-lat foot	3.8		120				10	

*Indicates abnormal value

Summary of ENMG findings

Motor nerve conduction of the deep portion of the right fibular nerve is absent with stimulation of the fibular nerve in the popliteal fossa but normal motor conduction findings with stimulation of the fibular nerve just below the head of the fibula or just above the ankle. Right superficial fibular

Results of EMG Studies

Muscle	*Insertional Activity*	*Spontaneous Activity*	*Motor Units*	*Interference Patterns*
R ext dig brev	Normal	None	**None***	**None***
R ext dig long	Normal	None	**None***	**None***
R ant tib	Normal	None	**None***	**None***
R peroneus long	Normal	None	Normal	**Single unit***
R short BIC FEM	Normal	None	Normal	Full
R abd HAL	Normal	None	Normal	Full
R Post TIB	Normal	None	Normal	Full
R gastroc	Normal	None	Normal	Full
R quadriceps	Normal	None	Normal	Full

sensory conduction study with stimulation just proximal to the ankle, and recording over the dorsum of the right foot was normal. Normal left fibular and right tibial nerve motor conduction studies. The right tibial H-reflex response latency was normal. Right sural sensory response latency was normal while the amplitude of the sural sensory response was near the low limits of normal.

EMG study of the right lower extremity shows complete absence of motor unit recruitment in muscles innervated by the deep portion of the fibular nerve, with severely reduced interference pattern in the muscles innervated by the superficial motor branch of the fibular nerve. The EMG findings at rest, and with volitional contractions of the short head of the biceps femoris muscle were normal with full interference patterns.

Impression of ENMG Findings

EMG/NCV findings as listed above are consistent with a complete conduction interruption of the deep branch of the fibular nerve and near complete interruption of the superficial fibular nerve. The location of the lesion is between the head of the right fibula and the popliteal fossa, and is likely to be just proximal to the head of the fibula where the fibular nerve lies just beneath the skin and is readily exposed to external trauma. At this time, it cannot be determined whether the lesion is neuropraxic in nature (e.g., conduction block) or axonotmetic (e.g., axonal disruption with denervation). Recommend repeat study in three weeks to evaluate for EMG denervation changes in the fibular innervated muscles and presence or absence of motor and sensory action potentials with nerve stimulation distal to the head of the fibula.

Discussion

The above study is a clear example of a near complete peripheral nerve lesion. The nerve conduction findings reveal normal nerve conduction in the fibular nerve branches distal to the head of the fibula. With stimulation proximal to the head of the fibula motor nerve conduction responses are absent; a finding consistent with either complete conduction block or a complete disruption of fibular motor axons to EDB. EMG findings revealed no ability to voluntarily activated motor units in any muscles innervated by the fibular nerve. An important finding in this case was the normal EMG findings in the short head of the biceps femoris. The muscle receives its fibular nerve innervation prior to the fibular nerve entering the popliteal fossa. If subsequent study in three weeks revealed spontaneous electrical activity (fibrillation potentials or positive sharp waves) at rest in fibular innervated musculature, one could then classify the lesion as axonotmetic. These spontaneous potentials become evident only after the fibular motor axons have degenerated, and the denervated muscle fibers undergo the characteristic excitability changes associated with loss of innervation. In addition, if the lesion is complete axonotmetic in nature, stimulation of the fibular nerve distal to the site of the lesion would not evoke any motor response from the EDB in the motor conduction study or any sensory response from the dorsum of the foot in the sensory nerve conduction study.

Case 4: Low Back Injury (Rule out Nerve Root Lesion)

History from Patient Interview

Patient is a 42-year-old female with a long history of episodic low back and right leg pain which has usually resolved with rest, medication, and home exercises. Her current bout of pain started 3 months ago while lifting at work. She noted immediate minor low back pain, which did not limit her mobility. Upon awakening the next morning, she was in severe pain and unable to move because of low back and right leg pain. The pain in her leg is worse with flexion motions and extends to her ankle and foot. She notes a sense of numbness along the right lateral foot border. She reports that the leg feels weak, but in no particular pattern. She denies any loss of bowel or bladder control. Pain arises with coughing or sneezing and radiates into her leg.

Clinical Examination

The patient ambulates slowly, with slight limp on right. Posture examination reveals trunk held rigidly and slightly shifted to left. The trunk range of motion is limited in all planes, but with pain greatly increased with flexion and right rotation. Strength is difficult to assess secondary to pain with testing, but is grossly intact and at least 4/5 throughout the lower extremities. Deep tendon reflexes are intact at quadriceps and left triceps surae; right triceps surae response is absent. Sensation is decreased over the right lateral aspect of the foot. Sitting and supine straight leg-raise tests were positive.

Results

Nerve Conduction Velocity Studies

	Latency (ms)		**Distance (mm)**		**Conduction Velocity (m/s)**		**Amplitude (μV)**	
Nerve	Right	Left	Right	Left	Right	Left	Right	Left
Fibular motor								
Ankle—EDB	4.2		80				5,600	
Fibular neck	10.2		300		50		5,400	
Popliteal		12.0	120		55		5,200	
F-wave	46.0							
Fibular superficial sensory								
Lateral fibula	3.6			120				20
Tibial motor								
Ankle—AH	4.4	4.6	100	100			6,400	12,000
Popliteal	12.2	12.2	400	410	51	54	5,800	11,000
H-reflex	Absent[a]	27.4						
Sural sensory								
Calf–lateral foot	3.8		14				16	

EDB, extensor digitorum brevis; AH, abductor hallucis.
[a]Indicated abnormal value.

EMG Studies

Muscle	Insertional Activity	Spontaneous Activity	Motor Units	Interference Pattern
Right VM	Normal	None	Normal	Full
Right TA	Normal	None	Normal	Full
Right EH	Normal	None	Normal	Full
Right EDB	Normal	None	Normal	Full
Right AH	Increased	+Sharp waves	Frequent polyphasics, fibrillations	Decreased
Right gastrocnemius	Increased	+Sharp waves	Frequent polyphasics	Decreased
Right GM	Increased	+Sharp waves	Frequent polyphasics	Decreased
Left gastrocnemius	Normal	None	Normal	Full
Left GM	Normal	None	Normal	Full
Right paraspinals				
L3–L4	Normal	None	Normal	
L4–L5	Normal	None	Normal	
L5–S1	Increased	+Sharp waves	Occasional polyphasics	
S1–S2	Increased	+Sharp waves	Frequent polyphasics, fibrillations	
Left paraspinals				
S1–S2	Normal	None	Normal	

AH, abductor hallucis brevis; VM, vastus medialis; TA, tibialis anterior; EH, extensor hallucis longus; EDB, extensor digitorum brevis; GM, gluteus maximus.

Summary of ENMG Findings

EMG/nerve conduction velocity study as listed above is consistent with a lesion at or about the right S1 nerve root level, with changes consistent with axonal degeneration.

Impression of ENMG Findings

Nerve conduction studies of right fibular and tibial motor nerves and left tibial motor nerves were normal. Normal sensory responses of the right superficial fibular and sural nerves were recorded. Patient had absent H-reflex on the right; left H-reflex had normal latency.

EMG study showed increased spontaneous activity in the right S1 myotomal distribution, including the paraspinal musculature, along with an increased percentage of polyphasic motor units in the same distribution. Muscles outside of the S1 distribution were normal.

Discussion

This study illustrates findings consistent with a nerve-root lesion. In the case of single nerve-root lesions, nerve conduction velocities will be normal with normal-to-borderline normal evoked motor response amplitudes. Sensory responses will usually be normal, even in the clinical absence of sensation. This is a result of the lesion being proximal to the dorsal root ganglion. The presence of positive sharp waves and fibrillation potentials indicates that the nerve fibers have undergone Wallerian degeneration. The presence of polyphasic motor units indicates that the surviving nerve fibers are reinnervating the denervated muscle fibers, via collateral sprouting. The unilateral loss of the H-reflex fits with the clinical picture of an absent ankle deep tendon reflex.

SUMMARY

This chapter has addressed the ENMG examination and its uses in establishing a differential diagnosis of neuromuscular disorders. Both modern procedures in ENMG and classical approaches to electrophysiologic examination and evaluation have been described. The objective was to provide an understanding of the procedures as well as an appreciation for the meaning of the results of ENMG studies. Findings from ENMG can be used in conjunction with a spectrum of other clinical tests to assist in establishing a diagnosis and subsequent comprehensive plan of care, including medical, surgical and rehabilitative procedures. The chapter has emphasized that the results of ENMG examination should never be used alone to define the site, extent, or nature of pathology. That is, the results of electrophysiological tests are not diagnostic when viewed in isolation. Education and training in musculoskeletal and neuromuscular evaluation is prerequisite for the performance and interpretation of the ENMG examination. Clinical competence in the actual performance ENMG may be attained by further study and extensive clinical practice, preferably under the guidance of an experienced practitioner in the field. For those interested in developing competence in ENMG, guidelines have been established by several organizations, including the Section on Clinical Electrophysiology of the American Physical Therapy Association (Alexandria, Virginia) and the American Association of Electrodiagnostic Medicine (Rochester, Minnestota).

Disclaimer: The opinions, views, and comments contained within this chapter are those of the authors and do not reflect the official position of the United States government, the Department of Defense, or the United States Navy.

SELF-STUDY QUESTIONS

For answers, see Appendix B.

1. Compare and contrast the intracellular and extracellular recording techniques used to monitor activity in nervous and muscular tissues.
2. What are nine clinically important questions that may be answered by the findings of nerve conduction studies?
3. Describe the placement of stimulation and recording electrodes for a median motor nerve conduction study.
4. Compare and contrast the orthodromic and antidromic sensory nerve conduction techniques for the median nerve.
5. List the nerves commonly tested in motor nerve conductions and in sensory nerve conduction studies.
6. What types of neuromuscular disorders can produce a measurable reduction in the amplitude of the (i) compound motor action potential or (ii) compound sensory nerve action potential?
7. Identify two abnormal conditions that may reduce nerve conduction velocity.
8. List two factors (not technique related or pathological) that may influence conduction velocity (speed of action potential propagation) in peripheral nerves.
9. Define neuropraxia, axonotmesis, and neurotmesis.

10. What electrical potentials are noted in normal muscle during voluntary contraction?

11. What types of EMG potentials are considered abnormal findings during an examination in a muscle at rest and during voluntary, isometric contraction?

12. Compare and contrast EMG and NCV findings for a neuropraxic versus an axonotmetic injury. How would these findings change with time (1 day, 5 days, and 21 days postinjury)?

13. What is an F-wave, and what is thought to occur that gives rise to this pattern?

14. Identify five conditions that may give rise to an increase in the latency of the F-wave response.

15. a. What is the name of the test that is analogous to the Achilles tendon reflex test?
b. Identify the components of the stretch reflex pathway that are associated with this test.

16. The blink reflex test examines the integrity of which two cranial nerves?

17. How would the results of blink reflex testing differ between a unilateral Bell palsy and chronic inflammatory, demyelinating, polyneuropathy that compromises cranial nerve function?

18. What is the purpose of somatosensory evoked potential testing? Describe the pathways examined during this form of electrophysiological examination.

19. What is the purpose of motor evoked-potential testing? Describe the pathways examined during this form of electrophysiological examination.

20. Name two clinical tests of cutaneous sensory function.

21. List the contraindications/precautions to performing ENMG examination.

22. List 10 questions that a clinician might ask during a patient interview that would be helpful in elucidating the underlying cause of a neuromuscular disorder.

23. List eight signs of neuromuscular dysfunction that may be observed during routine clinical examination.

24. What are the typical types of findings in nerve conduction studies in an individual with mild and moderate carpal tunnel syndrome?

25. Draw a diagram of the brachial plexus and label all five terminal branches, all supraclavicular branches, and all infraclavicular branches.

REFERENCES

1. Kimura J. Principles of nerve conduction studies. In: Kimura, J. *Electrodiagnosis of Diseases of Nerve and Muscle*. 2nd ed. Philadelphia: F.A. Davis; 1989, 79–80.
2. NIOSH. *Performing Motor and Sensory Neuronal Conduction Studies in Adult Humans: A NIOSH Technical Manual*. NIOSH Publication No. 90-113. Washington, DC: National Institute for Occupational Safety and Health; 1990:8.
3. Ma DM, Liveson JA. *Nerve Conduction Handbook*. Philadelphia: F.A. Davis; 1983.
4. Chaudhry V, Cornblath DR, Mellits ED, et al. Inter- and intra-examiner reliability of nerve conduction measurements in patients with diabetic neuropathy. *Ann Neurol*. 1991;30:841–843.
5. Bromberg MB, Jaros L. Symmetry of normal motor and sensory conduction measurements. *Muscle Nerve*. 1998;21:498–503.

6. Olney RK. AAEM Minimonograph no. 38. Neuropathies in connective tissue disease. *Muscle Nerve* 1992;15:531–542.
7. NIOSH. *Performing Motor and Sensory Neuronal Conduction Studies in Adult Humans: A NIOSH Technical Manual*. (NIOSH) Publication No. 90-113. Washington, DC: National Institute for Occupational Safety and Health; 1990:12-15.
8. Wilbourn AJ. Sensory nerve conduction studies. *J Clin Neurophysiol.* 1994;11:584–601.
9. Nielsen RP, Skurja M, Greathouse DG, et al. Electrophysiological differentiation of brachial Plexus Injuries. *J Clin Electrophysiol.* 1998;10:2–22.
10. Falck B, Stalberg E. Motor nerve conduction studies: measurement principles and interpretation of findings. *J Clin Neuorphysiol.* 1995;12:254–279.
11. Sunderland S. *Nerve Injuries and Their Repair.* Edinburgh: Churchhill Livingstone; 1991.
12. Fisher MA. AAEM Minimonograph no. 13. H reflexes and F waves: physiology and indications. *Muscle Nerve*. 1992;15:1223–1233.
13. Fisher MA, Hoffen B, Hultman C. Normative F-wave values and the number of recorded F waves. *Muscle Nerve.* 1994;17:1185–1189.
14. Gill NW, Ruediger TM, Gochis RD, et al. Test-retest reliability of the ulnar F-wave minimum latency in normal adults. *Electromyogr Clin Neurophysiol.* 1999;39:195–200.
15. Weber F. The diagnostic sensitivity of different F-wave parameters. *J Neurol Neurosurg Psychiatr* 1998;65:535–540.
16. Rivner MH. F-wave studies: limitations. *Muscle Nerve.* 1998;1101–1104.
17. Marchini C. et al. Median nerve F-wave study derived by flexor carpi radialis. *Electromyogr Clin Neurophysiol.* 1998;38:451–453.
18. Papathanasiou ES, Zamba E, Papacostas SS. Radial nerve F-waves: normative values with surface recording of the extensor indicis muscle. *Clin Neurophysiol.* 2001;112:145–152.
19. Andersen H, et al. F-wave latency, the most sensitive nerve conduction parameter in patients with diabetes mellitus. *Muscle Nerve.* 1997;20:1296–1302.
20. Fraser JL, Olney RK. The relative diagnostic sensitivity of different F-wave parameters in various polyneuropathies *Muscle Nerve.* 1992;15:912–918.
21. Andersen H, Stalberg E, Falck B. F-wave latency, the most sensitive nerve conduction parameter in patients with diabetes mellitus. *Muscle Nerve.* 1997;20:1296–1302.
22. Fisher MA. The contemporary role of F-wave studies. *Muscle Nerve.* 1998;21:1098–1101.
23. Toyokura M. F-wave duration in diabetic polyneuropathy. *Muscle Nerve.* 1998;21:246–49.
24. Dumitru D. *Electrodiagnostic Medicine.* Philadelphia: Hanley and Belfus; 1994:747.
25. Aminoff MJ. *Electromyography in Clinical Practice.* 3rd ed. New York: Churchhill Livingstone; 1998.
26. Oh SJ. *Electromyography—Neuromuscular Transmission Studies.* Baltimore, Md:Williams & Wilkins; 1988.
27. Bromberg MB. Electromyographic (EMG) findings in denervation. *Crit Rev Phys Rehabil Med.* 1993;5:83–127.
28. Kimura J. Techniques and normal findings. In: Kimura J. *Electrodiagnosis in Diseases of Nerve and Muscle: Principles and Practice.* 2nd ed. Philadelphia: F.A. Davis; 1989:227–248.
29. Kimura J. Techniques and normal findings. In: Kimura J. *Electrodiagnosis in Diseases of Nerve and Muscle: Principles and Practice.* 2nd ed. Philadelphia: F.A. Davis; 1989:249–274.
30. Kraft GH. Fibrillation potential amplitude and muscle atrophy following peripheral nerve injury. *Muscle Nerve.* 1990;13:814–821.
31. Aminoff MJ. Chapter 5. General aspects of needle electrograph. *Electromyography in Clinical Practice.* 3rd ed. New York:Churchhill Livingstone; 1998:63–65.
32. Mitsikostas DD, Karandreas N, Coutsopetras P, et al. Fasciculation potentials in healthy people. *Muscle Nerve.* 1998;21(4):533–535.
33. Bromberg MB. Electromyographic (EMG) findings in denervation. *Crit Rev Phys Rehabil Med.* 1993;5:83–127.

34. Aminoff MJ. *Electromyography in Clinical Practice*. 3rd ed. New York: Churchhill Livingstone; 1998:70.

35. Harper CM, Thomas JE, Cascino TL, Litchy WJ. Distinction between neoplastic and radiation-induced brachial plexopathy, with emphasis on the role of EMG. *Neurology*. 1989;39:502–506.

36. Aminoff MJ. *Electromyography in Clinical Practice*. 3rd ed. New York: Churchhill Livingstone; 1998:79.

37. Parry CBW. Strength-duration Curves. In Litch S, ed. *Electrodiagnosis and Electromyography*. Baltimore, Md: Waverly Press; 1971:241–271.

38. Ritchie AE. *Peripheral Nerve Injuries*. Special Report, Sen. Med. Res. Council. London: H.M. Stationery Office; 1954.

39. Adrian ED. The electrical reactions of muscle before and after nerve injury. *Brain*. 1916;39:1–33.

40. Oester YT, Licht S. Routine Electrodiagnosis. In: Licht S, ed. *Electrodiagnosis and Electromyography*. Baltimore, Md: Waverly Press; 1971.

41. Bell-Krotoski J, Weinstein S, Weinstein C. Testing sensibility, including touch-pressure, two-point discrimination point localization and vibration. *J Hand Ther*. 1993;6:114–123.

42. Dellon AL. *Evaluation of Sensibility and Re-education of Sensation in the Hand*. Baltimore, Md: Williams & Wilkins; 1981.

43. Lister G. *The Hand: Diagnosis and Indications*. Edinburgh: Churchill Livingstone; 1977: 73.

44. Kendall FP, McCreary EK, Provance PG. *Muscle Testing and Function*. 4th ed. Baltimore, Md:Williams & Wilkins; 1993.

SUGGESTED READING

Brooke MH. *A Clinician's View of Neuromuscular Diseases*. Baltimore, Md: Williams & Wilkins; 1986.

Brown WM. *The Physiological and Technical Basis of Electromyography*. Stoneham, Mass: Butterworth; 1984.

Chusid J, McDonald JJ. *Correlative Neuroanatomy and Functional Neurology*. Los Altos, Calif: Lange Medical Publications; 1967.

Dawson DM, Hallett M, Millender LH. *Entrapment Neuropathies*. Boston: Little, Brown & Co.; 1983.

Hoppenfeld S. *Orthopaedic Neurology*. Philadelphia: JB Lippincott; 1977.

Kimura J. *Electrodiagnosis in Diseases of Nerve and Muscle: Principles and Practice*. New York: Oxford University Press, 2000.

Leffert RD. *Brachial Plexus Injuries*. New York: Churchill Livingstone; 1985.

Oh SJ. *Clinical Electromyography: Nerve Conduction Studies*. Baltimore, Md: University Park Press; 1984.

Schaumburg HH, Spencer PS, Thomas PK. *Disorders of Peripheral Nerves*. Philadelphia: F.A. Davis; 1983.

Smorto MP, Basmajian JV. *Electrodiagnosis*. New York: Harper & Row; 1977.

APPENDIX A

Peripheral Neuroanatomy of the Upper and Lower Extremities

Andrew J. Robinson

CLINICAL NEUROANATOMY OF THE UPPER EXTREMITIES

The sensory and motor innervation of the upper extremities and shoulder girdle in humans typically arises from the anterior primary rami of the four lower cervical spine levels (C5, C6, C7, C8) and the first thoracic spine level (T1). As these nerve roots exit the intervertebral foramina, nerve axons unite, separate, and recombine to form the complex network of nervous tissue called the *brachial plexus* (Fig. A.1). The brachial plexus is structurally divided into roots, trunks, divisions, and cords. The C5 to C6 nerve roots unite to form the *upper trunk*, the C7 nerve root forms the *middle trunk*, and the C8 to T1 nerve roots unite to form the *lower trunk*. At times, the C4 nerve root may contribute to the upper trunk and the T2 nerve root may contribute to the lower trunk. Each trunk of the brachial plexus subsequently divides into *anterior* and *posterior divisions*. The six divisions of the trunks next form the three cords of the brachial plexus.

The anterior divisions of the upper and middle trunk form the *lateral cord*, and the anterior division of the lower trunk becomes the *medial cord*. The posterior divisions of the upper, middle, and lower trunks merge to form the *posterior cord*. The medial cord does not usually receive contributions from the C7 nerve root or middle trunk.

The peripheral nerves that innervate the upper extremity and shoulder girdle may be organized in terms of where they arise from the brachial plexus. The cords of the brachial plexus continue into the arm and give rise to the five major peripheral nerves that innervate the upper arm, forearm, and hand. These five nerves (musculocutaneous, axillary, radial, median, and ulnar) are called the *terminal branches* of the brachial plexus. The nerves that arise from the plexus roots and trunks that lie proximal to the clavicle are called the *supraclavicular branches*. The nerves that arise from plexus components distal to the clavicle (cords) arising from and proximal to the terminal branches are called the *infraclavicular branches*.

Four nerves branch from the brachial plexus above the clavicle. The *long thoracic nerve,* which innervates the serratus anterior muscle that produces scapular protraction, is formed by the small branches from the C5 to C7 nerve roots just after they exit the intervertebral foramen. The *dorsal scapular nerve,* which innervates the rhomboid and levator scapulae musculature,

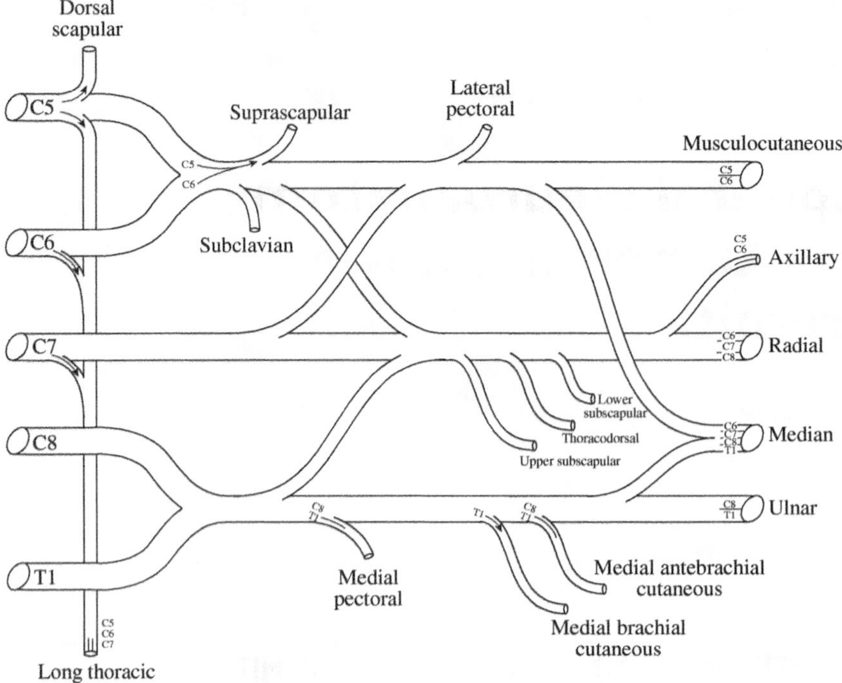

Figure A.1. Brachial plexus formed by cervical and thoracic nerve roots and divided into trunks, divisions, and cords. Peripheral nerves that innervate the shoulder girdle branch from every level of the brachial plexus: dorsal scapular; suprascapular; lateral pectoral; axillary; thoracodorsal; subscapular; medial pectoral; and long thoracic.

arises directly from the C5 nerve root. The *suprascapular nerve* originates from the upper trunk and passes posteriorly to innervate the supraspinatus and infraspinatus muscles of the scapula. These muscles hold the head of the humerus in the glenoid fossa and control lateral rotation of the arm. The *subclavian nerve* also branches from the upper trunk and innervates the subclavius muscle.

Six nerves arise from the cords of the brachial plexus below the clavicle. The *lateral pectoral* and *medial pectoral* nerves arise from the lateral and medial cords, respectively, near the point where these cords are formed from the anterior divisions of the trunks. The lateral pectoral nerve innervates the sternocostal portion of the pectoralis major, and the medial pectoral nerve innervates the inferior portion of the pectoralis major and the pectoralis minor. Together these nerves control humeral adduction and internal rotation. The posterior cord gives rise to three infraclavicular branches: the *upper subscapular, thoracodorsal* and *lower subscapular,* nerves. The upper subscapular innervates the superior portion of the subscapularis, and the lower subscapular innervates the inferior portion of the subscapularis, as well as the teres major. These muscles contribute to humeral internal rotation and adduction. The thoracodorsal nerve innervates the latissimus dorsi that produces humeral internal rotation and humeral extension. Two sensory nerves arise from the medial cord of the brachial plexus. These two nerves, the *medial brachial cutaneous* nerve and the *medial antebrachial cutaneous* nerve, innervate the skin of the upper medial arm and medial forearm, respectively.

As noted above, five terminal branches of the brachial plexus project from the cords of the brachial plexus. The *musculocutaneous* nerve (Fig. A.2) arises from the lateral cord to innervate the coracobrachialis, biceps, and brachialis muscles. The *lateral antebrachial cutaneous* nerve is a continuation of the musculocutaneous nerve that innervates the skin of the lateral forearm. The *axillary* and *radial* nerves (Fig. A.3) arise from the posterior cord of the plexus. The axillary nerve

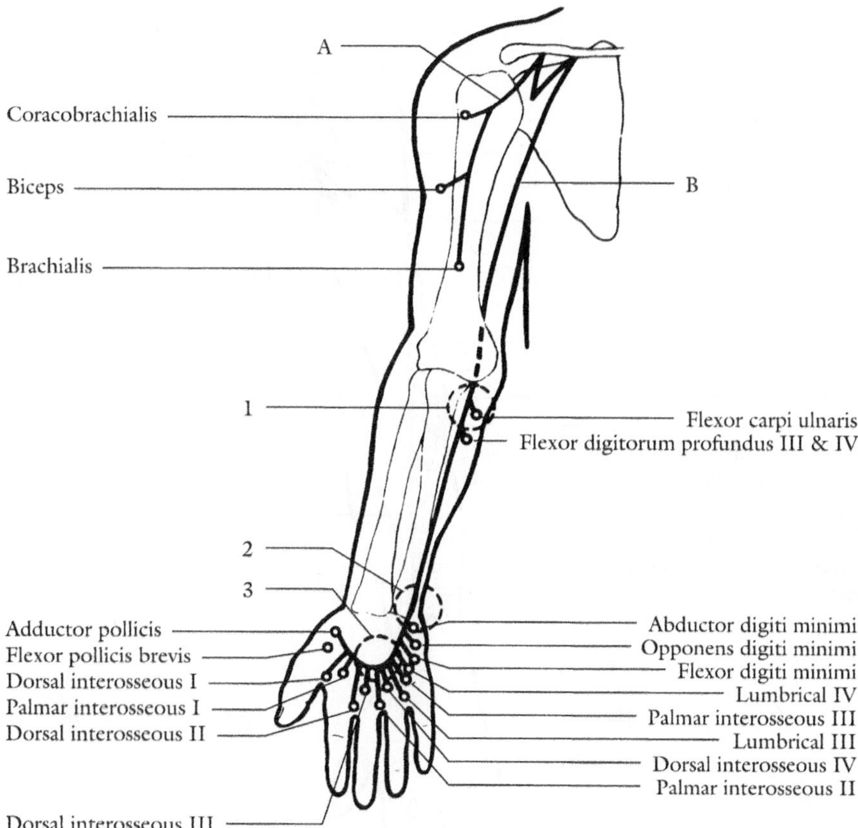

Figure A.2. Muscular innervation by the musculocutaneous **(A)** and ulnar **(B)** nerves, including common sites of compression or injury at *1*, ulnar groove; *2*, canal of Guyon'; and *3*, palm. (Reprinted with permission from Kimura J. *Electrodiagnosis of Diseases of Nerve and Muscle*. Philadelphia: F.A. Davis; 1989.)

supplies the deltoid and teres minor muscles to control humeral flexion, abduction, and extension. The axillary nerve also supplies sensory innervation to the skin overlying the deltoid muscle.

The *radial nerve* supplies both sensation and muscle innervation to the posterior arm and forearm. The radial nerve innervates the triceps and passes posterior to the humerus to innervate the supinator, anconeous, wrist, and finger extensor muscles, as well and the long abductor and extensors of the thumb. At the supinator muscle the radial nerve divides into the *posterior interosseus* (deep radial) and *superficial radial* nerves. The deep radial innervates the finger extensor and the thumb abductor extensor muscles, while the superficial radial innervates the skin of the posterior and lateral aspect of the hand and the dorsal surface of the thumb.

The *median nerve* is a terminal branch of the plexus formed from branches from both the lateral and medial cords. The lateral cord component of the median nerve contributes fibers originating from C6 to C7 nerve-root levels. The medial cord contributes axons to the median nerve that originate from the C8 and T1 nerve roots. The median nerve travels with the ulnar in the groove between the biceps and triceps on the medial side of the upper arm. At about the middle of the upper arm, the median and ulnar nerves diverge, with the median traveling just medial to the biceps tendon and the ulnar nerve traveling to the ulnar notch and cubital tunnel. All of the muscles innervated by the median nerve are below the elbow (Fig. A.5). In the forearm, after innervating and passing through the pronator teres muscle, the median nerve innervates the flexor carpi radialis and palmaris longus and sends off a motor branch called the *anterior*

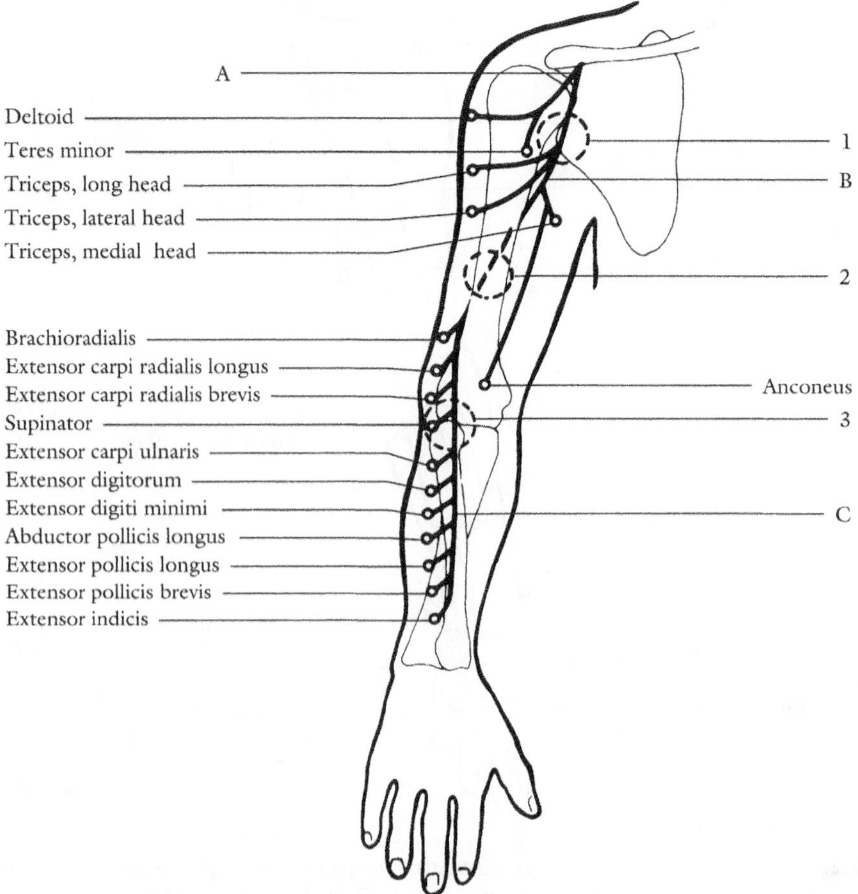

Figure A.3. Muscular innervation by the axillary nerve **(A)** and radial nerve **(B)** with common sites of injury (dashed circles) at *1*, spiral groove and *2*, elbow. (Reprinted with permission from Kimura J. *Electrodiagnosis of Diseases of Nerve and Muscle*. Philadelphia: F.A. Davis; 1989.)

interosseous nerve. The anterior interosseous nerve innervates the flexor digitorum profundus to the index and long fingers, flexor pollicis longus, and pronator quadratus muscles. The main trunk of the median nerve passes through a fibrous arch in the flexor digitorum superficialis and supplies innervation to the superficial finger flexor musculature (flexor digitorum superficialis) and continues into the hand. In the hand, the median nerve innervates the muscles of the thenar eminence (abductor pollicis brevis, flexor pollicis brevis, and opponens pollicis), as well as the first and second lumbricals.

The median nerve sends sensory branches only to the hand. The sensory distribution of the median nerve is mainly to the volar surface of first through third digits and lateral one-half of the fourth finger. Sensation to the skin at the base of the thenar eminence is via the median *palmar cutaneous* nerve, which arises from the median nerve above the wrist and is external to the carpal tunnel.

The medial cord becomes the ulnar nerve just distal to the branching of the medial cord to the median nerve. The *ulnar nerve* is formed, in most cases, by the axons from C8 and T1 nerve roots. The ulnar nerve alone supplies sensation to the ventral and dorsal medial hand, including the hypothenar eminence, the little finger, and the medial half of the ring finger.

As the ulnar nerve reaches the elbow, motor innervation is provided to the flexor carpi ulnaris. The ulnar nerve then passes through the ulnar groove to dive into the cubital tunnel between the

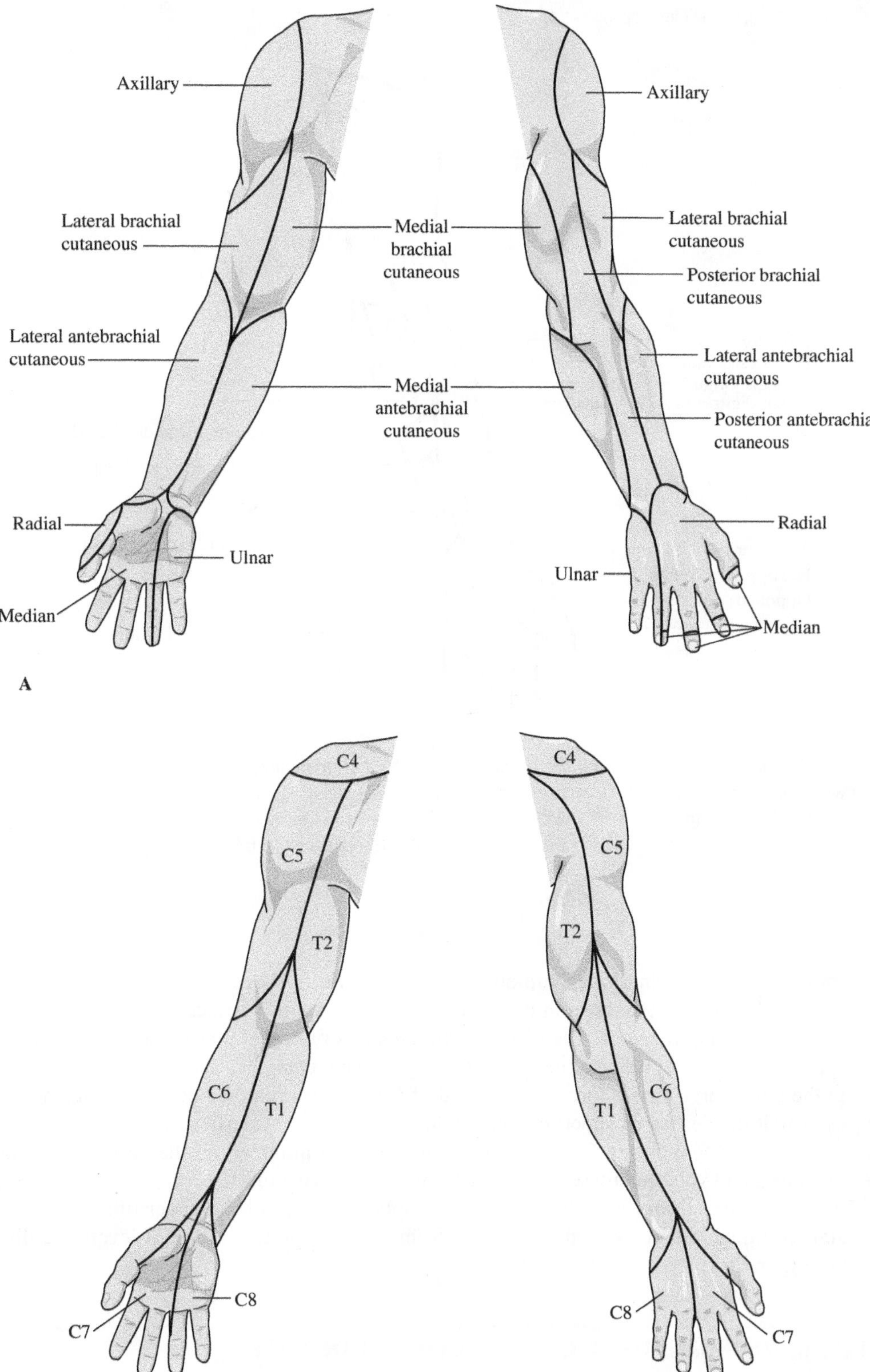

Figure A.4. The cutaneous sensory innervation of the upper extremities by **(A)** individual peripheral nerves and **(B)** spinal nerve-root level.

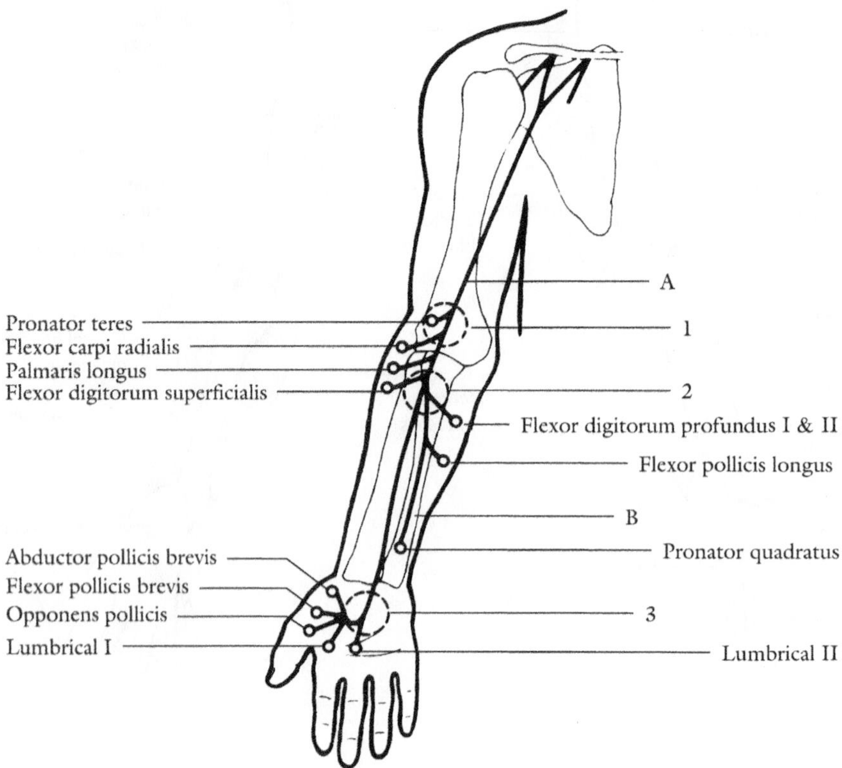

Figure A.5. Muscular innervation by the median nerve **(A)** and branching anterior interosseous **(B)** along with common sites of nerve compression (dashed circles) including *1*, within the pronator teres; *2*, at the branch point for anterior interosseous nerve, and *3*, at the carpal tunnel. (Reprinted with permission from Kimura J. *Electrodiagnosis of Diseases of Nerve and Muscle*. Philadelphia: F.A. Davis; 1989.)

heads of the flexor carpi ulnaris, a common point of entrapment. Above the wrist, the *ulnar dorsal cutaneous nerve* arises. It passes from the ulnar nerve on the ventral surface of the forearm to the dorsal medial aspect of the hand. The *ulnar palmar cutaneous nerve* also arises within the forearm and supplies sensory innervation to the base of the hypothenar eminence and palm.

As the ulnar nerve passes through the canal of Guyon between the hook of the hamate and the pisiform, it divides into a superficial and a deep branch. The superficial branch supplies the hypothenar eminence muscles, including the abductor digiti minimi, and the deep branch supplies the dorsal and volar interossei and adductor pollicis brevis muscles.

The cutaneous sensory distribution of the peripheral nerves of the upper limb, as well as the cutaneous innervation by neurons arising from various spinal nerve root levels are illustrated in Figure A.4.

CLINICAL NEUROANATOMY OF THE LOWER EXTREMITY

The innervation of the lower extremities is provided by nerve fibers derived from the first lumbar to third sacral levels of the spinal cord. The spinal cord nerve roots from these levels combine to form the lumbar (Fig. A.6) and sacral plexuses (Fig. A.7). The lumbar plexus is composed

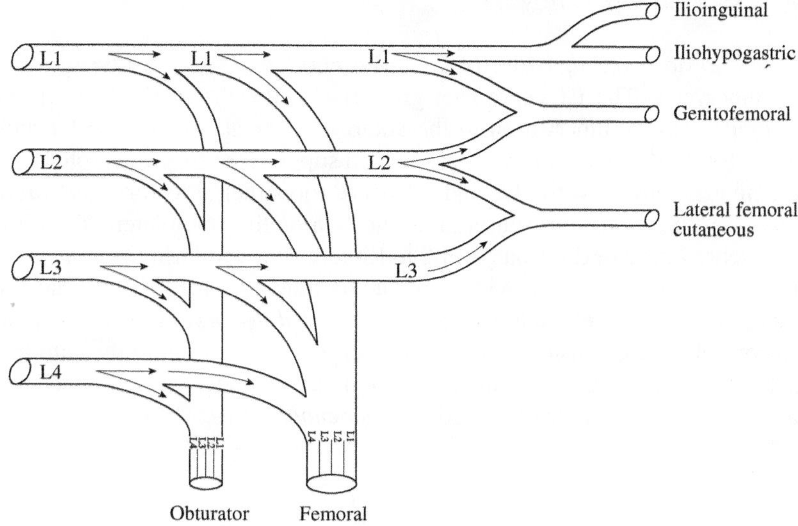

Figure A.6. Components of the lumbar plexus with the major terminal branch the femoral nerve.

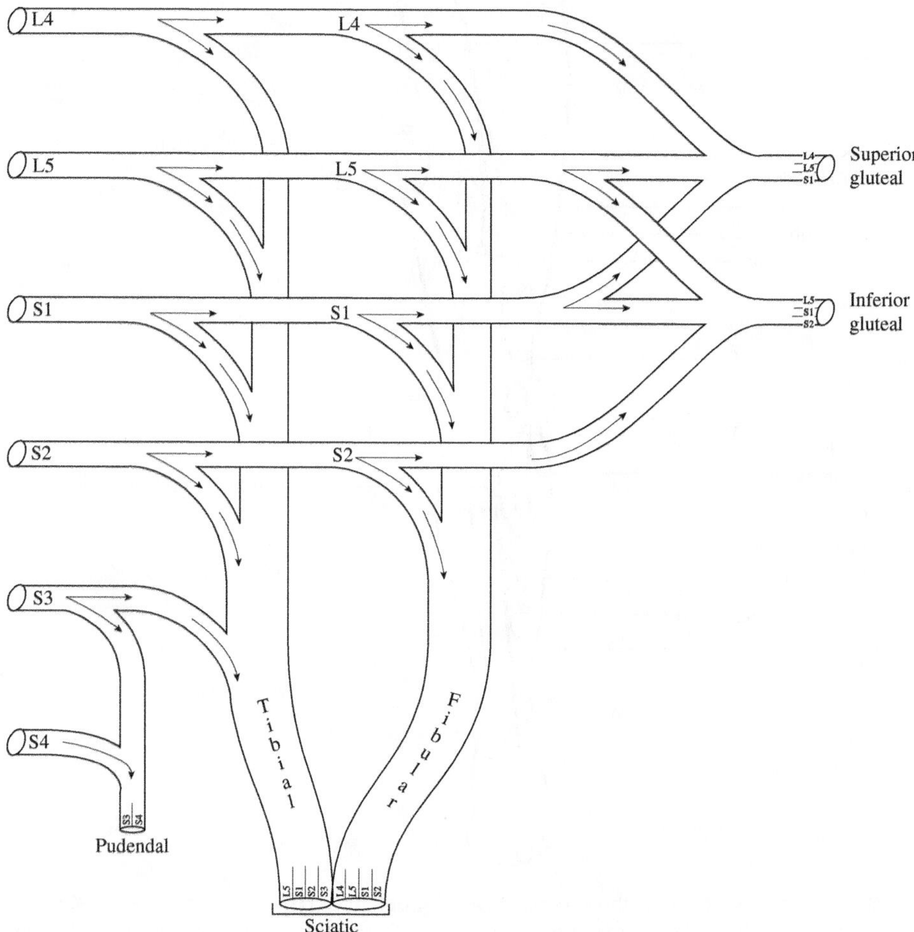

Figure A.7. Components of the sacral plexus with the major terminal branch the sciatic nerve.

primarily of the *anterior rami divisions* of L1 to L4 nerve roots and lies deep to the iliopsoas muscle that it innervates. The L1 nerve root gives rise to the *ilioinguinal* and *iliohypogastric nerves* that provide sensory innervation to the anterior lower abdomen. The L1 and L2 nerve roots combine to form the *genitofemoral nerve*, which supplies sensory and motor innervation to the external genitalia. Similarly, the L2 and L3 nerve roots merge to form the *lateral femoral cutaneous nerve*, serving cutaneous sensation to the skin on the anterolateral thigh from the hip to the knee. Branches (anterior divisions) of L2 to L4 roots unite to form the *obturator nerve* that innervates the hip adductors and provides cutaneous innervation to the medial thigh. Other branches (posterior divisions) of L2 to L4 form the *femoral nerve* (Fig. A.8) that innervates the quadriceps to control knee extension and provides sensory innervation to the anterior and some of the medial thigh. In addition, the terminal extension of the femoral nerve projecting to the skin of the medial aspect of the lower leg is called the *saphenous nerve.*

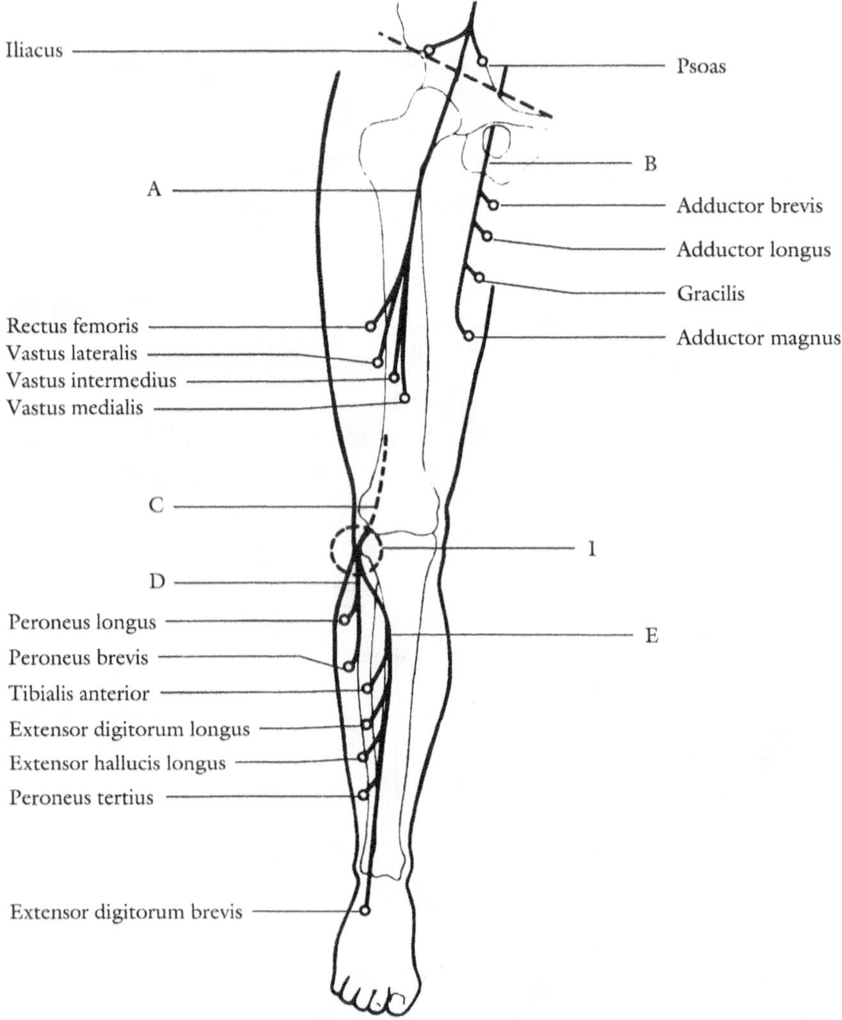

Figure A.8. Muscular innervation by the femoral nerve **(A),** obturator **(B),** common peroneal **(C),** superficial peroneal **(D),** and deep fibular **(E)** nerves, with common site of compression (dashed circles) at the head of the fibula (*1*). (Reprinted with permission from Kimura J. *Electrodiagnosis of Diseases of Nerve and Muscle.* Philadelphia: F.A. Davis; 1989.)

The lower lumbar (L4, L5) and upper sacral (S1 to S3) roots unite form the sacral plexus, which gives rise to five major nerves that provide motor and sensory innervation to the lower limbs. The L4 to S1 nerve roots project branches to form the *superior gluteal nerve* that innervates the gluteus medius to control hip abduction, while the L5 to S2 nerve roots project to form the *inferior gluteal nerve* that innervates the gluteus maximus which controls hip extension. The *sciatic nerve* (Fig. A.9) is formed from the L4 to S2 nerve roots. From the anterior and posterior components of S1 to S3, the *posterior femoral cutaneous nerve* arises, innervating the skin on the posterior thigh to the level of the knee. The anterior divisions of the L4 to S2 roots form the *tibial division* of the sciatic nerve, and the posterior components of L4 to S2 form the *peroneal* (fibular) *division* of the sciatic nerve.

The S2, S3, and S4 nerve roots also give rise to the *pudendal nerve.* The pudendal nerve innervation includes the external anal sphincter, the pelvic floor muscles, and urethral sphincter. The pudendal nerve hence controls urinary and fecal continence.

The sciatic nerve (Fig. A.9) passes through the sciatic notch and subsequently beneath the piriformis muscle. The sciatic has no cutaneous supply above the knee and passes down the thigh

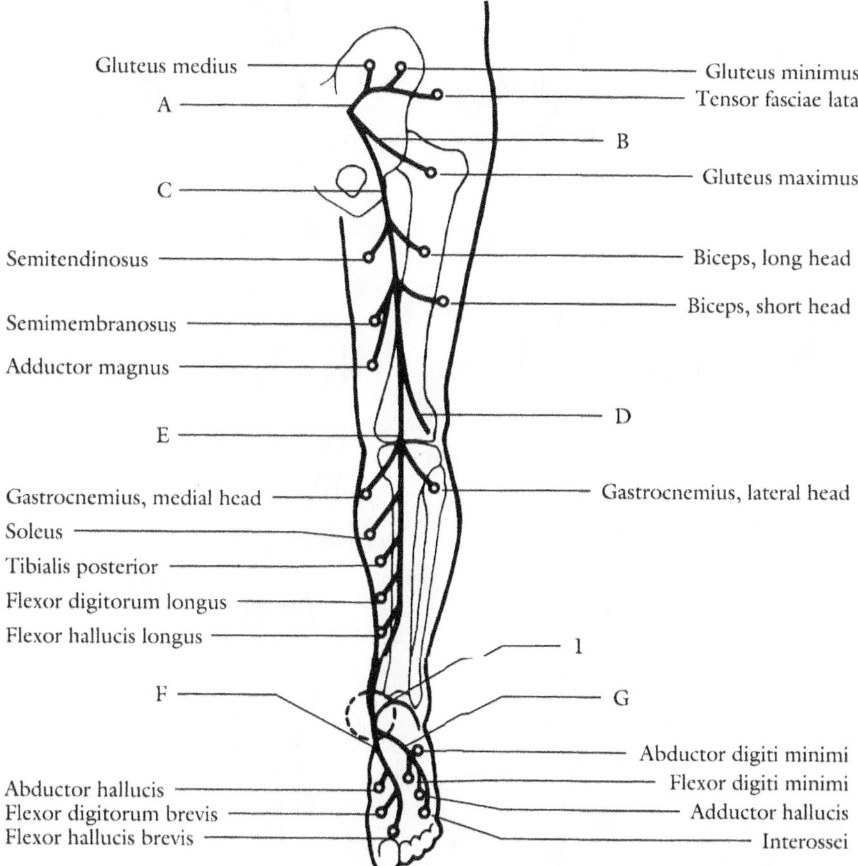

Figure A.9. Muscular innervation by the superior gluteal **(A),** inferior gluteal **(B),** sciatic **(C),** common peroneal (fibular) **(D),** tibial **(E),** medial plantar **(F),** and lateral plantar **(G)** nerves. Also shown is the common site of compression (*1*) for the tibial nerve at the tarsal tunnel. (Reprinted with permission from Kimura J. *Electrodiagnosis of Diseases of Nerve and Muscle*. Philadelphia: F.A. Davis; 1989.)

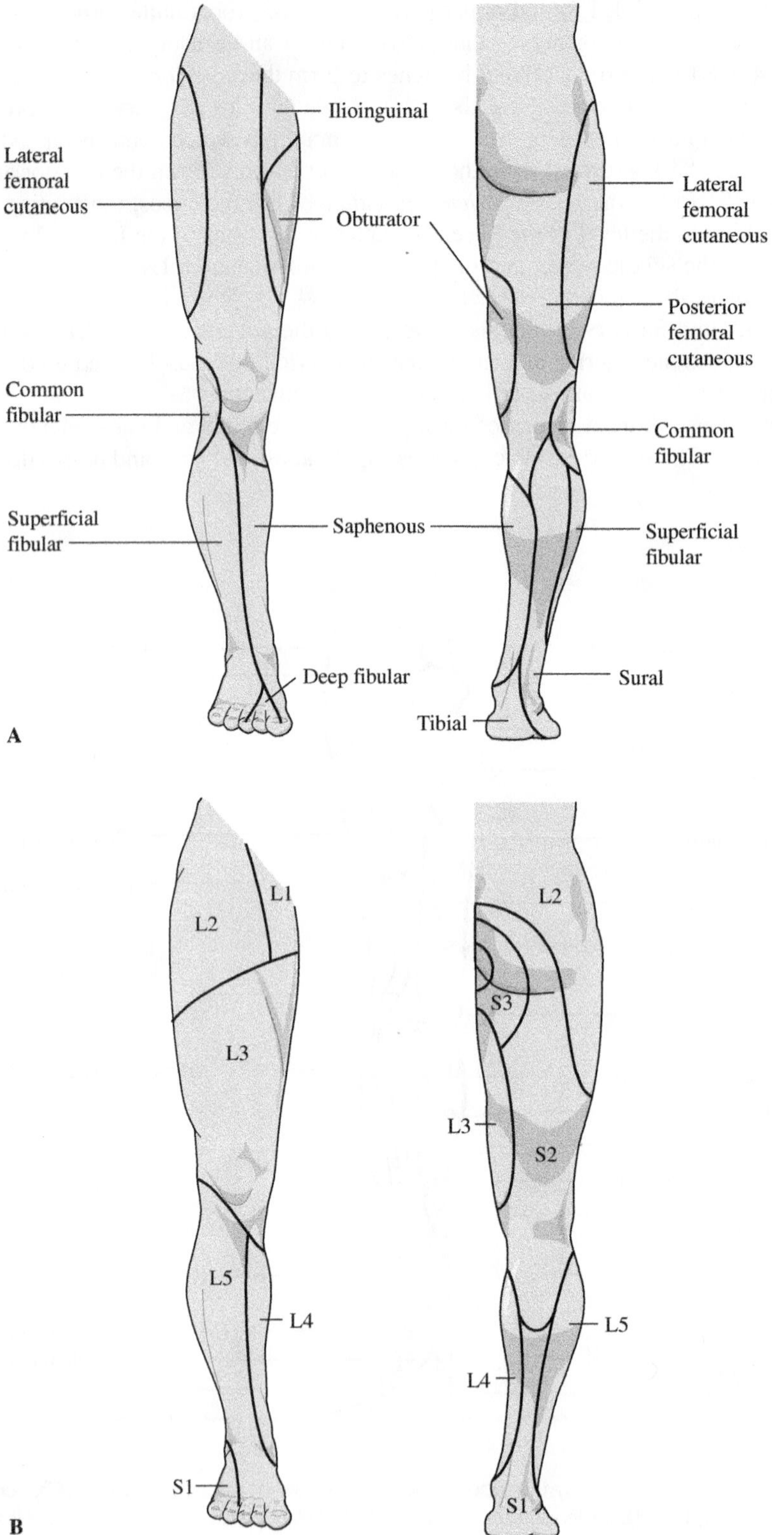

Figure A.10. Sensory innervation of the lower extremity. **A:** Peripheral nerve dermatomes. **B:** Cervical nerve root dermatomes.

deep to the hamstring muscles. The tibial division innervates all of the hamstrings except the short head of the biceps femoris, which is innervated by the peroneal division. At the knee, the *tibial nerve* supplies branches to the medial and lateral gastrocnemius, soleus, and other smaller muscles. As the nerve continues into the lower leg, it branches to the posterior tibialis, flexor digitorum longus, and flexor hallicis longus muscles and gives an additional branch to the soleus in the lower leg. A branch from the tibial nerve unites with a branch from the peroneal (fibular) nerve to form the *sural nerve,* innervating the skin on the lateral foot.

The continuation of the tibial nerve, after giving off muscular branches in the lower leg, winds around under the medial malleolus and passes through the tarsal tunnel formed by a triangular ligamentous structure extending from the medial malleolus to the heel. Distal to the tarsal tunnel, the tibial nerve divides. The *medial plantar nerve* supplies the abductor hallucis brevis, the flexor hallucis brevis, and first lumbrical muscles. It then supplies sensory receptors to the skin on the medial plantar aspect of the foot and first three digits. The *lateral plantar nerve* branches to the quadratus plantae and abductor digiti minimi quinti muscles, and then divides into a superficial and a deep component. The superficial component supplies the lateral interossei and flexor digiti quinti muscles and the skin on the lateral plantar aspect of the foot. The deep branch supplies all other deep muscles of the foot.

The peroneal (fibular) division of the sciatic nerve, after branching to the short head of the biceps femoris muscle, supplies the skin over the upper anterolateral leg and then divides into superficial and deep branches after passing around the neck of the fibula. The *superficial peroneal* (fibular) *nerve* innervates the peroneus longus and brevis, and then continues as the medial dorsal and intermediate dorsal cutaneous nerves. These supply the lower lateral leg and dorsal surface of the foot, with the exceptions of the lateral fifth digit (sural) and the web space between the first and second digit (deep peroneal).

The *deep peroneal* (fibular) *nerve* gives branches to the anterior tibialis, extensor digitorum longus, extensor hallucis longus, and possibily peroneus tertius muscles. In the foot, it supplies the extensor digitorum brevis muscle, and then terminates in the first dorsal interosseous muscle and supplies the skin over the web space between the first and second toes of the foot. The cutaneous innervation by lower extremity peripheral nerves and by axons arising from the lumbar and sacral nerve roots are shown in Figure A.10.

APPENDIX B

Answers to Self-study Questions

CHAPTER 1

1. (a) voltage; (b) electromotive force; (c) electrical potential difference
2. current
3. resistance
4. impedance
5. (a) cathode; (b) anode
6. (a) cations; (b) anions
7. anode; cathode
8. (a) voltage (V); (b) resistance (R); (c) current (I)
9. current
10. increase
11. (a) pulse current (PC); (b) alternating current (AC); (c) direct current (DC)
12. waveform
13. (a) ampere; (b) volt; (c) ohm; (d) farad; (e) ohm; (f) siemens; (g) pulses per second (pps); (h) hertz (Hz); (i) ampere (mA or μA); (j) millisecond (ms) or microsecond (μs); (k) coulomb; (l) seconds
14. (a) rectangular, symmetric, alternating current; (b) rectangular, unbalanced, asymmetric, biphasic, pulsed current; (c) sinusoidal, unbalanced, asymmetric, biphasic, pulsed current; (d) twin-spike, monophasic pulsed current

15.

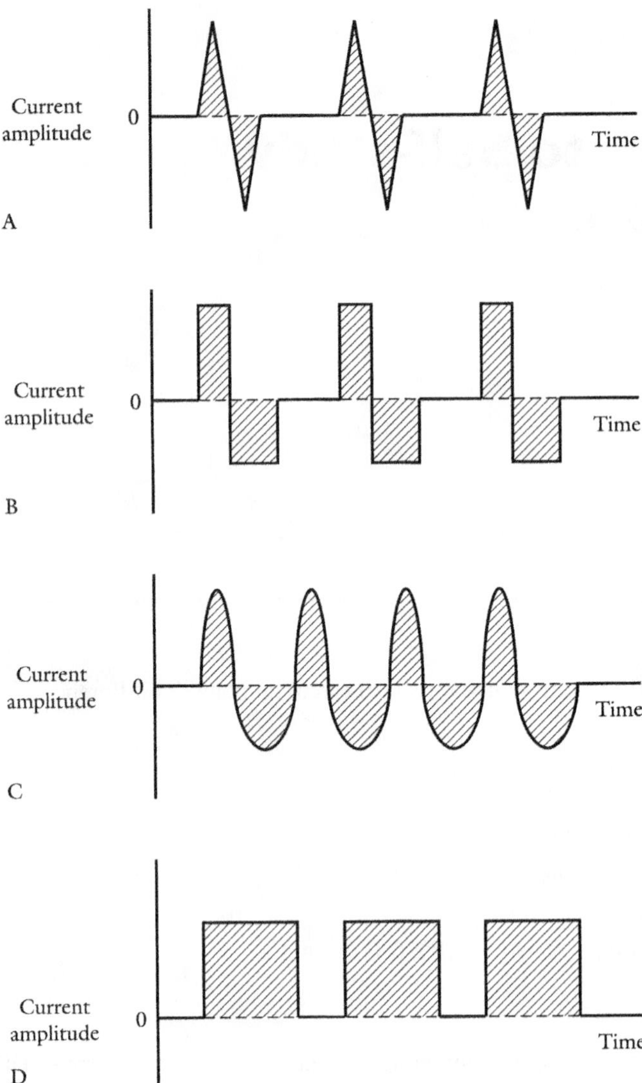

16. (a) phase duration; (b) pulse duration; (c) interpulse interval; (d) rise time; (e) decay time; (f) pulse charge; (g) phase charge

17. 25%

18. Ramp up: the time in seconds over which the amplitude of stimulation is gradually increased during the initial portion of the on time of stimulation. Ramp down: the time in seconds over which the amplitude of stimulation is gradually decreased during the final seconds of the on time of stimulation.

19. Burst: a series of groups of pulses or groups of alternating current cycles delivered at a specified frequency over a specified time interval.

20. Amplitude modulations are sequential, intermittent, or variable variations in the peak amplitude of a series of pulses or AC waveforms.

CHAPTER 2

1. The power supply of the stimulator is either a direct current source or an alternating current source. DC power supplies provide low voltages (1.5 V to 9.0 V), most commonly from batteries that chemically store electrical charge. Conventional AC power supplies provide 115 V, 60 Hz, sinusoidal, symmetric, alternating current or "line current" available from outlets in most home and commercial wiring systems.
2. amplitude control
3. (a) analog; (b) digital
4. (a) Allows selection of the waveform shape (rectangular, sinusoidal, etc.); (b) controls the number of seconds over which the amplitude of stimulation is automatically increased (or decreased) to a preset amplitude; (c) allows selection of the number of seconds a pattern of stimulation is passed to a patient and the number of seconds during which stimulation ceases; (d) allows selection of the time period (ms or μs) from the onset of a single pulse to the end of that pulse; (e) allows selection of the number of pulses per second to be delivered in continuous or interrupted trains of pulses; (f) allows selection of the number of bursts (brief trains of pulses) per second to be delivered; (g) allows selection and adjustment of the peak (or peak-to-peak) magnitude of stimulus waveforms; (h) allows selection of relative timing of stimulation on two or more stimulation channels; usually allows user to set two channels of stimulation on and off simultaneously or alternately on and off.
5. (a) pulse amplitude controls for each of the two separate channels available for stimulation; regulates amplitude of pulses produced; (b) on time/off time controls; allows user to adjust duration of stimulation and duration of no stimulation as stimulator automatically cycles on and off; (c) ramp time control to adjust the number of seconds over which the amplitude rises to a preset level; (d) frequency control; adjusts pulse frequency for both channels; (e) pulse duration control; adjusts the time from the onset to the end of each pulse delivered; (f) waveform selector; allows selection of either rectangular monophasic pulsed current, rectangular symmetric biphasic pulsed current, or rectangular unbalanced, asymmetric biphasic pulsed current; (g) channel output controls; for selection of both channels producing continuous train of pulses without interruption (continuous), both channels cycling on and off simultaneously (synchronous), or output channels cycling on and off alternately (reciprocal).
6. Surface electrodes serve as the interface between the electrical stimulator and the subject so that driving forces produced by the stimulator may produce movement of charged particles in the tissues. Electrodes differ in construction, size, shape, impedance, and durability.
7. Two
8. Monopolar electrode orientation: one electrode of a single stimulating circuit placed in the region where a therapeutic effect is desired, with the second electrode of the circuit positioned away from the target region. Bipolar orientation: both surface electrodes from a stimulator channel are placed over the target area. Quadripolar electrode orientation: both electrodes from two separate stimulating circuits are positioned in the primary target area for stimulation. Refer to Figures 2.13 through 2.15 for diagrams of these electrode configurations.

9.

Characteristics	*TENS Device*	*NMES Device*
No. of output channels	Two	Two
No. of amplitude controls	Two	Two
On time:off time controls	No	Yes
Frequency controls	Yes	Yes
Pulse duration controls	Yes	Sometimes
Synchronous/reciprocal modes	Rarely	Yes
Ramp modulation control	Automatic	Yes
Frequency modulation	Usually	No
Pulse duration modulation	Occasionally	No

10. Sinusoidal, symmetric alternating current, generally at frequencies of 1,000 to 4,000 Hz

11. Twin-spike, monophasic, pulsed current

12. A point stimulator employs a very small "active" electrode designed to stimulate trigger points or acupuncture points and generally includes a sensing feature to allow the user to locate points on the skin of low impedance. TENS and NMES portable units have no sensing feature and are designed to be used with pad surface electrodes.

13. Two channels of stimulation are used with two electrodes for each channel. Electrodes are usually oriented such that the current induced by one channel intersects ("interferes with") the current produced by the second channel.

14. Iontophoresis devices produce direct current and usually have only amplitude controls and a treatment timer. In addition, a meter is generally included to monitor stimulator output. They are designed to produce only very low amplitudes of DC for the delivery of medication and cannot be used for stimulation of electrically excitable nerve and muscle tissues.

15. The two-prong supply plug does not connect the electrical device chassis directly to ground as is the case with the three-prong plug, which should be used with all electrical instruments.

16. A ground fault is the passage of current to ground by a pathway other than through power supply lines. A GFI monitors the current carried to an electrical device and the current returning from the device. If the supply and return currents differ by more than 3 to 5 mA, the GFI trips and stops power supply to the device.

17. All switches, dials, push buttons, pressure-sensitive switches, and other types of stimulator controls; meters, auditory and visual signals; connections at stimulator or electrode interface; wires, broken-lead insulation, power plugs, power outlets; electrodes. Every stimulator applied clinically should receive regular inspections by a qualified biomedical technician.

18. Skin damage may occur in DC applications due to the alkaline or acidic reactions that occur beneath the electrodes or in response to the coagulation of capillaries that may occur beneath the anode.

19. Electrodes are not removed while stimulation is occurring because the density of current beneath an electrode increases as less and less contact is made with the skin. This increased current density might produce an uncomfortable or undesirable response in the patient.

20. Some short-wave diathermies with poorly shielded cables and wires may produce an electromagnetic field strong enough to induce currents in the leads of the electrical stimulation system, producing a potentially harmful response.

CHAPTER 3

1. (a) Sodium and potassium; (b) sodium is higher in concentration in the extracellular fluid; potassium is higher in concentration in the intracellular fluid
2. The sodium–potassium pump consists of special membrane-bound proteins that use energy in the form of ATP to actively transport sodium ions out of the cell while simultaneously moving potassium ions into the cell in a 3:2 ratio.
3. (a) permeability of the membrane; (b) electrochemical gradients (forces) acting on the ions
4. voltage-gated sodium and potassium channel proteins
5. See Figure 3.3 A.
6. Sensory, motor, and autonomic sensory axons mediate sensations such as touch, pain, and movement. Motor axons produce contraction in skeletal muscles. Autonomic axons regulate blood flow and sweating.
7. Orthodromic propagation of action potentials occurs in the same direction as occurs with physiologic activation—that is, toward the central nervous system in sensory fibers and away from the central nervous system in motor fibers. Antidromic propagation of action potentials occurs opposite to that normally occurring in peripheral axons—that is, toward the central nervous system in motor fibers and away from the central nervous in sensory fibers.
8. (a) diameter of the axons; (b) presence of myelination
9. (a) ventral horn of the spinal cord; (b) dorsal root ganglion
10. Epineurium: protects nerve fibers from compressive forces; perineurium: provides much of elasticity and tensile strength to peripheral nerve; endoneurium: contains Schwann cells and endoneurial fluid
11. (a) muscle fiber; (b) myofibrils; (c) actin; (d) myosin; (e) troponin; (f) tropomyosin
12. Mitochondria are where oxidative metabolism of glucose takes place to produce ATP for energy-requiring processes in cells such as protein synthesis and muscle contraction
13. The sarcoplasm reticulum serves as a storage site for intracellular calcium ions. The calcium ions are released into the intracellular fluid when action potentials invade the t-tubules.
14. T-tubules carry muscle action potentials to the interior of muscle fibers, where these action potentials initiate the release of calcium ions from the sarcoplasmic reticulum.
15. The motor unit consists of the alpha motoneuron cell body, its axon, and all of the muscle fibers innervated by that axon. Muscle has three types of motor units: fast twitch, fatigable (FF), fast twitch, fatigue resistant (FR), and slow twitch, very fatigue resistant (S). Type FF units are used least in ordinary contractions, but are capable of producing very high forces. Type FR units are used moderately and produce less contraction force. Type S units are used the most frequently in voluntary contractions, but produce the least amount of force.
16. The strength–duration curve represents all of the stimulus–duration combinations that are just sufficient to activate a particular type of nerve fiber. The curve indicates that threshold levels of stimulation may be achieved by using high-amplitude, very short-duration stimuli progressively to very low-amplitude, long-duration stimuli.
17. Excitation contraction: (i) alpha motoneuron action potential produces the release of the neurotransmitter acetylcholine. (ii) Acetylcholine diffuses to motor end-plate and binds with receptors. (iii) Receptor proteins open sodium channels in muscle membrane and sodium moves into muscle fiber. (iv) Sodium-induced depolarization triggers voltage-gated sodium and potassium channels to open. (v) Muscle action potential is produced and propagates along membrane entering t-tubules. (vi) Action potential invasion of t-tubules causes lateral cisternae of sarcoplasmic reticulum to release calcium ions. (vii) Calcium ions

diffuse in sarcoplasm and bind with troponin molecules on thin filaments. (viii) Calcium binding to troponin causes tropomyosin to change shape and move away from binding sites on actin for myosin. (ix) Myosin heads on thick filaments bind to actin molecules and thin filaments. (x) Myosin heads swivel while attached to actin, initiating the contraction.

18. (a) rate coding: the frequency of activation of muscle fibers; (b) recruitment: the number of muscle fibers or motor units activated

19. (a) amplitude of stimulus; (b) duration of stimulus

20. frequency of stimulation

21. (a) Sensory-level stimulation: electrical stimulation at levels sufficient to activate only superficial cutaneous Aβ sensory nerve fibers and generally giving rise to a tingling or "pins and needles" sensation; (b) motor-level stimulation: electrical stimulation at levels sufficient to activate alpha motoneuron axons and/or muscle fibers directly resulting in some form of muscle contraction; (c) noxious-level stimulation: electrical stimulation at levels sufficient to activate peripheral pain fibers (Aδ or C fibers) and give rise to the perception of pain

22. Aβ

23. (a) tapping; (b) tingling (pins and needles)

24. (a) twitch; (b) tetanic

25. (a) size (diameter) of axons; (b) location of the axons with respect to the stimulating electrodes

CHAPTER 4

1. Pain: an unpleasant sensory and emotional experience associated with actual or potential tissue damage, or described in terms as such. Hyperalgesia: an increased pain response to a normally noxious (painful) stimulus. Allodynia: pain in response to normally innocuous (non-painful) stimuli or activities. Referred pain: pain felt outside the area of injury but not associated with a response to the applied stimuli.

2. Acute pain is protective and serves as a warning sign that the body is experiencing actual or potential tissue damage, usually the result of an injury that can be pinpointed to time and place; it occurs immediately at the time of injury and usually goes away once healing is completed. Chronic pain is nonprotective and serves no biological purpose, outlasts normal tissue healing time, is greater than would be expected from the extent of the injury, and occurs in the absence of identifiable tissue damage.

3. See Figure 4.3 and Table 4.2; the simplified three-neuron pain pathway is a valuable concept in clinical neurological examination to assess the ability of individuals to perceive and localize painful stimuli applied to the skin in various areas.

4. Sensory discriminative component of pain is concerned with the quality (i.e., burning, sharp, dull), location, duration, and intensity (or magnitude), and is mediated by the spinothalamic tract to primary and secondary somatosensory cortexes; motivational–affective component of pain is concerned with the unpleasantness of pain (e.g., nauseating, sickening) and motivational tendency toward escape or attack and is mediated by the spinothalamic tract to the anterior cingulate and the anterior insular cortex; cognitive–evaluative dimension is based on past experience and on outcome of different response strategies (annoying, miserable, unbearable), and the pathway for mediation of this dimension of the pain experience is not clearly established.

5. Primary pain afferents are unipolar (also known as psuedounipolar) neurons with cell bodies located either in the dorsal root ganglia (for trunk and extremities) or the trigeminal ganglia (for the head). The peripheral processes of these neurons are axons of either the Aδ (type III) or C (type IV) size class that extend into the peripheral tissues (e.g., skin, muscle, joint) and internal organs (e.g., bladder, intestinal tract). The central processes project into the spinal cord or brainstem where they synapse (directly or indirectly) on spinal cord pain-transmission neurons in the dorsal horn, trigeminal pain-transmission neurons in the brainstem, or motoneurons in the ventral horn.

6. Serotonin, bradykinin, substance P, hydrogen ions, potassium ions
7. Activation of nociceptors in the skin gives rise to fast pain (also known as first pain) and/or slow pain (also known as second pain). Fast pain arises when the skin is pinched or pricked with a pin and is thought to be mediated by Aδ (type III) nociceptive afferents. Slow pain is often described as a burning sensation and persists after the painful stimulus is removed and is thought to mediated by C (Type IV) nociceptive afferents. Activation of muscle or joint pain afferents results in diffuse, difficult to localize, aching pain, or deep, cramplike pain and is thought to mediated by C (Type IV) nociceptive afferents arising from these tissues.
8. Excitatory neurotransmitters released from primary afferent nociceptors are numerous and include glutamate, substance P, and calcitonin gene-related peptide (CGRP). Glutamate binds to the AMPA, kainite, NMDA, or metabotropic glutamate receptors that are ion channels that open upon binding of glutamate to allow positively charged ions, sodium and/or calcium to enter the neuron, producing a transient depolarization of the neuron. Substance P binds to NK1 (neurokinin 1) receptors and increases activity and responsiveness of dorsal horn pain transmission neurons. CGRP activates metabotropic receptors that use protein kinases to produce long-lasting excitatory changes in spinal cord nociceptive neurons.
9. See Table 4.5.
10. Spinal cord pain-transmission neurons receive convergent synaptic input from primary pain afferents arising from both somatic tissues (skin, muscle, joint, etc.) and visceral structures (internal organs). Referred pain arises when activation of nociceptors in one type of tissue, such as an internal organ (e.g., heart, gall bladder), is misinterpreted as painful in another type of tissue, such as skin. Thus, the input sent supraspinally is misinterpreted at the cortical level.
11. Sensitization in primary pain afferents is characterized by increased spontaneous activity, a decrease in threshold of response to noxious stimuli, an increase in responsiveness to the same noxious stimuli, the response of nociceptors to normally nonpainful stimuli, and/or an increase in receptive field size. Sensitization of nociceptors may be produced by chemical substances released with tissue injury or inflammation such as substance P, cytokines, prostaglandins, leukotrienes, and hydrogen ions.
12. Sensitization of spinal cord pain-transmission neurons may arise due to (i) prolonged synaptic transmission between primary afferent nociceptors and second-order dorsal horn neurons; (ii) a reduction in inhibitory neurotransmitter activity in the dorsal horn; or (iii) the release of chemicals from glial cells that excite pain transmission neurons and/or enhance pain neurotransmitter release from primary nociceptive afferents.
13. The gate-control theory of pain proposed that large diameter, non-nociceptive primary afferent fibers send input to the dorsal horn and interfere with the transmission of pain between nociceptors and dorsal horn neurons by inhibiting or "gating" activity in nociceptors. The theory also suggested that this inhibitory spinal gating effect was under control descending from higher brain centers and was activated by both cognitive and subconscious activity at these supraspinal centers.
14. Presynaptic inhibition of excitatory neurotransmitter release from the central processes of nociceptors and post-synaptic inhibition of spinal pain transmission neurons.
15. Spinothalamic tract, the postsynaptic dorsal column pathway, the spinomesencephalic and the spinorecticular pathways

16. Descending modulation of pain transmission can be produced by the activation of numerous areas of the brain and brainstem, including but not limited to the midbrain periaqueductal gray (PAG), the rostral ventral medial medulla (RVM), and the lateral pontine tegmentum. Anatomically, the PAG sends projections to the RVM and the lateral pontine tegmentum. The RVM and lateral pontine tegmentum then project axons to the spinal cord and reduce dorsal horn pain neuron activity and ultimately the perception of pain.
17. The central nervous system contains "endogenous substances" with analgesic properties like opioids of natural or synthetic origin. The endogenous opioids include β-endorphins, methionine- and leucine-enkephalin, endomorphin 1 and 2, and dynorphin A and B, each of which has a distinct anatomical distribution and activates specific receptors. β-endorphins are found in hypothalamic neurons and in the anterior and intermediate lobes of the pituitary. Neurons in the hypothalamus send β-endorphin projections to the PAG and can "turn on" the descending inhibitory pathways Release of β-endorphin from the pituitary also occurs with vigorous exercise and stress. Since there is an increase in the number of opioid receptors on the peripheral terminals of primary afferent fibers after inflammation, the increased plasma concentrations of β-endorphin likely produce their pain-inhibiting effects peripherally.

    Enkephalins, endomorphins, and dynorphins are found in neurons in the brain and dorsal horn in areas known to be involved in analgesia such as the PAG, RVM, and dorsal horn of the spinal cord. Activation of opioid receptors with selective agonists, systemically or locally in the PAG, RVM or spinal cord produces analgesia. Dorsal horn neurons containing the neurotransmitter enkephalin produce both presynaptic inhibition of primary afferent nociceptors and postsynaptic inhibition of dorsal horn neurons.
18. High-frequency TENS (sensory and motor) activates descending inhibitory pathways from the RVM to the spinal cord to produce analgesia by activation of acetylcholine and δ-opioid receptors in the spinal cord. See Table 4.7. In contrast, low-frequency TENS (sensory and motor) activates descending inhibitory pathways from the RVM to the spinal cord to produce analgesia by activation of serotonin, acetylcholine, and μ-opioid receptors in the spinal cord.
19. Noxious intensity TENS uses multiple mechanisms (opioid and nonopioid), but likely involves activation of descending inhibitory pathways from the brainstem, RVM, PAG, and SRD to produce inhibition utilizing opioid, serotonin, and/or noradrenergic receptors in the spinal cord.
20. Either high or low frequency TENS is more effective in reducing primary hyperalgesia if given in combination with acute administration of morphine or clonidine.

CHAPTER 5

1. Electrical stimulation for pain control should be used when pain is no longer providing a protective response but instead contributing to the maintenance of abnormal function and inhibiting therapeutic progression.
2. Where is your pain?

   When did the pain start?

   Was the onset of pain sudden or gradual?

   What activities initiate or worsen your pain?

   How do you relieve your pain?

   Has the pain changed since it began?

3. Pain questionnaires: sickness impact profiles, Oswestry Low Back Pain Questionnaire, McGill Pain Questionnaire

   Pain drawings to describe the location and quality of pain

   Visual analog scale to assess the intensity and unpleasantness of pain

   Magnitude estimation

   Monitoring of drug (e.g., analgesic, antiinflammatory) intake

   Monitoring of daily activities
4. Sensory-level stimulation: fixed pulse frequency of 50 to 100 pps, fixed pulse duration or phase duration of 20 to 50 μs, amplitude adjusted to achieve perceptible tingling (paresthesia) beneath the electrodes, treatment time of 20 to 60 minutes, stimulation used as frequently as necessary. Motor-level stimulation: fixed pulse frequency of 2 to 4 pps or bps, pulse duration of >150 μs, amplitude of stimulation adjusted to achieve strong visible muscle contraction, treatment duration of 30 to 45 minutes, treatment two to four times per day. Noxious-level stimulation: fixed frequency of 1 to 5 pps, pulse duration of 1 ms to 1 s, amplitude increased until pain is perceived in response to stimulation, treatment time is seconds to minutes per stimulation site, often stimulate several points (acupuncture points or trigger points), treatment usually once per day.
5. Modulation of pulse amplitude, pulse duration, and/or pulse frequency is used to avoid accommodation (the reduction in perception) to the stimulation.
6. Sensory-level stimulation is usually perceived by the patient as very comfortable; response to sensory-level stimulation is at times an immediate decrease in the perception of pain; and conventional TENS may be used as needed throughout the day.
7. Electrodes are most commonly placed around or over the site of pain in sensory-level TENS. The objective of this placement is to activate large diameter axons (Aβ axons in skin and subcutaneous tissues) that activate the spinal cord gating mechanism that impairs pain transmission between primary pain afferents and spinal cord pain transmission neurons. Optimal stimulation sites have not been definitively established for sensory-level TENS for specific pain syndromes.
8. Arachnoiditis, failed cervical and low back syndrome, complex regional pain syndrome, peripheral nerve injury, postamputation pain syndrome, postherpetic neuralgia
9. Presence of demand-type cardiac pacemakers, sleep apnea monitors such as ECG monitors and ECG alarms, implanted stimulator, or other electromedical devices where TENS currents may interfere with function. Patients with known heart disease. Stimulation over fluid-filled organs or areas of marked edema. Undiagnosed pain syndromes. Electrode placement that causes current through the head. Use in pregnant women (safety of TENS devices for use during pregnancy or delivery has not been established).
10. Allergic reaction to tape, electrodes, or gels; skin irritation or electrode burn under electrode.
11. Several options available to the clinician, including changing the level of TENS (sensory vs. motor vs. noxious), changing the frequency of TENS (high frequency vs. low frequency), and changing the location of electrodes.
12. No studies of the clinical effectiveness of this mode of stimulation demonstrate a better pain-controlling effect than sham stimulation.
13. Too few studies with sufficient rigor for subject randomization, objective outcome variables, and explanation of relevant TENS parameters exist to make definitive conclusions on the benefits of TENS for chronic pain.
14. Rheumatoid arthritis, osteoarthritis, and myofascial trigger point syndromes
15. Rheumatoid arthritis, osteoarthritis, myofascial trigger point syndromes, and diabetic neuropathy

16. A measureable, observable, or perceived reduction in pain that may not be directly attributable to stimulation. The placebo effect is relevant to TENS since pain reduction in TENS may occur in part through the power of suggestion.
17. The study used a 4-week trial of electrical stimulation: HFTENS (80 to 100 pps) for 2 weeks, followed by 2 weeks of LFTENS (2–4 pps) with the third 2-week trial at the self-selected favorite. Others in the study were randomly given either sham electrical stimulation, electrical stimulation and exercise, or sham electrical stimulation and exercise. Electrodes were placed over the area of pain. Exercise was more effective than electrical stimulation, and electrical stimulation was no more effective than placebo. No statistically significant differences were found in any outcome between the subjects with true or sham TENS after 2 weeks, 4 weeks, or at 3 months after treatment had been withdrawn.
18. This study compared the pain control effectiveness of HFTENS, sham-TENS with individuals in a control group. A preassessment of pain severity was performed using a VAS. Patients recorded pain complaints for both intensity and unpleasantness on a VAS every 2 hours for 10 weeks. The subjects followed up with ratings for 3-day periods at 11 wks, 22 weeks, and 34 weeks after treatment. The HFTENS group demonstrated statistically significant reduction in pain ratings before and after treatment of greater than 40% compared to 17% in the sham TENS group. Over the 10-week treatment period of two 30-minute treatments weekly, the pretreatment pain complaints were reduced in the HFTENS group only. The effectiveness of TENS treatment continued into the 11th week following cessation of the actual TENS treatment. Both the TENS and sham-TENS groups demonstrated greater pain relief than the control group at 22 and 34 weeks.
19. Reporting of the methods used and numbers of subjects recruited have frequently been inadequate. Rarely have descriptions included the specification of the electrical stimulation unit, electrode number, size and location, current intensity, and clear descriptions of stimulation frequency or modulation. The measurement methods and data for different analgesic outcomes have often been absent or ill defined.
20. A growing body of work supports the consideration of TENS for primary dysmenorrheal pain, especially when typical pharmacological agents are not tolerated or desired.

CHAPTER 6

1. Stimulation characteristics:

    Amplitude: to at least 60% MVIC of muscle being stimulated

    Pulse/phase duration: 200 to 300 μs

    Frequency of stimulation: 65 to 80 pps

    On:off times of stimulation: 10 s on (excluding any ramp time) and 50 to 120 s off

   NMES training program characteristics:

    Number of contractions per training session: 10

    Number of training sessions per week: 3
2. (a) Increased muscle strength; (b) resistance to fatigue increases
3. Carrier frequency: 2,500-Hz sine wave

   Burst frequency: 50 bps

   On:off times of stimulation: 15 s on (includes 5 s ramp), 50 s off

   15 contractions daily at supramaximal contraction intensity
4. 30 to 100 pps

5. The frequencies have been found to be effective in NMES for strengthening in clinical populations.
6. fatigue
7. Superimposing a supramaximal stimulation burst on a MVIC allows the clinician to determine if the patient is truly maximally activating the tested muscle.
8. Pulse duration: at least 200 μs

   Frequency: variable 30 to 100 pps or bps

   Amplitude: capable of producing 100% MVIC contraction in the target muscle, with sufficient reserve amplitude available to present a continually increasing training dose
9. directly correlated
10. not correlated
11. Over the carotid bodies; in areas of peripheral vascular disorders; over the trunk of pregnant females; in close proximity to diathermy devices; over the eyes; over skin injuries; over the thoracic region, where it may interfere with function of vital organs such as the heart; in close proximity to demand cardiac pacemakers; in regions of the phrenic nerve or urinary bladder
12. Caused by a noxious stimuli below the level of the T_6 or lower spinal cord lesion. Increased blood pressure, sweating, headachce, increased spasticity, bradycardia. This is a medical emergency and potentially life threatening.
13. Skin burns beneath the electrodes
14. Patients unable to provide clear feedback, such as infants, those with senility, or those unable to follow commands or understand the process. A pregnant woman should not receive NMES in the vicinity of the fetus.
15. Volitional activation of the muscle by the patient, indicating whether a patient is capable at full voluntary contraction of muscle.
16. Muscle activation tells how much of the muscle a patient is able to volitionally use. If activation is low, the patients will benefit from NMES to activate their muscle fibers until they are able to do so themselves.
17. Waveform shape; stimulation frequency increase the ramp time
18. Current evidence suggests that portable stimulators may be just as effective as clinical stimulators.
19. Amplitude: supramaximal intensity with observation of muscle contraction

    Frequency: 1 to 200 Hz

    Pulse/phase duration: 40 μs to 16 s

    On:off times of stimulation: 5 to 10 s on (excluding any ramp time): 2 to 5 s off
20. Strengthening of the muscle in the absence of volitional activation. Long pulse durations are believed to most resemble the normal activity of the motoneuron. Supra maximal stimulation activates all or nearly all muscle fibers.
21. Similar to NMES for strengthening, it allows the external stimulus to activate and strengthen the muscle fibers. However, it is done in the absence of neural innervation until the nerve regenerates. It does not inhibit axonal sprouting.
22. Increase the off time.
23. Hypertension or hypotension, because autonomic responses may adversely affect blood pressure control in the patient. NMES in areas of excessive adipose tissue may result in a skin burn. Such patients must be monitored carefully.

24. (a) Strong contraction with the sensation between the two electrodes. Encouragement and reassurance about the procedure. (b) Single pin-prick sensation.
25. Amplitude controls; pulse amplitude and pulse/phase duration controls; frequency controls; on:off controls; ramp controls; treatment duration timer increments

CHAPTER 7

1. Neuromuscular electrical stimulation that produces a functionally useful movement.
2. Sensory integration theory and dynamical systems theory
3. Avoid placing electrodes over scratches or open wounds. Clients should be able to provide clear feedback regarding the level of stimulation. Avoid using NMES in areas of peripheral vascular disorders such as deep vein thrombosis. Avoid using NMES in people with uncontrolled hypertension/hypotension. Avoid using NMES in the regions of demand-type cardiac pacemakers and bladder, phrenic, or spinal cord stimulators.
4. Spinal cord injury, cerebral vascular accident (stroke), cerebral palsy, multiple sclerosis, and traumatic brain injury
5. Strength and range of motion
6. Flexibility in adjusting pulse-duration, frequency, and amplitude.
7. Orthotic bracing 16 or 23 hours per day until bone maturity is reached.
8. Supraspinatus and posterior deltoid
9. (i) Most slings are not effective at reducing or preventing glenohumeral joint subluxation. (ii) The slings that are effective in reducing glenohumeral joint subluxation promote nonuse of the affected arm and hold the elbow joint in a flexed posture that may increase the risk of contracture development.
10. Middle deltoid
11. Between 4 and 7 hours per day
12. EMG-triggered NMES of the involved side wrist and finger extensors with simultaneous performance of voluntary wrist and finger extension of the less involved side
13. Yes. Cauraugh et al. (8) and Caraugh and Kim (42) showed that 360 EMG-triggered NMES contractions performed over a 2-week period (2 sessions per day of 30 contractions performed 3 times per week) produced improvements in hand function.
14. Lateral pinch grasp and palmar grasp
15. C5 to C6 motor level.
16. The Bionic Glove was difficult to don and doff independently, small shifts in the electrode position could drastically change function, and the rigidity of the hand portion of the glove made it difficult to handle small objects.
17. Increased overground walking velocity and decreased physiological cost index
18. Burridge et al. (53) did not monitor stimulator use or report if the participants were required to use the stimulator in a standardized fashion, such as for 20 minutes of stimulated dorsiflexion assist during continuous walking.
19. Technological limitations in activating three or more muscle groups in appropriate patterns for gait in the clinical environment; having the appropriate number of support personnel to efficiently carry out the training task.
20. Use of partial body weight supported treadmill locomotion and stimulating a flexion withdrawal reflex to get multi-muscle activation for swing-phase assist during gait

21. Standing is produced by bilaterally stimulating the quadriceps femoris, gluteus maximus, and lumbar paraspinals (if the patient has trunk instability). Stepping is produced by stimulating a flexion withdrawal reflex in the leg that is to be advanced, followed by stimulation of the quadriceps femoris to produce terminal knee extension during the end of the swing phase.
22. Placement of electrodes over the antagonists of spastic muscle to produce reciprocal inhibition or placement of electrodes directly over the spastic muscles to antidromically produce Renshaw cell mediated inhibition of motoneurons to spastic muscles.

CHAPTER 8

1. A chronic wound is one that fails to heal within the expected time for the underlying etiology. A chronic wound may also be defined as one that does not heal in the expected sequence of repair in terms of time, appearance, and response to aggressive and appropriate treatment.
2. Inflammatory phase: characterized by the body's initial responses to a wound, including hemostasis (stopping bleeding), autolysis (removal of damaged cellular debris), and phagocytosis (to fight bacteria). Proliferative phase: characterized by cellular activity that leads to formation of a granulation tissue (fibroplasia), new epithelial layer (re-epithelialization), the development of a new vascular supply (neovascularization, angiogenesis), and wound contraction. Remodeling phase: characterized by the degradation of the collagen formed in the initial two phases of healing with a replacement and proliferation of new collagen.
3. Some systemic medications (e.g., corticosteroids, aspirin, and indomethacin) suppress inflammatory phase response. Some topical medications (e.g., iodine) can kill cells that produce healing. Malnutrition reduces supply of nutrients to healing wound. Prolonged pressure or stretch reduces capillary blood supply to tissues. Infection counteracts healing processes. Immunodeficiency impairs inflammatory response to infection. Smoking impairs supply of nutrients and oxygen and removal of carbon dioxide and wastes by reducing capillary circulation to wound. Dryness or necrotic tissue impedes migration of cells in inflammatory and proliferative phases of healing.
4. Pressure sores: compression of tissues reduces tissue blood perfusion and produces tissue necrosis. Arterial insufficiency ulcers: arteriosclerosis, arterial occlusion (e.g., thrombosis), arterial disruption. Venous insufficiency ulcers: sustained venous hypertension, venous valvular dysfunction. Diabetic ulcers: tissue trauma in insensate area, peripheral vascular disease.
5. Stage I: nonblanchable erythema of intact skin, the heralding lesion of skin ulceration. In individuals with darker skin, discoloration of the skin, warmth, edema, induration, or hardness may also be indicators. Stage II: partial-thickness skin loss involving the epidermis or dermis, or both. The ulcer is superficial and presents clinically as an abrasion, blister, or shallow crater. Stage III: full-thickness skin loss involving damage or necrosis of subcutaneous tissue, which may extend down to but not through the underlying fascia. The ulcer presents clinically as a deep crater with or without undermining of adjacent tissue. Stage IV: full-thickness skin loss with extensive destruction, tissue necrosis, or damage to muscle, bone, or supporting structures (such as tendon, joint capsule) and may be associated with undermining or sinus tracts.
6. Galvanotaxis: the attraction of electrically charged (positively or negatively charged) cells toward an electrical conductor of opposite polarity. Augmentation of collagen synthesis and proliferation of fibroblasts. Stimulation of angiogenesis and wound microperfusion. Killing or impeding the growth of bacteria in the wound. Enhancing the rate of epithelialization. Enhancing blood flow to wounds.

7. Removal of necrotic tissue; management of wound infection
8. a. Direct current (DC) is the continuous, unidirectional flow of charged particles for greater than one second.

    Amplitude of current: 200 to 800 mA; <1,000 mA
    Treatment duration: 1 to 2 hours
    Treatments per day: 1 to 3 per day
    Number of treatments days/ week: 5 to 7 per week

    b.

Type of Current	*HVPC*	*Rectangular Monophasic PC*
Pulse amplitude	100–200 V peak	30–35 mA peak
Pulse duration	100 μs	150 μs
Pulse frequency	30–130 pps	64–128 pps
Mode	Continuous	Continuous
Treatment duration	30–60 min	30 min
No. of treatments/day	1–2	2
Treatment frequency	5–7 days/wk	7 days/wk

9. One electrode directly over the wound opening and a second electrode 15 to 30 cm proximal to the wound.
10. Pulse amplitude: Strong sensory level; just below motor level
    Pulse duration: 100 μs
    Pulse frequency: 50 pps
    Mode: Continuous
    Treatment duration: 30 minutes
    Number of treatments/day: 3
    Treatment frequency: 5 to 7 days/week
11. One electrode just proximal to the wound and the second electrode just distal to the wound
12. Stimulators are not readily available from commercial manufacturers.
13. Osteomyelitis or malignancy in or around the wound; patients with cardiac conductivity disorders; presence of any implanted stimulation device; reduction of cutaneous sensation; adverse reactions (e.g., bleeding); zinc, mercury, or silver in topical medications on the wound
14. Applications of electrical stimulation for wound care in large numbers of subjects with wound of the same type of class; studies where the dosage of stimulation is controlled in terms of the density of current (current per unit area of the wound electrode) over predetermined periods of time

CHAPTER 9

1. More than 13 million adults in the United States are affected by incontinence; incontinence is twice as common in women as men, and 1 in 10 Americans over the age of 65 are affected by incontinence.
2. The anal sphincter, the superficial perineal muscles, the urogenital diaphragm, and the pelvic diaphragm

3. The hypogastric nerve innervates both the detrusor muscle of the bladder and the internal urethral sphincter. Activation of the hypogastric nerve neurons produces detrusor muscle relaxation and internal urethral sphincter contraction. The pelvic nerve innervates the detrusor muscle and activation of this nerve produces detrusor contraction. The pudendal nerve innervates the urogential diaphragm and activity in the pudendal axons produces contraction in the urogenital diaphragm.
4. Symptoms of urinary dysfunction include but are not limited to: incontinence, postmicturition dribbling, frequency, slow voiding, difficulty in initiating voiding, sense of urgency and pain at rest or during voiding.
5. Stress: involuntary leakage with effort, exertion, sneezing, or coughing. Urge: involuntary leakage accompanied by or immediately preceded by urgency. Mixed: involuntary leakage associated with urgency and also with exertion, effort, sneezing, or coughing. Overflow: unexpected leakage of small amounts of urine due to a full bladder. Functional: untimely urination because of physical disability, external obstacles, or problems in thinking or communicating that prevent a person from reaching a toilet. Transient: leakage that occurs temporarily because of a condition that will pass (e.g., infection, medication).
6. Supportive, hypertonic, and incoordination
7. Weakness impairment; endurance impairment; pain and hypertonic impairment; coordination impairment
8. At least partial innervation of the pelvic floor muscles; intact reflexes (intact sensation and motor innervation of the PFM implies intact reflexes); ability of the client to feel the electrical stimulation; cognitive ability to understand the procedure.
9. Contraindications/precautions to electrical stimulation include: acute perineal infections (vaginal, urethral, bladder, rectal); patients that have pessaries (a internal devise to support a displaced uterus, bladder, or rectum), as many have metal parts; atrophic vaginitis; patients with reduced ability to perceive the sensation associated with stimulation; heavy menstrual flow.
10. Sensory-level stimulation applied vaginally or rectally activates the afferent (sensory) branch of the pudendal nerve of the S2 to S4 nerve roots. Central connections of these afferents activate pudendal efferent neurons. Pudendal nerve axon activation leads to contraction in the muscle fibers of the urogenital diaphragm that increases urethral closure pressure and decreases the incidence of incontinence.
11. Electrodes should: be compatable with specific stimulator used; be comfortable for the patient; produce no significant adverse tissue reaction; be placed appropriately for the particular stimulation intervention chosen. Providers should consider the type of conductive material (metal or carbon-filled silicone) in the electrode; the arrangement of conductive surfaces (horizontal or circumferential) on electrodes; the electrode shape (dumbbell and cylindrical); and the electrode size for each individual treated.

    Other considerations related to electrodes include: all internal electrodes are single user and cannot be transferred from patient to patient; electrodes should be easy to use by patients and easily cleaned (follow manufacturer's recommendations for cleaning); high-volt pulsed current is delivered through the Sohn's electrode used rectally or vaginally (this electrode is intended for multiple use and is autoclaved after each patient); patients should be instructed to inspect the electrode for cracks before using; lead wires should be durable, resist cracking and be long enough to facilitate ease of electrode insertion; Lubrication on the electrode is best with water-soluble gel, warm water, or other commercial electroconductive gels approved for internal use.
12. To inhibit the bladder so that symptoms of urgency, frequency, and urge incontinence are relieved.

13. Hypertonus dysfunction results from increased tension in the pelvic floor muscles causing musculoskeletal pain and/or other dyfunctions related to inability to relax the PFM such as as in urinary and fecal retention.
14. A collection of symptoms including pain, pressure, or discomfort in the rectum that is aggravated by sitting and often radiates to the coccyx, left gluteal area, vagina, and thighs
15. Percutaneous peripheral afferent nerve stimulation; sacral nerve stimulation; magnetic stimulation; clitoral nerve stimulation
16. Simple visualization of PFM contraction with a mirror; palpation (external or internal) of PFM contraction; vaginal weights; pressure biofeedback (manometry); electromyographic (EMG) biofeedback
17. Supportive dysfunction, hypertonus dysfunction, and incoordination dysfunction
18. To provide patients with more information about the electrical activity in the PFM during voluntary contraction and relaxation of these muscles, ultimately resulting in increased contraction of the PFM and decreased urinary incontinence
19. To provide patients with more information about the electrical activity in the PFM, ultimately reducing resting PFM tone and decreasing pain and functional impairments associated with excessive PFM tone
20. Elevated resting tone as reflected by increased electrical activity in the PFM at rest; irregular resting tone; slow derecruitment; slow peak microvolt (amplitude) readings; inconsistent contraction ability; increases in accessory muscle activity; poor holding capacity

CHAPTER 10

1. repulsion; anode; cathode
2. direct; 1.0; 4.0
3. amplitude; duration; mA·min
4. 40 mA·min; 80 mA·min
5. 10 additional minutes
6. cathode; NaOH, alkaline
7. Convenience; ease of application; possibly safer for the patient because of better skin conformance and chemical buffering techniques
8. 0.5; 1.0
9. False: increasing the concentration beyond the recommended level may not increase the amount of ions administered and may actually retard ion transfer.
10. negative; positive
11. decrease; less
12. Damaged or broken skin; decreased sensation; implanted electrical devices
13. anti-inflammatory; catabolic
14. Local anesthetics; salicylates; opioids
15. acetic acid; cathode

CHAPTER 11

1. Biofeedback is the use of electronic instrumentation to provide objective information (feedback) to an individual about a physiological function or response so that the individual becomes aware of his or her response. The individual then attempts to alter the feedback signal to modify the physiological response.

2. Advantages of EMG biofeedback are the speed and continuity with which the information is provided to the clinician and patient. The sensitivity, objectivity, accuracy, and quantitative nature of the feedback signal are also major advantages of EMG biofeedback. In addition, modern feedback devices can provide a variety of novel feedback signals that can serve to motivate the patient.
3. The selection of appropriate patients for the application of EMG biofeedback basically involves answering three simple questions: (i) Does the patient demonstrate a motor impairment that would suggest that the information provided by the feedback would be of benefit? (ii) Does the patient demonstrate the ability for voluntary control? (iii) Is the patient sufficiently motivated and cognitively aware to utilize the feedback information?
4. It may help the clinician determine the effectiveness of a particular intervention.
5. Size and number of active motor units, frequency of motor unit firing.
6. The larger the recording area, the greater the volume of muscle that is monitored, and hence the greater the EMG recorded. Similarly, the larger the interelectrode distance, the larger the volume of muscle that is monitored and the larger the EMG. Thus, to increase the specificity of the EMG recording electrodes, small recording areas and close interelectrode spacing could be used.
7. Cross-talk is a phenomenon in which the electrical activity from the targeted muscle is contaminated by the signal from surrounding muscles.
8. Subcutaneous electrodes allow precise identification of a single targeted muscle, allowing access to deeper muscles without interference from superficial layers of muscle. Furthermore, the signal received is not attenuated by skin, subcutaneous fat, and fascia. However, subcutaneous electrodes are more invasive to the patient and therefore not as acceptable. The effect of movement artifact also increases with the use of subcutaneous electrodes.
9. Movement artifact is the high-voltage, nonphysiological contamination of the EMG due to the physical perturbation of the electrodes, input cables, and wires.
10. It serves to reduce the movement artifact (<100 Hz) and electronic noise (>1,000 Hz). The frequency range used is therefore typically 100 Hz to 1,000 Hz.
11. Amplification; filtering; rectification; integration; level/threshold detection
12. Raw; processed; auditory; visual; continuous; threshold triggered
13. The raw output (i.e., amplified and filtered only) can give the experienced clinician considerable information regarding the source of the signal. That is, is it truly physiological or is it primarily noise that is being recorded? It is difficult to use the raw signal to document progress objectively or to identify targeted levels of recruitment for the patient.
14. Goals of training; level of control; available muscle mass; subcutaneous fat; movement artifact; cross-talk
15. Areas that have a higher concentration of adipose tissue must be avoided. The distance between the recording electrodes and muscle producing unwanted electrical activity must be maximized. The smallest interelectrode distance that is practical must be used.
16. EMG biofeedback can assist a patient in reaching his or her true ability, but it cannot cure neurological damage.
17. Clinical experience has shown that patients typically respond better to positive feedback.
18. Conditions of the task (e.g., type of terrain, level ground or hills); criteria for the patient (e.g., distance, use of assistive device)
19. EMG biofeedback may provide information to the patient and clinician about a muscle that is too weak to allow for a large amount of joint displacement.
20. Performance of a functional task without the use of the biofeedback

CHAPTER 12

1. The intracellular recording technique is used primarily in research laboratory experiments on very large axons or cell bodies by penetrating the excitable cell membrane with a glass microelectrode and placing a second recording electrode outside the cell. Hence, one electrode is intracellular and a second electrode is extracellular. This system records changes in transmembrane (across the membrane) potentials.

   In the extracellular recording technique, one or two small conductors (called recording electrodes) are placed near but outside nerve or muscle cells. These electrodes monitor the changes in ionic concentration outside of electrically excitable cells as action potentials propagate along membranes. The extracellular electrodes are used to monitor the electrical activity in many nerve or muscle fibers; hence, the electrical signals recorded are referred to as compound nerve or muscle action potentials. Refer to Figure 12.1 for graphs of voltage changes recorded using each technique.

2. Are peripheral nerve fibers compromised?

   Are sensory fibers, motor fibers, or both involved?

   What is (are) the location(s) of the peripheral lesion(s)?

   How many peripheral nerves are involved?

   Is the nerve involvement limited to one limb or is involvement bilateral?

   Are both upper extremity and lower extremity nerves involved?

   What is the magnitude of peripheral nerve involvement? Is the lesion partial or complete?

   Is the peripheral nerve impairment increasing or decreasing over time? Is there evidence for recovery or further degeneration?

   Does evidence for localized nerve block, axonal degeneration, or segmental demyelination exist?

   Does the pattern of nerve involvement suggest a localized (e.g., single nerve) or a widespread (e.g., polyneuropathy) disorder?

3. Active recording electrodes are placed over a muscle innervated by a terminal branch of the median nerve (e.g., abductor pollicis brevis). Reference recording electrode is placed distal to active electrode over muscle tendon insertion or over distal thumb joint. Ground electrode is placed on the dorsal surface of the hand over ulnar styloid. Stimulation electrodes may be placed over median nerve at the wrist no less than 8 cm proximal to the active recording electrode, at the elbow before the median nerve penetrates the pronator teres, or in the axilla immediately lateral and anterior to the brachial artery.

4. Orthodromic conduction technique in the median nerve: distal ring electrode is placed over the distal interphalangeal crease, and the more proximal ring electrode is placed over the midpoint of the proximal phalanx on the second or third digit. The more proximal electrode is connected to the cathodal output of the stimulator, and the more distal electrode is connected to the anode. Surface recording electrodes may be positioned directly over the median nerve at points where the nerve is close to the skin surface (just above the wrist, at the elbow, over the median nerve in the upper arm or axilla). A ground electrode is placed on the dorsum of the hand or over the styloid process of the ulna.

   Antidromic conduction technique in the median nerve: for the antidromic recording technique, the ring electrodes on the second or third digit are used as recording electrodes. Stimulation is provided at sites as described in the answer to question 3 for median nerve motor conduction studies.

5. In the upper extremity, for motor nerve conduction studies: median, ulnar, deep radial, axillary, suprascapular; for sensory nerve conduction studies: median, ulnar, superficial radial, medial antebrachial cutaneous (medial cutaneous of forearm), lateral antebrachial cutaneous (lateral cutaneous of forearm), dorsal ulnar cutaneous. In the lower extremity, for motor nerve conduction studies: tibial, deep fibular (peroneal), femoral; for sensory nerve conduction studies: tibial, superficial fibular (peroneal), sural, cutaneous.
6. (i) Degeneration of motor axons, conduction block in motor axons distal to the site of stimulation secondary to mechanical compression and/or demyelination, neuromuscular junction failure, muscle fiber disease or degeneration. Amplitudes of CMAPs may be reduced in neuropraxic, axonotmetic, or neurometic neuropathies or in a variety of muscle disorders. (ii) Degeneration of sensory axons, conduction block in sensory axons distal to the site of stimulation (antidromic technique) secondary to mechanical compression and/or demyelination.
7. Mechanical compression of nerve axons and demyelination of axons
8. Temperature of the limb examined (cool limbs have reduced nerve conduction velocity) and age of patient (conduction gradually decreases beyond the fifth decade of life and is lower than normal in children younger than 5 years)
9. Neuropraxia is characterized by localized conduction slowing with or without conduction block, no interruption of axon continuity, and no axonal degeneration. Axonotmesis is characterized by partial or complete disruption in axon continuity without significant damage to the connective tissue layers in the peripheral nerve. Neurotmesis is characterized by partial or complete axonal disruption accompanied by damage to one or more of the connective tissue layers within the peripheral nerve.
10. During needle insertion: insertional activity that stops at about the moment that needle movement stops; in skeletal muscle at rest: miniature end plate potentials, end-plate potentials and end-plate spikes; with mild contraction: biphasic or triphasic motor unit potentials; with strong contraction: full interference pattern
11. During needle insertion: insertional positive waves, prolonged insertional activity, reduced insertional activity; in muscle at rest: fibrillation potentials, positive sharp waves, fasciculation potentials, myotonic discharges, complex repetitive discharges, myokymic discharges; with mild contraction: no motor unit potentials, >15% polyphasic motor unit potentials, motor unit potentials with many turns, abnormally small or abnormally large amplitude motor unit potentials; with strong contraction: reduced or absent recruitment pattern
12. See Figures 12.15 and 12.16 and Table 12.3.
13. An F-wave is a compound muscle action potential recorded in response to stimulation of motor nerve fibers, which is thought to result from the antidromic propagation of action potentials in motor axons. The antidromically propagated potentials are thought to "reactivate" a small number of motor neurons, which then send these action potentials back to the muscle, causing the muscle contraction that is monitored as the F-wave.
14. Demyelinating polyneuropthies (e.g., Guillian-Barré syndrome), amyotrophic lateral sclerosis, myotonic dystrophy, entrapment neuropathies proximal to the stimulation site (e.g., thoracic outlet syndrome), brachial or lumbosacral plexopathy (e.g., radiation neuropathy).
15. (a) H-reflex test. (b) Components of the reflex pathway include Ia afferent axons from soleus, synaptic junction between Ia and soleus alpha motoneurons, Aα motor axons in tibial nerve to soleus, neuromuscular junction between tibial nerve and soleus, and soleus muscle fibers.
16. Opthalmic division of trigeminal nerve (cranial nerve V) and the facial nerve (cranial nerve VII)
17. In a unilateral Bell palsy, the ipsilateral R1 and R2 responses may be prolonged, while the contralateral R1 will be within normal limits. In a chronic inflammatory demyelination polyneuropathy, both the ipsilateral and contralateral blink reflex response may be prolonged.

18. Somatosensory evoked potential testing is used to examine conduction in the central nervous system somatosensory pathways and may provide insight into the conduction of the proximal segments of peripheral sensory axons. The pathways involved in SSEP testing include peripheral somatosensory axons (e.g., Aβ axons associated with touch-pressure sensation), the dorsal column-medial lemniscal pathway, and the somatosensory cortex.

19. Motor evoked potential testing is used to examine the integrity of descending voluntary motor pathways. Motor evoked potential testing involves activation of the motor cortex regions, transmission along lateral corticospinal pathways, transmission along peripheral motor axons, and activation of the skeletal muscles monitored during testing.

20. Semmes–Weinstein monofilament testing to determine psychophysical thresholds to touch and two-point discrimination testing.

21. Abnormal blood clotting factors/anticoagulant therapy; extreme swelling; dermatitis; uncooperative or confused patient; recent myocardial infarction; blood-transmittable disease (Creutzfeldt-Jakob disease); immunosuppression; central going lines; pacemakers or other implanted medical devices; hypersensitivity to stimulation (open wounds, burns)

22. What are the individual's complaints? (e.g., pain, tingling sensation, functional deficit, anesthesia, fatigue, weakness)

Are the symptoms/signs diffuse, or are they localized to one area or extremity?

Is an entire extremity involved or only one area?

Does the problem occur continuously, or are there certain times of the day or night?

Do any activities change the symptoms?

When did the symptoms/problems begin?

Did symptoms occur suddenly or gradually?

Did an accident or injury precipitate the problem(s)?

Have the problems worsened or improved?

Do any family members or coworkers have similar problems?

What medications are you taking currently?

What are your work activities?

23. Signs of neuromuscular disorders include:

Atrophy (localized vs. diffuse)

Trophic or temperature changes in the skin

Differences in appearance of the extremities (e.g. skin color, skin texture, girth)

Joint deformities or limitations in joint movement

Functional abnormalities or limitations (e.g., gait deviations, balance disorders, asymmetry of upper extremity/lower extremity movement)

Muscle weakness (unilateral vs. bilateral; upper vs. lower limbs vs. trunk)

Reflex changes (decreased, increased, or asymmetric)

Sensory disturbances (nerve root dermatome vs. peripheral nerve dermatome distribution)

24. In mild carpal tunnel syndrome, the most common finding is an increase in the sensory distal latency between the wrist and thumb, index, long, and ring fingers with an increase in transcarpal conduction time to >1.7 ms. Amplitudes of sensory responses in the digits may or may not be significantly reduced. Motor axon conduction is spared, and amplitudes of CMAPs recorded from the abductor pollicis brevis are within normal limits. In moderate carpal tunnel syndrome, compromise (prolonged distal latencies with or without reduced amplitudes of responses) is detected in the conduction of both sensory and motor axons of the median nerve. Electromyographic examination does not provide evidence of loss of motor axons to the abductor pollicis brevis.

25.

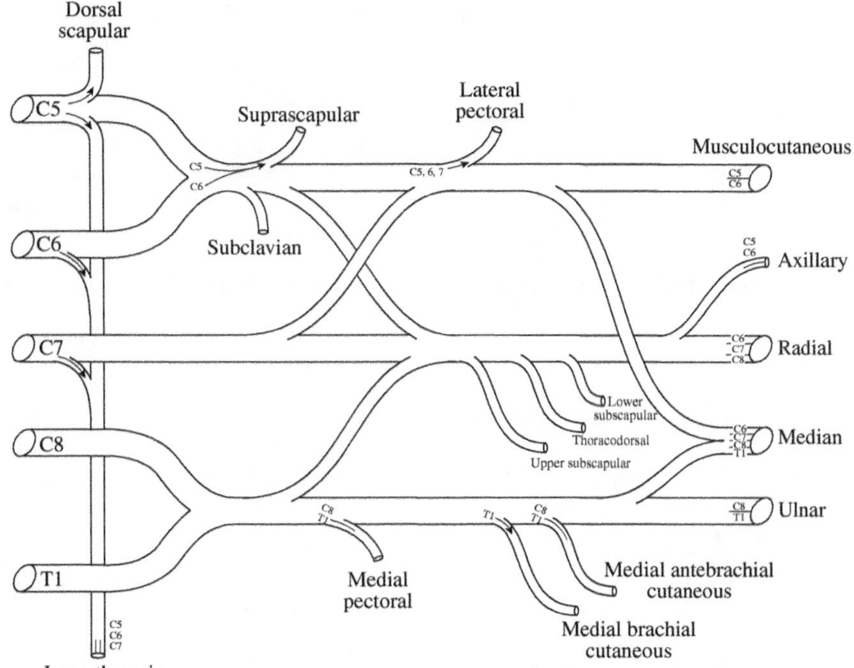

Dorsal scapular
C5
C6
C7
C8
T1
Suprascapular
Lateral pectoral
Musculocutaneous
Subclavian
Axillary
Radial
Lower subscapular
Thoracodorsal
Upper subscapular
Median
Ulnar
Medial pectoral
Medial antebrachial cutaneous
Medial brachial cutaneous
Long thoracic

Index

B

C

D

F

N

O

P

U

V

W

Z